WORKBOOK

PREHOSPITAL
EMERGENCY CARE

10th Edition

WORKBOOK

Edward B. Kuvlesky, NREMT-P, AAS
Craig N. Story, EMT-P, MPA

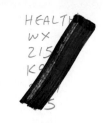

PREHOSPITAL
EMERGENCY
CARE

10th Edition

WITHDRAWN

Joseph J. Mistovich, MEd, NREMT-P
Chairperson and Professor
Department of Health Professions
Youngstown State University
Youngstown, Ohio

Keith J. Karren, PhD
Professor Emeritus
Department of Health Science
Brigham Young University
Provo, Utah

Medical Editor
Howard A. Werman, MD

Legacy Author
Brent Q. Hafen, PhD

PEARSON

Boston   Columbus   Indianapolis   New York   San Francisco   Upper Saddle River
Amsterdam   CapeTown   Dubai   London   Madrid   Milan   Munich   Paris   Montreal   Toronto
Delhi   Mexico City   São Paulo   Sydney   Hong Kong   Seoul   Singapore   Taipei   Tokyo

Publisher: Julie Levin Alexander
Publisher's Assistant: Regina Bruno
Editor-in-Chief: Marlene McHugh Pratt
Senior Acquisitions Editor: Sladjana Repic
Program Manager: Lois Berlowitz
Development Project Manager: Sandra Breuer
Editorial Assistant: Kelly Clark
Director of Marketing: David Gesell
Executive Marketing Manager: Brian Hoehl
Marketing Specialist: Michael Sirinides
Marketing Assistant: Crystal Gonzalez
Team Lead for Brady and Health Professions: Cynthia
  Zonneveld
Project Manager: Julie Boddorf
Production Editor: Arun Pragash Albert, S4Carlisle Publishing
  Services
Manufacturing Manager: Vincent Scelta
Manufacturing Buyer: Nancy Maneri
Editorial Media Manager: Amy Peltier
Media Project Manager: Ellen Martino
Creative Director: Andrea Nix
Senior Art Director: Maria Guglielmo
Cover Designer: Christine Cantera
Cover Image: Mark Ide
Composition: S4Carlisle Publishing Services
Printer/Binder: RR Donnelley
Cover Printer: RR Donnelley

Credits and acknowledgments borrowed from other sources
and reproduced, with permission, in this textbook appear on the
appropriate pages within the text.

Notice on Trademarks Many of the designations by manufac-
turers and sellers to distinguish their products are claimed as
trademarks. Where those designations appear in this book, and
the publisher was aware of a trademark claim, the designations
have been printed in initial caps or all caps.

Notice on Care Procedures It is the intent of the authors
and publisher that this text book be used as part of a formal
EMT education program taught by qualified instructors and
supervised by a licensed physician. The procedures described in
this text book are based on consultation with EMT and medical authorities. The authors and publisher have taken care to
make certain that these procedures reflect currently accepted
clinical practice; however, they cannot be considered absolute
recommendations.

The material in this text book contains the most current
information available at the time of publication. However,
federal, state, and local guidelines concerning clinical practices,
including, without limitation, those governing infection control
and universal precautions, change rapidly. The reader should
note, therefore, that the new regulations may require changes in
some procedures. It is the responsibility of the reader to become
thoroughly familiar with the policies and procedures set by federal, state, and local agencies as well as the institution or agency
where the reader is employed. The authors and the publisher
of this text book and the supplements written to accompany it
disclaim any liability, loss, or risk resulting directly or indirectly
from the suggested procedures and theory, from any undetected
errors, or from the reader's misunderstanding of the text. It is
the reader's responsibility to stay informed of any new changes
or recommendations made by any federal, state, or local agency
as well as by the reader's employing institution or agency.

Notice on Gender Usage The English language has historically
given preference to the male gender. Among many words, the
pronouns "he" and "his" are commonly used to describe both
genders. Society evolves faster than language, and the male pronouns still predominate in our speech. The authors have made
great effort to treat the two genders equally, recognizing that a
significant percentage of EMTs are female. However, in some in-
stances, male pronouns may be used to describe both males and
females solely for the purpose of brevity. This is not intended to
offend any readers of the female gender.

Notice on "Case Studies" The names used and situations de-
picted in the case studies throughout this text are fictitious.

Notice on Medications The authors and the publisher of this
book have taken care to make certain that the equipment, doses
of drugs, and schedules of treatment are correct and compatible
with the standards generally accepted at the time of publication.
Nevertheless, as new information becomes available, changes
in treatment and in the use of equipment and drugs become
necessary. The reader is advised to carefully consult the
instruction and information material included in the page insert
of each drug or therapeutic agent, piece of equipment, or
device before administration. This advice is especially important
when using new or infrequently used drugs. Prehospital care
providers are warned that use of any drugs or techniques must
be authorized by their medical director, in accord with local laws
and regulations. The publisher disclaims any liability, loss, injury,
or damage incurred as a consequence, directly or indirectly, of
the use and application of any of the contents of this book.

PEARSON

6 16

ISBN-13: 978-0-13-337188-8
ISBN-10:   0-13-337188-3

Edward B. Kuvlesky, NREMT-P, AAS, a graduate of Youngstown State University, is a field supervisor at Indian River County Fire Rescue, Indian River County, Florida.

Craig N. Story, EMT-P, MPA, is the former EMS program director at Polk Community College in Winter Haven, Florida. Craig is the director of evening programs at Florida Southern College in Lakeland. He is in the final stages of completing his PhD at the University of South Florida in Tampa.

Contents

Introduction

Welcome to the *Prehospital Emergency Care, Tenth Edition Workbook*. We have combined our writing skills and our knowledge as prehospital health care professionals and educators to produce a highly functional supplement for you. This is a self-instructional workbook, written to reinforce key concepts presented in the textbook. You can work on the chapters at your own pace and monitor your progress and understanding by checking the *Answers to Chapter Exercises* and rereading text pages indicated in the answer key.

The content of the three special sections that appear in many chapters is as follows: *Medical Terminology* presents a chart of chapter-relevant medical terms that are frequently used in emergency care. The chart provides a pronunciation for each term; breaks the term into a defined prefix, root, and suffix; and ends with a definition of the whole term. Questions following the chart reinforce the meanings and often highlight how the term might be used in an emergency situation. *Documentation Exercise* presents a real-life emergency-call scenario that is longer and more detailed than the *Case Study* scenarios, including detailed vital signs and other physical exam and patient history information that you would gather on such a call. A few questions to check your understanding of the scenario follow. The final piece of the exercise is a blank prehospital care report form that you will fill out, using information from the scenario, as if you were the EMT who had responded to that call. Note that *no answers* are provided in the form of a completed PCR. There will be differences in the way that each student completes the form, especially in the narrative segment. We recommend that after you fill out the document to the best of your ability, you discuss it with fellow students and your instructor to help you sharpen your documentation skills.

Great effort has been made to provide high-quality multiple-choice questions (with a few fill-ins here and there) because this is the accepted format of most standardized tests, such as a state exam or the National Registry exam. The *Course Review Self-Test* (covering all chapters in the text) is entirely in multiple-choice format. The test items for the various chapters are in scrambled order, as they might be on a major standardized or national test. However, the chapter each item relates to and the text page on which the information was covered is identifiable by consulting the *Answers to Course Review Self-Test*.

We have provided detachable *Medication Cards* containing information about the six medications that the EMT can administer or assist the patient in administering, with on-line or off-line approval from medical direction.

The authors and the publisher have worked diligently to produce the finest study supplement possible. We welcome any comments that you may have regarding this workbook and ask that you address your suggestions to the publisher. We wish you much success in your studies and as an EMT.

Ed Kuvlesky
Craig Story

Emergency Medical Care Systems, Research, and Public Health

STANDARD

Preparatory (Content Areas: EMS Systems, Research); **Public Health**

COMPETENCIES

Applies fundamental knowledge of the EMS system, safety/well-being of the EMT, medical/legal and ethical issues to the provision of emergency care.

Uses simple knowledge of the principles of illness and injury prevention in emergency care.

OBJECTIVES

After reading this chapter, you should be able to:

1-1. Define key terms introduced in this chapter.
1-2. Describe the key historical events that have shaped the development of the emergency medical services (EMS) system, including:
    a. Lessons learned in trauma care from experiences in the Korean and Vietnam conflicts
    b. Publication of *Accidental Death and Disability: The Neglected Disease of Modern Society*
    c. Highway Safety Act of 1966
    d. Emergency Medical Services System Act of 1973
    e. Public CPR courses
    f. Publication of the *National Emergency Medical Services Education and Practice Blueprint*
    g. Publication of *EMS Agenda for the Future* and *The EMS Education Agenda for the Future: A Systems Approach*
    h. Development of *National EMS Core Content*, *National EMS Scope of Practice Model*, and *National EMS Education Standards*
    i. The Institute of Medicine report *The Future of EMS Care: EMS at the Crossroads*
1-3. Briefly explain each of the components of the Technical Assistance Program Assessment Standards:
    a. Regulation and policy
    b. Resource management
    c. Human resources and training
    d. Transportation
    e. Facilities
    f. Communications
    g. Public information and education

h. Medical direction

i. Trauma systems

j. Evaluation

1-4. Discuss the differences between 911 and non-911 EMS access systems, including the features and benefits of 911 systems.

1-5. Compare and contrast the scopes of practice of the following levels of EMS providers:

a. Emergency Medical Responder (EMR)

b. Emergency Medical Technician (EMT)

c. Advanced Emergency Medical Technician (AEMT)

d. Paramedic

1-6. Explain the importance of the EMT's understanding of the health care resources available in the community.

1-7. Give examples of how EMTs can carry out each of the following roles and responsibilities:

a. Personal safety and the safety of others

b. Patient assessment and emergency care

c. Safe lifting and moving

d. Transport and transfer of care

e. Record keeping and data collection

f. Patient advocacy

1-8. Describe the expectations of EMTs in terms of each of the following professional attributes:

a. Appearance

b. Knowledge and skills

c. Physical demands

d. Personal traits

e. Maintaining certification and licensure

1-9. Discuss the purposes of medical direction/oversight in the EMS system.

1-10. Describe the purpose of quality improvement/continuous quality improvement programs in EMS.

1-11. Explain the EMT's roles and responsibilities in quality improvement.

1-12. Identify activities in EMS that pose a high risk of mistakes and injuries.

1-13. Discuss steps that you can take to minimize mistakes and injuries in EMS.

1-14. Discuss the steps of evidence-based decision making.

1-15. Explain the limitations of evidence-based decision making in EMS.

1-16. Describe the relationship between EMS and public health.

1-17. List the ten greatest public health achievements in the United States in the 20th century.

▌KEY IDEAS

This chapter describes the EMS system and the roles and responsibilities of the EMT. Emphasis is placed on the personal safety of the EMT and the safety of other rescuers.

■ Prehospital care is provided by the Emergency Medical Services (EMS) system. Each state manages its EMS system in its own way, using federal guidelines.

■ EMS, fire, and law enforcement services may be accessed in many areas by the universal access number 911 and in other areas by non-911 numbers.

■ The four levels of emergency medical service practitioners identified in the *National EMS Scope of Practice Model* are Emergency Medical Responder (EMR), Emergency Medical Technician (EMT), Advanced Emergency Medical Technician (AEMT), and Paramedic.

■ The health care system includes the EMS system, emergency departments, and specialized care facilities such as trauma, burn, obstetrical, pediatric, poison, stroke, cardiac, spine injury, and hyperbaric centers.

■ The roles and responsibilities of the EMT include personal safety; the safety of others; maintaining vehicle and equipment readiness; emergency vehicle operation; patient assessment and emergency medical care; safe lifting and moving; transport and transfer of the patient; recordkeeping and data collection; patient advocacy; providing emotional support to the patient, relatives, and others at the scene; integrating the EMS service with other emergency and nonemergency services; resolving the emergency incident; maintaining medical and legal standards; providing administrative support; enhancing professional development; and developing and maintaining community relations. Your first priority is your own safety, then the safety of other rescuers. Once the scene is safe, the patient's needs are your priority.

■ The professional attributes required of the EMT are knowledge and skills, a professional appearance, good health, a calm and reassuring personality, leadership abilities, good judgment, moral character, stability and adaptability, resourcefulness, an ability to listen, and an ability to cooperate with others.

■ Every EMS system must have a physician medical director who is legally responsible for the clinical and patient care aspects of the system.

■ The goal of quality improvement is to identify aspects of the system that can be improved and to implement programs to improve identified shortcomings.

▌ TERMS AND CONCEPTS

1. Write the number of the correct term next to each definition.

1. EMS system
2. EMT
3. Advanced Emergency Medical Technician (AEMT)
4. Paramedic
5. Emergency Medical Responder (EMR)
6. Prehospital or out-of-hospital care

_____ a. Provides the highest level of prehospital care, including advanced assessments, formation of a field impression, and invasive and drug interventions

_____ b. The first person on the scene who has emergency care training

_____ c. An organization that coordinates emergency care as part of the continuum of health care

_____ d. Care provided prior to transport to the hospital

_____ e. Performs the responsibilities of an EMT with the addition of the use of advanced airway devices, monitoring of blood glucose levels, initiation of intravenous and intraosseous infusions, and administration of a select number of medications

_____ f. Provides basic emergency medical care and transportation to patients who access the EMS system, including advanced oxygen therapy and ventilation equipment, pulse oximetry, use of automatic blood pressure monitoring equipment, and limited medication administration

▌ CONTENT REVIEW

1. The roles and responsibilities of the EMT include
   a. insertion of intravenous lines.
   b. controlling life-threatening situations.
   c. decompressing the chest cavity.
   d. reading and interpreting electrocardiograms.

2. The EMT's responsibilities for scene safety include
   a. personal safety first, then other rescuers'/bystanders' safety, then patient safety.
   b. other rescuers'/bystanders' safety first, then personal safety, then patient safety.
   c. personal safety first; the EMT has no responsibility for the safety of others.
   d. patient safety first, then other rescuers'/bystanders' safety, then personal safety.

3. The responsibility for maintaining an EMT's certification or licensure to practice is the responsibility of the
   a. system's medical director.
   b. system's training officer.
   c. the EMT.
   d. system's shift supervisor.

4. The risk of being struck by traffic at nighttime scenes is
   a. seldom a risk for the EMT or other emergency responders.
   b. reduced by wearing dark clothing and waving a flare from side to side.
   c. reduced by wearing reflective clothing and providing adequate scene lighting.
   d. an assumed risk that is "just a part of the job."

5. You are responding to the scene of a shooting. The dispatcher advises you that law enforcement is also responding. Upon arrival, you observe a large crowd of people who appear to be fighting. The patient is lying next to the crowd. Law enforcement has not yet arrived. You should next
   a. be alert to any threat and approach the patient.
   b. retreat to a safe area and await law enforcement arrival.
   c. exit the vehicle and await law enforcement arrival.
   d. remain in the vehicle and await law enforcement arrival.

6. A process of internal and external reviews and audits of all aspects of an emergency medical system is called which of the following?
   a. Chart review
   b. Quality improvement
   c. Medical command
   d. Medical control

7. Which of the following statements is true with regard to evidence-based medicine?
   a. It makes little or no use of previously published medical research.
   b. It focuses on research to evaluate evidence of care activities that improve patient outcomes.
   c. Because of federal regulations and mandates, it evaluates only evidence of validity.
   d. It uses the large amount of research conducted in prehospital care to make treatment decisions.

8. During a routine physical examination, your personal physician informs you that he is interested in becoming the medical director for the service that you work for. He asks you to describe the medical director's responsibilities. Which of the following best describes the important responsibilities of the medical director?
   a. Is minimally involved in EMS education programs and refresher courses
   b. Is only responsible for providing on-line medical direction
   c. Develops, establishes, and monitors EMS guidelines for EMS personnel
   d. Is only responsible for providing off-line medical direction

9. Which statement best describes the relationship between the EMT and the EMS system medical director?
   a. The prehospital care rendered by the EMT is not governed or controlled by the medical director.
   b. All care rendered by the EMT is considered an extension of the medical director's authority.
   c. The in-hospital care rendered by the EMT is considered an extension of the medical director's authority.
   d. The medical director advises the on-scene paramedic, who guides the EMT.

10. To be effective as an EMT, you must have the personality characteristics in the following list. Using a 1–5 rating system (5 is the highest), rate your own personality characteristics.

    _____ Pleasant personality (ability to get along with others, reassuring and calming voice and manner)

    _____ Leadership ability (takes control, sets priorities, able to give clear directions)

    _____ Good judgment (able to make appropriate decisions quickly in unsafe or stressful conditions)

    _____ Good moral character (high ethical standards)

    _____ Stability (able to deal with feelings openly and honestly)

    _____ Resourcefulness and improvisation (able to adapt to change quickly and use resources effectively)

    _____ Ability to listen (able to hear with careful attention to verbal and nonverbal clues)

    _____ Cooperativeness (able to act as a leader while working with others)

11. The EMT is responsible for the patient's privacy and valuables. The EMT should also honor patient requests, if possible. The term that best describes these responsibilities is
    a. EMS advocacy.
    b. patient's rights.
    c. EMS rights.
    d. patient advocacy.

12. Some patient care activities are considered high-risk activities that put the patient at risk for greater injury, medical mistakes, or furthering existing injury. Mark each item in the following list that is considered a high-risk activity with the letter H.

    _____ Failing to immobilize or improper immobilization of a spine-injured patient

    _____ Ambulance crash during transport of a patient to a medical facility

    _____ Lifting and moving patients

    _____ Transfer of care between emergency responders or between the receiving medical facility personnel

    _____ Communication that leads to misunderstanding

13. EMS is part of the public health system and plays an integral role in carrying out its mission. List four roles that EMS commonly performs with regard to improving public health.

    1. _____

    2. _____

    3. _____

    4. _____

14. Which of the following is a common function of state EMS agencies?
    a. Funding for local EMS medical direction
    b. Coordinating local response plans
    c. Regulation of the statewide EMS system
    d. Dispatching local response agencies

15. Cell phones are responsible for approximately what percentage of all 911 calls?
    a. 40 percent
    b. 50 percent
    c. 60 percent
    d. 70 percent

▌ CASE STUDY

It's 1:00 in the morning, and you have been dispatched to a single-vehicle auto crash. You wipe the sleep from your eyes and prepare to respond to the call. The dispatcher informs you that law enforcement is on the scene, and there is one patient who has a possible head injury. A fire/rescue truck is also responding to the call. The car has struck a power pole just over the top of a steep hill.

1. Which has the primary responsibility for traffic control at this scene?
    a. Fire/rescue department
    b. EMS/ambulance service
    c. Power company
    d. Law enforcement

2. Which has the primary responsibility for extrication/rescue at this scene?
    a. Fire/rescue department
    b. EMS/ambulance service
    c. Power company
    d. Law enforcement

3. Which has the primary responsibility for patient care and transport?
    a. Fire/rescue department
    b. EMS/ambulance service
    c. Power company
    d. Law enforcement

Law enforcement is on the scene controlling traffic as you arrive. The fire/rescue crew and power company have stabilized potential hazards. You evaluate the patient and determine that he has minor injuries and is in stable condition. While you are transporting the patient to the hospital, the patient asks you to please call his wife and let her know he is okay.

4. Which statement best describes the most appropriate action to take in response to the patient's request to call his wife and explain what has happened?
    a. Tell him that you can't take the time to call her.
    b. Tell him you will call her if you get a chance.
    c. Explain that this is not a part of your responsibilities.
    d. Call the patient's wife and explain what has happened.

5. What information is *most likely* to be used by EMS system administration for quality improvement audits on this call?
   a. Prehospital care report of call
   b. Feedback from crews on scene
   c. Feedback from the patient involved
   d. Feedback from the patient's wife

6. Which of the following creates the greatest potential hazard at this scene?
   a. Highway traffic
   b. Gasoline leak
   c. Power lines
   d. Violent bystander

Workforce Safety and Wellness of the EMT

▌STANDARD

Preparatory (Content Areas: Workforce Safety and Wellness); **Medicine** (Infectious Diseases)

▌COMPETENCIES

Applies fundamental knowledge of the EMS system, safety/well-being of the EMT, medical/legal and ethical issues to the provision of emergency care.

Applies fundamental knowledge to provide basic emergency care and transportation based on assessment findings for an acutely ill patient.

▌OBJECTIVES

After reading this chapter, you should be able to:

2-1. Define key terms introduced in this chapter.

2-2. Given a description of a patient or family member's behavior, identify the stage of grief it most likely represents.

2-3. Explain the principles for interacting with patients and family members in situations involving death and dying.

2-4. Give examples of situations that EMS providers may find stressful.

2-5. Compare and contrast the characteristics of acute, delayed, and cumulative stress reactions.

2-6. Recognize signs and symptoms of stress reactions.

2-7. Describe lifestyle changes you can make to help you deal with stress.

2-8. Describe responses your friends and family may have to your work in EMS.

2-9. Describe changes in the work environment that can help you manage job-related stress.

2-10. Discuss the components of a comprehensive system of critical incident stress management.

2-11. Describe measures you can take to protect yourself from exposure to diseases caused by pathogens and accidental and work-related injury.

2-12. Give examples of diseases caused by each of the different types of pathogens (bacteria, viruses, fungi, protozoa, and helminths).

2-13. Describe the Standard Precautions that must be taken to protect health care workers from exposure to infectious diseases.

2-14. Describe the personal protective equipment that may be used by EMS personnel.

2-15. Explain the role of immunizations and tuberculosis testing in maintaining good health.

2-16. Discuss the risks and preventive measures for specific infectious diseases of concern to EMTs, including:
  a. Hepatitis B
  b. Hepatitis C
  c. Tuberculosis
  d. Acquired immune deficiency syndrome
  e. Severe acute respiratory syndrome
  f. West Nile virus
  g. Infections due to multidrug-resistant organisms

2-17. Explain the risks and measures that can be taken to protect yourself against the following hazards:
  a. Hazardous materials
  b. Hazardous rescue situations
  c. Traffic-related injuries
  d. Violence and crime

2-18. Describe the components of physical and mental wellness.

KEY IDEAS

This chapter provides an overview of ways you can safeguard your emotional and physical well-being while providing emergency care.

- Your ability to recognize and effectively deal with stressful situations is as essential to your well-being as it is to that of your patients and their family members.

- The highly charged environment of emergency care requires that you recognize the warning signs of stress and remedy them before stress results in burnout.

- Scene safety includes practicing Standard Precautions to protect yourself from a communicable disease, wearing appropriate personal protective equipment at the scene of accidents and illness, recognizing common infectious diseases, and practicing strategies to prevent work-related injuries.

TERMS AND CONCEPTS

1. Write the number of the correct term next to each definition.
   1. Burnout
   2. Critical incident stress management (CISM)
   3. Standard Precautions
   4. Sterilization
   5. Personal protective equipment (PPE)

   _____ a. State of exhaustion and irritability

   _____ b. Strict infection control measures based on the presumption that all blood and body fluids are infectious

   _____ c. A process to deal with stress encountered by the EMT

   _____ d. Items worn to guard against injury or disease transmission

   _____ e. Use of chemical or physical substances to kill all surface microorganisms

CONTENT REVIEW

1. Which of the following is one of the five emotional stages that dying patients may experience?
   a. Repression
   b. Denial
   c. Regression
   d. Confusion

2. Beside each of the following actions that you might take when dealing with a dying patient, family member, or bystander, write "A" for an appropriate action or "I" for an inappropriate action.

   _____ a. Talk to the unresponsive patient as if the patient is fully alert.

   _____ b. Always remove family members from the area or room during resuscitation efforts.

   _____ c. If a critically injured or ill patient asks you, "Am I going to die?" respond by saying, "Everything is going to be OK," or "You are going to be OK."

   _____ d. If a dying patient wants a message delivered to survivors, always listen carefully and deliver any message the patient conveys.

3. As an EMT, you should be alert to recognize warning signs of stress. Which of the following may signal stress?
   a. Irritability; loss of appetite; loss of interest in work
   b. Calm demeanor and renewed interest in work
   c. Planning long-term recreational events with family or friends
   d. Ability to get along well with coworkers and friends; able to make decisions

4. A session held prior to a critical incident stress debriefing (CISD) that helps to vent emotions and gather information is which of the following?
   a. Defusing
   b. Critical incident
   c. Peer support
   d. Follow-up service

5. Microorganisms that can spread disease by a person's contact with blood, inhalation of airborne droplets, or touching contaminated objects are generally referred to as
   a. pathogens.
   b. viruses.
   c. bacteria.
   d. fungi.

6. Which of the following is considered the single most important way to prevent the spread of infection?
   a. Hand washing
   b. Sterilizing reusable equipment
   c. Bagging contaminated laundry
   d. Placing sharp objects in a container

7. Before attempting rescue or patient care in a situation such as a hazardous material or biological agent incident, a high-angle rescue, or a white-water rescue, the EMT should usually
   a. contact the emergency service supervisor for instructions.
   b. consult with law enforcement personnel prior to acting.
   c. call for specialized rescue teams or experts.
   d. quickly enter the emergency scene.

8. Number the following steps in the proper order from 1 to 5 for providing emergency care at a scene involving possible hazardous materials.

  _____ a. Provide patient assessment and emergency care.

  _____ b. Look for and compare placards or signs to *DOT Hazardous Materials: The Emergency Response Guidebook.*

  _____ c. Make sure that the scene is controlled by a specialized hazardous materials team before you enter.

  _____ d. Use binoculars to try to identify hazards before approaching the scene.

  _____ e. Put on appropriate protective clothing, such as a self-contained breathing apparatus and a "hazmat" suit.

9. If you suspect potential violence at an emergency scene, you should
   a. request law enforcement assistance before entering the scene.
   b. enter cautiously and call for law enforcement assistance if needed.
   c. first remove patients from the scene and then call for police assistance.
   d. first secure the scene and then begin patient assessment and care.

10. If you are providing emergency care at a crime scene, you should take precautions to preserve the chain of evidence by
    a. waiting to start treatment until all evidence has been collected by law enforcement.
    b. not disturbing the scene unless necessary to provide care.
    c. immediately removing the patient from the scene to begin care.
    d. contacting medical oversight for permission to enter the scene.

11. A hepatitis B infection
    a. will always cause symptoms such as fever or headache.
    b. is only transmitted by direct contact such as shaking hands.
    c. is a minor medical ailment that resolves itself over a few days.
    d. may be prevented by obtaining a vaccination.

12. Which statement best describes the action to take if the EMT suspects exposure to the hepatitis B virus?
    a. Arrange for an immediate injection of hepatitis B immunoglobulin (HBIG).
    b. Arrange with your personal physician for an immediate hepatitis B vaccination.
    c. Report the incident to your supervisor and follow your local exposure control policy.
    d. Contact the Centers for Disease Control and Prevention for the latest treatment recommendations.

13. Tuberculosis
    a. is of little consequence due to its low rate of incidence in the United States.
    b. requires that self-contained breathing apparatus (SCBA) be worn by the EMT.
    c. spreads by droplets from the cough of a patient and from the patient's infected sputum.
    d. is a serious but not a highly infectious disease.

14. The Occupational Safety and Health Administration (OSHA) respiratory protective standards for emergency response personnel include the use of a _____ when in contact with tuberculosis patients.
    a. self-contained breathing apparatus (SCBA)
    b. surgical mask
    c. HEPA or N-95 respirator
    d. J350 mask

15. Which of the following has been identified as a mode of transmission of the human immunodeficiency virus (HIV), which causes acquired immune deficiency syndrome (AIDS)?
    a. Direct contact with an infected person, such as shaking hands
    b. Exposure to coughing or sneezing by an infected person
    c. Indirect contact, such as with eating utensils or bed linens used by an infected person
    d. Sexual contact with an infected person

16. Which statement is most correct regarding AIDS?
    a. It results from destruction of the body's hormonal balance.
    b. It is caused by a virus that destroys the body's ability to fight infections.
    c. It always presents signs and symptoms.
    d. It is easier to contract via occupational exposure than is hepatitis B.

17. You are transferring a patient from one medical facility to another and notice on the patient's transfer orders that he has hepatitis C. You know that hepatitis C
    a. can be prevented by obtaining a vaccination.
    b. is the most common bloodborne infection in the United States.
    c. is easily transmitted via mucous membranes.
    d. causes no symptoms in about 10 percent of patients.

18. You and an EMT student intern are transporting a suspected severe acute respiratory syndrome (SARS) patient from a local hospital to a regional medical center for specialized treatment. The patient has a fever of 102°F, is coughing heavily, and generally states that he "aches all over." You and the EMT student intern are wearing gloves, eye protection, a surgical mask, and a cover gown. What other action should you take to best protect yourself and your EMT intern?
    a. Remove the surgical mask from the patient to improve communication.
    b. Look for signs of fever and respiratory symptoms for 48 hours.
    c. Avoid touching your eyes, nose, or mouth with your gloved hands.
    d. Avoid washing your hands after glove removal to limit droplet spread.

19. You are at the station between calls watching TV with a coworker. A report comes on describing an outbreak of West Nile virus in your community. Your partner asks you what the signs and symptoms of West Nile virus are. Which response best describes severe signs and symptoms?
    a. Vision loss, headache, stiff neck, and muscle weakness
    b. Excessive thirst, yellow vision, and slurred speech
    c. Inability to urinate, nausea, and dizziness
    d. Dyspnea and difficulty in swallowing

20. Multidrug-resistant organisms
    a. are commonly encountered in patients at health spas, resorts, and pools.
    b. are considered to be of little threat or consequence to EMTs.
    c. are never transmitted by person-to-person contact.
    d. include MRSA, VRE, PRSP, and DRSP.

❙ CASE STUDY

It's early afternoon, and you have just finished cleaning out the jump kit from a prior call when the alarm bell sounds. You are called to a scene at a railroad yard where one of the workers is trapped from the waist down between two rail cars. Specialty rescue teams are en route, and the patient's wife, who has been called by his coworker, has just arrived at the scene. Your patient is responsive. He tells you that he knows that as soon as they separate the cars, he will die. He asks that you leave him alone with his wife and that you do nothing heroic to try to intervene.

1. Of the five stages of emotional response to death and dying, which stage does your patient seem to be exhibiting regarding his imminent death?
   a. Denial
   b. Anger
   c. Depression
   d. Acceptance

2. The situation described would be
   a. considered a high-stress incident.
   b. a routine part of the EMT's job.
   c. something the EMT must learn to live with.
   d. considered an average incident.

As predicted, as soon as the cars are separated, your patient rapidly loses responsiveness and becomes pulseless and apneic. He has sustained massive open crush injuries to his abdomen and pelvis. There is nothing that can be done to save his life, and he dies. In the days following this incident, you begin to have trouble sleeping and often have nightmares. You are having trouble concentrating, and your heart pounds every time you get dispatched on a call.

3. Your partner suggests that the EMS personnel who responded to this incident should attend a stress management session. Who should *not* participate in the session?
   a. Police personnel
   b. Communications personnel
   c. Emergency department personnel
   d. Patient's family

4. Beside each of the following actions, write "A" for an appropriate action or "I" for an inappropriate action to be taken to mitigate the potential effects of stress.

   _____ a. Drink one or two beers each night when off duty to relieve stress.

   _____ b. Avoid any exercise for at least two months following a high-stress incident.

   _____ c. Avoid sharing details of stressful events with family, friends, or coworkers.

   _____ d. Request a rotation in duty to a busier station to put the stressful event into perspective.

Medical, Legal, and Ethical Issues

CHAPTER

3

STANDARD

Preparatory (Content Area: Medical/Legal and Ethical)

COMPETENCY

Applies fundamental knowledge of the EMS system, safety/well-being of the EMT, medical/legal and ethical issues to the provision of emergency care.

OBJECTIVES

After reading this chapter, you should be able to:

3-1. Define key terms introduced in this chapter.

3-2. Differentiate between the concepts of *scope of practice* and *standard of care*.

3-3. Given a scenario, determine whether you would have a duty to act.

3-4. Explain your duties with respect to patients, your partner, yourself, and your equipment.

3-5. Describe the intent of Good Samaritan laws.

3-6. Explain each of the following legal protections for EMTs:
   a. Sovereign immunity
   b. Statutes of limitations
   c. Contributory negligence of the patient

3-7. Explain the EMT's legal obligations with respect to medical direction.

3-8. Differentiate between the concepts of ethics and morals.

3-9. Describe the ethical responsibilities of EMTs.

3-10. Given a scenario presenting an ethical dilemma, discuss the consequences of various decisions and actions.

3-11. Explain each of the following types of consent:
   a. Informed consent
   b. Expressed consent
   c. Implied consent
   d. Consent to treat minors
   e. Involuntary consent

3-12. Compare and contrast the typical provisions and prehospital applications of each of the following types of advance directives:
  a. Do not resuscitate order
  b. Living will
  c. Durable power of attorney
  d. Physician orders for life-sustaining treatment

3-13. Given a scenario in which a patient has an advance directive, determine the appropriate action to be taken.

3-14. Given a scenario in which a patient refuses care, discuss the actions you should take.

3-15. Differentiate between criminal and civil liability.

3-16. Explain the concept of negligence.

3-17. Give examples of ways you can avoid each of the following tort claims:
  a. Abandonment
  b. Assault
  c. Battery
  d. False imprisonment/kidnapping
  e. Defamation

3-18. Explain patients' rights and your legal and ethical responsibilities concerning confidentiality and privacy.

3-19. Describe COBRA and EMTALA provisions as they apply to EMS.

3-20. Give examples of ways you can protect yourself legally in transport and transfer situations.

3-21. Describe special considerations for patients who are potential organ donors.

3-22. Identify presumptive signs of death.

3-23. Identify situations in which law enforcement or the medical examiner's / coroner's office should be contacted.

3-24. Discuss special considerations in responding to potential crime scenes.

3-25. Describe situations in which the EMT may be mandated to make a report, such as suspected abuse, crimes, and infectious diseases.

▎ KEY IDEAS

The EMT provides patient care in an increasingly complex legal and ethical environment. Important ethical and legal concepts are described in this chapter.

- The EMT's scope of practice, or the actions and care that are legally allowed by the state in which the EMT is providing care, is determined by the National Highway Traffic Safety Administration's *National EMS Scope of Practice Model*, the *National EMS Education Standards*, state law, regulations, and local policies.

- The standard of care describes the care expected of a "reasonably prudent" EMT or how an EMT with similar training in a similar situation would perform. This encompasses what is often called "the reasonable person standard or test." The standard of care is established by EMT textbooks, the care expected by other EMTs in the community or region, local and state protocols, the National Highway Traffic Safety Administration's *National EMS Education Standards*, and the EMS system's operating policies and procedures.

- Your legal obligation to provide service for a patient is called the "duty to act." Duties to your patient, yourself, your partner, and your equipment are also important concepts.

- Good Samaritan laws are generally designed to protect an individual from liability for acts performed in good faith unless those acts constitute gross negligence. The law provides limited protection for the EMT and varies from state to state.

- Your best defense to lawsuits is prevention. Always render care to the best of your ability, always work within your scope of practice and within the standard of care, always behave in a professional manner, and ensure that you are covered by adequate liability insurance. If you keep your patients' best interests in mind when rendering care, you will seldom, if ever, go wrong.

- The EMT's legal right to function is contingent upon medical direction.

- A conscious, competent, and rational adult has the right to refuse treatment or transportation.

- Permission to care for a patient is called "consent." You must obtain consent from every patient prior to treatment. There are five forms of consent: informed, expressed, implied, minor, and involuntary consent.

- Informed consent is provided when the patient is informed of the care to be provided and understands the associated risks and potential consequences of refusing treatment or transportation.

- Common types of advance directives are a living will, a do not resuscitate (DNR) order, a health care durable power of attorney (health care proxy), and physician orders for life-sustaining treatment (POLST). As a general rule, you should consider initiating treatment immediately so that if the issue cannot be resolved, you will not be held negligent for not providing care or delaying treatment. Contact medical direction for instructions on how to proceed, and continue treatment until the problem has been resolved.

- Document refusals of care completely and accurately. Make sure that the patient is competent—an adult who is lucid (oriented to person, place, and time) and capable of making an informed decision—and not under the influence of drugs or alcohol, consult medical direction, and try again to persuade the patient to accept treatment prior to departing the scene.

- Four items must be demonstrated in a successful negligence action: (1) The EMT had a duty to act. (2) The EMT breached that duty to act. (3) The patient suffered an injury or harm that is recognized by the law as a compensable injury. (4) The injury was the result of the breach of the duty (proximate cause).

- Common intentional torts in EMS are abandonment, assault, battery, false imprisonment or kidnapping, and defamation (slander and libel).

- The Health Insurance Portability and Accountability Act (HIPAA) of 1996 protects the privacy of patient health care information and provides the patient with control over how the information is used. Information obtained when treating a patient must be kept confidential.

- The Consolidated Omnibus Budget Reconciliation Act (COBRA) and the Emergency Medical Treatment and Active Labor Act (EMTALA) are federal regulations designed to ensure the public's access to emergency health care regardless of their ability to pay. Avoid potential liability by never making a decision to transport to a specific medical facility based on the patient's ability to pay.

- Appropriate crime scene actions include the following: take one way in and out, touch or move only what is required to care for the patient, document anything unusual, do not cut through knots or bullet or stab holes in the patient's clothing, and preserve evidence in sexual assault cases.

- Law enforcement should be notified in cases of abuse, injuries related to a crime, and drug-related injuries. Follow your state laws.

- When dealing with difficult legal or ethical issues, always put the welfare of the patient first.

▌ TERMS AND CONCEPTS

1. Write the number of the correct term next to each definition.
   1. Advance directive
   2. Duty to act
   3. Expressed consent
   4. Implied consent
   5. Minor consent
   6. Scope of practice
   7. Battery
   8. Good Samaritan law
   9. Informed consent

10. Slander
11. Tort
12. Physician orders for life-sustaining treatment (POLST)

_____ a. Permission obtained from a parent or legal guardian for emergency treatment of a patient who is under legal age

_____ b. The assumption that an unresponsive patient would agree to emergency treatment

_____ c. Permission that must be obtained from every conscious, mentally competent adult before emergency treatment may be provided

_____ d. Written instructions regarding future resuscitation and care, such as living wills, DNR orders, and health care proxies

_____ e. The obligation to care for a patient who requires it

_____ f. The actions and care that are legally allowed to be provided by a health care provider

_____ g. A wrongful act, injury, or damage

_____ h. The act of touching a patient unlawfully

_____ i. Generally protects a person from liability for acts performed in good faith unless those acts constitute gross negligence

_____ j. Spoken defamation

_____ k. Permission obtained when the patient is provided information related to the care and consequences of care

_____ l. Used in patients with serious or terminal illness who are not expected to survive for longer than one year

❙ CONTENT REVIEW

1. Which of the following determines the EMT's scope of practice?
   a. The EMT's capability to perform medical procedures
   b. The National EMS Act of 1999
   c. National EMS Educational Standards
   d. The Federal Medical Practice Act

2. On a call, you begin to dress the severely bleeding wound of an adult patient who has told you to go away and leave her alone. The patient appears competent. You can legally be charged with which of the following?
   a. Breach of duty
   b. Negligence
   c. Abandonment
   d. Battery

3. Which of the following provides some protection from liability for emergency care provided in good faith?
   a. Code of ethics
   b. Malpractice act
   c. Good Samaritan law
   d. Emergency care statute

4. Emergency care that is expected of any EMT under similar circumstances is known as which of the following?
   a. Standard of care
   b. Code of care
   c. Patient care guidelines
   d. Emergency care guidelines

5. Under the law, to care for a conscious, competent, adult patient, you must receive which of the following?
   a. Consent from the wife or husband of the patient
   b. The patient's expressed or implied consent
   c. Prior consent from medical oversight
   d. Consent that is written and witnessed

6. A 10-year-old is critically injured. The parents cannot be located. Treatment can be initiated under which of the following forms of consent?
   a. Implied consent
   b. Expressed consent
   c. Minor consent
   d. Incapacitated consent

7. Under the law, in order to refuse treatment, a *patient* must
   a. be mentally competent.
   b. be free of any life-threatening injuries or conditions.
   c. sign a form releasing the EMT from liability.
   d. have a witness to the refusal-of-treatment form.

8. Which of the following is considered a valid indication of refusal of care from a competent adult?
   a. Nodding the head "yes" before treatment begins
   b. Pushing you away after treatment has begun
   c. Shrugging the shoulders
   d. Questioning the health care provider

9. Stopping care without ensuring that another health care professional with equivalent or better training will take over is called which of the following?
   a. Neglect
   b. Abandonment
   c. Refusal
   d. Battery

10. Confidential patient information may be released only under certain circumstances. Which of the following is one of these circumstances?
    a. While off duty, another EMT asks you about patient care information.
    b. Your spouse asks you what happened at a neighbor's house.
    c. A lawyer calls you and demands information related to the incident.
    d. A health care provider needs to know this information in order to continue medical care.

11. Your legal obligation to provide service to a patient while you are on duty (and, in some states, even while you are off duty) is known as
   a. the Good Samaritan law.
   b. duty to act.
   c. scope of practice.
   d. advance directive.

12. You are on the scene where a patient is refusing treatment and transport to the hospital. You are unsure whether the patient is able to make a rational decision. You should
   a. transport the patient against his wishes.
   b. have the patient sign a refusal-of-care form.
   c. contact medical direction for a consultation.
   d. have a family member sign the refusal.

13. A willful threat to a patient that can occur without actual touching is called
   a. battery.
   b. false imprisonment.
   c. slander.
   d. assault.

14. The HIPAA, as it relates to the EMT, includes which of the following general provisions?
   a. Limits on disclosure of patient information, training on specific policies, requirements for specific treatments provided, and timelines for reporting violations
   b. Limits on disclosure of patient information, training on specific policies, obtaining patient signatures, and the assignment of an EMS privacy officer
   c. Limits on patients' rights to information, patient training on specific policies, timelines for reporting violations, and the assignment of an EMS privacy officer
   d. Limits on patients' rights to information, training on specific policies, and requirements for specific treatments provided

15. COBRA and EMTALA are both federal regulations designed to
   a. reduce potential errors associated with interfacility patient transfers.
   b. help patients pay for needed emergency medical care and rehabilitation.
   c. ensure public access to emergency care regardless of ability to pay.
   d. limit the legal liability exposure of EMS systems by providing limits of liability.

16. State laws that allow a parent to relinquish custody of an unharmed infant to a proper authority are generally referred to as
   a. Abandoned Infant Acts.
   b. Jason's Act(s).
   c. the Infant Relinquishment Act(s).
   d. Baby Safe Haven Law(s).

CASE STUDY 1

It's 4:00 in the morning, and you have been dispatched to care for a patient complaining of chest pain. Upon arrival, you observe a male patient who appears to be in his mid-60s. He looks pale and sweaty. However, he appears to be alert and is able to give you his name, address, day of the week, and time of day. He describes his pain as severe but refuses to be treated or transported to the hospital. You describe the need for medical care to the patient. While you are explaining this information to him, he repeatedly cups his hand behind his ear and asks, "What? What are you telling me?" Unexpectedly, your partner asks the patient to sign a refusal-of-care release form. The patient signs the form quickly and hands it back. Your partner looks at you and says, "Let's go!"

1. What is the most important concern you should have relating to this patient's refusal of treatment?
   a. The patient's mental competence
   b. The patient's understanding of the possible consequences of refusal
   c. The patient's signing the release without reading it
   d. Lack of professional courtesy if you second-guess your partner's suggestion to go

2. Your next action in this situation should be to
   a. leave as soon as the refusal form has been signed.
   b. encourage the patient to seek help if additional symptoms develop.
   c. have a witness sign the refusal form along with the patient.
   d. try again to persuade the patient to accept treatment.

▌CASE STUDY 2

You are employed as an EMT for a public EMS agency. Your partner, Joe, and you are dispatched to a call for a child who is choking. You are dispatched at 3:00 P.M. You have about a 10-block response to the scene. En route, your unit runs out of gas. You look at Joe. Joe gives you a blank stare and says, "I guess I forgot to fill it up!" A secondary unit responds to the call and arrives in 10 minutes. You learn later that the secondary unit arrived on scene and quickly removed a piece of hot dog from the child's airway. The child suffered permanent brain damage because of this incident.

1. The following are four items that must be demonstrated to be successful in a negligence action. Place a Y for yes or an N for no next to each item to determine if negligence occurred in this case.

   _____ a. The EMTs had a duty to act.

   _____ b. The EMTs breached the duty to act.

   _____ c. The patient suffered an injury.

   _____ d. The injury was the result of the negligence of the EMTs.

Documentation

▌ STANDARD

Preparatory (Content Area: Documentation)

▌ COMPETENCY

Applies fundamental knowledge of the EMS system, safety/well-being of the EMT, medical/legal and ethical issues to the provision of emergency care.

▌ OBJECTIVES

After reading this chapter, you should be able to:

4-1. Define key terms introduced in this chapter.

4-2. Describe each of the following purposes served by the prehospital care report (PCR):
   a. Continuity of patient care
   b. Administrative uses
   c. Legal document
   d. Education and research
   e. Evaluation and continuous quality improvement (CQI)

4-3. Describe characteristics, including advantages and disadvantages, of both paper and computer-based (electronic) PCR formats.

4-4. Explain the purposes of the U.S. Department of Transportation (DOT) minimum data set for PCRs.

4-5. List the elements of the DOT minimum data set for PCRs.

4-6. Describe the purpose and contents of each of the following sections of a PCR:
   a. Administrative data
   b. Patient demographics and other patient data
   c. Vital signs
   d. Narrative
   e. Treatment

4-7. Give examples of each of the following types of PCR narrative information:
   a. Chief complaint
   b. Pertinent history
   c. Subjective information
   d. Objective information
   e. Pertinent negatives

4-8. Use common abbreviations and medical terminology accurately in PCRs.

4-9. Explain each of the following legal concerns with respect to the PCR:
   a. Confidentiality
   b. Allowed distribution of the PCR or information included in it
   c. Documenting a patient's refusal of treatment
   d. Falsification of the PCR
   e. Correction of errors

4-10. Discuss how to handle each of the following situations with respect to the PCR:
   a. Transfer of patient care when returning to service prior to completing the PCR
   b. Multiple-casualty incidents (MCIs)
   c. Special reporting situations, such as infectious disease exposure and suspicion of abuse or neglect

4-11. Accurately and completely record pertinent patient and EMS call information using the SOAP, CHART, and CHEATED methods.

▌ KEY IDEAS

The focus of this chapter is the written documentation of patient care. Documenting all of your encounters with patients is an essential part of your job as an EMT. Key ideas and concepts include the following:

- Documentation serves many functions. Among them are ensuring continuity of care and establishing a baseline of patient status; administrative uses, such as billing and insurance information; and acting as a legal record of assessment, care given, and patient response.

- Documentation may also be used for educational, research, and continuous quality improvement purposes. It is important to include any other information that may be a local or state requirement.

- The most traditional format for the patient care report is the written prehospital care report (PCR). An alternative format that is used and accepted widely is the computerized direct data entry report. Both are designed to provide a complete and accurate picture of your contact with the patient.

- Documentation is governed by two basic rules: "If it wasn't written down, it wasn't done," and "If it wasn't done, don't write it down."

▌ TERMS AND CONCEPTS

1. Write the number of the correct term next to each definition.
   1. Minimum data set (MDS)
   2. Pertinent negatives
   3. Prehospital care report (PCR)
   4. Triage tag

   _____ a. Document containing only key patient information, used during a multiple-casualty incident

   _____ b. Signs and symptoms that might be expected in certain situations but that the patient denies

   _____ c. Information that the U.S. Department of Transportation recommends all patient care reports include

   _____ d. Documentation of an EMT's contact with a patient

CONTENT REVIEW

1. The *primary* reason for high-quality documentation is
   a. as a resource for quality improvement review.
   b. to assist in the preparation of patient bills.
   c. to ensure high-quality patient care.
   d. as a resource in malpractice suits.

2. The documentation provided in the PCR
   a. typically becomes a part of the patient's permanent medical record.
   b. is of little use in a lawsuit brought against the EMT.
   c. is seldom created in an electronic form.
   d. may not be used for preparing bills or for submission to insurance.

3. The use of accurate and synchronous clocks is
   a. seldom important in EMS documentation.
   b. critical for proper EMS documentation.
   c. only important for dispatch purposes.
   d. only important for medical information.

4. The narrative section of the patient care report should include the patient's chief complaint, the SAMPLE history, and
   a. your diagnosis of the patient's problem.
   b. physical assessment findings.
   c. all remarks made by bystanders.
   d. your conclusions about the incident.

5. Which of the following would be considered a pertinent negative for a patient who was the unrestrained driver of a car involved in a serious motor vehicle accident?
   a. The patient complains of abdominal pain.
   b. The patient reports that it hurts to take a deep breath.
   c. The patient denies back and/or neck pain.
   d. The patient denies any allergies to food or drugs.

6. At least _____ set(s) of vital signs should be taken and recorded on all patient transports.
   a. one
   b. two
   c. three
   d. four

7. Under most state and federal laws, you may *not* provide confidential information about a patient
   a. when reporting to another health care provider when transferring care.
   b. in response to questions from friends of the patient.
   c. when providing information to the police as part of a criminal investigation.
   d. if you are subpoenaed to appear in court and provide information in a legal case.

8. When dealing with a patient who has refused treatment,
   a. document your explanation of possible consequences of failing to accept care, and have the patient sign the form acknowledging refusal of treatment.
   b. only discuss the situation with the patient, as required by patient privacy provisions.
   c. the call is generally less involved and easier to document.
   d. issues of patient competency are rarely a concern of the EMT.

9. Objective information is
   a. a sign.
   b. a symptom.
   c. based on an individual's perception.
   d. symptoms the patient denies having.

10. Which of the following best describes the appropriate way to correct an error on the written patient care report discovered while the report is being written?
   a. Use correction fluid to cover the incorrect entry.
   b. Use multiple heavy lines to block out the incorrect entry.
   c. Draw a single line through the incorrect entry and initial it.
   d. Report the error verbally but do not alter the report.

11. Which of the following are commonly used for patient care reports in a multiple-casualty incident?
   a. Triage tags
   b. Casualty codes
   c. Regularly used patient care reports
   d. Multiple-casualty forms

12. Which of the following situations may require additional, special documentation by the EMT?
   a. Suspected abuse of a child or an elderly patient
   b. Patient care provided to a patient complaining of chest pain
   c. Patient care given to patients in motor vehicle accidents
   d. Patient care provided to a patient with difficulty breathing

13. The Department of Transportation has designated certain information on the PCR to be the MDS. Select the item that is *not* part of the MDS and that you would *not* be likely to see on a PCR form.
   a. Crew member names
   b. Chief complaint
   c. Patient's next of kin
   d. Pulse rate

14. When writing the PCR, you may use approved abbreviations to help document your findings. In each space, write the abbreviation that stands for the given term.

a	Pt	Rx	TID
$\bar{c}$	q	$\bar{s}$	Tx
PO	QID	STAT	x

   _____ a. Four times a day

   _____ b. Times

_____ c. Before

_____ d. Patient

_____ e. Prescription

_____ f. Every

_____ g. Treatment

_____ h. With

_____ i. Immediately

_____ j. Without

_____ k. Orally, by mouth

_____ l. Three times a day

15. The mnemonics SOAP, CHART, and CHEATED are often used by EMS personnel to
   a. determine the level of responsiveness or mental status.
   b. describe the patient's mechanism of injury.
   c. convey the pertinent negatives as described by the patient.
   d. organize the information on the PCR.

16. When using any of the following mnemonics—SOAP, CHART, or CHEATED—you know that the "A" refers to
   a. arrival on scene.
   b. actions on scene.
   c. absent physical findings.
   d. assessment.

CASE STUDY

You get dispatched to the local high school on a report of a fall. Upon arrival at the school, you report to the office, where you find that your patient slipped on a wet floor and "twisted his ankle." Your 50-year-old patient is Mr. Henderson, the school principal. He says, "I'm sorry you were sent out for nothing. I'm more embarrassed than hurt." You introduce yourself and ask if you can check him over anyway, so long as you're here. He agrees.

On your primary assessment, you find him to be alert and oriented, having no apparent difficulty breathing, and in no apparent distress. You see no signs of bleeding. Mr. Henderson lets your partner check his pulse, which is strong and regular. His skin is pink, warm, and dry.

During your focused physical exam, you find that Mr. Henderson's right ankle, which he reports is "a little sore," is markedly swollen, discolored, and very tender to gentle palpation. His foot is slightly pale but warm to the touch. His pedal pulse is present, and he has good sensation and motion. Vital signs: blood pressure 138/78 mmHg, pulse 68 beats per minute, and respirations 18 per minute and adequate; PaO_2 is 96% on room air. Skin is still normal, as are pupils. You complete your history and find that Mr. Henderson has no allergies and takes no medications. He denies any medical problems, loss of consciousness, or any other injuries. He had soup and a sandwich for lunch about a half hour ago. He says that he has felt fine all day but slipped on some water on the floor as he was leaving the cafeteria.

You urge Mr. Henderson to allow you to splint his ankle and transport him to the hospital so he can get X-rays to see if his ankle is broken. He refuses, saying, "Thanks for checking me out, but you guys have to be available for real emergencies. I've already called my wife, and she's on her way to take me to the doctor. She ought to be here in 10 minutes or so. Bad enough that I fell down in front of half the school. There's no way I'm going out of here on that stretcher." You agree that he's stable enough to be transported by car but remind him that he shouldn't bear any weight on his ankle until he's been seen by the doctor. You also remind him that if any problems arise or if he changes his mind, he should call 911.

1. In the space provided, write the narrative section of the patient care report for this call.

2. Before leaving the scene, what else should you do?
   a. Have the patient read the patient care report and sign the refusal form.
   b. Call medical control and have the patient speak to the physician.
   c. Direct the patient to contact his own physician for advice.
   d. Contact the patient's wife in an attempt to have her convince him to be transported.

3. While walking toward your ambulance, a coworker of Mr. Henderson approaches you. The coworker is visibly upset. Explaining that he is the safety officer for the school, he asks you what happened to Mr. Henderson and if he is injured. How should you respond to the safety officer?
   a. Explain that, legally, you cannot discuss the call because of patient confidentiality rights.
   b. Discreetly discuss the call only in general terms, not disclosing anything specific about the injuries.
   c. Do not discuss the call, but allow him to read the PCR because it is public information.
   d. Because he is the safety officer, you may disclose all of the information you have about the patient.

Communication

❙ STANDARD

Preparatory (Content Areas: EMS System Communication; Therapeutic Communication)

❙ COMPETENCY

Applies fundamental knowledge of the EMS system, safety/well-being of the EMT, medical/legal and ethical issues to the provision of emergency care.

❙ OBJECTIVES

After reading this chapter, you should be able to:

5-1. Define key terms introduced in this chapter.

5-2. Discuss the purposes and characteristics of each of the following EMS system communication components:
   a. Base station
   b. Mobile radios
   c. Portable radios
   d. Digitalized radio equipment
   e. Mobile data terminals
   f. Cell phones

5-3. Describe the responsibilities of the Federal Communications Commission.

5-4. Explain the importance of EMS system communication equipment maintenance.

5-5. Given a radio transmitter/receiver, demonstrate the standard ground rules for radio communications.

5-6. List key points in an EMS call at which you should communicate with dispatch.

5-7. Deliver a concise, organized radio report that clearly conveys essential information to medical direction or the receiving facility.

5-8. Describe the process of receiving and confirming an order from medical direction over the radio.

5-9. Identify situations in which you should make additional contact with medical direction or the receiving facility after providing an initial radio report.

5-10. Given a scenario, deliver an oral report to transfer care of the patient to a receiving facility or another EMS provider.

5-11. Given a scenario, demonstrate effective communication that enhances team dynamics.

5-12. Discuss the advantages and disadvantages of using radio codes.

5-13. Convert back and forth between military time and standard clock times.

5-14. Communicate using commonly used radio terms.

5-15. Describe the components of the communication process.

5-16. Discuss factors that can enhance or interfere with effective communication.

5-17. Give examples of each of the following techniques of therapeutic communication:

    a. Clarification

    b. Summary

    c. Explanation

    d. Silence

    e. Reflection

    f. Empathy

    g. Confrontation

5-18. Given a scenario, engage in an effective communication process with a patient.

5-19. Recognize the potential messages that may be communicated via nonverbal behaviors.

5-20. Describe the uses, advantages, and disadvantages of open-ended and closed questions.

5-21. Analyze your communications with a patient in a scenario to recognize the following pitfalls in communication:

    a. Leading or biased questions

    b. Interrupting the patient

    c. Talking too much

    d. Providing false assurance

    e. Giving inappropriate advice

    f. Implying blame

5-22. Discuss considerations for each of the following situations:

    a. Communicating with a patient's family

    b. Getting a noncommunicative patient to talk

    c. Interviewing a hostile patient

    d. Cross-cultural communications

    e. Language barriers

    f. Communicating with children and elderly patients

KEY IDEAS

This chapter focuses on the role of communications in the delivery of emergency medical services. A good understanding of EMS communications skills and equipment is essential to your success as an EMT. Reliable communications systems are critical to all aspects of an EMS call. Key concepts include the following:

■ Standard components of an emergency communications system include a base station and mobile or portable transmitters/receivers. Additional components, such as repeaters and digitalized encoders and decoders, are used to enhance communication capabilities within an EMS system.

■ The Federal Communications Commission (FCC) has jurisdiction over all radio operations in the United States, including those used by EMS systems.

■ Communications within an EMS system depend on adhering to basic rules of radio communication at all times.

■ Effective team communication improves how the team accomplishes its goals and also improves the quality of services provided to the patients and the community.

■ SBAR is a mnemonic for situation, background, assessment, and recommendation and is used as a method of organizing communications with medical direction.

■ Digital data terminals receive dispatch information and transmit critical information back to dispatch.

■ Patients with special needs, such as the hearing impaired, children, and the elderly, require special consideration to ensure effective communication at the scene of an emergency.

TERMS AND CONCEPTS

1. Write the number of the correct term next to each definition.

    1. Base station
    2. Decoder
    3. Encoder
    4. Repeater
    5. Mobile (digital) data terminal
    6. Open-ended question
    7. Leading question
    8. Haptics
    9. Ethnocentrism
    10. Culture
    11. SBAR

    _____ a. Device that converts sound waves into digital codes for transmission

    _____ b. The central dispatch and coordination area of an EMS communications system

    _____ c. Devices that receive transmissions from one source and rebroadcast them at a higher power on another frequency

    _____ d. Device that recognizes and responds to only certain codes imposed on a radio broadcast

    _____ e. Receives and transmits digital dispatch information

    _____ f. The study of touching

    _____ g. Questions that allow the patient to give a detailed response in his own words

    _____ h. The thoughts, communications, actions, and values of racial, ethnic, religious, or social groups

    _____ i. The view that one culture's way of doing things is the right way and any other way is inferior

    _____ j. Questions that suggest an answer guided by the individual who is asking the question

    _____ k. Method of organizing communications with medical direction

CONTENT REVIEW

1. An EMS base station
    a. generally uses a low output of between 50 and 75 watts of transmission power.
    b. should be located in a low-lying area, free from potentially damaging high winds.
    c. does not require close proximity to the hospital that serves as the medical command center.
    d. serves as a dispatch and coordination area and is in contact with other system elements.

2. Repeaters are used within an EMS communications system to allow
    a. communications over a wide geographical area.
    b. significant reductions in operating costs.
    c. communication with medical direction.
    d. communications to be transmitted through the air via cells.

3. Cell phones within an EMS system
   a. usually have poor sound quality.
   b. seldom become overwhelmed during disaster situations.
   c. are usually difficult to maintain and are cost prohibitive.
   d. often improve communication privacy.

4. One role of the FCC in EMS communications systems is to
   a. purchase base-station radio equipment.
   b. license base stations.
   c. serve as a repeater for base-station operations.
   d. conduct radio operations training for EMS personnel.

5. Which of the following is a "ground rule" for radio operations?
   a. Use the radio just as if you were talking on a telephone.
   b. Keep transmissions brief, organized, and to the point.
   c. Never listen for other radio traffic before transmitting.
   d. Don't waste valuable airtime by repeating back orders or information.

6. The role of dispatch in an EMS communications system is to obtain information about the nature of the emergency, direct the appropriate emergency service(s) to the scene, and
   a. notify the medical command center of the request for service.
   b. alert the local news media to provide essential information.
   c. provide the caller with instructions about what to do until help arrives.
   d. contact the medical director to provide a link for medical direction.

7. In addition to communicating with dispatch to acknowledge the dispatch information, to advise dispatch that you are en route, and again while en route to report your estimated time of arrival at the scene, number the following list in the proper order from 1 to 5 to show the other times that you should communicate with dispatch.

   _____ To announce your arrival back at base
   _____ To announce your arrival on scene and request further assistance
   _____ To announce you are "clear" and available for another call
   _____ To announce your arrival at the hospital
   _____ To announce your departure from the scene and your estimated hospital arrival time

8. When communicating with medical direction, you should use a standard format that includes your unit identification and service level; the patient's age, sex, and chief complaint; a brief, pertinent history of the present illness, including scene assessment and mechanism of injury; past major illnesses; and
   a. the name of the patient's insurance provider.
   b. a detailed description of the patient's past illnesses.
   c. a comprehensive description of the findings of the physical exam.
   d. the patient's mental status.

9. After receiving an order or instructions from medical direction, dispatch, or other medical personnel, you should
   a. always say thank you before you "sign off."
   b. repeat the instructions word for word.
   c. click your "press to talk" button twice to signal your understanding.
   d. acknowledge the instructions by saying "10-4."

10. If you receive orders from medical direction that do not appear to be appropriate, you should always
    a. question the order to clarify if there has been a misunderstanding.
    b. follow the orders as given by medical direction.
    c. double-check with your partner before following the orders.
    d. request to speak with someone else.

11. When interacting with bystanders or other EMRs when you arrive on the scene, you should
    a. obtain permission from police and fire personnel before beginning patient care.
    b. obtain complete information from on-scene emergency providers before making patient contact.
    c. ask for information about what happened and what care has been given.
    d. quickly and loudly point out any errors in treatment provided by on-scene emergency providers.

12. Your patient is a non-English-speaking traveler in your community. Which of the following is an appropriate action in this situation?
    a. See if a companion or a bystander can interpret.
    b. Talk loudly and slowly to make yourself understood.
    c. No action is necessary—nothing can be done in this circumstance.
    d. Draw pictures to communicate with the non-English speaker.

13. You are working in an EMS system that utilizes radio codes. Which statement best describes an advantage of radio codes?
    a. They provide clear, concise information.
    b. They lengthen radio airtime.
    c. They are generally understood by the patient.
    d. They are regulated by the Federal Communications Commission.

14. Which of the following statements is accurate regarding Ten-Codes?
    a. They are the primary code system used by EMS systems.
    b. They are published by the FCC.
    c. They are generally understood by the patient.
    d. They are less favored than the use of standard English.

15. To ensure accuracy and synchronicity, most EMS systems use military time rather than standard A.M. and P.M. designations. Choose the military time that correctly represents 8:32 P.M. standard time.
    a. 0832 hours
    b. 1832 hours
    c. 2032 hours
    d. 2232 hours

▌ CASE STUDY

You were dispatched to the carousel on the playground at 1031 Bruce Road for an injured child. Your partner notifies dispatch of your arrival. You note no signs of danger as you park the ambulance and put on your personal protective equipment. As you approach the group gathered near a picnic table, you can hear the sound of a child crying. You introduce yourself to the woman holding the crying child on her lap and ask what happened and what you can do to help. The mother of your patient, Mrs. Smith, thanks you for coming so quickly and tells you that her son, Mikey, tripped while running and cut his chin. She says he did not lose consciousness. Mikey's crying has quieted, and he's watching you closely. You ask him if you can look at his chin. He nods his permission. His mother removes the washcloth that she had been using to control the bleeding. You observe an approximately 1-inch laceration. You explain what you are going to do, and then, as you gently apply a sterile dressing and bandage to Mikey's injury, you reassure him quietly. He tells you that he is 3 years old and has a dog and three big sisters. He also says he never rode in an "ambliance." You see no other signs of injury.

Your partner obtains a set of baseline vitals. Mikey's blood pressure is 80/68 mmHg. His heart rate is strong, at 80 beats per minute. His respirations are 28 per minute, full and adequate. His skin is slightly flushed, warm, and moist. His capillary refill is less than 2 seconds. His pupils are normal and equal in size and reactivity, and the SpO$_2$ is 96% on room air. You obtain a history. When asked, Mikey says his chin "hurts bad." He denies neck or back pain and is alert and oriented to person, place, and time. His mother reports that he is a healthy child who takes no medications and has no known allergies. Mikey tells you that he had a Popsicle in the car on his way to the park. Mrs. Smith says that they arrived about an hour ago and that Mikey was fine before he fell as he ran to get on the carousel. You secure Mikey in the child restraint seat on the stretcher in the back of the ambulance and then help Mrs. Smith get settled and secured to the jump seat. You perform the reassessment on Mikey, finding him still completely alert and oriented. His dressing remains dry. His vital signs are essentially unchanged. You radio the hospital with your report.

In the space provided, write the report you would give orally at the following times:

1. Arrival on scene (to dispatch):

2. En route to the hospital (to the receiving hospital):

3. At the hospital when you transfer care:

Lifting and Moving Patients

▌ STANDARD

Preparatory (Content Area: Workforce Safety and Wellness)

▌ COMPETENCY

Applies fundamental knowledge of the EMS system, safety/well-being of the EMT, medical/legal and ethical issues to the provision of emergency care.

▌ OBJECTIVES

After reading this chapter, you should be able to:

6-1. Define key terms introduced in this chapter.

6-2. Explain the importance of always using proper techniques when lifting, carrying, and moving patients and equipment.

6-3. Define the term *body mechanics*.

6-4. Demonstrate each of the four principles of body mechanics listed in the text when lifting and moving patients and equipment.

6-5. Explain the roles of proper body posture and physical fitness in preventing injuries resulting from lifting and moving patients.

6-6. Describe considerations in teamwork and communication with partners and patients when lifting and moving patients.

6-7. Apply the general guidelines for lifting and moving patients that are described in the text.

6-8. Discuss the advantages, disadvantages, and steps of each of the following lifting and moving techniques and processes:
   a. Power lift
   b. Power grip
   c. Squat lift
   d. One-handed equipment carrying
   e. Reaching
   f. Log roll
   g. Pushing and pulling

6-9. Differentiate between scenarios in which emergency, urgent, and nonurgent moves are indicated.

6-10. Given a scenario, demonstrate an appropriate moving technique to be used, including:

a. Armpit-forearm drag

b. Shirt drag

c. Blanket drag

d. Rapid extrication

e. Direct ground lift

f. Extremity lift

g. Direct carry

h. Draw sheet method

6-11. Demonstrate the steps required to securely "package" a patient for transport.

6-12. Describe the proper use, advantages, disadvantages, and limitations of each of the following pieces of equipment used in lifting and moving patients:

a. Wheeled stretcher

b. Portable stretcher

c. Stair chair

d. Backboard

e. Scoop stretcher

f. Basket stretcher

g. Flexible stretcher

h. Devices for bariatric patients

6-13. Given a scenario involving any of the following types of patients, demonstrate proper positioning of the patient:

a. Unresponsive patient

b. Patient with chest pain or difficulty breathing

c. Patient with known or suspected spinal injury

d. Patient in shock

e. Patient with nausea or vomiting

f. Patient in third trimester of pregnancy

g. Infant or toddler

h. Elderly patient

i. Patient with a physical disability

6-14. Discuss special considerations when preparing patients for air medical transport.

6-15. Discuss special considerations when using a neonatal isolette.

▌ KEY IDEAS

This chapter presents proper methods of lifting and moving patients and equipment. It is not enough to know this material. You need to use the information every day and on every response.

- Proper use of body mechanics for safe lifting can greatly decrease injuries. The four basic principles of body mechanics are as follows: (1) Keep the weight of the object close to the body. (2) To lift a heavy object, use the leg, hip, and gluteal muscles plus contracted abdominal muscles. (3) "Stack" shoulders over hips, hips over feet. (4) Reduce the height or distance that an object must be lifted.

- Poor posture can fatigue your back and promote injury.

- Communication and teamwork are essential to safe lifting and moving.

- It is important to be able to perform the following techniques: power lift, squat lift, one-handed equipment-carrying technique, stair chair technique, reaching techniques, and pushing and pulling techniques.

▌ TERMS AND CONCEPTS

1. Write the number of the correct term next to each definition.

1. Emergency move
2. Nonurgent move
3. Lordosis
4. Kyphosis
5. Power grip

_____ a. Stomach is too anterior and the buttocks are too posterior

_____ b. Performed when no immediate threat to life exists

_____ c. Palm and fingers in complete contact with the object and fingers bent at same angle

_____ d. Shoulders are rolled forward, which results in fatigue on the lower back

_____ e. Performed when there is an immediate danger to the patient or rescuer

CONTENT REVIEW

1. You are much more likely to injure your back when performing which task?
   a. Reaching a great distance to lift a light object
   b. Reaching a short distance to lift a heavy object
   c. Reaching up to shoulder height to lift a light object
   d. Lifting a light object while keeping it close to you

2. You are preparing to move a heavy object. Which muscles will provide the most power with the greatest degree of safety?
   a. Leg, hip, and gluteal muscles
   b. Back and shoulder muscles
   c. Chest and arm muscles
   d. Abdominal and intercostal muscles

3. The body mechanics principle called "stacking" means
   a. stacking objects to be lifted one on top of the other.
   b. keeping your shoulders, hips, and feet in vertical alignment.
   c. eliminating curvature from your spine.
   d. staying under an object being lifted overhead.

4. To help prevent injury and manage stress, you should follow a physical fitness program that includes what four ingredients?

   _____

   _____

   _____

   _____

5. When performing a power lift, which of the following is correct?
   a. Stand to the side of the object and lift the hips before the upper body.
   b. Turn feet inward, lock knees, and lift the hips before the upper body.
   c. Lock the back and lift the upper body before the hips.
   d. Bend forward at the waist and lift the upper body before the hips.

6. When performing the squat lift with a weak leg or ankle, you should
   a. place the weaker leg slightly behind your good leg.
   b. place the weaker leg slightly in front of the good leg.
   c. place the weaker leg beside and parallel with the good leg.
   d. not use the squat lift with a weak leg.

7. You are preparing to carry a heavy tool using the one-handed equipment-carrying technique. You know that you should avoid
   a. leaning to the opposite side.
   b. bending your knees.
   c. locking your back.
   d. bending at the hips.

8. You and your partner are preparing to navigate stairs using a stair chair. You should
   a. tilt the stair chair forward.
   b. position the patient facing the stairs.
   c. keep one hand on the railing.
   d. use a spotter to direct and navigate.

9. If you have to reach for an object that is greater than _____ from your body, you should reposition yourself closer to the object.
   a. 5 inches
   b. 10 inches
   c. 20 inches
   d. 3 feet

10. When you need to push or pull an object, which of the following is correct?
    a. Push rather than pull, and keep the load at knee level.
    b. Push rather than pull, and keep the load between the hips and shoulders.
    c. Pull rather than push, and keep the load at shoulder level.
    d. Pull rather than push, and keep the load at hip level.

11. In which of the following situations would use of the rapid extrication technique be inappropriate?
    a. The patient presents with loss of sensation and motor response to the lower extremities.
    b. The patient is bleeding severely; the vehicle appears unstable and may slide down a ravine.
    c. The patient seems uninjured, but there appears to be smoke coming from the vehicle and there is a strong smell of gasoline.
    d. The patient has stopped breathing, and a weak central pulse is palpated on the neck.

12. You and your partner have decided to utilize the two-person carry to move your patient. Which of the following is correct pertaining to the two-person carry?
    a. The stronger EMT should be placed at the foot of the stretcher.
    b. The EMT at the foot end of the patient faces the EMT at the head end.
    c. The EMT at the foot end of the stretcher walks forward while calling out obstacles.
    d. The EMT at the head is required to walk backwards, which may increase the risk of injury.

13. When carrying a supine patient on stairs, you should
    a. carry the patient headfirst up the steps; therefore, the EMT at the head end moves backward up the steps.
    b. walk backward down the stairs carrying the patient headfirst, while the EMT at the feet guides the patient.
    c. utilize the stair chair or tracked stair chair device to transition the steps using a spotter to look for obstacles.
    d. allow the patient free movement of his hands to aid in balance while moving the patient up or down the stairs.

14. Power cots
    a. typically weigh less than a traditional stretcher.
    b. are not capable of being outfitted with a power loading system.
    c. increase the spinal loading associated with repetitive movements.
    d. decrease the spinal loading associated with repetitive movements.

CASE STUDY

You and your partner, Kyle, work in an East Coast community and are dispatched to a guarded beach for an injured surfer. As you and Kyle approach the scene, you are met by the lifeguard captain, Vicky. She explains that the patient has deeply lacerated his leg and will need to be carried across the beach and over the dune line to the parking lot. Fortunately, there is a ramp that leads to a boardwalk, and a set of stairs connects the boardwalk to the parking lot. Vicky says that she has three lifeguards who can assist with moving the patient. Kyle suggests a four-corner carry with the wheeled stretcher in the up position (legs fully extended), thus reducing the chance of dropping the patient. If the carriers need a break, this position will allow the stretcher to rest on the extended wheels without lowering the patient to ground level, thus reducing the chance of injury. You commend Kyle for his foresight and planning.

1. After the patient has been loaded and you are ready to move him, you instruct the rescuers on the corners of the stretcher to
   a. keep their backs leaning to the opposite side of the patient to compensate the weight.
   b. keep their backs locked and stay as close to the stretcher as possible, avoiding leaning.
   c. relax their back muscles and bend at the waist to keep the stretcher moving forward.
   d. grip the stretcher handles with only their fingers, avoiding contact between palms and handles.

2. As you and the team reach the boardwalk, you instruct them to
   a. continue to carry the stretcher because once you are in motion, stopping will result in fatigue.
   b. continue to carry the stretcher because it is important that the patient receive a smooth ride.
   c. lower the stretcher onto its wheels so the stretcher does part of the work, with the rescuers at the back pushing it along the boardwalk.
   d. lower the stretcher onto its wheels so the stretcher does part of the work, with the rescuers at the front pulling it along the boardwalk.

3. As you reach the stairs, your team takes a brief break. You instruct your team to lower the stretcher (legs retracted) so the wheels won't catch on the stairs. You should also instruct them to
   a. have a spotter at the bottom to help guide them.
   b. flex the body at the hips and not the waist.
   c. keep the weight and arms close to the body.
   d. All of these.

4. You and Kyle will use the power-lift technique to lift the stretcher into the up position. Regarding the power lift, which of the following is *not* correct?
   a. This technique is not recommended for use with heavy patients.
   b. This technique offers you the best defense against injury.
   c. This technique protects the patient with a safe and stable move.
   d. This technique is useful for rescuers with weak knees or thighs.

Anatomy, Physiology, and Medical Terminology

┃ STANDARDS

Anatomy and Physiology; Medical Terminology

┃ COMPETENCIES

Applies fundamental knowledge of the anatomy and function of all human systems to the practice of EMS.

Uses foundational anatomical and medical terms and abbreviations in written and oral communication with colleagues and other health professionals.

┃ OBJECTIVES

After reading this chapter, you should be able to:

7-1. Define key terms introduced in this chapter.

7-2. Explain the importance of knowledge of anatomy and physiology to patient assessment and care.

7-3. Define the terms *anatomy* and *physiology*.

7-4. Describe each of the following terms of position:
  a. Anatomical position
  b. Supine
  c. Prone
  d. Lateral recumbent
  e. Fowler's position
  f. Semi-Fowler's position
  g. Trendelenburg position
  h. Shock position

7-5. Identify each of the following anatomical terms:
  a. Midline
  b. Sagittal plane
  c. Frontal plane
  d. Transverse plane
  e. Midaxillary line
  f. Midclavicular line
  g. Anterior and posterior
  h. Dorsal and ventral
  i. Right and left

j. Superior and inferior

k. Medial and lateral

l. Proximal and distal

m. Plantar

n. Palmar

o. Abdominal quadrants: right upper quadrant, left upper quadrant, left lower quadrant, right lower quadrant

7-6. State the function of each of the following musculoskeletal system structures:

a. Skeletal muscle

b. Tendons

c. Ligaments

d. Bone

7-7. Describe each of the following components of the skeleton, including its location, the bones that make it up, and its function:

a. Skull

   i. Cranium

   ii. Face

b. Spinal column

   i. Cervical spine

   ii. Thoracic spine

   iii. Lumbar spine

   iv. Sacral spine

   v. Coccyx

c. Thorax

   i. Sternum (including manubrium, body, and xiphoid process)

   ii. Ribs

d. Pelvis

   i. Ilium and iliac crest

   ii. Ischium

   iii. Pubis

   iv. Acetabulum

e. Upper extremities

   i. Clavicle

   ii. Scapula, including acromion process

   iii. Humerus

   iv. Radius

   v. Ulna, including olecranon process

   vi. Carpals

   vii. Metacarpals

   viii. Phalanges

f. Lower extremities

   i. Femur

   ii. Patella

   iii. Tibia, including medial malleolus

   iv. Fibula, including lateral malleolus

   v. Tarsals, including the calcaneus

   vi. Metatarsals

   vii. Phalanges

7-8. Demonstrate each of the following joint movements:

a. Flexion and extension

b. Adduction and abduction

c. Circumduction

d. Pronation and supination

7-9. Describe each of the following types of joints:
    a. Ball-and-socket
    b. Hinge
    c. Pivot
    d. Gliding
    e. Saddle
    f. Condyloid

7-10. Differentiate between skeletal (voluntary), smooth (involuntary), and cardiac muscle.

7-11. Identify the basic functions of the respiratory system.

7-12. Identify the following structures of the respiratory system:
    a. Upper airway: nose, mouth, pharynx, nasopharynx, larynx
    b. Lower airway: trachea, bronchi, bronchioles, alveoli
    c. Epiglottis
    d. Lungs
    e. Pleura
    f. Diaphragm

7-13. Identify important differences in respiratory system anatomy in children.

7-14. Describe the basic mechanics and physiology of normal ventilation, respiration, and oxygenation, including:
    a. Inhalation and exhalation
    b. Use of intercostal muscles and diaphragm
    c. Negative and positive pressure
    d. Nervous system control of respiration
    e. Alveolar/capillary exchange of oxygen and carbon dioxide
    f. Capillary/cell exchange of oxygen and carbon dioxide

7-15. Identify characteristics of both adequate and inadequate breathing.

7-16. List the functions of the circulatory (cardiovascular) system.

7-17. Describe the anatomy and physiology of the heart to include:
    a. Location and size
    b. Tissue layers
    c. Chambers
    d. Valves
    e. Blood supply
    f. Blood flow through the heart
    g. Conduction system

7-18. Discuss the anatomy and physiology of the blood, circulation, perfusion, and metabolism to convey basic comprehension of:
    a. Arteries and arterioles
    b. Capillaries
    c. Veins and venules
    d. Blood composition
    e. Perfusion and capillary exchange
    f. Cell metabolism

7-19. Describe the basic functions of the nervous system.

7-20. Differentiate between the structural components and basic functions of the central nervous system and peripheral nervous system.

7-21. Differentiate between the functional divisions of the peripheral nervous system:
    a. Voluntary (somatic) nervous system
    b. Involuntary (autonomic) nervous system
      i. Sympathetic division
      ii. Parasympathetic division

7-22. Describe the basic role of the reticular activating system (RAS) and cerebral hemispheres in consciousness and unconsciousness.

7-23. Explain the overall function of the endocrine system.

7-24. Discuss the location and general function of each of the following components of the endocrine system:
  a. Thyroid gland
  b. Parathyroid glands
  c. Adrenal glands
  d. Gonads
  e. Islets of Langerhans of the pancreas, insulin, and glucagon
  f. Pituitary gland

7-25. Describe the general actions of epinephrine and norepinephrine on $beta_1$, $beta_2$, $alpha_1$, and $alpha_2$ receptors of the sympathetic nervous system.

7-26. List the general functions of the integumentary system.

7-27. Identify the structures of the integumentary system, including the epidermis, dermis, and subcutaneous layer.

7-28. Describe the basic anatomy and physiology of each of the following structures of the digestive system:
  a. Stomach
  b. Pancreas
  c. Liver
  d. Gallbladder
  e. Small intestine (duodenum, jejunum, ileum)
  f. Colon

7-29. List the basic structure and function of the organs of the urinary or renal system to include:
  a. Kidneys
  b. Ureters
  c. Urinary bladder
  d. Urethra

7-30. State the basic structure and function of the organs of the male and female reproductive systems:
  a. Male
    i. Testes
    ii. Accessory glands
    iii. Penis
  b. Female
    i. Ovaries
    ii. Fallopian tubes
    iii. Uterus
    iv. Vagina
    v. External genitalia

7-31. Explain the importance of knowledge of medical terminology in communication among health care team members.

7-32. Apply knowledge of common prefixes, suffixes, and roots to interpret medical terms.

▌ KEY IDEAS

This chapter introduces basic terminology and concepts of the anatomy and physiology of the human body—information that you will need to help you determine when the body is functioning normally and when it is not, and to help you communicate with other health care providers.

■ The EMT must be able to identify the following positions: normal anatomical position, supine, prone, lateral recumbent, Fowler's.

■ The EMT must be able to define descriptive terms such as *midline, midclavicular line, midaxillary line, plantar,* and *palmar.*

- The EMT must be able to define the terms *anterior, superior, dorsal, lateral,* and *distal* and their opposites—*posterior, inferior, ventral, medial,* and *proximal.*
- The EMT must be able to understand and describe the anatomy and physiology of the following body systems: musculoskeletal, respiratory, circulatory, nervous, endocrine, and skin.
- The EMT must be able to identify and locate the central and peripheral pulse points.

▌MEDICAL TERMINOLOGY

Term	Prefix	Word Root Combining Form	Suffix	Definition
cerebrospinal (SAIR-uh-bro-SPI-nul)		cerebr/o (cerebrum, brain); spin (spine)	-al (pertaining to)	Referring to the brain and spinal cord. Example: *cerebrospinal fluid,* a cushion of fluid around the brain and spinal cord.
dermis (DER-mis)		derm/a/is (skin)		The middle layer of the skin. (The layers of the skin from outer- to innermost are the epidermis, the dermis, and the subcutaneous layer.)
epidermis (EP-uh-DER-mis)	epi- (upon, over, above)	derm/a/is (skin)		The outermost layer of the skin above the dermis.
epiglottis (EP-uh-GLOT-is)	epi- (upon, over, above)	glottis (the sound- producing area of the larynx)		A small, leaf-shaped flap of tissue located above the glottis, which covers the entrance of the larynx.
hypoperfusion (HY-po-per-FYU-zhun)	hypo- (below, under, deficient)	perfusion (delivery of oxygen and other nutrients to the cells)		The insufficient delivery of oxygen and other nutrients to the body's cells. Also called *shock.*
interpleural (in-ter-PLUR-ul)	inter- (between)	pleur (relating to the pleura, the membranes that line the lungs and thorax)	-al (pertaining to)	Pertaining to the area between the visceral and parietal pleura. Example: *interpleural space,* a tiny space with negative pressure, which allows the lungs to stay inflated.
intervertebral (in-ter-VER-tuh-brul)	inter- (between)	vertebra (segment of the spinal column)	-al (pertaining to)	Pertaining to the area between two vertebrae. Example: *intervertebral disk,* a fluid-filled pad between two vertebrae.

Term	Prefix	Word Root Combining Form	Suffix	Definition
midaxillary (mid-AX-uh-lair-e)	mid- (center)	axil (armpit)	-ary (pertaining to)	Refers to the center of the armpit. Example: *midaxillary line,* an imaginary line extending downward from the center of either armpit.
midclavicular (mid-klav-IK-yu-ler)	mid- (center)	clavicle (collarbone)	-ular (pertaining to)	Refers to the center of the collarbone (clavicle). Example: *midclavicular line,* an imaginary line extending downward from the center of either collarbone.
myocardium (MY-o-KAR-de-um)		my/o (muscle); card/ium (heart)		The cardiac muscle that makes up the middle layer of the walls of the heart.
nasopharynx (NA-zo-FAIR-inks)		nas/o (nose); pharynx (throat)		Nasal portion of the pharynx, situated above the soft palate.
pericardium (PAIR-uh-KAR-de-um)	peri- (around)	card/ium (heart)		Double-walled sac that encloses and supports the heart.
physiology (FIZ-e-OL-uh-je)		physi/o (nature)	-logy (study of)	The study of the function of the living body and its parts.
subcutaneous (SUB-kyu-TAY-ne-us)	sub- (below, under, beneath)	cut (skin)	-aneous (pertaining to)	Pertaining to the layer of fatty tissue just below the dermis.

1. The word root *physi/o* in the medical term *physiology* means
   a. nature.
   b. study of.
   c. lung.
   d. spleen.

2. The prefix *inter-* in the medical term *intervertebral* translates to
   a. above.
   b. below.
   c. between.
   d. under.

3. The prefix *epi-* in the medical term *epiglottis* means
   a. leaf-shaped.
   b. over, above.
   c. two, double.
   d. separation.

4. A medical term that ends with the suffix *-logy*, as in *physiology*, indicates
  a. study of.
  b. tension.
  c. condition.
  d. pertaining to.

5. The medical term *subcutaneous* contains the word root *cut*. This relates to the
  a. brain.
  b. finger.
  c. breast.
  d. skin.

6. In each space, write the prefix, word root, or suffix that matches the definition.

  axil   my/o

  card/ium   perfusion

  glottis   peri

  hypo   pleur

  inter   vertebra

  _____ a. Delivery of oxygen and other nutrients to the cells

  _____ b. Relating to muscle

  _____ c. The sound-producing area of the larynx

  _____ d. Segment of the spinal column

  _____ e. Below, under, deficient

  _____ f. Relating to the heart

  _____ g. Around (an object)

  _____ h. Referring to the armpit

  _____ i. Referring to the lining of the lung and thorax

  _____ j. Between (objects)

TERMS AND CONCEPTS

1. In each space, write the term described by the statement. Not all terms will be used.

  Anterior   Midline

  Distal   Normal anatomical position

  Inferior   Posterior

  Lateral   Prone

Medial	Superior
Midaxillary	Transverse line
Midclavicular	Frontal or coronal plane
Sagittal plane	Midsagittal plane
Transverse plane	

_____ a. An imaginary line drawn horizontally through the waist to divide the body into superior and inferior planes

_____ b. The back or toward the back

_____ c. Lying on the stomach

_____ d. Above, toward the head

_____ e. Position in which the patient is standing erect, facing forward, with arms down at the sides and palms forward

_____ f. Refers to the center of the armpit

_____ g. Below, toward the feet

_____ h. Refers to the side, left, or right of the midline, or away from the midline of the body

_____ i. The front or toward the front

_____ j. Distant or far from the point of reference

_____ k. An imaginary line drawn vertically through the middle of the patient's body, dividing it into right and left planes

_____ l. A vertical plane that runs lengthwise and divides the body into right and left halves

_____ m. The plane that divides the body into two equal halves

_____ n. The plane that divides the body into front and back halves

_____ o. The plane that is parallel with the ground and divides the body into upper and lower halves

▌ CONTENT REVIEW

1. When you are describing an injury to the right chest, *right* refers to
   a. your right, while facing the patient.
   b. your right, while facing away from the patient.
   c. the patient's right, regardless of position.
   d. your right, while in a prone position.

2. Fill in each term of direction on the appropriate line.

Anterior
Distal
Inferior
Lateral
Medial
Midaxillary
Midline
Palmar
Plantar
Posterior
Proximal
Superior

A _____
B _____
C _____
D _____
E _____
F _____
G _____
H _____
I _____
J _____
K _____
L _____

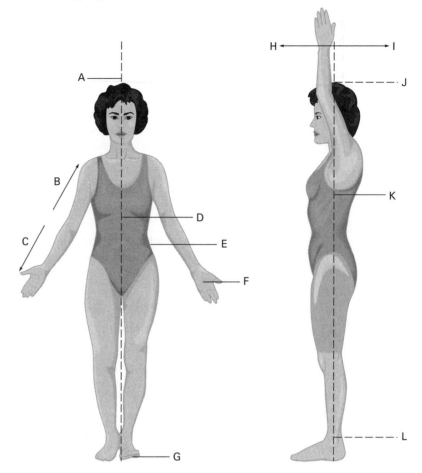

3. The emergency physician confirms that your patient has sustained a *bilateral femur* fracture. This would indicate
   a. both right and left thighbones are fractured.
   b. both right and left forearm bones are fractured.
   c. there are two fractures of one forearm bone.
   d. there are two fractures of one thighbone.

4. Describing the location of your patient's burns as *posterior thigh* would indicate
   a. the back of the thigh.
   b. the front of the thigh.
   c. the inner side of the thigh.
   d. the outer side of the thigh.

5. You place a patient on his side so fluids can drain from his mouth. In what position have you placed him?
   a. Supine
   b. Prone
   c. Lateral recumbent or recovery position
   d. Fowler's position

6. The section of the spinal or vertebral column that the ribs are attached to is which of the following?
   a. Cervical spine
   b. Lumbar spine
   c. Sacral spine
   d. Thoracic spine

7. Which section of the spine is most prone to injury?
   a. Cervical spine
   b. Lumbar spine
   c. Sacral spine
   d. Thoracic spine

8. Shoulder and hip joints are _____, the kind of joint that permits the widest range of motion.
   a. hinged joints
   b. condyloid joints
   c. gliding joints
   d. ball-and-socket joints

9. Which muscle type is responsible for deliberate movements such as walking and chewing?
   a. Cardiac muscles
   b. Smooth muscles
   c. Skeletal muscles
   d. Involuntary muscles

10. In the unresponsive patient, what anatomical structure may not properly seal the airway, permitting vomit or other liquids to enter the trachea?
    a. Diaphragm
    b. Epiglottis
    c. Bronchi
    d. Larynx

11. What occurs when the diaphragm and the intercostal muscles contract, increasing the size of the thoracic cavity?
    a. Air flows out of the lungs; exhalation.
    b. Air flows into the lungs; inhalation.
    c. Air flows rapidly in, then out, in a sneeze.
    d. Air flows out in an involuntary cough.

12. When assessing the infant or child, you know that
    a. the infant's or child's trachea is larger than that of an adult.
    b. the infant's or child's tongue takes up proportionally more space in the pharynx.
    c. infants and children rely more heavily on the abdominal muscles for breathing.
    d. the infant's or child's head is proportionally smaller in relation to the body.

13. Inadequate breathing for the adult patient may be characterized by
    a. warm, dry skin.
    b. a rate of 12–20 breaths per minute.
    c. equal chest expansion.
    d. use of accessory muscles during breathing.

14. Fill in each skeletal term on the appropriate line.

A _____
B _____
C _____
D _____
E _____
F _____
G _____
H _____
I _____
J _____
K _____
L _____
M _____
N _____
O _____
P _____
Q _____
R _____
S _____
T _____
U _____
V _____
W _____
X _____
Y _____
Z _____
AA _____
BB _____
CC _____
DD _____
EE _____
FF _____
GG _____
HH _____
II _____

Calcaneus	Frontal bone	Occipital bone	Sternum
Carpals	Greater trochanter	Parietal bone	Symphysis pubis
Cervical vertebra	Humerus	Patella	Tarsals
Clavicle	Iliac crest	Pelvic girdle	Temporal bone
Coccyx	Ilium	Phalanges	Tibia
Cranium	Mandible	Radius	Ulna
Elbow	Maxilla	Ribs	Xiphoid process
Femur	Metacarpals	Sacrum	Zygomatic bone
Fibula	Metatarsals	Scapula	

15. Carbon dioxide is exchanged for oxygen through the walls of the capillaries at which of the following?
    a. Alveoli and cells
    b. Alveoli and bronchi
    c. Arteries and veins
    d. Bronchi and cells

16. The heart is composed of four chambers. The two upper chambers, called _____, receive blood from the veins. The two lower chambers, called _____, pump blood out to the arteries.
    a. pericardium/myocardium
    b. arterioles/venules
    c. aortas/valves
    d. atria/ventricles

17. Which component of the blood is responsible for defending against infection?
    a. Platelets
    b. Plasma
    c. Red blood cells
    d. White blood cells

18. Pulses felt at different points on the body are classified as central or peripheral. Which of the following is considered to be a central pulse?
    a. Radial
    b. Brachial
    c. Carotid
    d. Tibial

19. The delivery of oxygen and other nutrients to the cells, through adequate circulation of blood through the capillaries, is known as which of the following?
    a. Diastolic circulation
    b. Systolic circulation
    c. Hypoperfusion
    d. Perfusion

20. The central nervous system consists of which of the following?
    a. Brain and spinal cord
    b. Brain and heart
    c. Medulla and brain
    d. Spinal cord and vertebrae

21. Which is considered to be the master gland, located at the base of the brain?
    a. Adrenal
    b. Pituitary
    c. Thyroid
    d. Parathyroid

22. Which best describes the anatomy and physiology of the skin?
    a. The epidermis contains the blood vessels, sweat glands, oil glands, and nerves.
    b. The skin consists of three layers, with the epidermis consisting of mostly fatty tissue.
    c. The skin is the second-largest organ of the body and consists of two layers, the epidermis being the thicker layer.
    d. The skin is the largest organ of the body, protects the body against bacteria, and regulates temperature.

23. Your partner asks you to place the patient in a Semi-Fowler's position. Which of the following best describes the Semi-Fowler's position?
    a. On the left side with knees flexed
    b. Flat on the back with knees bent
    c. On the back with the legs elevated 12 inches
    d. On the back with the torso elevated less than 45 degrees

24. Decreasing the diameter of the blood vessels, which will increase resistance and make it harder for blood to pass through them, resulting in an increase in pressure, is known as
    a. vasoconstriction.
    b. vasodilation.
    c. bronchoconstriction.
    d. bronchodilation.

25. The mechanical process primarily based on changes in pressure inside the chest that cause air to flow into or out of the lungs is known as
    a. respiration.
    b. oxygenation.
    c. pronation.
    d. ventilation.

26. The muscle that contributes 60–70 percent of the effort to breathe is known as the
    a. intercostal.
    b. diaphragm.
    c. epiglottis.
    d. abdominal.

27. Which of the following pulse sites represents feeling the mechanical contraction of the heart and not the pressure wave of blood, and thus does not provide an assessment of the effectiveness of the heart or blood volume?
    a. Carotid
    b. Brachial
    c. Apical
    d. Femoral

28. About 97 percent of the oxygen carried in the blood is carried on the surface of red blood cells by attaching to which of the following?
    a. White blood cells
    b. Plasma
    c. Corpuscles
    d. Hemoglobin

29. For cells to function correctly, they require energy. The main source of energy comes from the cell's metabolizing
    a. glucose.
    b. carbon dioxide.
    c. amino acids.
    d. thiamine.

30. The hormone epinephrine contains all four properties ($alpha_1$, $alpha_2$, $beta_1$, and $beta_2$). Which of the following properties would cause the skin to become cool, pale, and diaphoretic from vasoconstriction in the skin?
    a. Alpha$_1$
    b. Alpha$_2$
    c. Beta$_1$
    d. Beta$_2$

31. Which nerve exits the spinal cord at the cervical spine between C3 and C5 and stimulates the contraction of the diaphragm?
    a. Optic nerve
    b. Phrenic nerve
    c. Sciatic nerve
    d. Tidal nerve

32. Which two components of the nervous system control consciousness and must be intact and functioning for your patient to be awake?
    a. Mesencephalon and the ganglion system
    b. Pons and the phrenic nervous system
    c. Medulla oblongata and the sympathetic nervous system
    d. Cerebral hemisphere and the reticular activating system

33. Which organ contains the islets of Langerhans, which are responsible for producing insulin?
    a. Pancreas
    b. Liver
    c. Kidney
    d. Appendix

34. Which solid organ is located in the left upper quadrant of the abdomen, helps with filtration of the blood, and serves as a reservoir of blood that the body can use in an emergency?
    a. Small intestine
    b. Adrenal gland
    c. Spleen
    d. Gallbladder

35. Urine is carried from the kidneys to the bladder through which structure(s)?
   a. Ureters
   b. Urethra
   c. Duodenum
   d. Hepatic ducts

❙ CASE STUDY

You are a student EMT riding with an ambulance unit. At 1400 hours, the unit is dispatched to a car-versus-tree crash. As you approach the scene, you notice a heavily damaged auto. The scene appears to be under control by police and rescue personnel. The experienced EMT reminds you to wear your personal protective equipment (PPE). You find the patient lying supine with a police officer supporting his neck.

1. Define the supine position.

_____

_____

The patient appears to be unresponsive. The senior EMT states that he has conducted the primary assessment and will manage the airway while his partner retrieves the equipment to stabilize the spine. "You need to do a rapid physical exam," he tells you. You know that this means a head-to-toe exam for obvious injuries. The senior EMT supervises as you examine the head and neck. Then, as you cut away the patient's shirt, you note a large laceration to the center of the chest area above the nipple on the patient's right (your left as you face him). Further examination reveals a deformity to the upper arm (patient's left, your right) close to the shoulder.

2. How would you describe the lacerated chest?
   a. Large laceration to the right midclavicular line superior to the right nipple
   b. Large laceration to the right midaxillary line superior to the right nipple
   c. Large laceration to the right midclavicular line inferior to the right nipple
   d. Large laceration to the left midclavicular line superior to the left nipple

3. How would you describe the arm injury?
   a. Deformity to the proximal end of the left humerus
   b. Deformity to the proximal end of the right radius/ulna
   c. Deformity to the proximal end of the left calcaneus
   d. Deformity to the distal end of the left humerus

After exposing the lower body, you find that both right and left thighs are grossly deformed. You find a puncture wound on the left thigh away from the midline and close to the knee.

4. How would you describe the injuries?
   a. Right and left thigh area deformity with a puncture wound to the left medial thigh proximal to the patella
   b. Bilateral femoral region deformity with a puncture wound to the left lateral thigh proximal to the patella
   c. Bilateral femoral region deformity with a puncture wound to the left ventral area distal to the greater trochanter
   d. Bilateral femoral region deformity with a puncture wound to the left dorsal area distal to the patella

The patient is secured to a spine immobilization device and loaded onto the wheeled stretcher.

While transporting the patient to the hospital, the senior EMT commends you on your knowledge of anatomy and anatomical terms.

Pathophysiology

▌ STANDARD

Pathophysiology

▌ COMPETENCY

Applies fundamental knowledge of the pathophysiology of respiration and perfusion to patient assessment and management.

▌ OBJECTIVES

After reading this chapter, you should be able to:

8-1. Define key terms introduced in this chapter.

8-2. Explain the importance of understanding basic pathophysiology.

8-3. Differentiate between the processes of aerobic and anaerobic cellular metabolism, including explanations of:
   a. The amount of ATP produced
   b. Removal of by-products of metabolism

8-4. Describe the consequences of failure of the cellular sodium/potassium pump.

8-5. Explain the concept of perfusion, including the physical and physiological components necessary to maintain perfusion.

8-6. Describe the composition of ambient air.

8-7. Apply Boyle's law to ventilation.

8-8. Explain how changes in compliance of the lungs and chest wall and changes in airway resistance affect ventilation.

8-9. Describe the consequences of loss of contact between the parietal and visceral pleura.

8-10. Explain the concept of minute ventilation.

8-11. Differentiate between minute ventilation and alveolar ventilation.

8-12. Describe the roles of chemoreceptors, lung receptors, and the nervous system in the control of ventilation.

8-13. Explain the concept of the ventilation/perfusion (VQ) ratio.

8-14. Describe the transport of oxygen and carbon dioxide in the blood.

8-15. Explain the exchange of gases across the alveolar/capillary membrane and the exchange of gases between capillaries and cells.

8-16. Describe the composition of blood, including the function of plasma and the formed elements.

8-17. Explain the effects of changes in hydrostatic pressure and plasma oncotic pressure on the movement of fluid between the circulatory system and interstitial spaces.

8-18. Discuss factors that affect cardiac output, including heart rate, stroke volume, myocardial contractility, preload, and afterload.

8-19. Describe the concept of systemic vascular resistance and its relationship to blood pressure and pulse pressure.

8-20. Summarize the local, neural, and hormonal factors that regulate blood flow through the capillaries.

8-21. Explain the regulation of blood pressure by baroreceptors and chemoreceptors.

8-22. Explain the relationship between ventilation, perfusion, and cellular metabolism.

▌KEY IDEAS

The most fundamental purpose of emergency care is to restore or sustain the basic requirement for life: a patient's cellular perfusion. This chapter describes basic human pathophysiological processes related to cellular perfusion of cells with oxygen and glucose, and connects these concepts to essential treatment and assessment findings.

- Cellular metabolism (cellular respiration) is the process where the body breaks down molecules of glucose and produces energy for normal cell function. There are two types of cellular metabolism: aerobic and anaerobic.

- Perfusion is the delivery of oxygen, glucose, and other substances to the cells and the elimination of waste products. Adequate perfusion requires the components of the delivery system to work properly. These components are the composition of the ambient air, a patent airway, the mechanics of ventilation, regulation of ventilation, the ventilation/perfusion (VQ) ratio, transport of oxygen and carbon dioxide, blood volume, pump function of the myocardium, systemic vascular resistance, microcirculation, and blood pressure.

- Ambient air at sea level contains approximately 79 percent nitrogen, 21 percent oxygen, 0.9 percent argon, and 0.03 percent carbon dioxide.

- One of the most important and basic emergency care procedures is maintenance of the patient's airway. An airway obstruction can occur at several anatomical levels in both the upper and lower airway, including the nasopharynx, oropharynx, posterior pharynx, epiglottis, larynx, trachea, and bronchi.

- Boyle's law helps to explain the "mechanical process" of ventilation. Compliance is a measure of the ability of the chest wall and lungs to stretch, distend, and expand. Airway resistance is related to the ease of flow of air down the conduit of airway structures leading to the alveoli.

- Minute ventilation, also known as *minute volume*, is the amount of air moved in and out of the lungs in one minute. It is determined by multiplying the tidal volume by the frequency of ventilation in one minute. Minute ventilation = tidal volume (V_T) × frequency of ventilation (f/minute).

- Alveolar ventilation is the amount of air moved in and out of the alveoli in one minute. Alveolar ventilation = (tidal volume – dead air space) × frequency of ventilation/minute.

- Breathing is mostly an involuntary process that is controlled by the autonomic nervous system via chemoreceptors, lung receptors, and respiratory centers in the brain stem.

- The VQ ratio describes the dynamic relationship between the amount of ventilation the alveoli receive and the amount of perfusion through the capillaries surrounding the alveoli.

- Oxygen must be continuously delivered by the blood to the cells for normal cellular metabolism to occur. Carbon dioxide, the by-product of aerobic metabolism, must be carried back to the lungs, where it is blown off in exhalation. A disturbance in the transport system may lead to cellular hypoxia, where there is a lack of available oxygen to the cells, and hypercarbia, where the carbon dioxide is building up in the blood.

- One factor that determines adequate blood pressure and perfusion is blood volume. An adult has approximately 70 mL of blood for every kilogram (2.2 lb) of body weight.

- Adequate blood pressure and perfusion requires the myocardium to work effectively as a pump. The heart's ability to pump is typically expressed as *cardiac output*, defined as the amount of blood ejected by the left ventricle in one minute.

- The systolic blood pressure is a measure of cardiac output. The diastolic blood pressure is a measure of the systemic vascular resistance. The body's compensation is geared toward maintaining pressure inside the vessels and perfusion of the cells.

- The blood pressure is derived by multiplying two major factors: cardiac output and systemic vascular resistance. Blood pressure (BP) = cardiac output (CO) × systemic vascular resistance (SVR).

▌ TERMS AND CONCEPTS

1. Write the number of the correct term next to each definition.

   1. Aerobic metabolism
   2. Apneustic center
   3. Alveolar ventilation
   4. Chemoreceptors
   5. Dead air space
   6. Deoxyhemoglobin
   7. Airway resistance
   8. Boyle's law
   9. Glycolysis
   10. J-receptors
   11. Plasma oncotic pressure
   12. Preload
   13. Ventilation/perfusion (VQ) ratio

   _____ a. The breakdown of a molecule of glucose in the cell in the presence of oxygen to produce energy

   _____ b. The restriction of airflow that is related to the diameter of the airways

   _____ c. Anatomical areas in the respiratory tract where no gas exchange occurs, but air collects during inhalation

   _____ d. Is responsible for keeping fluid inside the vessel by exerting a "pull" effect

   _____ e. The respiratory center in the brain stem that intensifies and prolongs inhalation

   _____ f. The breakdown of glucose into pyruvic acid in the cells

   _____ g. The amount of air that enters the alveoli for gas exchange

   _____ h. Hemoglobin that does not have any oxygen molecules attached to it

   _____ i. The concept that the volume of a gas is inversely proportionate to its pressure

   _____ j. Found in the capillaries surrounding the alveoli and are sensitive to increases in the pressure in the capillary and cause rapid, shallow ventilation when stimulated

   _____ k. Constantly monitor the arterial content of oxygen, carbon dioxide, and the blood pH and stimulate a change in respiratory rate and depth

_____ l. The pressure generated in the left ventricle at the end of diastole (resting phase of the cardiac cycle)

_____ m. The dynamic relationship between the amount of ventilation that the alveoli receive and the amount of perfusion through the capillary surrounding the alveoli

❙ CONTENT REVIEW

1. The process that occurs when glucose crosses the cell membrane and is broken down into pyruvic acid is called
   a. cellular respiration.
   b. cellular metabolism.
   c. ATP transfer.
   d. glycolysis.

2. A series of reactions that produce energy *in the presence* of oxygen within the cell is called
   a. aerobic metabolism.
   b. glycolysis.
   c. ATP transfer.
   d. anaerobic metabolism.

3. A series of reactions that produce energy *without the presence* of oxygen in the cell is called
   a. aerobic metabolism.
   b. glycolysis.
   c. ATP transfer.
   d. anaerobic metabolism.

4. Failure of the intracellular sodium/potassium pump causes
   a. potassium to accumulate in the intracellular fluid.
   b. sodium to accumulate in the extracellular fluid.
   c. water to accumulate within the cell.
   d. the increased production of ATP.

5. Perfusion is described as
   a. the elimination of waste products from body cells in an efficient manner.
   b. the delivery of oxygen, glucose, and other substances to the cells and the elimination of waste products.
   c. the adequate functioning of only the following component parts: the mechanics of respiration, regulation of respiration, the VQ ratio, and blood volume.
   d. the delivery of oxygen, glucose, and other substances to the cells.

6. Which statement is most correct relating to patient oxygenation concepts?
   a. Ambient air at sea level contains 79 percent oxygen and has a partial pressure of 597 mmHg.
   b. The concentration of oxygen in the ambient air has little to no effect on the amount of oxygen that ends up in the blood.
   c. The partial pressure of oxygen is 159 mmHg at sea level.
   d. The FiO_2 is the fraction of oxygen delivered to a patient via a ventilation device such as a bag-valve-mask ventilator.

7. The carina is located at the _____ intercostal space anteriorly and at the _____ thoracic vertebra posteriorly.
   a. first/second
   b. third/second
   c. fourth/second
   d. second/fourth

8. Identify each of the following accessory muscles of respiration as muscles associated with inhalation or exhalation. Identify the accessory muscles of inhalation with an "I" and those associated with exhalation with an "E."
   _____ Sternocleidomastoid
   _____ Abdominal muscles
   _____ Scalene muscles
   _____ Pectoralis minor muscles
   _____ Internal intercostal muscles

9. The concept that the volume of gas is inversely proportionate to its pressure is called
   a. Henry's law.
   b. the pressure gradient.
   c. Boyle's law.
   d. isobaric pressure.

10. During inhalation, the _____ provides approximately _____ of the effort of breathing.
    a. diaphragm/30–40 percent
    b. diaphragm/60–70 percent
    c. internal intercostals/60–70 percent
    d. internal intercostals/80–90 percent

11. Two conditions that may require the use of accessory muscles to generate a greater force to fill and empty the lungs are higher _____ and poor _____.
    a. peripheral blood pressures/compliance
    b. pulse oximetry readings/airway resistance
    c. pulse oximetry readings/peripheral blood pressures
    d. airway resistance/compliance

12. Swelling from edema within the airway structures is the most common cause of
    a. decreased compliance.
    b. increased blood pressure.
    c. increased pulse oximeter readings.
    d. increased airway resistance.

13. A patient who has a tidal volume of 500 mL and is breathing at a rate of 12 times per minute has a minute volume of
    a. 6 liters/minute.
    b. 600 liters/minute.
    c. 60 liters/minute.
    d. 6,000 liters/minute.

14. What is the patient's alveolar ventilation in question 13?
    a. 4 liters/minute
    b. 4.2 liters/minute
    c. 40.2 liters/minute
    d. 4,200 liters/minute

15. Ventilatory rates of _____/minute or greater in the adult patient and greater than _____/minute in the pediatric patient are considered too fast to be sustainable and allow for adequate time for a normal tidal volume.
    a. 20/40
    b. 30/50
    c. 40/60
    d. 50/70

16. The central chemoreceptors
    a. are located near the respiratory center in the medulla.
    b. are most sensitive to the level of oxygen in the blood.
    c. are located in the aortic arch and the carotid bodies.
    d. become the primary stimulus for ventilation in patients with chronically high CO_2 levels.

17. Hypoxia becomes the main stimulus for ventilation rather than hypercarbia in patients with
    a. blepharoptosis.
    b. a history of cardiac problems.
    c. cirrhosis.
    d. chronic obstructive pulmonary disease (COPD).

18. The relationship between alveolar blood flow and alveolar airflow is called the
    a. VQ ratio.
    b. oxyhemoglobin ratio.
    c. Boyle/Warren ratio.
    d. gas/flow ratio.

19. Which statement is most correct regarding oxygen and carbon dioxide transport in the blood?
    a. Carbon dioxide is chiefly carried attached to hemoglobin.
    b. A hemoglobin molecule with oxygen attached is called *deoxyhemoglobin*.
    c. A hemoglobin molecule can carry up to two oxygen molecules.
    d. Oxygen is transported in the blood dissolved in plasma and attached to hemoglobin.

20. The majority of blood is found within the
    a. arterial system.
    b. venous system.
    c. pulmonary vessels.
    d. capillaries.

21. Plasma oncotic pressure
    a. exerts a "push" effect on intravascular fluids.
    b. if high, will promote a loss of vascular volume.
    c. exerts a "pull" effect on intravascular fluids.
    d. if low, will draw excessive fluid into the intravascular space.

22. Fill in the blanks of the following statements using either the term *increase* or *decrease*.

    1. A(n) _____ in stimulation by the sympathetic nervous system will increase the heart rate.

    2. A(n) _____ in stimulation by the sympathetic nervous system will decrease the heart rate.

    3. A(n) _____ in stimulation by the parasympathetic nervous system will decrease the heart rate.

    4. A(n) _____ in stimulation by the parasympathetic nervous system will increase the heart rate.

23. The Frank-Starling law of the heart states that
    a. the stretch of the muscle fiber at the end of systole determines the forces necessary to eject the blood contained within it.
    b. the stretch of the muscle fiber at the end of diastole determines the forces necessary to eject the blood contained within it.
    c. the stretch of the cardiac valve at the end of systole determines the forces necessary to eject the blood contained within it.
    d. the stretch of the pulmonary valve at the end of diastole determines the forces necessary to eject the blood contained within it.

24. Preload is
    a. the pressure generated in the right ventricle at the end of systole.
    b. the pressure generated in the right ventricle at the end of diastole.
    c. the pressure in the left ventricle generated at the end of diastole.
    d. the resistance in the aorta that must be overcome by contraction of the left ventricle to eject the blood.

25. Stroke volume is the amount of blood ejected by the _____ with each contraction.
    a. right atrium
    b. right ventricle
    c. left atrium
    d. left ventricle

26. Fill in the blanks of the following statements using either the term *increase* or *decrease*.

    1. A decrease in heart rate will _____ cardiac output.

    2. An increase in heart rate, if not excessive, will _____ cardiac output.

    3. A decrease in blood volume will _____ preload, _____ stroke volume, and _____ cardiac output.

    4. An increase in blood volume will _____ preload, _____ stroke volume, and _____ cardiac output.

    5. A decrease in myocardial contractility will _____ stroke volume and _____ cardiac output.

    6. An increase in myocardial contractility will _____ stroke volume and _____ cardiac output.

    7. Neural stimulation from the sympathetic nervous system will _____ heart rate, _____ myocardial contractility, and _____ cardiac output.

8. Neural stimulation from the parasympathetic nervous system will _____ the heart rate, _____ myocardial contractility, and _____ cardiac output.

9. Beta₁ stimulation from epinephrine will _____ heart rate, _____ myocardial contractility, and _____ cardiac output.

10. Beta₁ blockade (patient on beta blocker) will block beta₁ stimulation, _____ heart rate, _____ myocardial contractility, and _____ cardiac output.

11. An extremely high diastolic blood pressure will _____ the pressure in the aorta, requiring a more forceful contraction to overcome the aortic pressure and a higher myocardial workload, and may _____ the cardiac output and weaken the heart over time.

12. A reduction in diastolic blood pressure will _____ the pressure in the aorta, require a less forceful contraction to overcome the aortic pressure, and reduce the myocardial workload, and may improve the cardiac output of a weakened heart.

27. A narrow pulse pressure is defined as being
    a. the difference between systolic and diastolic blood pressure.
    b. less than 25 percent of the systolic pressure.
    c. less than 50 percent of the systolic pressure.
    d. less than 75 percent of the systolic pressure.

28. Fill in the blanks of the following statements using either the term *increase* or *decrease*.
    1. A(n) _____ in cardiac output will increase the blood pressure.
    2. A(n) _____ in cardiac output will decrease the blood pressure.
    3. An increase in the heart rate will _____ the cardiac output, which will _____ the blood pressure.
    4. A decrease in the heart rate will _____ the cardiac output, which will _____ the blood pressure.
    5. An increase in the stroke volume will _____ the cardiac output, which will _____ the blood pressure.
    6. A decrease in the stroke volume will _____ the cardiac output, which will _____ the blood pressure.
    7. An increase in systemic vascular resistance will _____ the blood pressure.
    8. A decrease in systemic vascular resistance will _____ the blood pressure.

CASE STUDY 1

You have been dispatched to the scene of a pediatric patient who was trapped for a few minutes in an abandoned refrigerator. While responding, you review the most likely physiological responses the patient will encounter.

1. Listed are the components necessary for adequate perfusion. Place a check mark next to each item that will be affected early in this patient's physiological response to this incident.
    _____ Composition of ambient air
    _____ Patent airway
    _____ Mechanics of ventilation
    _____ Regulation of ventilation

_____ VQ ratio
_____ Transport of oxygen and carbon dioxide by the blood
_____ Blood volume
_____ Pump function of the myocardium
_____ Systemic vascular resistance
_____ Microcirculation
_____ Blood pressure

2. For each item marked in question 1, describe the rationale for the patient's physiological response.

_____

_____

_____

_____

_____

_____

_____

_____

_____

_____

_____

CASE STUDY 2

You are on the scene with a 45-year-old man who was cutting firewood with a chain saw. The saw kicked back and struck the man in the medial aspect of his right leg just below his knee. The patient's vital signs are as follows: Pulse is 98 bpm regular and palpable; respirations are 16/minute; skin is pale, cool, and moist to touch; pupils are equal and reactive to light; blood pressure is 110/86; pulse oximetry is 98% on 15 lpm of oxygen. The patient is alert and oriented.

1. If this patient's tidal volume is 450 mL, what are his minute ventilation and alveolar ventilation?
   a. 72.0l/48.0l
   b. 720 mL/480 mL
   c. 7.2 l/4.8l
   d. 7.2 mL/4.8 mL

2. What is the patient's pulse pressure?
   a. 4
   b. 14
   c. 24
   d. 34

3. How do you determine if the pulse pressure is normal?
   a. A normal pulse pressure is greater than 25 percent of the systolic blood pressure.
   b. A normal pulse pressure is greater than 25 percent of the diastolic blood pressure.
   c. A normal pulse pressure is greater than 40 percent of the systolic blood pressure.
   d. A normal pulse pressure is greater than 40 percent of the diastolic blood pressure.

4. Listed are the components necessary for adequate perfusion. Place a check mark next to each item that will be affected early in this patient's physiological response to this incident.

_____ Composition of ambient air
_____ Patent airway
_____ Mechanics of ventilation
_____ Regulation of ventilation
_____ VQ ratio
_____ Transport of oxygen and carbon dioxide by the blood
_____ Blood volume
_____ Pump function of the myocardium
_____ Systemic vascular resistance
_____ Microcirculation
_____ Blood pressure

5. For each item marked in question 4, describe the rationale for the patient's physiological response.

_____

_____

_____

_____

_____

_____

_____

_____

_____

_____

_____

_____

Life Span Development

STANDARD

Life Span Development

COMPETENCY

Applies fundamental knowledge of life span development to patient assessment and management.

OBJECTIVES

After reading this chapter, you should be able to:

9-1. Define key terms introduced in this chapter.

9-2. Identify the age ranges associated with each of the following terms:
   a. Neonate
   b. Infant
   c. Toddler
   d. Preschooler
   e. School age
   f. Adolescent
   g. Early adulthood
   h. Middle adulthood
   i. Late adulthood

9-3. Describe the physiological changes that occur immediately after birth.

9-4. Discuss the key physical and psychosocial characteristics of individuals in each of the following age groups:
   a. Neonates and infants
   b. Toddlers
   c. Preschool-age children
   d. School-age children
   e. Adolescents
   f. Early adulthood
   g. Middle adulthood
   h. Late adulthood

KEY IDEAS

This chapter describes the changes that the human life will experience through different ages and stages and how that will affect the care you provide.

- Physical and psychosocial changes occur throughout a person's lifetime.

- Individuals mature at different rates, but most change occurs within time periods specific to different groups: infancy, toddler and preschool age, school age, adolescence, early adulthood, middle adulthood, and late adulthood.

  - Neonate (birth to 1 month)

  - Infancy (1 month–1 year) is a period of rapid growth and significant developmental changes. The following summarizes the changes and differences:

    - Physiological changes—normally weighs 3.0–3.5 kg; head is 25 percent of total body weight; airways are shorter, narrower, less stable, and more prone to obstruction than in the adult; nose breathers until four weeks; lungs prone to trauma from high ventilation pressures; susceptible to early respiratory fatigue; diaphragmatic breathers; rapid respiratory rates can lead to rapid heat and fluid loss; immune system is immature and susceptible to infections and disease; able to sense pain and touch but not localize pain; sunken fontanelles are an indicator of fluid dehydration.

    - Psychosocial changes—parent-dependent; communicates by crying when wet, hungry, or tired; allows parent to hold during assessment.

  - A toddler is a child who is 12–36 months of age. A preschooler is 3–6 years of age. The following summarizes the major changes and differences:

    - Physiological changes—by age 5, will have all primary teeth; increase in muscle mass; alveoli increase in number; more susceptible to minor respiratory and gastrointestinal infections; brain develops rapidly (90 percent of adult weight) along with motor skills; average toilet training occurs at 28 months.

    - Psychosocial changes—language is mastered by 36 months (simple phrases and sentences); separation anxiety at 18 months; play serves important role in development. Take extra time during assessment; allow the child to touch equipment before you use it; never lie to a child; and allow parents to stay with the child during assessment, if possible.

  - School-age children are 6–12 years of age. The following summarizes the major changes and differences:

    - Physiological changes—musculoskeletal system increases in density and grows larger; primary teeth are replaced with permanent teeth; read and write; some struggle with nocturnal enuresis.

    - Psychosocial changes—attend school and make friends outside the home; interact more with adults and other children; same-sex friendships are important; capable of fundamental reasoning and developing problem-solving skills; concept of self, self-esteem, and morals are developed; understand concepts associated with pain, illness, and death/loss; able to identify public safety personnel as capable of helping them in a crisis.

  - Adolescence is a period of time from 12–18 years of age. The following summarizes the major changes and differences:

    - Physiological changes—most experience a rapid 2–3-year growth spurt; muscle and bone growth is nearly complete by age 18; puberty occurs (may begin at age 10 in girls/age 12 in boys).

    - Psychosocial changes—family conflicts arise and revolve around the belief that they are invulnerable and the focus of attention; want to be treated as adults but are incapable of making adult decisions; prefer privacy during examination and would prefer interview in private (obtain parent's consent); develop identity; antisocial or self-destructive behaviors may occur at eighth or ninth grade; depression and suicide are more common in this age group than any other; concerned about body image and comparison with peers; those that engage in sexual activity feel invulnerable to risks associated with unsafe sex practices.

- Early adulthood is a stage of development from age 20–40 years. The following summarizes the major changes and differences:
    - Physiological changes—peak physical conditioning is reached between 19 and 26 years; accidents are the leading cause of death in this age group.
    - Psychosocial changes—assume more responsibility and become more independent; develop relationships and begin families; childbirth is most common in this age group; finish school and establish careers.
- Middle adulthood occurs from age 41–60 years. The following summarizes the major changes and differences:
    - Physiological changes—body systems functioning at high level with varying degrees of degradation based upon disease and lifestyle decisions; more susceptible to chronic illnesses and diseases (diabetes and arthritis); cardiovascular health and cancer becomes an issue; weight gain is easy and loss difficult; vision and hearing changes occur; women experience menopause.
    - Psychosocial changes—individuals reach personal goals and reach out to help others; some question lack of goal accomplishment; many delay seeking medical attention.
- Late adulthood refers to the period after age 61. The following summarizes the major changes and differences:
    - Physiological changes—the incidence of illness and disease increases with age, most body systems become less efficient.
    - Psychosocial changes—must face new challenges; reflect on lives; may feel isolated; 95 percent of older adults live in communities adapted to their needs; some feel ashamed to ask for help or assistance; can lead to decline in well-being and self-worth; many experience the death or dying of their companions.

▌ TERMS AND CONCEPTS

1. Write the number of each term next to its definition.

    1. Nocturnal enuresis
    2. Maximum life span
    3. Adolescence
    4. Menopause
    5. Toddler
    6. Fontanelles
    7. Puberty
    8. Infancy
    9. Life expectancy
    10. Preschooler
    11. Reflex

    _____ a. Theoretically the longest period of time for an organism to live

    _____ b. The period in which the sexual organs mature

    _____ c. A child who is 12–36 months of age

    _____ d. The period of time when a person is 12–18 years of age

    _____ e. Involuntary bed-wetting at night

_____ f. A child who is 3–6 years of age

_____ g. The average length of years of life remaining based on the individual's year of birth

_____ h. The permanent end of menstruation and fertility, which usually occurs in a woman's late 40s or 50s

_____ i. An instantaneous and involuntary movement resulting from a stimulus

_____ j. Soft spots on a baby's head that allow the head to pass through the birth canal during delivery

_____ k. The stage of development ranging from 1 month to 1 year of age

| CONTENT REVIEW

1. An infant's
   a. head is equal to 50 percent of its total body weight.
   b. birth weight is normally 2.0–2.5 kg.
   c. lung tissue is very fragile and is prone to trauma from excessive pressure during ventilation.
   d. alveoli are greater with increased collateral ventilation.

2. By the age of 2 months, an infant should be able to
   a. sit without assistance.
   b. crawl and creep on hands and knees.
   c. put objects into containers.
   d. recognize familiar faces.

3. A toddler
   a. is 3–6 years of age.
   b. is 12–36 months of age.
   c. will have a normal heart rate of 130–150 beats per minute.
   d. will typically have a systolic blood pressure of 110–130 mmHg.

4. By the age of 3, a child should be able to
   a. stand on one foot for more than 10 seconds.
   b. walk alone and begin to run.
   c. hop, jump, swing, climb, and do somersaults.
   d. dress and undress without assistance.

5. When assessing a toddler or preschooler,
   a. communicate quickly and concisely to save time.
   b. prevent the parent from staying with the child during the assessment.
   c. allow the child to touch the equipment before you use it.
   d. avoid upsetting the child by using half-truths when necessary.

6. Early adulthood
   a. is the stage of development from 20–60 years of age.
   b. is the stage of development from 20–40 years of age.
   c. is a stage with a low childbirth rate.
   d. is a stage associated with more psychological problems than other groups.

7. What stage of development do the following characteristics most closely describe?
   Sleep cycle is disrupted, lung elasticity is diminished, workload and size of the heart increases, pain perception is diminished, and metabolism and insulin production are decreased.
   a. Adolescence
   b. Early adulthood
   c. Middle adulthood
   d. Late adulthood

8. Depression and suicide are more common for this age group than any other age group.
   a. Adolescence
   b. Early adulthood
   c. Middle adulthood
   d. Late adulthood

Complete the following chart that reviews normal vital signs throughout the life span.

Stage of Development	Respirations (average in breaths per minute)	Pulse (average in beats per minute)	Blood Pressure (average in mmHg)	Temperature (°F)
Infancy: At birth	40–60	9. _____	70 systolic	98–100
Infancy: Neonate	30–40	100–160	10. _____	98–100
Infancy: At one year	20–30	100–120	90 systolic	11. _____
Toddlers	20–30	80–130	70–100 systolic	98.6–99.6
Preschoolers	12. _____	80–120	80–110 systolic	98.6–99.6
School age	20–30	13. _____	80–120 systolic	98.6
Adolescence	14. _____	55–105	100–120 systolic	98.6
Early adulthood	16–20	70	120/80	98.6
Middle adulthood	16–20	70	15. _____	98.6
Late adulthood	Depends on patient's physical and health status	Depends on patient's physical and health status	Depends on patient's physical and health status	98.6

CASE STUDY

You have been dispatched to a local skateboard park located in a large warehouse in a revitalized area of down-town. The caller, the manager of the skateboard park, says that he has a young male patron who is depressed. Upon arrival at the scene, you observe a male who appears to be about 15 years of age sitting on the edge of a large ramp inside the warehouse. Your partner takes the patient's vital signs and reports the following: Pulse is 70 bpm strong and regular, respirations are 14/minute and regular and full, the blood pressure is 100/80, and the temperature is 98.6°F.

1. The patient's
   a. pulse is not appropriate for the patient's stage of development.
   b. respirations are not appropriate for the patient's stage of development.
   c. blood pressure is appropriate for the patient's stage of development.
   d. temperature is not appropriate for the patient's stage of development.

2. Given this patient's stage of development, which of the following is the patient most likely to report or display?
   a. Has little or no conflicts with his family
   b. Prefers his parent or parents to be present during the evaluation
   c. Does not believe that he is the "center of attention"
   d. Participates in risky behaviors

3. A large crowd has gathered around the patient during your early assessment. The patient seems reluctant to answer your questions or interact with you at all. You should consider
   a. asking your partner to take a history because the patient seems to dislike you.
   b. delaying history taking until after his arrival at the hospital.
   c. having a friend ask items required to take a history.
   d. moving the patient to an area where privacy can be attained.

CHAPTER 9 SCENARIO: DOCUMENTATION EXERCISE

Read the following scenario and think about how you would document this call if you were the EMT who responded to the scene. Then answer the multiple-choice questions and fill in the sample prehospital care report, basing your documentation on information from the scenario.

It is 6 P.M. on a bright, sunny Sunday late afternoon. You are reading an interesting article about the EMT's role in providing public health to local communities that was written by a paramedic you work with. The alarm sounds. "Unit 17, respond to the Presbyterian Assisted Living Facility at 16 Lake Hunter Drive, cross street Cresap Avenue, for patient that is confused. Time out 18:02 hours." Your partner, Harvey, advises dispatch that you are responding. You arrive on the scene at 18:07 and advise dispatch of your arrival. You park in a circular drive in front of a huge, multistory, institutional green building that houses a large number of retirees. An older gentleman waves his hand to catch your attention just as you put the vehicle in park. You gather your jump kit, stretcher, and other gear and head to the door where he is waiting for you. You quickly introduce yourself and your partner and ask why the ambulance was called. The gentleman replies, "I'm working the front desk and got a call from Mrs. Johnson, the aide on the second floor. She told me that Mr. Savage in room 205 is acting strangely and would I please call for an ambulance. That is really all I know." You thank him, take the elevator to the second floor, and arrive at the patient's room.

The door is open. You knock on the door and announce your arrival. You enter the front room of the apartment and observe an elderly man who you guess to be in his mid-80s sitting upright in a chair. He looks up and makes eye contact with you as you enter the well-kept and tidy room. His skin color looks normal, and no abnormal respiratory sounds are heard as you approach the patient. He appears to be in minor distress and continues to look at you as you approach. Mrs. Johnson is sitting in a chair next to the patient. You kneel down next to him and say, "Good afternoon, Mr. Savage. We are EMTs, and we are here to help you. Can you tell me what happened today?" You do this as Harvey talks to Mrs. Johnson to get a quick history of what happened. At the same time, you reach down and monitor Mr. Savage's pulse. It is regular, strong, and full, and his skin is warm and dry. No odor is noted on his breath. Mr. Savage replies, "There is really nothing wrong

with me at all. Mrs. Johnson overreacts to everything. I just started taking a new blood pressure medication, and it made me a little dizzy. That's all. I'm really just fine."

Harvey returns and begins to take the patient's vital signs. You continue taking the patient history and conducting the physical exam. "Are you allergic to any medications, Mr. Savage?" you ask. He replies, "No, I'm not." You ask Mr. Savage what medications he is currently taking. He replies confidently, "Well, I just started taking Lopressor 100 mg once a day. I just started taking it this afternoon." You next ask, "Mr. Savage, other than the high blood pressure, have you been sick before or have you been treated for any other medical problems?" He quickly responds, "Nope, I'm in great health really, just a bit of high blood pressure. Not too bad for an old guy, huh?" You reply, "You're right, Mr. Savage. You look like you're in great shape!" You ask about his last meal and he tells you that he last ate at about 5 P.M. in the small cafeteria located downstairs. You next ask Mr. Savage to tell you more about the dizziness. He says, "Well, I was just fine when I went down to supper. I took my Lopressor pill with me and took it just before I ate. I had a great meal. A plate full of vegetables and a large salad and I cheated a bit by getting a root beer float. I don't do that very often! I came back upstairs, and Mrs. Johnson came in to check on me. I was sitting down and I guess that I stood up too quickly, because it made me dizzy and I sat back down. I told Mrs. Johnson I was dizzy and she called downstairs and said to get an ambulance here right away. I told her not to, that I was fine. That's all."

Harvey calls out the vital signs: Pulse 72 strong and regular, respirations 18 and regular, blood pressure is 144/98, pupils are equal and reactive, and the SpO_2 is 98%. You follow up with a few other questions. Mr. Savage tells you this has not happened to him before and that his doctor told him he might get dizzy from taking the blood pressure medication. He denies any pain or discomfort and specifically denies chest pain, a headache, and any numbness or tingling in his extremities.

Harvey conducts a neurological exam and there are no significant findings. The pulses are equal and present bilaterally in all extremities. You ask if Mr. Savage would like to be transported to the hospital for evaluation and treatment. Mr. Savage declines and says that he will call his doctor in the morning and let her know what happened. You explain the risks and consequences of refusing care. Mr. Savage understands and continues to refuse transport. You remind Mr. Savage to call if the dizziness or other symptoms occur and to be sure to call the doctor in the morning. Mr. Savage signs a refusal-of-care form, and you remind him again to call for help if needed. Mr. Savage thanks you and Harvey and apologizes for the inconvenience. You tell him, "That's our job, Mr. Savage!" You head back downstairs and report to dispatch that you are back in service at 1830.

1. Mr. Savage is in late adulthood. You know that patients in this life stage
   a. generally will not feel ashamed to ask for assistance if needed.
   b. don't experience isolation or feel alone.
   c. live on fixed incomes and must make difficult financial decisions.
   d. experience minimal gastrointestinal changes.

2. Conducting the neurological exam on Mr. Savage
   a. was unnecessary and a waste of critical time.
   b. was unnecessary and should have been conducted only if he was transported.
   c. was appropriate given Mr. Savage's chief complaint.
   d. was appropriate only if Mr. Savage had some history of traumatic injury.

3. What additional action should have been performed?
   a. Palpate Mr. Savage's abdomen.
   b. Auscultate Mr. Savage's breath sounds.
   c. Examine Mr. Savage's posterior back.
   d. Evaluate Mr. Savage's blood glucose level.

EMERGENCY TRIP SHEET

TRIP #
MEDIC #
BEGIN MILES
● MILES
CODE___/___ PAGE___/___
UNITS ON SCENE

BILLING USE ONLY

DAY	
DATE	
RECEIVED	
DISPATCHED	
EN-ROUTE	
ON SCENE	
TO HOSPITAL	
AT HOSPITAL	
IN-SERVICE	

NAME	SEX M F DOB ___/___/___
ADDRESS	RACE
CITY	STATE	ZIP
PHONE ( ) -	PCP DR.
RESPONDED FROM	CITY
TAKEN FROM	ZIP
DESTINATION	REASON
SSN - -	MEDICARE #	MEDICAID #
INSURANCE CO	INSURANCE #	GROUP #
RESPONSIBLE PARTY	ADDRESS
CITY	STATE	ZIP	PHONE ( ) -
EMPLOYER

CREW	CERT	STATE #

TIME	ON SCENE (1)	ON SCENE (2)	ON SCENE (3)	EN-ROUTE (1)	EN-ROUTE (2)	AT DESTINATION
BP						
PULSE						
RESP						
SpO$_2$						
ETCO$_2$						
EKG						

IV THERAPY
SUCCESSFUL Y N # OF ATTEMPTS _____
ANGIO SIZE _____ ga.
SITE _____
TOTAL FLUID INFUSED _____ cc
BLOOD DRAW Y N INITIALS

INTUBATION INFORMATION
SUCCESSFUL Y N # OF ATTEMPTS _____
TUBE SIZE _____ mm
TIME _____ INITIALS _____

MEDICAL HISTORY
●ICATIONS
ALLERGIES
C/C
EVENTS LEADING TO C/C
ASSESSMENT
TREATMENT

CONDITION CODES		▨		▨	

TREATMENTS

TIME	TREATMENT	DOSE	ROUTE	INIT

GCS	E___ V___ M___ TOTAL =
GCS	E___ V___ M___ TOTAL =

HOSPITAL CONTACTED

CPR BEGUN BY B P TIME BEGUN	
AED USED Y N BY:	
RESUSCITATION TERMINATED - TIME	

EMS SIGNATURE

(   ) OSHA REGULATIONS FOLLOWED

Airway Management, Artificial Ventilation, and Oxygenation

▌ STANDARD

Airway Management, Respiration, and Artificial Ventilation (Content Areas: Airway Management; Respiration; Artificial Ventilation)

▌ COMPETENCY

Applies knowledge (fundamental depth, foundational breadth) of general anatomy and physiology to patient assessment and management in order to assure a patent airway, adequate mechanical ventilation, and respiration for patients of all ages.

▌ OBJECTIVES

After reading this chapter, you should be able to:

10-1.   Define key terms introduced in this chapter.
10-2.   Distinguish between the terms *respiration, ventilation, pulmonary ventilation, external respiration, internal respiration,* and *cellular ventilation.*
10-3.   Relate the anatomy and physiology of the respiratory system to ventilation and respiration.
10-4.   Recognize signs of mild to moderate and severe hypoxia.
10-5.   Explain differences between adults and children in the signs of hypoxia.
10-6.   Describe the relationship between airway status and mental status.
10-7.   Give examples of conditions that can lead to impaired ventilation and respiration.
10-8.   Describe how partial or complete obstruction of the airway leads to hypoxia.
10-9.   Describe differences between adults and children in the anatomy and physiology of the respiratory system.
10-10. Explain the causes of each of the following abnormal upper airway sounds:
   a. Snoring
   b. Crowing
   c. Gurgling
   d. Stridor
10-11. Demonstrate each of the following procedures necessary for airway assessment and correction:
   a. Opening the mouth of an unresponsive patient
   b. Suctioning the mouth

   c. Head-tilt, chin-lift maneuver

   d. Jaw-thrust maneuver

   e. Insertion of an oropharyngeal airway

   f. Insertion of a nasopharyngeal airway

   g. Positioning a patient for control of the airway

10-12. Describe the performance requirements for fixed suction devices.

10-13. Compare the function of fixed and portable suction devices.

10-14. Compare the use of rigid and soft suction catheters.

10-15. Explain special considerations to be kept in mind when suctioning patients, including signs of hypoxia and patients with copious amounts of vomit that cannot be quickly suctioned.

10-16. Describe the indications, advantages, disadvantages, precautions, uses, and limitations of oropharyngeal and nasopharyngeal airways.

10-17. Distinguish between patients with adequate and inadequate breathing by considering the following:

   a. Minute ventilation

   b. Alveolar ventilation

   c. Inspection of the chest

   d. Patient's general appearance

   e. Regularity of breathing

   f. Flaring of the nostrils

   g. Patient's ability to speak

   h. Airflow

   i. Breath sounds

10-18. Identify patients with indications for supplemental oxygen and positive pressure ventilation.

10-19. Describe the physiological differences between spontaneous and positive pressure ventilation.

10-20. Distinguish between adequate and inadequate positive pressure ventilation.

10-21. Demonstrate each of the following procedures for artificial ventilation:

   a. Mouth-to-mouth and mouth-to-mask ventilation

   b. Delivery of positive pressure ventilations with a bag-valve-mask device (one-person and two-person), with a flow-restricted, oxygen-powered ventilation device, and with an automatic transport ventilator

10-22. Differentiate between the duration and volume of ventilation for patients with and without pulses.

10-23. Explain the significance of avoiding gastric inflation when administering positive pressure ventilation.

10-24. Describe indications and methods for administering positive pressure ventilations to a patient who is breathing spontaneously.

10-25. Discuss the indications, contraindications, and methods for administering continuous positive airway pressure (CPAP) or bilevel positive airway pressure (BiPAP).

10-26. Discuss the hazards of overventilation.

10-27. Discuss special considerations of airway management and ventilation for the following:

   a. Patients with stomas or tracheostomy tubes

   b. Infants and children

   c. Patients with facial injuries

   d. Patients with foreign body airway obstructions

   e. Patients with dental appliances

10-28. Describe the properties of oxygen.

10-29. Differentiate between the various sizes of oxygen cylinders available.

10-30. Describe the hazards associated with oxygen use and safety precautions to be observed when using oxygen or handling oxygen cylinders.

10-31. Describe the regulation of oxygen pressures, including the uses of high-pressure and therapy regulators.

10-32. Discuss the use of oxygen humidifiers.

10-33. Discuss the administration of oxygen by nonrebreather mask, nasal cannula, simple face mask, partial rebreather mask, Venturi mask, and tracheostomy mask.

KEY IDEAS

In this chapter, your knowledge of the respiratory system and airway management will be put to use. After completion of this chapter, you should be able to establish and maintain an airway, as well as ensure effective ventilation and oxygen administration. It is important to do the following:

- Review the anatomy and physiology of the respiratory system in both adults and infants/children.
- Understand the two manual methods of opening an airway, and explain the circumstances in which each should be used.
- Understand that the EMT may insert an oropharyngeal or nasopharyngeal airway adjunct to assist in establishing and maintaining an open airway, and understand the circumstances in which each should be used.
- Understand how to assess for adequate or inadequate ventilation.
- Know the methods that the EMT can use to ventilate the patient artificially, and understand the advantages and disadvantages of each.
- Know the techniques for ventilating patients with and without suspected spinal injury.
- Know the signs that indicate the patient is being ventilated adequately.
- Describe the appropriate procedure for initiating oxygen therapy, including preparing the equipment, and the steps for discontinuing oxygen administration.

MEDICAL TERMINOLOGY

Term	Prefix	Word Root Combining Form	Suffix	Definition
bilateral (bi-LAT-uh-rul)	bi- (two, double)	later (side)	-al (pertaining to)	On both sides
bradypnea (brad-ip-NEE-uh)	brady- (slow)	pnea (to breathe, or breathing)		A breathing rate slower than the normal rate
cyanosis (si-uh-NO-sis)		cyan (dark blue)	-osis (condition of)	A bluish color of the skin and mucous membranes that indicates poor oxygenation of tissues
deoxygenated (de-OK-suh-jun-ate-id)	de- (down, away from)	oxy (oxygen); gen (formation, produce)	-ate (use, action); -ed (indicates adjective formed from verb)	Containing low amounts of oxygen, as with venous blood
hemoglobin (HEE-muh-glo-bin)		hem/o (blood); globin (globule)		A complex protein molecule found on the surface of the red blood cell that is responsible for carrying a majority of the oxygen in the blood
hypoxia (hi-POX-ee-uh)	hyp/o- (below, deficient)	oxy (oxygen)	-ia (condition of)	A reduction of oxygen delivery to the tissues

Term	Prefix	Word Root Combining Form	Suffix	Definition
laryngectomy (lair-in-JEK-tuh-me)		laryng (larynx)	-ectomy (surgical excision)	A surgical procedure in which a patient's larynx is removed
nasopharynx (NAY-zo-FAIR-inks)		nas/o (nose); pharynx (pharynx, throat)		Nasal portion of the pharynx, situated above the soft palate
oropharynx (OR-o-FAIR-inks)		or/o (mouth); pharynx (pharynx, throat)		Portion of the pharynx that extends from the mouth to the oral cavity at the base of the tongue
tachypnea (tak-ip-NEE-uh)	tachy- (fast)	pnea (to breathe or breathing)		A breathing rate faster than the normal rate
tracheostomy (tray-kee-OS-tuh-me)		trache/o (trachea)	-stomy (new opening)	A surgical opening in the trachea into which a tube is inserted for the patient to breathe through

1. The prefix *bi-* in the medical term *bilateral* means
   a. two, double.
   b. before.
   c. slow.
   d. half.

2. *Cyan,* the word root in *cyanosis,* indicates
   a. to suck in.
   b. hollow air sac.
   c. dark blue.
   d. to the right.

3. The suffix *-ectomy* in the medical term *laryngectomy* indicates
   a. pertaining to the epiglottis.
   b. surgical excision.
   c. inflammation or infection.
   d. sound production.

4. The word root *trache/o* in the medical term *tracheostomy* means
   a. traction.
   b. trachea.
   c. tract.
   d. transition.

5. The suffix *-stomy* when used in the term *tracheostomy* relates to a(n)
   a. structure.
   b. tube.
   c. contraction.
   d. opening.

TERMS AND CONCEPTS

1. In each space, write the number of the term described by the statement. Not all terms will be used.

1. Agonal respirations	12. Nasal cannula
2. Alveoli	13. Nasopharynx
3. Bradypnea	14. Nonrebreather mask
4. Cricoid cartilage	15. Oropharyngeal airway
5. Cyanosis	16. Oropharynx
6. Epiglottis	17. Oxygenated
7. Esophagus	18. Pleura
8. Hemoglobin	19. Retractions
9. Hypopnea	20. Tachypnea
10. Hypoxia	21. Tidal volume
11. Mucous membrane	22. Tracheostomy

_____ a. A breathing rate slower than the normal rate

_____ b. Gasping respirations that have no pattern and occur infrequently

_____ c. Two layers of connective tissue that surround the lungs

_____ d. Air sacs in the lungs; point of gas exchange with the pulmonary capillaries

_____ e. Bluish color of skin and mucous membranes that indicates poor oxygenation

_____ f. Depressions seen in the neck, above the clavicles, between the ribs, or below the rib cage from excessive muscle use during breathing

_____ g. A surgical procedure that creates a stoma in the neck for the patient to breathe through

_____ h. Volume of air inhaled and exhaled in one respiration

_____ i. A breathing rate faster than the normal rate

_____ j. Molecule that carries oxygen in the blood

_____ k. Portion of the pharynx that extends from the mouth to the base of the tongue

_____ l. A reduction of oxygen delivery to the tissues

_____ m. Portion of the pharynx that extends from the nostrils to the soft palate

_____ n. Passage for foods and liquids to enter the stomach

_____ o. Flap of tissue that closes over the trachea during swallowing

_____ p. Oxygen delivery device that includes a one-way valve and reservoir and can deliver up to 100 percent oxygen

_____ q. Semicircular hard plastic device that is inserted into the mouth and holds the tongue away from the back of the pharynx

_____ r. Inadequate tidal volume in a breathing patient

CONTENT REVIEW

1. Which anatomical feature may cause more frequent airway obstruction in infants and children than in adults?
   a. The nose and mouth are proportionally larger.
   b. The cricoid cartilage is wider and more rigid.
   c. The tongue takes up relatively more space.
   d. The diaphragm and external intercostal muscles are less developed.

2. Fill in each term naming a structure of the upper airway on the appropriate line.

   Cricoid cartilage
   Epiglottis
   Esophagus
   Larynx
   Mandible
   Nasal cavity
   Nasopharynx
   Oropharynx
   Soft palate
   Thyroid cartilage
   Tongue
   Trachea
   Vocal cords

   A _____
   B _____
   C _____
   D _____
   E _____
   F _____
   G _____
   H _____
   I _____
   J _____
   K _____
   L _____
   M _____

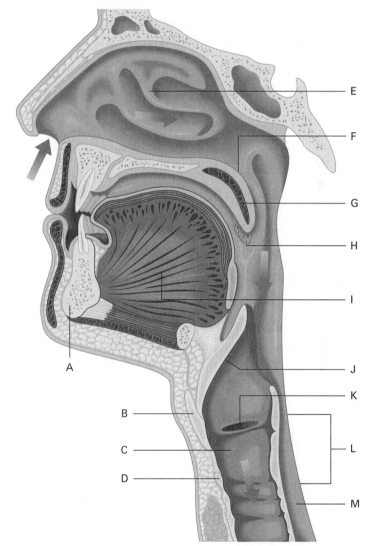

3. A major muscle of breathing that separates the chest cavity from the abdominal cavity is which of the following?
   a. Diaphragm
   b. Alveolus
   c. Visceral pleura
   d. Bronchiole

4. The point at which the trachea bifurcates (splits) into the right and left mainstem bronchi is termed the
   a. larynx.
   b. carina.
   c. pleura.
   d. bronchiole.

5. While inspecting an injured patient's mouth, you find broken teeth in the oropharynx, and suctioning equipment is not immediately available. You should
   a. perform five quick abdominal thrusts.
   b. perform five back blows with your hand.
   c. sweep the mouth with your index finger.
   d. sit the patient up to help secure the airway.

6. Describe the steps to perform the head-tilt, chin-lift maneuver.

   _____

   _____

   _____

   _____

   _____

7. When treating a patient with a suspected spinal injury, which method of opening the airway should be used?
   a. Jaw-thrust maneuver
   b. Head-tilt, chin-lift maneuver
   c. Lateral-flexion maneuver
   d. Hyperextension maneuver

8. To help prevent obstruction of the trachea when performing the head-tilt, chin-lift maneuver on infants or children, the head should be placed in which position?
   a. Flexed
   b. Tilted
   c. Extended
   d. Neutral

9. When suctioning, you should use what type of Standard Precautions?
   a. Gloves
   b. Mask
   c. Protective eyewear
   d. All of these

10. Your patient is unresponsive and has a large amount of vomitus in the oropharynx. Which suction catheter should be used?
    a. English catheter
    b. French catheter
    c. Hard catheter
    d. Soft catheter

11. Suction should only be applied for _____ seconds in the adult patient and _____ seconds for infants and children.
    a. 20/10
    b. 20/5
    c. 15/5
    d. 10/5

12. You are preparing to suction the patient with inadequate breathing who is producing large amounts of frothy secretions that are continuous and require constant suctioning. You should
    a. suction for 15 seconds, provide oxygen by nonrebreather mask for 15 seconds, and repeat.
    b. suction for 15 seconds, provide oxygen by nonrebreather mask for 5 minutes, and repeat.
    c. suction for 15 seconds, provide positive pressure ventilation for 2 minutes, and repeat.
    d. suction for 15 seconds, provide positive pressure ventilation for 10 minutes, and repeat.

13. You have decided to use an oropharyngeal airway on a deeply unresponsive patient. How would you measure for the proper size?
    a. Measure the airway from the tip of the patient's nose to the tip of the earlobe.
    b. Measure the airway from the patient's earlobe to the bottom of the angle of the jaw.
    c. Measure the airway from the level of the front teeth to the angle of the jaw.
    d. Oropharyngeal airways should not be used if the patient is deeply unresponsive.

14. After selecting the correct-size nasopharyngeal airway and lubricating the airway with a water-soluble lubricant, the airway should be inserted into the larger nostril until
    a. the patient gags, and then pull back slightly.
    b. resistance is met or bleeding occurs.
    c. the flange rests on the flare of the nostril.
    d. the bevel comes in contact with the septum.

15. Cells that are not receiving an adequate amount of oxygen are suffering from
    a. hypoxia.
    b. hypoventilation.
    c. hyperperfusion.
    d. hemoglobin.

16. You must assess your patient for adequate or inadequate breathing. Briefly describe what you would observe about the following four factors in a patient who is breathing adequately.
    a. Rate _____
    b. Rhythm _____
    c. Quality _____
    d. Depth _____

17. Which of the following is a late and significant sign of hypoxia?
    a. Headache
    b. Hypertension
    c. Cyanosis
    d. Restlessness

18. What are the normal respiratory rate limits for the following patients?

    Adult: _____ to _____ respirations a minute

    Child: _____ to _____ respirations a minute

    Infant: _____ to _____ respirations a minute

19. From the following answers, choose the one that best indicates that your patient is breathing adequately.
    a. Bilateral chest rise
    b. Tachypnea
    c. Bradypnea
    d. Agonal breathing

20. You are treating a medical patient who is responding to painful stimuli with moaning. His breathing is adequate. The best method to protect this patient from aspirating is to
    a. place the patient on a nonrebreather mask at 15 lpm.
    b. place the patient in a modified lateral (recovery) position.
    c. insert an oropharyngeal airway.
    d. apply cricoid pressure while he is in a supine position.

21. After auscultating the chest of an elderly patient who has fallen out of bed, you note that the breath sounds on both sides are dramatically decreased. You should
    a. place the patient back in bed.
    b. administer oxygen by a nonrebreather mask.
    c. provide positive pressure ventilation.
    d. help the patient to a sitting position.

22. Which of the following statements regarding the use of cricoid pressure (Sellick maneuver) is correct?
    a. It cannot be used in the deeply unresponsive apneic patient.
    b. It collapses the trachea against the cervical vertebrae.
    c. You may be asked to perform when assisting with endotracheal intubation.
    d. It can be used in the patient with an altered mental status.

23. Exhaled breath contains about
    a. 21 percent oxygen.
    b. 16 percent oxygen.
    c. 5 percent oxygen.
    d. 0.05 percent oxygen.

24. You are preparing to ventilate your patient with the pocket mask. Which of the following is an advantage of performing mouth-to-mask ventilations with the pocket mask?
    a. The mask eliminates direct contact with the patient.
    b. There is no need for the use of an oral airway.
    c. Nearly 100 percent oxygen concentration can be reached.
    d. The device eliminates the need to watch for chest rise.

25. When ventilating the apneic patient with a pulse using the bag-valve mask (BVM), the adult patient should be ventilated every _____ seconds, and the infant and child should be ventilated every _____ seconds.
    a. 5–6/3–5
    b. 2–3/3–5
    c. 8–10/5–6
    d. 3–5/5–6

26. Fill in the parts of the BVM unit on the appropriate lines.

Bag

Face mask

Intake valve/oxygen-reservoir valve

Nonrebreathing patient valve

Oxygen reservoir

Oxygen-supply connecting tube

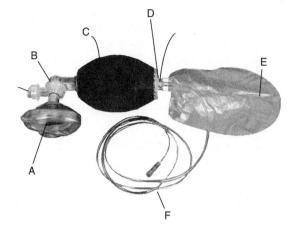

A _____

B _____

C _____

D _____

E _____

F _____

27. The BVM with a reservoir, when attached to an oxygen source, can deliver nearly 100 percent oxygen. What percentage of oxygen is delivered to the patient by BVM without an oxygen source?
  a. 61 percent
  b. 41 percent
  c. 21 percent
  d. 11 percent

28. Which of the following is a desirable feature of the BVM?
  a. It allows a single operator to maintain a tight mask seal easily.
  b. It allows delivery of ventilations enriched from an oxygen source.
  c. It can be easily taught to the emergency medical responder (EMR) and layperson.
  d. It protects the airway from regurgitation of vomitus.

29. Your patient is experiencing agonal breathing, and you suspect a spinal injury. You should
  a. perform a head-tilt, chin-lift maneuver to open the airway, then ventilate.
  b. pull on the head to align the airway, then ventilate.
  c. establish in-line stabilization and perform a jaw-thrust maneuver, then ventilate.
  d. establish in-line stabilization, but do not ventilate because the patient is breathing.

30. From the following, choose the correct statement pertaining to use of the flow-restricted, oxygen-powered ventilation device (FROPVD).
  a. It is unnecessary to use an airway adjunct while in use.
  b. It is the ventilation of choice for children and infants.
  c. Gastric distention is a rare side effect.
  d. The EMT is unable to feel lung compliance during ventilation.

31. When ventilating with the FROPVD, the trigger or button on the valve should be released
  a. as soon as the chest begins to rise.
  b. after the chest has risen fully.
  c. after the audible alarm sounds.
  d. after 5 to 7 seconds of activation.

32. While ventilating a patient with the FROPVD, the chest does not rise adequately. You should *first*
   a. depress the trigger or button up to twice as long.
   b. follow foreign body airway obstruction maneuvers.
   c. reevaluate the position of the head, chin, and mask seal.
   d. use an alternative means to ventilate the patient.

33. To determine the correct tidal volume and rate for the automatic transport ventilator (ATV), you should
   a. watch the stomach rise and fall.
   b. consult with medical direction.
   c. set the inspiration time for 10 seconds.
   d. estimate the tidal volume by observing the pulse oximeter.

34. Although there are different sizes of oxygen tanks, when full, all contain the same pressure, which is
   a. approximately 1,000 pounds per square inch.
   b. approximately 2,000 pounds per square inch.
   c. approximately 3,000 pounds per square inch.
   d. approximately 4,000 pounds per square inch.

35. Which of the following, when it comes into contact with oxygen under pressure, may cause an explosion to occur?
   a. Ambient air
   b. Petroleum jelly
   c. All adhesive tapes
   d. Sterile water

36. Which type of pressure regulator has only one gauge, which registers the content of the oxygen tank?
   a. Therapy regulator
   b. Treatment regulator
   c. High-pressure regulator
   d. Continuous-flow regulator

37. You are preparing to change the oxygen tank to a full one. To remove any dust or debris, before placing the yoke of the pressure regulator onto the oxygen cylinder, you should
   a. tap the valve with the yoke of the regulator.
   b. wipe the valve stem with a clean, damp cloth.
   c. quickly open and shut the valve on the cylinder.
   d. gently rinse the valve under running water.

38. You have transferred your patient over to the receiving facility staff. When discontinuing the oxygen administration to the patient, you should
   a. turn off the oxygen, then remove the mask from the patient's face.
   b. remove the mask from the patient's face, then turn off the oxygen.
   c. hyperoxygenate the patient for 5 minutes, then remove the mask.
   d. turn off the oxygen, then ask the patient to breathe for 2 minutes.

39. While preparing to administer oxygen to your patient, you know that the liter flow typically needed to keep the reservoir bag filled on the nonrebreather mask is
   a. 2 liters per minute.
   b. 5 liters per minute.
   c. 10 liters per minute.
   d. 15 liters per minute.

40. You are attempting to treat a child with a nonrebreather mask, but the child will not tolerate the mask and pushes it away from his face. What is the recommended way to continue the treatment?
   a. Hold the mask on the face while diverting the child's attention.
   b. Ask the parent to hold the mask on the face until the child accepts the mask.
   c. Have someone familiar with the child hold the mask close to the child's face.
   d. Administer the oxygen by using an FROPVD.

41. Which of the following best describes external respirations?
   a. The mechanical process of moving air in and out of the lungs
   b. The gas exchange process that occurs between the cells and the systemic capillaries
   c. The process that breaks down glucose in the presence of oxygen and produces high amounts of energy in the form of ATP
   d. The gas exchange process that occurs between the alveoli and the surrounding pulmonary capillaries

42. The proper liter flow range for the nasal cannula is commonly set at _____ liters per minute.
   a. 1–6
   b. 8–10
   c. 15
   d. 22–44

43. The only mask recommended for oxygen delivery in the prehospital setting is which one of the following?
   a. Simple face mask
   b. Partial rebreather mask
   c. Nonrebreather mask
   d. Venturi mask

44. If your patient's dentures are securely in place, before ventilating, you should
   a. remove them to achieve a better mask seal.
   b. remove them to avoid the danger of breaking them in the mouth.
   c. leave them in the mouth so they will not be misplaced.
   d. leave them in the mouth to achieve a better mask seal.

45. You arrive on the scene and find a 62-year-old male lying on the garage floor. The police indicate that this is an attempted suicide. They indicate that the patient had the car running in the garage with all the doors shut. As you assess the patient, you note that he is breathing at 24 times per minute with adequate volume. Your partner attaches the pulse oximeter prior to your placing the patient on oxygen. You would anticipate the SpO_2 reading to be
   a. less than 70%.
   b. approximately 90%.
   c. 93–95%.
   d. close to 100%.

46. In the healthy patient, chemoreceptors in the brain sense changes in _____ levels and send impulses to the respiratory muscles to increase or decrease the rate and depth of respirations, thus controlling the respiratory effort.
   a. hydrogen
   b. carbon dioxide
   c. oxygen
   d. nitrogen

47. The patient suffering from a condition known as chronic obstructive pulmonary disease (COPD) typically has chronically high carbon dioxide levels. Thus, the chemoreceptors must rely on which of the following to regulate breathing?
   a. Carbon monoxide
   b. Oxygen
   c. Nitrogen
   d. Hydrogen

48. You are assessing a patient who displays signs of hypoxia. You immediately assess the airway for adequacy of breathing. The patient presents with poor tidal volume and tachypnea, with an SpO_2 of 91%. You should next
   a. apply oxygen by nasal cannula 4 lpm.
   b. apply oxygen via nonrebreather mask 10 lpm.
   c. provide positive pressure ventilations.
   d. provide blow-by oxygen at 100 percent.

49. Which of the following positions may lead to inadequate ventilations and severe hypoxia by pushing the abdominal contents upward against the diaphragm, limiting its movement?
   a. Supine
   b. Recovery
   c. Semi-Fowler's
   d. Prone

50. You are preparing to suction your patient using a rigid (Yankauer) catheter. You know that the tip of the catheter may stimulate the vagus nerve, causing the patient to become
   a. bradycardic.
   b. apneic.
   c. tachypneic.
   d. hypovolemic.

51. You are assessing the adequacy of your patient's breathing. What two variables must you know before you can assess the breathing accurately?
   a. Respiratory rate and tidal volume
   b. Respiratory volume and minute rate
   c. Spirometer volume and respiratory effort
   d. Oximeter reading and minute volume

52. You have assessed your patient and determined that he is breathing 12 times a minute with an inadequate tidal volume. You should immediately increase the tidal volume by
   a. instructing the patient to increase his breaths per minute by breathing faster.
   b. delivering a ventilation with the BVM when the patient begins to breathe in.
   c. placing the patient in the tripod position and coaching him to use accessory muscles.
   d. delivering smaller-volume breaths at an increased minute rate using the BVM.

53. You are providing ventilations to a pulseless adult patient using the laryngeal mask airway (LMA). What ventilation rate should this patient receive?
    a. 3–5 ventilations per minute
    b. 5–7 ventilations per minute
    c. 8–10 ventilations per minute
    d. 12–14 ventilations per minute

54. You are preparing to provide ventilations to your apneic newborn patient with a pulse. At what rate should you ventilate this patient?
    a. 10–12 ventilations per minute
    b. 12–20 ventilations per minute
    c. 20–30 ventilations per minute
    d. 40–60 ventilations per minute

55. You are attempting to ventilate your pulseless and apneic trauma patient; the jaw thrust is ineffective in opening the airway. You should
    a. continue to apply the jaw thrust until the airway is maintained.
    b. perform the head-tilt, chin-lift maneuver to ventilate the patient.
    c. call for ALS backup and wait for their arrival to perform an emergency airway intervention.
    d. place the patient in the coma or left lateral recumbent position and transport immediately.

56. You are preparing to ventilate your adult patient, who is breathing at a rate of 40 breaths per minute (tachypnea), which leads to an inadequate tidal volume (hypopnea). You should
    a. ventilate at the patient's rate, then slowly adjust the rate to one breath every 5–6 seconds.
    b. continue to ventilate at the patient's rate until the respiratory effort spontaneously decreases.
    c. ventilate at a lower than normal rate—every 8–12 seconds—until the patient's rate decreases.
    d. provide ventilations of one breath every 5–6 seconds, then increase the rate to every 3–4 seconds.

57. You are preparing to ventilate your adult stoma patient with the BVM. Which of the following is an acceptable practice when ventilating the adult stoma patient?
    a. When suctioning, insert a soft suction catheter approximately 6 to 8 inches.
    b. Perform a head-tilt, chin-lift, or jaw-thrust maneuver to manage the airway.
    c. Select a mask—usually the child or infant mask—to fit securely over the stoma.
    d. Administer the ventilation over a 3- to 4-second period, watching for abdominal rise.

58. You have responded to a report of a child choking on a toy. You find the responsive child choking but moving air when inhaling and exhaling. You should
    a. perform a head-tilt, chin-lift maneuver to clear the airway.
    b. instruct the patient to cough to try to dislodge the object.
    c. administer abdominal thrusts to expel the object from the airway.
    d. instruct the mother to perform a blind finger sweep of the mouth.

59. You are preparing your patient for the use of continuous positive airway pressure (CPAP). In which position should you place your patient?
    a. Supine
    b. Semi-Fowler's
    c. Prone
    d. Left lateral recumbant

60. While treating your elderly congestive heart failure (CHF) patient with CPAP, you note that the patient's Glasgow Coma Scale (GCS) deteriorates to 10 and he is no longer able to understand your commands. Your next immediate action should be to
    a. perform a stroke evaluation test and place the patient onto his left side, providing oxygen via nasal cannula.
    b. increase the CPAP pressure by 20 cmH^{2}O until the patient's response improves, and then reassess the patient's GCS.
    c. reassess the patient, and then place into a supine position while continuing the CPAP treatment.
    d. immediately remove the CPAP device and provide positive pressure ventilations with a BVM.

61. You are treating your patient with CPAP. After reassessing your patient, which of the following indicates that your patient is responding positively to the treatment?
    a. Increase in respiratory rate, increase in heart rate, decrease in SpO_2 reading, decrease in blood pressure
    b. Increase in respiratory rate, decrease in heart rate, increase in SpO_2 reading, increase in blood pressure
    c. Decrease in respiratory rate, decrease in heart rate, increase in SpO_2 reading, a reduction in cyanosis and accessory muscle use
    d. Decrease in respiratory rate, increase in heart rate, decrease in SpO_2 reading, increase in accessory muscle use

62. Which of the following patients should receive supplemental oxygen therapy?
    a. A 34-year-old patient who has had an anxiety attack, breathing 28 times each minute with a SpO_2 of 99%
    b. A 50-year-old who has a painful swollen leg after falling off a chair; SpO_2 is 96%; skin is warm and dry
    c. An 8-year-old who has abdominal pain, is breathing normally with skin that is warm and dry, and exhibits no signs of hypoxemia
    d. A 72-year-old who was involved in a motor vehicle accident; no outward signs of injury; skin is slightly pale, cool, and diaphoretic; blood pressure 102/88.

▌ CASE STUDY 1

While you are placing your blanket on your bunk at the station in preparation for bed, the alerting system sounds. "Unit One, respond to 10930 Heltman for an elderly woman short of breath." You and your partner, Nancy, recognize the location as a local church. As you walk in, a member of the clergy directs you to the back of the church, where you find a woman sitting bolt upright in a tripod position, obviously very anxious. You introduce yourselves to the patient, and she replies with gasping breaths, "I'm Mary. Help me. I can't breathe." You reassure her and, anticipating possible respiratory arrest, call for paramedic backup from another station.

1. From your brief interaction with Mary, what indications lead you to believe she is experiencing serious respiratory distress? (Name at least three.)

   _____

   _____

   _____

2. At this time, which of the following would be the most appropriate treatment for Mary?
   a. Nasal cannula at 6 liters per minute
   b. Venturi mask at 10 liters per minute
   c. Simple face mask at 10 liters per minute
   d. Nonrebreather mask at 15 liters per minute

A friend of Mary's tells you that Mary has emphysema (COPD) and sometimes has to be on oxygen at home. As you assess Mary's breathing sounds, you detect a gurgling noise and then notice a pink frothy secretion coming from her mouth. Nancy advises you that Mary's respiratory rate is 36 per minute.

3. Which suction catheter and technique would be most appropriate for Mary in this situation?
   a. Use a rigid catheter, insert the catheter without suction, and apply suction for 15 seconds.
   b. Use a rigid catheter, insert the catheter with suction, and suction for 20 seconds.
   c. Use a French catheter, insert into the mouth without suction, and apply for 15 seconds.
   d. Use a soft catheter, insert into the mouth without suction, and apply for 20 seconds.

It becomes apparent that Mary's breathing is inadequate and that positive pressure ventilation is needed. You decide to use the BVM, with you and Nancy delivering the ventilations. Before using the mask and the associated airway adjuncts, Nancy explains the procedure to Mary.

4. Keeping in mind that Mary is still slightly responsive, which of the following adjuncts and techniques is most appropriate for her at this time?
   a. Oropharyngeal airway inserted by using the 180-degree-turn advancing technique
   b. Oropharyngeal airway inserted by using a tongue-depressor technique
   c. Nasopharyngeal airway inserted bevel first until the flange rests on the nostril
   d. Nasopharyngeal airway inserted flange first until the bevel rests on the nostril

Despite your best team efforts, Mary becomes unresponsive and is no longer breathing on her own. Her pulse can be felt and is bounding. Dispatch advises you that the estimated time of arrival for the paramedic backup unit is less than one minute.

5. What should you and Nancy do, now that Mary is not breathing on her own?
   a. Start cardiopulmonary resuscitation (CPR) until the paramedic unit arrives.
   b. Continue to ventilate and suction the patient as you did when she was responsive.
   c. Continue to ventilate the patient, but because she is unresponsive, suction is not needed.
   d. Roll the patient to clear the airway and start CPR immediately.

CASE STUDY 2

You and your partner, Joshua, are dispatched to a construction site where there is a report of a young female worker who fell from the third floor. Dispatch advises you that Engine Company 4 and a paramedic backup unit from your system are both responding. Your unit arrives on scene. As you approach the patient, a coworker states that the patient fell headfirst from the third floor onto the dirt where she lies now. Another worker tells you that the patient was unconscious when he rolled her from her stomach to her back. As you visually examine the patient, you notice that she is breathing with agonal respirations and is bleeding freely from the mouth.

1. In this situation, how would you open the mouth and airway?
   a. In-line stabilization with the hyperextension/head-lift maneuver
   b. In-line stabilization with the head-tilt, chin-lift maneuver
   c. In-line stabilization with the jaw-thrust maneuver
   d. In-line stabilization with the crossed-finger technique

2. After opening the mouth and airway, you find a copious amount of blood, with teeth in the oropharynx. How should you remove the foreign material?
   a. Turn the patient's head to the side to permit drainage.
   b. Roll the patient to a prone position and finger sweep.
   c. Suction using the soft or French catheter.
   d. Suction using the rigid or hard catheter.

The patient's agonal respirations are clearly inadequate. With the oral airway in place, Joshua will stabilize the patient's head and hold the BVM in place while you squeeze the bag to ventilate the patient. You squeeze the bag, but the patient's chest does not rise.

3. Which of the following may cause the chest not to rise with ventilations?
   a. Incorrect position of the head and chin
   b. Air escaping from around the mask
   c. Airway obstruction
   d. Any or all of these may cause a failure.

After reevaluating and adjusting your patient and airway technique, the patient's chest is rising and falling normally with every squeeze of the bag. The backup paramedic unit arrives, with the engine company following. The paramedic lieutenant, Moser, states, "This type of airway problem can be very difficult to control. You did a good job." You and Joshua assist the paramedics with spinal immobilization and give them your report. Joshua assists the paramedics further on the way to the hospital.

Baseline Vital Signs, Monitoring Devices, and History Taking

▌ STANDARD

Assessment (Content Areas: Secondary Assessment; Monitoring Devices; History Taking)

▌ COMPETENCY

Applies scene information and patient assessment findings (scene size-up, primary and secondary assessment, patient history, and reassessment) to guide emergency management.

▌ OBJECTIVES

After reading this chapter, you should be able to:

11-1. Define key terms introduced in this chapter.

11-2. Explain the importance of taking and recording a patient's vital signs over a period of time to identify problems and changes in the patient's condition and of accurately documenting the vital signs and patient history.

11-3. Perform the steps required to assess the patient's breathing, pulse, skin, pupils, blood pressure, and oxygen saturation and consider the patient's overall presentation when interpreting the meaning of vital sign findings.

11-4. Differentiate between normal and abnormal findings when assessing a patient's breathing, to include the respiratory rate, quality of respirations, rhythm of respirations, and signs that may indicate respiratory distress or respiratory failure.

11-5. Differentiate between normal respiratory rates for adults, children, infants, and newborns, and evaluate the need to administer treatment based on assessment of a patient's breathing.

11-6. Auscultate breath sounds to determine the presence of breath sounds, equality of breath sounds, and the presence and likely underlying causes of abnormal breath sounds.

11-7. Assess the pulse at various pulse points and consider the patient's age and level of responsiveness when selecting a site to palpate the pulse.

11-8. Differentiate between normal and abnormal findings when assessing a patient's pulse, to include the pulse rate, quality of the pulse, and rhythm of the pulse.

11-9. Associate pulse abnormalities with possible underlying causes and describe the changes in the pulse associated with pulsus paradoxus.

11-10. Recognize normal and abnormal findings in the assessment of skin color, temperature, condition, capillary refill, and color of the mucous membranes and associate abnormal skin findings with potential underlying causes.

11-11. Explain factors that can affect capillary refill findings.

11-12. When assessing the pupils, recognize dilation, constriction, inequality, and abnormal reactivity and associate abnormal findings with potential underlying causes.

11-13. In relation to blood pressure measurement, explain systolic and diastolic blood pressure, consider normal values for age and gender, find the pulse pressure, and identify potential causes of abnormal findings or changes.

11-14. Compare palpation and auscultation of blood pressure as to processes, useful findings, and documentation and discuss how technique and selection of equipment can affect the accuracy of readings.

11-15. Demonstrate assessment of orthostatic vital signs.

11-16. Given a patient scenario, determine the frequency with which vital signs should be reassessed.

11-17. Explain what pulse oximetry measures, use pulse oximetry to help determine the need for supplemental oxygen, and describe factors and limitations in interpreting pulse oximetry findings.

11-18. Describe the correct procedure for noninvasive blood pressure monitoring.

11-19. Describe the processes for controlling the scene, achieving a smooth transition of care, and reducing the patient's anxiety.

11-20. Determine a patient's chief complaint.

11-21. Given a scenario, efficiently elicit an adequate patient history using closed-ended and open-ended questions and active listening techniques.

11-22. Use the mnemonics SAMPLE and OPQRST to ensure a complete prehospital patient history.

11-23. React appropriately when asking questions about sensitive topics or when caring for patients who present special challenges to history-taking and assessment.

KEY IDEAS

This chapter focuses on the critical EMT skills of obtaining a patient history, using monitoring equipment, and taking vital signs. These skills are key elements of assessing the patient, measuring the patient's response to prehospital emergency care, and providing essential information for hospital personnel.

- Baseline vital sign measurements are your first assessments related to respiration; pulse; skin color, condition, and temperature; pupils; blood pressure; and pulse oximetry. All subsequent measurements of these "signs of life" will be compared to your initial baseline.

- Respiration assessment includes rate, which is assessed by determining the number of breaths per minute, and quality. *Respiratory quality* refers to how much air is moving in and out with each breath (tidal volume), and how well it is moving.

- *Pulses* are pressure waves generated by each heartbeat that can be felt in an artery that is near the skin surface. Pulses are assessed for rate (the number of heartbeats per minute) and quality (strength and regularity). In the adult patient, a rapid pulse (greater than 100 bpm) is called *tachycardia*, while a slow pulse (less than 60 bpm) is called *bradycardia*.

- The skin provides many important clues about the patient's status. When assessing the patient's skin, you should note its color, condition, and temperature.

- Capillary refill is considered a more reliable sign of circulatory status in infants and younger children than in older children or adults.

- The size, equality, and reactivity of the patient's pupils can provide helpful information and clues about what might be wrong with your patient.

- Blood pressure is assessed by using a sphygmomanometer to measure the amount of pressure exerted against the arterial walls when the left ventricle of the heart contracts (systolic pressure) and when the left ventricle of the heart is at rest (diastolic pressure). Blood pressure is measured in millimeters of mercury (mmHg). The pulse pressure is the difference between the systolic and diastolic blood pressures.

- Comparing the pulse and blood pressure in a patient who is supine and then standing is called *testing orthostatic vital signs (tilt test)*. An increase in the pulse by 10–20 bpm and a decrease in the systolic blood pressure by 10–20 mmHg may indicate significant blood or fluid loss.

- The pulse oximeter is used to detect hypoxia and to monitor airway management and oxygen therapy. An SpO$_2$ reading of 97–100% is normal, while in a compromised patient, a reading of less than 94% may indicate hypoxia and require oxygen and ventilation. Inaccurate readings may be produced by hypoperfusion states (shock), hypothermia, excessive patient movement, the patient's use of nail polish, carbon monoxide, or anemia. Inaccurate readings may also be produced during some seizures or in cigarette smokers.

- Vital signs should be taken and recorded as often as necessary to provide proper care. Generally, reassessing vital signs every 15 minutes is reasonable for a stable patient, but an unstable patient requires vital signs taken every 5 minutes.

- Obtaining a medical history for your patient can be done easily using the acronym SAMPLE to remind you to ask about and record information about signs and symptoms, allergies, medications, pertinent past history, last oral intake, and events leading to the injury or illness.

- When obtaining a patient history, use active listening techniques. These include facilitation, reflection, clarification, an empathetic response, confrontation, and interpretation.

- Assessment activities may embarrass your patients or make them anxious, so it is important that you reassure them and make every effort to maintain their dignity.

- You will use monitoring equipment to gather additional assessment information not obtainable in the traditional physical exam, such as the amount of glucose in the blood or amount of hemoglobin saturated with oxygen.

MEDICAL TERMINOLOGY

Term	Prefix	Word Root Combining Form	Suffix	Definition
auscultation (OS-kul-TAY-shun)		auscultat (to listen to)	-ion (process)	Listening with a stethoscope
bradycardia (brad-uh-KAR-de-uh)	brady- (slow)	card (heart)	-ia (condition of)	A slow heart rate, less than 60 beats per minute
cyanosis (si-uh-NO-sis)		cyan (dark blue)	-osis (condition of)	A bluish color of the skin and mucous membranes that indicate poor oxygenation of tissues
diastolic (dye-us-TOL-ik)		diastol (expansion)	-ic (pertaining to)	The blood pressure that occurs during the relaxation phase of the heart cycle; the bottom number of the blood pressure reading
sphygmomanometer (sfig-mo-mah-NOM-uh-ter)		sphygm/o (pulse); meter (measuring instrument)		Instrument used to measure blood pressure
systolic (sis-TOL-ik)		systol (contraction)	-ic (pertaining to)	The blood pressure that occurs during the contraction phase of the heart cycle; the top number of the blood pressure reading
tachycardia (tak-uh-KAR-de-uh)	tachy- (fast)	card (heart)	-ia (condition of)	A rapid heart rate, more than 100 beats per minute

1. In each space, write the prefix, word root, or suffix that matches the definition.

auscultat	ic
brady	osis
card	sphygm/o
cyan	systol
diastol	tachy

_____ a. Contraction

_____ b. Pulse

_____ c. Expansion

_____ d. Fast

_____ e. To listen to

_____ f. Pertaining to

_____ g. Slow

_____ h. Heart

_____ i. Dark blue

_____ j. Condition of

TERMS AND CONCEPTS

1. Write the number of the correct term next to each definition.

1. Auscultation
2. Diastolic blood pressure
3. Palpation
4. Signs
5. Stridor
6. Symptoms
7. Systolic blood pressure
8. Pulse pressure
9. Tachycardia
10. Bradycardia

_____ a. A harsh, high-pitched airway sound

_____ b. Assessment by listening with a stethoscope

_____ c. Assessment by feeling

_____ d. Conditions that you can observe

_____ e. Pressure in the arteries when the heart's left ventricle contracts

_____ f. Pressure in the arteries when the heart's left ventricle rests

_____ g. Conditions that must be described by the patient

_____ h. In the adult, a pulse rate less than 60 beats per minute

_____ i. The difference between the systolic and diastolic blood pressures

_____ j. In the adult, a pulse rate greater than 100 beats per minute

CONTENT REVIEW

1. There are six vital signs that are commonly assessed by the EMT. Which vital sign is missing from the following list?

   Respiration

   Pulse

   Pupils

   Blood pressure

   Pulse oximeter

   a. Neurological check
   b. Core temperature
   c. Skin
   d. Electrocardiogram (ECG)

2. Respiration is usually assessed by counting the number of respirations
   a. in a 15-second period and multiplying by 4.
   b. in a 20-second period and multiplying by 3.
   c. in a 30-second period and multiplying by 2.
   d. in a 60-second period.

3. Chest wall motion of about a 1-inch expansion, no use of accessory muscles of breathing, and an exhalation of about twice the length of the inhalation. These indications describe which respiration pattern or type?
   a. Normal
   b. Shallow
   c. Labored
   d. Noisy

4. Assessing the quality of a patient's respirations provides the EMT with what critical information?
   a. How much air is moving and how well it is moving
   b. Only how much air the patient is moving
   c. Only how well the air is moving in and out of the patient
   d. An indication of the patient's perfusion status

5. Fill in the name of each pulse on the appropriate line.

   Brachial

   Carotid

   Dorsalis pedis

   Femoral

   Posterior tibial

   Radial

   A _____

   B _____

   C _____

   D _____

   E _____

   F _____

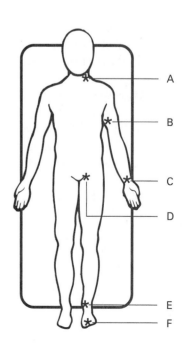

CHAPTER 11 Baseline Vital Signs, Monitoring Devices, and History Taking **93**

6. In most cases, to assess your patient's pulse, palpate the artery and count the number of beats
   a. for 15 seconds and multiply by 4.
   b. for 20 seconds and multiply by 3.
   c. for 30 seconds and multiply by 2.
   d. for 60 seconds.

7. To assess the pulse of your six-month-old patient, you should initially check the _____ pulse.
   a. carotid
   b. brachial
   c. radial
   d. femoral

8. For the six-month-old patient, what would be considered an average resting pulse rate?
   a. 60 beats per minute
   b. 80 beats per minute
   c. 100 beats per minute
   d. 130 beats per minute

9. In terms of pulse quality, which of the following would be considered normal for an adult?
   a. Weak and irregular at 70 beats per minute
   b. Strong and regular at 70 beats per minute
   c. Bounding and irregular at 70 beats per minute
   d. Thready and regular at 70 beats per minute

10. Which of the following may be a sign of extreme vasoconstriction or blood loss?
    a. Pale conjunctiva
    b. Red nail beds
    c. Blue-gray oral mucosa
    d. Yellow skin

11. When assessing skin color in infants, children, and dark-skinned people, the EMT should additionally check the
    a. posterior portion of both forearms.
    b. tops of both feet.
    c. palms of the hands and the soles of the feet.
    d. base of the neck.

12. How would you assess the relative skin temperature of your patient?
    a. Assess by placing the palm of your hand on the patient.
    b. Assess by using your forearm.
    c. Assess by placing the back of your hand on the patient.
    d. Assess by using the fingertips of your right hand.

13. Which of the following is a sign of normal skin condition?
    a. Clammy
    b. Wet
    c. Cool
    d. Dry

14. Which of the following is a correct upper limit for capillary refill time assessed at normal room temperature?
    a. 3 seconds for infants and children
    b. 2 seconds for female patients
    c. 5 seconds in the elderly
    d. 2 seconds for male patients

15. When assessing the patient's pupils with a light, which of the following is commonly initially assessed?
    a. Halo effect
    b. Corneal status
    c. Sensitivity to light
    d. Reactivity

16. Blood pressure is a reflection of the pressure in which of the following?
    a. Ventricles
    b. Arteries
    c. Veins
    d. Capillaries

17. When evaluating a patient's blood pressure, it is important to understand that
    a. the systolic blood pressure is determined by auscultation of the last sound.
    b. the diastolic blood pressure is determined by auscultation of the first sound.
    c. the blood pressure when using a sphygmomanometer is always reported as an odd number.
    d. a pulse pressure less than 25 percent of the systolic blood pressure is considered to be a narrow pulse pressure.

18. Which of the following is the average blood pressure for a 34-year-old female?
    a. 124/82
    b. 134/82
    c. 124/94
    d. 134/94

19. When measuring a patient's blood pressure by auscultation, you need
    a. a sphygmomanometer and your fingertips.
    b. a sphygmomanometer and a penlight.
    c. a sphygmomanometer and a stethoscope.
    d. only a sphygmomanometer.

20. Number the following steps in the proper order—from 1 to 6—for measuring a patient's blood pressure by auscultation, once you have selected and applied the proper-sized sphygmomanometer.

    _____ a. Note the systolic and diastolic sounds.

    _____ b. Deflate the cuff at 2 mmHg per second.

    _____ c. Palpate the radial pulse, inflate to 70 mmHg, and increase by 10 mmHg until the radial pulse is no longer palpable. Note the number and deflate the cuff.

    _____ d. Inflate the cuff 30 mmHg above the noted number.

    _____ e. Place the stethoscope in your ears.

    _____ f. Position the patient's arm.

21. In a stable patient, vital signs should be taken every _____ minutes.
    a. 5
    b. 10
    c. 15
    d. 20

22. Identify which element of the SAMPLE history applies to each of the following statements by writing S, A, M, P, L, or E, according to the key.

    S   Sign or symptom

    A   Allergies

    M   Medications

    P   Pertinent past history

    L   Last oral intake

    E   Events leading to the illness or injury

    _____   a. Medical alert tag notes "reacts to penicillin."

    _____   b. Patient ate large meal two hours ago.

    _____   c. Patient complains of nausea.

    _____   d. Patient requires insulin daily to control diabetes.

    _____   e. Patient diagnosed with emphysema 10 years ago.

    _____   f. Patient has chest pain that radiates down the left arm.

    _____   g. Mother reports that patient gets rashes from poison ivy.

    _____   h. Patient was outside shoveling snow.

    _____   i. Obvious deformity noted in right lower leg.

    _____   j. Patient has taken only small amounts of liquids since early morning.

    _____   k. Patient takes aspirin two to three times each day for arthritis pain.

    _____   l. Husband says patient has had epilepsy since head injury last year.

23. A paramedic asks you to help him test orthostatic vital signs on a patient you are both treating. This test is conducted to help determine if
    a. the patient has experienced a neurological emergency.
    b. the patient has a cardiac problem.
    c. significant blood or fluid loss has occurred.
    d. the patient has significant hypoxia.

24. Pulse oximetry
    a. is a method of detecting hypoxia in patients.
    b. that has a reading of 97% eliminates the potential of hypoxemia in a patient.
    c. provides an accurate reading in shock and hypothermia patients.
    d. readings are always accurate if the patient is wearing fingernail polish.

25. A 65-year-old male patient presents with severe respiratory distress. The patient is leaning slightly forward and is displaying excessive abdominal muscle use in an effort to breathe. This most likely indicates the patient is
   a. struggling to inhale.
   b. reacting normally.
   c. struggling to exhale.
   d. reacting to an acute abdominal disorder.

26. A mnemonic used to evaluate the patient's chief complaint or symptoms is OPQRST. List what each letter represents.

   O _____

   P _____

   Q _____

   R _____

   S _____

   T _____

CASE STUDY

As you read the following scenario, remember that vital signs and the history are key elements of patient assessment and provide essential information for hospital personnel.

It is about 10 P.M. on a Thursday night, and you are talking to your shift supervisor about conducting a training program at next month's shift meeting. The alarm sounds. "Rescue One, respond to a difficulty breathing at 1600 Osban Street, cross street New Jersey Avenue." You find your 60-year-old male patient sitting up in bed with his wife at his bedside. Mr. Baker is in obvious distress and reports that he can't breathe. He is breathing at a rate of 26 breaths per minute. He is using accessory muscles of his neck and shoulders, and you hear wheezing and gurgling with each breath. You find that his radial pulse is weak and irregular at a rate of 50 beats per minute. His skin is slightly cyanotic, cool, and moist. Using your penlight, you assess his pupils and find them to be equal, reactive, and of normal size. You auscultate his blood pressure at 80/50 mmHg, and his SpO_2 reading is 90%.

1. How would you describe this patient's respiratory status?
   a. Normal respiratory status
   b. Minor respiratory distress
   c. Moderate respiratory distress
   d. Severe respiratory distress

2. What might Mr. Baker's skin color, temperature, and condition indicate in this situation?
   a. Hyperperfusion
   b. Normal perfusion
   c. Hypoperfusion and liver failure
   d. Hypoperfusion and inadequate oxygenation

3. What is the relationship between Mr. Baker's pulse and his blood pressure?
   a. The pulse rate is bradycardic and may be responsible for the lowered blood pressure.
   b. The pulse rate is tachycardic and may be responsible for the lowered blood pressure.
   c. The relationship is normal, given Mr. Baker's age.
   d. The relationship is normal, given Mr. Baker's respiratory status.

While your partner starts Mr. Baker on oxygen, you begin to get his history from his wife. Mrs. Baker is upset and very worried about her husband. She tells you that he had a heart attack five years ago and takes Digoxin (a medication to strengthen his heart's contractions) and Lasix (a water pill) daily. Mr. Baker also occasionally takes nitroglycerin for episodes of chest pain, but she says that he denied having chest pain today. Although she told him that he shouldn't, he shoveled snow this morning and since then has been increasingly short of breath. He did not eat supper and only ate a bowl of soup at lunch. Mrs. Baker says that her husband has no allergies.

4. Identify the elements of the SAMPLE history found in this scenario.

   S _____

   A _____

   M _____

   P _____

   L _____

   E _____

5. Based on his current status, how frequently should you reassess Mr. Baker's vital signs?
   a. Every 5 minutes
   b. Every 10 minutes
   c. Every 15 minutes
   d. Every 20 minutes

Scene Size-Up

▌ STANDARD

Assessment (Content Area: Scene Size-Up)

▌ COMPETENCY

Applies scene information and patient assessment findings (scene size-up, primary and secondary assessment, patient history, and reassessment) to guide emergency management.

▌ OBJECTIVES

After reading this chapter, you should be able to:

12-1. Define key terms introduced in this chapter.

12-2. Explain the purposes and goals of performing a scene size-up on every EMS call.

12-3. Given a scenario, identify key findings in the scene size-up related to:

　a. Taking Standard Precautions

　b. Identifying possible scene hazards

　c. Identifying the mechanism of injury or nature of illness

　d. Determining the number of patients

　e. Determining the need for additional resources

12-4. Describe the dynamic nature of scenes and scene size-up.

12-5. Utilize dispatch information and information determined on arrival at the scene to assess scene safety.

12-6. Discuss types of situations that may require a call for additional or specialized resources.

12-7. Describe scenes you are likely to encounter and points to consider before entering such scenes, including crash scenes, other rescue scenes, crime scenes, and barroom scenes as well as potential hazards in approaching any vehicle and its passengers.

12-8. Discuss measures necessary to protect the patient, protect bystanders, control the scene, and maintain situation awareness.

12-9. Discuss factors involved in determining a mechanism of injury.

12-10. Discuss factors involved in determining the nature of the illness.

12-11. Discuss factors involved in determining the number of patients.

KEY IDEAS

This chapter covers the importance of proper scene size-up. Because the prehospital environment can be hostile and uncontrolled, it is extremely important to follow basic guidelines and use good sense when working as an EMT. It is imperative that the EMT pay close attention to the scene size-up on every call. By doing so, you may save your life, as well as that of your partner and patient.

- The EMT must ensure the safety of the EMS crew first, and then that of the patient and bystanders.
- Note scene characteristics, such as blood and other hazards, that may require the use of personal protective equipment (PPE) and Standard Precautions.
- Survey the total scene before entering, look for hazards that make the scene unstable, and do not enter if you are not trained to stabilize the hazards.
- The scene size-up consists of evaluating the five components in a stepwise manner: taking necessary Standard Precautions and other personal protection precautions, evaluating the scene for safety hazards, determining the mechanism of injury (MOI) or the nature of illness (NOI), determining the number of patients, and determining the need for additional resources.
- Beware of low-oxygen, toxic-substance, and confined-space areas, such as sewers, caverns, wells, manholes, silos, and closed storage areas. Never enter unless you are certain that it is safe.
- Never enter a known crime scene until it has been secured by the police. Be cautious and ready to retreat.
- At a crime scene, take steps to help preserve evidence. However, remember that your primary concern is treating the patient.
- Limit potential exposure to hazards by practicing recommendations suggested in the text.
- While on the scene of vehicle crashes, prevent emergency personnel and the EMT from being struck by traffic by practicing scene safety recommendations suggested in the text.
- The EMT must be prepared to call upon additional specialized rescue resources to ensure not only his own well-being, but also the successful rescue of the patient.
- Note whether the patient's problem is traumatic or medical in nature.
- The trauma scene size-up includes determining the MOI.
- The medical scene size-up requires collecting evidence that may help identify the NOI.
- Determine the number of patients and call for additional resources, if needed, prior to making contact with the patient.
- The scene size-up is a dynamic process that requires the EMT to assess and reassess the emergency scene continuously for potential hazards.

TERMS AND CONCEPTS

1. For each patient care situation described, indicate if it is a traumatic (T) or a medical (M) condition.

_____ a. 6-inch laceration to the right anterior forearm

_____ b. Gunshot wound to the right chest at nipple level on the midaxillary line

_____ c. Shortness of breath with audible wheezing on expiration

_____ d. Burn to the right anterior aspect of the thigh

_____ e. Ingestion of 20 to 30 capsules of an unknown medication

_____ f. Hot, dry, flushed skin

2. Write the number of the correct term next to each definition.

   1. Index of suspicion
   2. MOI
   3. NOI
   4. Scene safety
   5. Scene size-up

   _____ a. An overall assessment of the scene to which an EMT has been called

   _____ b. An anticipation that certain types of accidents and mechanisms will produce specific types of injuries

   _____ c. Factor involved in producing an injury to a patient, including the strength, direction, and nature of the force that caused the injury

   _____ d. Steps taken to ensure the safety and well-being of the EMT, coworkers, patients, and bystanders

   _____ e. The type of medical condition or complaint from which a patient is suffering

CONTENT REVIEW

1. One of the first goals of an EMT responding to a scene is scene safety. With this goal in mind, the EMT is concerned with the well-being of which of the following?
   a. The EMTs, patients, and bystanders
   b. The EMTs and patients only
   c. The EMTs only
   d. The patients only

2. Ensuring scene safety begins
   a. after patient contact is made.
   b. after arrival at the scene.
   c. while approaching the scene.
   d. while receiving dispatch information.

3. The EMT must use different levels of Standard Precautions. Which Standard Precaution device should be used with every patient contact when there is a chance of coming into contact with blood, other body fluids, or mucous membranes?
   a. Protective gown
   b. Eye protection
   c. Protective gloves
   d. HEPA or N-95 respirator

4. To help protect the patient's privacy from onlookers and to control bystanders, it is most effective to
   a. ask some of the bystanders to turn their backs to the patient while holding an unfolded bedsheet at shoulder height.
   b. advise the bystanders to immediately leave the scene or you will be forced to notify the police.
   c. request that the police immediately remove the bystanders from the scene.
   d. request that the police arrest curious bystanders for interfering with the patient's confidentiality.

5. As you arrive on the perimeter of a motor vehicle crash scene, you notice that there appear to be more patients than your unit can effectively handle. You should *first*
   a. proceed to the scene and evaluate the patients' needs.
   b. proceed to the patients and begin treatment.
   c. isolate the scene until law enforcement arrives.
   d. call for additional resources.

6. You are at the scene of a motor vehicle crash where power lines are lying across the vehicle. Which statement is correct?
   a. Consider all power lines to be energized until a power company representative advises you they are not.
   b. If the power lines are not arcing or smoking, you may assume that the lines are safe and not energized.
   c. You should approach the vehicle and remove the wires by using a wooden or fiberglass pole.
   d. If a local firefighter states, "The power was cut by the fire department," you can assume that it is safe.

7. If you are called to a vehicle crash involving a steep grade, and you are not trained to deal with this situation, you should
   a. improvise and use whatever means are immediately available to reach the vehicle.
   b. notify your dispatcher of the situation and wait for a properly trained rescue crew.
   c. call out to the patients in the vehicle and ask them to try to exit the vehicle.
   d. notify your dispatcher of the situation, and then proceed to try to reach the vehicle.

8. Upon arrival at a known crime scene, you should
   a. advise dispatch that you are entering the scene.
   b. enter the scene to reach the patient, exercising extreme caution.
   c. wait for police, and enter the scene as the police arrive.
   d. enter the scene only after it has been secured by police.

9. When approaching a residence, what is the correct way to knock on the door?
   a. Knock while standing in front of the door.
   b. Knock while standing off to the hinged side.
   c. Knock while standing off to the knob side.
   d. Knock and then turn your head to the side.

10. Which of the following is considered a mechanism of injury?
    a. A large-caliber gunshot
    b. A large laceration to the head
    c. A deformed and swollen wrist
    d. Hot and dry skin

CASE STUDY 1

It's Saturday night, and each Saturday night is family night at your station. Family members are all invited for supper. You are washing dishes and cleaning up the kitchen when the alarm sounds. You are dispatched to a possible shooting in the parking lot of the Cheap-O Motel, a local establishment known for its violent clientele. As you are en route, dispatch advises you that the police are on the scene and that the scene is secure. The police are requesting EMS to expedite; the patient is critical. Advanced life support (ALS) backup has been dispatched but is delayed.

1. As you approach the scene, you should
   a. advise dispatch and respond to the scene with the lights and siren on.
   b. advise dispatch and respond to the scene with only the lights on.
   c. stage your vehicle outside the scene until scene safety is confirmed.
   d. respond to the scene with lights and siren, when several block from the scene turn off lights and siren and continue to the scene.

2. As you arrive on scene, a police officer advises you that a second victim has just been located who has also been shot. You should *first*
   a. treat and transport both patients to the best of your abilities.
   b. immediately call for additional transporting units.
   c. treat and transport the most critical patient, then return for the other.
   d. treat both patients, then call for an additional unit to transport.

You start to treat one of the shooting victims, an unresponsive 32-year-old male with multiple large-caliber gunshot wounds to the chest. As you cut the clothes off the patient, being careful not to cut through the bullet holes, a small-caliber handgun falls from his pants pocket.

3. You should
   a. immediately pick up the gun by the barrel so you don't disturb fingerprints on the grip and take it to the nearest police officer.
   b. pick up the gun by putting a pencil through the trigger guard and place it in your ambulance until the police are available.
   c. not touch the gun but immediately advise the police of the situation.
   d. quickly kick the gun away with your foot.

While you are treating your patient, a crowd has begun to form and is becoming agitated and hostile. A young man picks up a bottle and throws it in your direction. It strikes the pavement with a frighteningly loud crash several feet away from you.

4. You should
   a. ask the crowd to please stand back or you will have them arrested.
   b. not let the crowd divert your attention, and keep on working.
   c. retreat temporarily until the police can give you support.
   d. leave the scene and request that police transport the patient.

CASE STUDY 2

You are reviewing and studying for your EMT refresher course. You have been enjoying the section on medical emergencies when the alarm startles you. You are dispatched to 100 Cherry Lane for an elderly woman who is not feeling well. You immediately get under way, and en route, you ask the dispatcher to call the residence back to gain more information. The dispatcher states that the original caller was an elderly male, and the only information he gave was that his "wife has had a cough for months and is not feeling well." The dispatcher advises that there is no further information available because now no one is answering the phone.

1. List at least three details dispatch relayed, and explain what each detail may tell you about the scene or the patient.

An elderly man answers the door and thanks you for being so prompt. You ask him, "What seems to be the problem this evening?" He replies, "My wife hasn't felt well for months, and she is always coughing." You ask, "Has your wife been diagnosed as having tuberculosis?" The man replies, "I'm not sure, but she has been sick for some time."

2. What type of Standard Precautions should you take?
   a. After entering the house, both EMTs should put on gloves and protective eyewear.
   b. After entering the house, only the EMT who is treating should put on gloves and protective eyewear.
   c. Before entering the house, both EMTs should put on gloves and an N-95 or a HEPA respirator.
   d. Before entering the house, both EMTs should put on gloves, eye protection, and an N-95 or a HEPA respirator.

   You introduce your partner and yourself to the patient, and your partner radios dispatch to inform them that patient contact has been made and that you are OK. You explain to the patient that the mask you are wearing is a precaution you take when a patient is coughing a lot. When you ask the patient to tell you why she had her husband call the ambulance, the patient replies, "I've been coughing uncontrollably for the past week. I need relief." The patient says she has not seen a doctor about her condition and doesn't know what may be causing it. She denies having any other symptoms, but you make a note of some clues in the environment that you will report to the hospital staff: a thermometer on the nightstand and pink-tinged tissues in a wastebasket by the bed, indications that the patient may be running a fever and coughing up blood-tinged sputum. You gather a couple of bottles of over-the-counter cough medications that the patient has been taking in an effort to control her cough and bring them to the hospital.

3. While you are transporting this patient to the hospital, which of the following would be appropriate?
   a. Because the patient and the scene present signs of tuberculosis (TB), you continue to wear the respirator and advise the hospital of the precaution.
   b. The patient and the scene present signs of TB, but because TB is not contagious, you take off the N-95 or HEPA respirator.
   c. Because the patient has not received a doctor's diagnosis of TB, you take off the N-95 or HEPA respirator.
   d. Because you are in the ambulance and not in the patient's house, the N-95 or HEPA respirator is not needed, and you take it off.

Patient Assessment

STANDARD

Assessment (Content Areas: Scene Size-Up; Primary Assessment; History Taking; Secondary Assessment; Monitoring Devices; Reassessment)

COMPETENCY

Applies scene information and patient assessment findings (scene size-up, primary and secondary assessment, patient history, and reassessment) to guide emergency management.

OBJECTIVES

After reading this chapter, you should be able to:

13-1. Define key terms introduced in this chapter.

13-2. Explain the importance of developing a systematic patient assessment routine and list the four main components of the patient assessment.

13-3. List the steps of the scene size-up.

13-4. State the main purpose of the primary assessment and list the components of the primary assessment.

13-5. Explain how forming and revising a general impression of the patient spans the entire patient assessment process.

13-6. Determine if a patient is injured or ill and obtain the chief complaint.

13-7. Identify immediate life threats during the general impression.

13-8. Given a variety of patient scenarios, differentiate those who do and do not need spinal stabilization, demonstrate how to establish in-line stabilization, and demonstrate patient positioning for assessment.

13-9. Using the AVPU method, assess and document the level of responsiveness.

13-10. Determine airway status in responsive patients and those with an altered mental status, demonstrate methods of establishing and maintaining an open airway, and recognize indications of partial airway occlusion.

13-11. Assess the rate and quality of breathing; determine if the patient has absent, inadequate, or adequate breathing; provide positive pressure ventilation in the patient with absent or inadequate breathing.

13-12. Assess oxygenation as determined by the SpO_2 level in the patient who is breathing adequately.

13-13. Assess the circulation to include assessing the pulse, identifying and controlling major bleeding, and assessing perfusion through skin color, temperature, and condition and capillary refill, and recognize and begin treatment for shock.

13-14. Discuss establishing patient priorities by evaluating critical findings to the airway, breathing, or circulation to determine if a patient is unstable and a candidate for rapid secondary assessment and immediate transport to the hospital.

13-15. Describe performing the secondary assessment using an anatomical approach, including steps for assessing the following:
   a. Head
   b. Neck
   c. Chest
   d. Abdomen
   e. Pelvis
   f. Lower extremities
   g. Upper extremities
   h. Posterior body

13-16. Describe performing the secondary assessment using a body systems approach.

13-17. Summarize assessment of the vital signs during the secondary assessment.

13-18. Discuss obtaining a history during the secondary assessment, including use of the SAMPLE and OPQRST mnemonics.

13-19. List the sequence in which the steps of the secondary assessment are generally performed for a trauma patient and define the following types of physical exam that can be chosen for a trauma patient:
   a. Rapid secondary assessment for a trauma patient
   b. Modified secondary assessment for a trauma patient

13-20. List the mechanisms of injury that have a high incidence of producing critical trauma and the special considerations for infants and children.

13-21. For the trauma patient with a significant mechanism of injury, discuss how to continue spinal stabilization, reasons to consider requesting advanced life support, and reasons to reconsider transport decisions.

13-22. Explain how to use the Glasgow Coma Scale (GCS) to rank the patient's level of consciousness and how to interpret the resulting GCS score.

13-23. Discuss how to conduct a rapid secondary assessment for a trauma patient with significant mechanism of injury, altered mental status, multiple injuries, or critical finding (unstable patient).

13-24. Discuss critical (unstable) findings, possibilities, and emergency care for the trauma patient associated with assessment of the head, neck, chest, abdomen, pelvis, extremities, posterior body, or baseline vital signs.

13-25. Explain the purpose and elements of the trauma score.

13-26. Discuss how to conduct a modified secondary assessment for a trauma patient with no significant mechanism of injury, altered mental status, multiple injuries, or critical finding (stable patient).

13-27. Explain circumstances when you should perform a complete, rather than a modified, secondary assessment on a trauma patient with no significant mechanism of injury.

13-28. Name the key differences in the secondary assessment for the responsive medical patient versus the unresponsive medical patient with regard to:
   a. Sequence of steps
   b. Appropriate type of physical exam (modified or rapid)

13-29. Explain how to conduct a secondary assessment for a medical patient who is not alert or is disoriented, is responding only to verbal or painful stimuli, or is unresponsive.

13-30. Discuss critical (unstable) findings, possibilities, and emergency care for the medical patient with an altered mental status associated with assessment of the head, neck, chest, or pelvic region.

13-31. Explain how to conduct a secondary assessment for a medical patient who is alert and oriented.

13-32. Explain the purposes of reassessment.

13-33. Explain how to conduct and to complete the reassessment.

| KEY IDEAS

Performing an accurate and reliable assessment is one of your most important functions as an EMT. All patient treatment and transport decisions will be based on the information gathered during the assessment. It is important to develop a consistent routine for assessing all patients. This chapter introduces basic assessment skills.

■ Patient assessment includes the scene size-up, primary assessment, secondary assessment, and reassessment. Communication and documentation are also key elements of patient assessment.

- The scene size-up includes taking necessary Standard Precautions, evaluating scene hazards, ensuring scene safety, determining the mechanism of injury or the nature of the illness, establishing the number of patients, and identifying the need for additional resources that may be required to manage the scene or the patient(s).

- The primary assessment is conducted on *all patients*. The main purpose of the primary assessment is to identify and manage immediately life-threatening conditions to the airway, breathing, oxygenation, and circulation. Be sure to assess and manage any immediate life threats to the airway, breathing, oxygenation, and circulation during the first 60 seconds after encountering the patient. The sequence is dictated by the presence of obvious life threats. The steps are (1) forming a general impression of the patient, (2) assessing the level of consciousness (mental status), (3) assessing the airway, (4) assessing breathing, (5) assessing oxygenation, (6) assessing circulation, and (7) establishing patient priorities for transport and further assessment and care.

- The secondary assessment has three major parts: physical exam (rapid or modified), baseline vital signs, and history. For a trauma patient or a medical patient with an altered mental status, the assessment is conducted in this sequence: (1) rapid secondary assessment, (2) baseline vital signs, and (3) history. For a trauma patient with no significant mechanism of injury and no altered mental status, it is conducted in this sequence: (1) modified secondary assessment, (2) baseline vitals, and (3) history. The sequence for a responsive medical patient who is alert and oriented is (1) history, (2) modified secondary assessment, and (3) baseline vital signs.

- The reassessment of the patient is conducted at frequent intervals, beginning immediately after the secondary assessment is conducted. The purposes of patient reassessment are to determine any changes in the patient's condition, to assess the effectiveness of your emergency care, and to intervene as necessary. The reassessment phase is a constant cycle of assess, intervene, and reassess.

MEDICAL TERMINOLOGY

Term	Prefix	Word Root Combining Form	Suffix	Definition
apnea (AP-nee-uh)	a- (no, not, without, lack of)	pnea (breathing)		The absence of breathing
dyspnea (DISP-nee-uh)	dys- (bad, difficult)	pnea (breathing)		Difficult or labored breathing
hemiplegia (hem-uh-PLEE-ja)	hemi- (half)	plegia (paralysis)		Paralysis of an arm and leg on one side of the body
icteric, icterus (ik-TAIR-ik, IK-ter-us)		icter (jaundice)	-ic (pertaining to); -us (condition of)	Yellow skin or sclera
paraplegia (pair-uh-PLEE-ja)	para- (beside)	plegia (paralysis)		Paralysis of both legs
quadriplegia (kwad-ruh-PLEE-ja)	quadri- (four)	plegia (paralysis)		Paralysis of both arms and both legs

1. In each space, write the prefix, word root, or suffix that matches the definition.

   a   ic   plegia

   dys   icter   pnea

   hemi   para   quadri

_____ a. Breathing

_____ b. Difficult

_____ c. No, not, without, lack of

_____ d. Jaundice

_____ e. Pertaining to

_____ f. Four

_____ g. Beside

_____ h. Half

_____ i. Paralysis

▌ TERMS AND CONCEPTS

1. Write the number of the correct term next to each definition.

   1. Apnea
   2. Aspiration
   3. AVPU
   4. Battle sign
   5. Cerebrospinal fluid
   6. Chief complaint
   7. Flail segment
   8. Patent
   9. Rapid secondary assessment
   10. Primary assessment
   11. Paradoxical motion
   12. Modified secondary assessment
   13. Flexion posturing

   _____ a. The patient arches the back and flexes the arms inward toward the chest. A sign of serious head injury. Also called _decorticate posturing._

   _____ b. Breathing a substance into the lungs.

   _____ c. Two or more adjacent ribs that are fractured in two or more places.

   _____ d. The patient's answer to the question, "Why did you call the ambulance?"

   _____ e. Black-and-blue discoloration to the mastoid area behind the ear, a late sign of skull or head injury.

   _____ f. The movement of a section of the chest in the opposite direction from the rest of the chest during respiration.

   _____ g. A physical exam that is focused on a specific site; performed on a responsive trauma patient with no significant mechanism of injury, no multiple injuries and no altered mental status, or on a medical patient who is responsive, alert, and oriented.

   _____ h. A head-to-toe physical exam that is swiftly conducted on a trauma patient who has a significant mechanism of injury, multiple injuries, or has an altered mental status; or on a medical patient who is unresponsive, not responsive to verbal stimuli or painful stimuli or not alert or oriented.

   _____ i. The portion of the assessment conducted immediately following scene size-up for the purpose of discovering immediately life-threatening conditions.

_____ j. Open; not blocked.

_____ k. The absence of breathing.

_____ l. Fluid that surrounds and cushions the brain and spinal cord.

_____ m. A mnemonic for alert, responds to verbal stimulus, responds to painful stimulus, unresponsive—to characterize levels of responsiveness.

CONTENT REVIEW

1. The patient assessment
   a. allows the EMT to manage all injuries and medical conditions completely.
   b. is conducted by the EMT, is comprehensive, and generates a complete patient medical history.
   c. requires a careful and complete physical exam of the patient.
   d. should be performed in a systematic manner on all patients.

2. The _____ and the _____ are the first two stages of performing a patient assessment.
   a. scene size-up / secondary assessment
   b. primary assessment / secondary assessment
   c. scene size-up / primary assessment
   d. primary assessment / physical exam

3. You have been dispatched to a scene where the patient's family is extremely hostile. A family member has made physical threats to you and your partner. Which of the following is the best action to take in this situation?
   a. Use scene-control techniques to regain control.
   b. Move as rapidly as possible to leave the scene.
   c. Request immediate law enforcement backup.
   d. Work back-to-back with your partner for protection.

4. You have arrived on the scene of a 25-year-old male who was struck by a car. The distraught driver of the car states that he was traveling about 30 miles per hour and his car struck the patient on his left side. The patient's head is turned to the side, his eyes are open, and he responds appropriately to your questions. He appears to be in moderate distress. A laceration to his forehead with minor bleeding is also observed. The next best action to take, given this information, is to
   a. open the patient's airway using the head-tilt, chin-lift maneuver.
   b. bring the head to a neutral in-line position while maintaining in-line stabilization of the head and neck.
   c. call for paramedic backup, and then open the patient's airway using the head-tilt, chin-lift maneuver.
   d. maintain the position of the head and provide in-line stabilization of the head and neck.

5. Once in-line stabilization of the head and neck is established, it must be maintained until
   a. a cervical spine immobilization device is applied.
   b. the modified secondary assessment has been completed.
   c. the patient is fully immobilized to a backboard.
   d. the patient is transferred to the care of hospital personnel.

6. A primary assessment
   a. must be completed prior to treatment of any life threats that may be discovered.
   b. does not necessarily need to be completed in a specific sequence to be effective.
   c. is performed on all patients, regardless of the mechanism of injury or nature of illness.
   d. is performed only on those patients who are critically injured or are critically ill.

7. Which of the following is the correct sequence for performing the primary assessment?
   1. Form a general impression.
   2. Assess circulation.
   3. Assess mental status.
   4. Assess airway.
   5. Assess breathing.
   6. Establish patient priorities.
   7. Assess oxygenation.

   a. 6, 4, 5, 2, 3, 7, 1
   b. 1, 4, 5, 2, 7, 3, 6
   c. 1, 3, 4, 5, 7, 2, 6
   d. 3, 4, 5, 7, 1, 2, 6

8. The patient's general age, the patient's sex, whether the patient seems ill or injured, and items you notice in the immediate environment can be obtained during which of the following steps of the primary assessment?
   a. General impression
   b. Assessment of breathing
   c. Assessment of mental status
   d. Establishment of patient priorities

9. Which question will best help you to establish a patient's chief complaint?
   a. "Where do you hurt?"
   b. "Can you take one finger and point to the pain?"
   c. "Does anything make the pain worse?"
   d. "Why did you call EMS today?"

10. On approach to a patient, you note that his eyes are closed. The sound of your voice causes the patient to open his eyes. This patient would be considered
    a. alert and oriented.
    b. alert and disoriented.
    c. alert and responsive to verbal stimuli.
    d. responsive to verbal stimuli.

11. Which of the following patients has the "highest" or best level of consciousness?
    a. A patient who grabs your hand when you elicit a pain response
    b. A patient who displays flexion posturing when you elicit a pain response
    c. A patient who mumbles incoherent words when you speak to her
    d. A patient who displays no action when you elicit a pain response

12. Which of the following is an appropriate method of eliciting a pain response in an unresponsive patient?
    a. Gracilis squeeze
    b. Trapezius pinch
    c. Needlestick
    d. Hair twist

13. Assessment of the airway in the responsive patient
    a. is accomplished by talking with the patient.
    b. is performed prior to the evaluation of mental status.
    c. is not necessary if the patient is looking at you.
    d. is performed as part of the scene size-up.

14. Unresponsive patients or patients with a severely altered mental status, such as those only responding to painful stimuli with flexion or extension, have a high incidence of airway occlusion due to
    a. uncontrolled coughing resulting in bronchoconstriction.
    b. relaxation of the muscles in the upper airway.
    c. spasm of the muscles in the upper airway.
    d. esophageal rupture resulting in epiglottic spasm.

15. Which partial airway obstruction sound is correctly paired with the appropriate management technique for resolving the obstruction?
    a. Gurgling respirations—quickly provide positive pressure ventilation
    b. Snoring respirations—use a head-tilt, chin-lift, or jaw-thrust maneuver
    c. Crowing respirations—provide deep suction of the airway
    d. Stridor—use a tongue blade to visualize for an airway obstruction

16. Which of the following is an early sign of hypoxia?
    a. Pink nail beds, conjunctiva, and oral mucosa
    b. Deteriorating or altered mental status
    c. Adequate chest wall movement with breathing
    d. Respirations at a rate of 20 per minute

17. Positive pressure ventilation may be delivered by a
    a. nasal cannula.
    b. partial rebreathing face mask.
    c. bag-valve-mask (BVM) device.
    d. nonrebreather face mask.

18. Which of the following statements is most correct regarding concepts related to evaluation of the patient's skin?
    a. In a cold environment, the vessels in the skin dilate to increase the blood flow to the skin.
    b. In a hot environment, the vessels in the skin constrict, causing the blood to be shunted to the core of the body.
    c. The alpha properties of circulating epinephrine cause the vessels in the skin to constrict, shunting blood away from the skin.
    d. Anemic, hypoxic patients will become cyanotic more rapidly than patients without anemia will.

19. When assessing the pulse in the primary assessment, determine
    a. the pulse rate in one minute.
    b. if the pulse is present or not.
    c. only the regularity of the pulse.
    d. only the strength of the pulse.

20. In order for a pulse to be palpable, the systolic blood pressure must be at least
    a. 40 mmHg.
    b. 50 mmHg.
    c. 60 mmHg.
    d. 70 mmHg.

21. Where is the least reliable place to check for skin color?
    a. Mucous membranes of the mouth
    b. Nail beds
    c. Mucous membranes that line the eyelids
    d. Under the tongue

22. Select the skin color that is correctly paired with a potential cause.
    a. Cyanotic: reduced tissue oxygenation
    b. Red: blood loss from internal or external causes
    c. Yellow: kidney failure
    d. Pale or mottled: hypertension or increased perfusion

23. Which of the following skin temperature and skin condition combinations is most commonly a sign of shock?
    a. Hot, dry skin
    b. Cool, dry skin
    c. Cold, dry skin
    d. Cool, clammy skin

24. If capillary refill at room temperature is _____ in the infant, child, or adult male, tissue perfusion may be inadequate. (Select the shortest time period that indicates inadequate perfusion.)
    a. greater than 1 second
    b. greater than 2 seconds
    c. greater than 3 seconds
    d. greater than 4 seconds

25. Your supervisor has asked you to assist with quality improvement (QI) by reviewing records of patient care. The supervisor wants you to determine if the following patients require rapid secondary assessment and immediate transport. Next to each patient description, write Y (yes) if rapid secondary assessment and immediate transport is required or N (no) if rapid secondary assessment and immediate transport is not required.

    _____ 1. An unresponsive diabetic who does not respond to painful stimuli

    _____ 2. A patient complaining of severe right lower abdominal pain

    _____ 3. A responsive patient complaining of minor chest discomfort with a blood pressure of 120/80

    _____ 4. A responsive patient with cool, clammy skin who collapsed at work

    _____ 5. A responsive patient with a minor cut on her leg

    _____ 6. A patient who was stung by a bee and looks ill

    _____ 7. A patient who is complaining of a headache and is unable to obey commands

    _____ 8. A patient complaining of shortness of breath

26. You have determined that a trauma patient requires rapid secondary assessment and immediate transport after completion of the primary assessment. You should next
    a. move the patient to the stretcher, then perform a rapid trauma assessment.
    b. perform a rapid secondary assessment, then move the patient to the stretcher.
    c. perform a modified secondary assessment (focused on specific injuries), then move the patient to the stretcher.
    d. move the patient to the stretcher, then perform a modified secondary assessment.

27. You did such a good job reviewing patient care reports for your supervisor that she has returned and asked you to perform additional QI reviews. The supervisor asks you to review reports to see if significant mechanisms of injury are present to justify a rapid secondary assessment. Next to each description, write Y (yes) if there is a significant mechanism of injury present or N (no) if there is not.

    _____ 1. A patient involved in a rollover collision

    _____ 2. An adult patient who fell from 3 feet

    _____ 3. A patient who was struck by a car

    _____ 4. A patient with a gunshot wound to the hand

    _____ 5. A patient whose impact causes deformity to a steering wheel

    _____ 6. A patient who was in the passenger seat of a vehicle in which the driver died

28. A significant mechanism of injury for an infant or child is a
    a. fall from a standing position.
    b. fall from a bicycle.
    c. bicycle collision with a motor vehicle.
    d. low-speed vehicle collision where the child was restrained.

29. Which of the following is the proper order for performing the secondary assessment in the trauma patient with a significant mechanism of injury or altered mental status?
    1. Rapid secondary assessment
    2. Modified secondary assessment
    3. Baseline vital signs
    4. History

    a. 2, 3, 4
    b. 1, 3, 4
    c. 3, 4, 1
    d. 3, 4, 2

30. Which of the following is the proper order for performing the secondary assessment in the trauma patient with no significant mechanism of injury, no multiple injuries, and no altered mental status?
    1. Rapid secondary assessment
    2. Modified secondary assessment
    3. Baseline vital signs
    4. History

    a. 3, 2, 4
    b. 4, 2, 3
    c. 1, 3, 4
    d. 2, 3, 4

31. You have responded to a traffic collision in which the adult patient sustained an injury to his head. He fails to open his eyes to pain, is unresponsive to verbal stimuli, and displays a flexor response (decorticate rigidity) to pain. What is the patient's Glasgow Coma Scale (GCS) score?
    a. 6
    b. 5
    c. 4
    d. 3

32. Which statement is most correct regarding patients with a head injury?
    a. A patient with a GCS score of less than 8 has a severe alteration in brain function.
    b. A normal response, which does not require immediate reporting in a patient with a head injury, occurs when the patient is unresponsive, then regains responsiveness for a short time, and then begins to exhibit a deteriorating mental status.
    c. Place is the first orientation to be lost in an altered mental status.
    d. Person is the first orientation to be lost in an altered mental status.

33. During the rapid trauma assessment, it is necessary to examine the patient for DCAP-BTLS. Write what each letter in DCAP-BTLS stands for.
    D _____
    C _____
    A _____
    P _____
    B _____
    T _____
    L _____
    S _____

34. There are five general techniques used during patient assessment. Which assessment technique is missing from this list?
    Inspect
    Palpate
    Auscultate (with a stethoscope)
    Listen

    a. Pelvic push
    b. Sensory check
    c. Neurological check
    d. Sense of smell

35. When assessing the neck during the rapid secondary assessment in the trauma patient, the EMT should inspect for
    a. tracheal articulation.
    b. carotid artery disease.
    c. jugular vein distention.
    d. laryngeal distortion.

36. Regarding assessing the chest for breath sounds during the rapid secondary assessment in the trauma patient, which statement is correct?
    a. Auscultation of the chest is not performed in the rapid secondary assessment.
    b. The EMT should auscultate the right and left chest at the base of the lungs only.
    c. The EMT should auscultate the right and left chest at the apex and base of the lungs.
    d. The EMT should auscultate the right and left chest at the apex of the lungs only.

37. When assessing the abdomen during the rapid secondary assessment, the EMT should palpate for
    a. tenderness.
    b. aortic compromise.
    c. crepitus.
    d. an unstable bowel.

38. During the rapid secondary assessment of the trauma patient, when should the EMT *not* palpate the pelvis?
    a. When the patient complains of pain in the pelvic region
    b. When the patient has a history of cardiovascular disease
    c. When the patient is under 12 or over 65 years of age
    d. When the patient complains of lower abdominal cramps

39. Following inspection and palpation of the extremities in the rapid secondary assessment of the trauma patient, the EMT should check for PMS. "PMS" refers to
    a. pulses, motor function, and sensation.
    b. pulses, motor function, and severity.
    c. pain, motor function, and sensation.
    d. pain, motor function, and severity.

40. In order to inspect the posterior body during the rapid secondary assessment of the trauma patient, the EMT should
    a. log-roll the patient while maintaining in-line stabilization.
    b. reach under the patient's body to palpate the spine.
    c. have the patient sit up so the back can be examined.
    d. not attempt to examine the posterior body.

41. When spinal injury is suspected, the cervical spine immobilization collar (CSIC) should be applied
    a. before the rapid secondary assessment is begun.
    b. after the head is assessed.
    c. after the neck is assessed.
    d. after the rapid trauma assessment is completed.

42. The vital signs should be reassessed and recorded every _____ minutes in the unstable trauma or medical patient.
    a. 15
    b. 10
    c. 8
    d. 5

43. During the secondary assessment, the EMT should obtain a history. The EMT can use the mnemonic SAMPLE. Write the type of information that each letter in SAMPLE stands for.

S _____

A _____

M _____

P _____

L _____

E _____

44. You are treating a responsive, alert, and oriented trauma patient who complains of a minor injury. There is no significant mechanism of injury or critical finding. During the modified secondary assessment, however, you develop a suspicion that more injuries may exist. Your next action should be to
   a. secure the patient to the stretcher and transport immediately.
   b. secure the patient to the stretcher and perform a rapid secondary assessment en route to the hospital.
   c. immediately perform a rapid secondary assessment.
   d. immediately perform a comprehensive physical exam.

45. Which of the following is the proper order for performing the secondary assessment in the responsive, alert, and oriented medical patient?
   1. Perform a modified secondary assessment.
   2. Obtain baseline vital signs.
   3. Perform a rapid secondary assessment.
   4. Obtain the history.

   a. 2, 3, 4
   b. 2, 4, 1
   c. 4, 2, 1
   d. 4, 1, 2

46. Which of the following is the proper order for performing the secondary assessment in the unresponsive medical patient?
   1. Perform a modified secondary assessment.
   2. Obtain baseline vital signs.
   3. Perform a rapid secondary assessment.
   4. Obtain the history.

   a. 2, 1, 4
   b. 3, 2, 4
   c. 1, 2, 4
   d. 4, 3, 2

47. During the rapid secondary assessment in the medical patient, the abdomen should be inspected for scars, discoloration, or distention. Palpate for which of the following?
   a. Tenderness, bowel obstruction, distention, and rigidity
   b. Deformity, tenderness, penetrations, and pulsating masses
   c. Rigidity, abdominal pain, distention, and lacerations
   d. Tenderness, rigidity, distention, and pulsating masses

48. When assessing the extremities during the rapid secondary assessment of the medical patient, be sure to check around the hands, feet, and ankles for
   a. peripheral edema.
   b. alterations in nail bed formation.
   c. jaundice.
   d. hepatic spots ("liver" spots).

49. Which baseline vital sign is missing from the following list?

   Respiration

   Pulse

   Skin

   Blood pressure

   Pulse oximetry

   a. Pupils
   b. Capillary refill
   c. GCS
   d. Chest auscultation

50. During the history for a medical patient who is alert and oriented, the OPQRST questions are asked to elicit more information about the patient's symptoms, especially pain. Write the type of information that each of the letters OPQRST stands for.

   O _____

   P _____

   Q _____

   R _____

   S _____

   T _____

51. The unresponsive medical patient should be transported in which position?
   a. Supine
   b. Prone
   c. Recovery
   d. Fowler

52. Which statement is most correct regarding patient medications?
   a. Gather prescription medications only.
   b. Gather prescription and over-the-counter medications.
   c. Gather over-the-counter medications only.
   d. It is not important to gather medications.

53. You have responded to a call for a medical patient who just "doesn't feel well." You should
   a. perform a modified secondary assessment of the neurological system.
   b. perform a detailed physical exam.
   c. perform a rapid secondary assessment.
   d. transport rapidly without additional interventions.

54. The _____ test is another way to assess for rebound tenderness and possible internal injury to abdominal organs.
   a. Michal
   b. Fermeni
   c. Warner
   d. Markle

55. Which statement is most correct regarding assessment or management of the medical patient?
   a. It is not important to determine the last oral intake when testing a patient's blood glucose level.
   b. A fasting blood glucose in the diabetic patient may be 12 to 14 mg/dL.
   c. If an unresponsive medical patient requires ventilation, put him in a lateral recumbent position.
   d. Pain is typically produced by ischemia, inflammation, infection, and obstruction.

| CASE STUDY 1

It is a Friday night and you have just completed a standby assignment at a local high school football game when you are dispatched to a motor vehicle crash. You determine that the scene is safe. You observe a car that has rolled over and has significant damage. The only patient was ejected from the vehicle. As you approach, you see that the patient is about 45 years old and looks severely injured. His eyes are closed and he looks pale. You direct your partner to provide in-line stabilization of the head and neck. The patient does not respond to your voice. He responds to a painful stimulus by arching his back and extending his arms and legs. His airway is open and clear; his breathing is shallow at 6 per minute. Your partner slides his finger up to palpate the carotid pulse and tells you that it is strong and regular.

1. What are the most appropriate actions to take given the information provided?
   a. Provide oxygen via a nonrebreather mask at 15 lpm, then check for pulses.
   b. Place a cervical spine immobilization collar and complete the primary assessment.
   c. Provide ventilation while maintaining in-line stabilization.
   d. Complete the primary assessment, and then provide oxygen via a nonrebreather mask at 15 lpm.

2. This patient will require
   a. a rapid secondary assessment and rapid transport to the hospital.
   b. a rapid secondary trauma assessment and a detailed physical exam conducted on scene.
   c. a focused secondary assessment and a detailed physical exam.
   d. a focused secondary assessment and components of the detailed physical exam.

3. You know that the patient's blood pressure is at least
   a. 80 mmHg.
   b. 70 mmHg.
   c. 60 mmHg.
   d. 50 mmHg.

CASE STUDY 2

You have just finished filling up the unit with fuel when you are dispatched to a house for an unknown medical emergency. You have taken Standard Precautions. The scene appears safe as you approach the older home. An elderly woman meets you at the door and says frantically, "George won't wake up! He takes a nap every afternoon, and I can't wake him up." In response to additional questioning, she tells you there is no trauma involved and her husband is the only patient. As you enter the room, you observe the patient (an approximately 70-year-old male) lying face up on his bed. You hear a snoring sound on inhalation and exhalation of each breath. He has a pillow behind his head, and his skin looks blue. There are no signs of trauma. His eyes remain closed in spite of your attempts to arouse him with your voice. The patient also fails to respond to a painful stimulus. You tell your partner to remove the pillow from behind the patient's head and open the airway. Your partner opens the airway and assesses the patient's breathing and oxygenation. You assess the patient's circulatory status.

1. For each item in the following list, write Y (yes) or N (no) to indicate if it is a potential clue to an airway problem in this patient.

    _____ a. The patient's wife was unable to wake the patient.

    _____ b. The patient's skin color is cyanotic.

    _____ c. The patient is unresponsive to painful stimulus.

    _____ d. A snoring sound is evident on inspiration and expiration.

    _____ e. A pillow is positioned under the patient's head.

2. What is the preferred method your partner should use to open the airway?
    a. Jaw-thrust maneuver
    b. Head-tilt, neck-lift maneuver
    c. Head-tilt, chin-lift maneuver
    d. Head-tilt maneuver

3. In this patient, which of the following would most likely require the EMT to provide positive pressure ventilation?
    a. Inadequate respiratory rate or inadequate tidal volume
    b. History of asthma or slow capillary refill
    c. Impaired lung capacity or high blood pressure
    d. Rapid heart rate or flushed skin color

4. Management of this patient should include
    a. a focused secondary assessment for a medical patient.
    b. a focused secondary assessment for a trauma patient.
    c. a rapid secondary assessment for a medical patient.
    d. a rapid secondary assessment for a trauma patient.

5. This patient's GCS score is
    a. 3
    b. 4
    c. 5
    d. 6

CASE STUDY 3

You are in the middle of studying for a promotional exam for your agency when you get a call for a man who cut his hand. You practice Standard Precautions as you leave the vehicle. Two young men greet you on the street. They yell, "Hurry up, man! Fred is gonna die!" The scene appears safe as you approach the residence located in a run-down neighborhood. As you are walking to the back of the house, you ask, "Why did you call EMS today?" One of the two replies, "Fred got mad at his girlfriend and put his fist through the window." You ask him if Fred is the only patient injured. He nods.

As you enter the backyard, you see the patient sitting on the back steps holding his arm. His girlfriend is yelling at him, then starts yelling at you: "He's not hurt! He doesn't need an ambulance!" "Knock it off!" the patient snaps at her. The patient, who appears to be about 25 years old, has a towel wrapped around his lower arm. He looks up in disgust as you approach. Obviously, his girlfriend is upsetting him, and he is upsetting her. His skin color is pink. He appears to be in minor distress. His shirt is covered with blood. He responds to your questions appropriately and relates the same story his friend told you. You ask your partner to get the baseline vitals. The patient's respirations are adequate. You check the patient's radial pulse; it feels strong and regular at about 90 per minute. The SpO$_2$ is 96%. His skin is warm and dry. On examination, you discover a large laceration on the anterior surface of the patient's wrist, which is bleeding moderately.

1. To maintain scene control, you should
   a. transport the patient rapidly from the scene.
   b. suggest a task for the girlfriend that will remove her from the immediate area.
   c. actively listen to the patient's description of the injury that occurred.
   d. order the girlfriend to leave the area at once.

2. The best method to initially control this patient's bleeding would be
   a. elevation.
   b. tourniquet.
   c. direct pressure.
   d. pressure points.

3. This patient would most likely require which of the following?
   a. Rapid secondary assessment followed by history, then vitals
   b. Rapid secondary assessment followed by vitals, then history
   c. Modified secondary assessment followed by vitals, then history
   d. Modified secondary assessment followed by history, then vitals

CASE STUDY 4

You have just left your main station after replacing some supplies when you are dispatched to a downtown office for a patient complaining of chest pain. You have taken Standard Precautions. The scene appears safe as you arrive in front of a local insurance company. Several employees are awaiting your arrival. You ask them, "Why did you call EMS today?" A young worker replies, "It's my boss. He says he is OK, but he doesn't look well at all. He told me his chest hurts." The worker tells you there is no trauma involved in this incident and the boss is the only patient.

As you enter a plush office, you observe the patient, who appears to be approximately 55 years old, leaning back in a large desk chair. He is pale, and your general impression is that he looks ill. There is no sign of trauma. You introduce yourself and ask the patient, "What seems to be the problem?" The patient replies, "Nothing, really. A little indigestion, maybe. I don't know why they called you, but I guess as long as you're here, you may as well check me out. My chest hurts. But I'm sure it must be something I ate." His breathing appears adequate. His radial pulse is weak and slow. His skin is cool and clammy. While you are obtaining a history, your partner obtains the baseline vital signs. He reports the following: respirations normal at 20 per minute; pulse weak and regular at 50 per minute; skin pale, cool, and moist; pupils equal and reactive; blood pressure 90/60; SpO_2 is 93%.

1. What history-taking method should you use on this patient?
   a. OPQRST questions only
   b. History using the mnemonic SAMPLE and including OPQRST questions
   c. SAMPLE history only
   d. DCAP-BTLS and SAMPLE history

2. Which of the following is the best question to ask to evaluate the quality of this patient's pain?
   a. Is the pain dull and squeezing?
   b. Where do you feel the pain?
   c. Can you take one finger and point to where the pain is located?
   d. How would you describe the pain?

3. The physical exam on this patient should be
   a. a rapid secondary assessment focused on the neck, chest, abdomen, and extremities.
   b. a rapid secondary assessment.
   c. a head-to-toe rapid trauma assessment.
   d. a detailed physical exam.

4. Appropriate management for this patient should include
   a. cardiopulmonary resuscitation (CPR).
   b. oxygen by nasal cannula to maintain an $SpO_2 > 94\%$.
   c. positive pressure ventilation and immediate transport.
   d. departing the scene, as the patient has refused treatment.

CASE STUDY 5

You are reviewing policies and treatment protocols with an EMT intern when a call comes in for a "sick child." You, your partner, and the EMT intern quickly respond to the call and arrive on the scene in less than 4 minutes. You have taken Standard Precautions. The scene appears safe as you arrive in front of a neatly kept home in a working-class neighborhood. As you enter the home, you observe the patient on a couch. The patient's mother tells you that the patient is 5 years old. He is lying on his back. He does not look at you as you enter the room. He looks pale, and your general impression is that he looks ill. His eyes appear to be sunken into the sockets. There is no sign of trauma, and the mother reports no traumatic event. You introduce yourself, gain consent, and ask the mother, "Why did you call EMS today?" The mother replies, "Ryan has been sick for the last week. He's been throwing up constantly." The patient does not respond to your voice, but he responds appropriately to pain. His breathing appears adequate at 20 per minute. The SpO_2 is 93%. His radial pulse is weak and rapid. His skin is cool and clammy.

1. You should next
   a. check for bleeding only.
   b. check the capillary refill and check for bleeding.
   c. check for pulse, motor, and sensory function in the extremities.
   d. check for a carotid pulse.

2. This patient should be given
   a. a modified secondary assessment focused on his abdomen.
   b. a modified secondary assessment focused on his chest.
   c. a focused secondary assessment detailed on his chest and abdomen.
   d. a head-to-toe rapid secondary assessment.

3. Regarding a transport decision, this patient should be considered
   a. a medium-priority patient.
   b. a high-priority patient.
   c. stable and should not be assigned to a category.
   d. a low-priority patient.

4. Your treatment for this patient should include
   a. oxygen by nasal cannula.
   b. oxygen by nonrebreather mask.
   c. insertion of an oropharyngeal airway.
   d. positive pressure ventilation by BVM.

Pharmacology and Medication Administration

▌ STANDARD

Pharmacology (Content Areas: Principles of Pharmacology; Medication Administration; Emergency Medications)

▌ COMPETENCY

Applies fundamental knowledge of the medications that the EMT may assist/administer to a patient during an emergency.

▌ OBJECTIVES

After reading this chapter, you should be able to:

14-1.   Define key terms introduced in this chapter.
14-2.   Describe the roles and responsibilities associated with administering and assisting patients with administration of medications.
14-3.   Differentiate between administration of medication and assisting a patient in taking his own medications.
14-4.   List the medications in the EMT's scope of practice.
14-5.   Differentiate between a drug's chemical, official, generic, and trade names.
14-6.   Demonstrate the proper administration of drugs by each of the following routes:
    a. Sublingual
    b. Oral
    c. Inhalation
    d. Intramuscular (epinephrine auto-injector only)
14-7.   Differentiate between the following medication forms:
    a. Tablet
    b. Liquid for injection
    c. Gel
    d. Suspension
    e. Fine powder for inhalation
    f. Gas
    g. Liquid for spray or aerosolization
14-8.   Explain the roles of off-line and on-line medical direction with regard to medication administration.

14-9. Adhere to the following key steps of medication administration:

    a. Obtain an order.

    b. Verify on-line orders.

    c. Select the proper medication.

    d. Verify the patient's prescription.

    e. Check the expiration date.

    f. Check for impurities and discoloration.

    g. Verify the form, route, and dose.

    h. Ensure that the "five rights" of medication administration are followed.

14-10. Document required information regarding medication administration.

14-11. Describe the reassessment of a patient after you have administered or assisted the patient in taking a medication.

KEY IDEAS

As an EMT, you will have the responsibility of administering certain medications carried on the EMS unit. You also may assist with the administration of certain prescribed medications that may be taken by the patient. Improper administration of these medications can result in dangerous or fatal consequences. It is vital that you be completely familiar with the medications and the proper procedures for administration. This chapter reviews these important concepts:

- You may *not* administer or assist with administration of any medication other than the medications covered in this chapter or in local protocol.

- The medications carried on the EMS unit that may be administered under the approval of medical direction are oxygen, oral glucose, aspirin, and activated charcoal.

- The medications prescribed for the patient that may be administered under the approval of medical direction are inhaled bronchodilators (prescribed metered-dose inhalers and small-volume nebulizers), nitroglycerin, and epinephrine.

- Medications can have up to four different names: chemical, generic, trade, and official. The EMT must be familiar with the generic and trade names.

- Drugs can be administered by the following common routes: sublingual, oral, inhalation, and injection (intramuscular).

- There are six essential terms related to each drug that the EMT may administer or assist with administration. The EMT must understand indications, contraindications, dose, administration, actions, and side effects.

- There are seven key steps to administering medications: obtain an order from medical direction; select the proper medication; verify the patient's prescription; check the expiration date; check for discoloration or impurities; verify the form, route, and dose; and provide documentation.

- The five "rights" of medication administration—right patient, right medication, right route, right dose, and right date (time)—provide an important reminder of the critical elements of administering medications to patients.

TERMS AND CONCEPTS

1. Write the number of the correct term next to each definition.

    1. Medication

    2. Drug

    3. Pharmacology

    4. Activated charcoal

    5. Aspirin

    6. Contraindications

7. Epinephrine
8. Metered-dose inhaler
9. Nitroglycerin
10. Oral glucose
11. Side effects

_____ a. A chemical substance that is used to treat or prevent a disease or condition

_____ b. Treatment with a substance that is used as a remedy for illness

_____ c. The study of drugs

_____ d. Dilates arterioles and veins and reduces the cardiac workload

_____ e. Situations when a drug should not be administered

_____ f. Administered to a patient with a history of diabetes with a low blood glucose level

_____ g. Commonly prescribed to patients with a history of asthma, emphysema, and chronic bronchitis

_____ h. Used to treat patients suffering from a severe allergic reaction

_____ i. Reduces platelets from forming clots

_____ j. Designed to absorb or bind to some ingested poisons

_____ k. Actions that are not desired and that occur in addition to the desired effects

CONTENT REVIEW

1. The EMT may not generally administer or assist in the administration of any medication other than the medications listed in this chapter. In addition, these drugs must be
   a. clearly identified by the official name on all prescriptions.
   b. clearly identified by the official or chemical name on all prescriptions.
   c. identified in local protocols as acceptable for the EMT to administer.
   d. only administered by oral or sublingual route.

2. Medications administered by the EMT are
   a. administered without medical direction.
   b. carried on the unit.
   c. only given by the oral or sublingual route.
   d. only those medications that are prescribed for the patient.

3. Which of the following is a medication that can be administered or assisted in administration by the EMT?
   a. Epinephrine
   b. Diazepam
   c. Lasix
   d. Lidocaine

4. You have responded to a patient complaining of chest pain. The patient states that his medication is upstairs on his dresser. Select the best response to this situation.
   a. Leave the patient momentarily to retrieve the patient's medication.
   b. Ask the patient to walk upstairs and retrieve the medication.
   c. Ask a family member to retrieve the medication.
   d. Help the patient up the stairs to retrieve the medication.

5. Which of the following is also known as the brand name of a drug?
   a. Trade name
   b. Generic name
   c. Chemical name
   d. Official name

6. Which of the following generic and trade names are *incorrectly* paired?
   a. Metaproterenol—Alupent, Metaprel
   b. Isoetharine—Serevent
   c. Epinephrine—Adrenalin
   d. Albuterol—Proventil

7. Which of the following generic and trade names are *incorrectly* paired?
   a. Nitroglycerin—Nitrostat
   b. Salmeterol—Ventolin
   c. Ipratropium—Atrovent
   d. Nitroglycerin spray—Nitrolingual Pumpspray

8. Medication that is placed or sprayed under the tongue is an example of medication given by which of the following?
   a. The inhalation route
   b. The intramuscular route
   c. The oral route
   d. The sublingual route

9. A suspension must be
   a. shaken before it is administered.
   b. given sublingually.
   c. inhaled.
   d. injected.

10. Situations when a drug should not be given are known as which of the following?
    a. Actions
    b. Contraindications
    c. Side effects
    d. Negative markers

11. What are the six essential items of medication information that the EMT should understand to ensure safe, proper, and effective medication administration?
    a. Indications, contraindications, dose, administration, actions, and side effects
    b. Indications, negative markers, dose, administration, actions, and side effects
    c. Indications, contraindications, dose, forms, prescriptions, and side effects
    d. Indications, negative markers, dose, administration, actions, and adverse actions

12. Which of the following is an example of a drug given by intramuscular injection?
    a. Alupent
    b. Epinephrine
    c. Glutose
    d. Isoetharine

13. Number the following key steps for administration of a medication in the proper order from 1 to 8.

_____ a. Document medication administration.

_____ b. Obtain an order from medical direction.

_____ c. Ensure selection of the proper medication.

_____ d. Check the expiration date.

_____ e. Verify the form, route, and dose.

_____ f. Verify the patient's prescription.

_____ g. Check for discoloration or impurities.

_____ h. Administer medication.

14. Which of the following is a source of information about a patient's prescription medication?
a. Package inserts
b. Wilson's Formulary Service
c. Doctors' Reference System
d. National Drug Guide

Complete the following chart.

Generic Name	Trade Name	Used For
Oxygen	**15.**	Wide range of emergencies
16.	Glutose, Insta-Glucose	**17.**
Activated charcoal	SuperChar, InstaChar, Actidose, LiquiChar	**18.**
Nitroglycerin	Nitrostat	**19.**
20.	Nitrolingual Pumpspray	**21.**
Epinephrine	**22.**	Allergic reactions
Albuterol	**23.**	Breathing difficulty associated with respiratory conditions
Metaproterenol	**24.**	**25.**
26.	Bronkosol, Bronkometer	**27.**
Salmeterol xinafoate	**28.**	Breathing difficulty associated with respiratory conditions
29.	Tornalate	**30.**
Levalbuterol	**31.**	Breathing difficulty associated with respiratory conditions
Pirbuterol	**32.**	**33.**
Terbutaline	**34.**	Breathing difficulty associated with respiratory conditions
Aspirin	**35.**	**36.**

CASE STUDY

You are helping an EMT intern study for an upcoming final exam when the alarm bell sounds. You respond to a call for a patient complaining of chest pain. You have completed the scene size-up and the primary assessment. The patient is a 56-year-old male who responds to painful stimuli only. The patient's wife tells you that he has been complaining of chest pain for the past two hours. He stopped talking just a few minutes before your arrival. A neighbor of the patient suggests that you give the patient her (the neighbor's) nitroglycerin. She takes it for a heart problem.

1. What is your best reaction to the neighbor's suggestion?
   a. Give the patient the neighbor's nitroglycerin.
   b. Contact the patient's personal physician for orders to administer the medication to the patient.
   c. Never administer medication to a patient unless it is prescribed and/or you are ordered to do so by medical direction.
   d. Take the medication with you and administer while en route to the hospital after checking the patient's vital signs.

2. Suppose that nitroglycerin prescribed to this patient is discovered on his person. *The nitroglycerin can and should be placed into the mouth of this patient.* Select the best response to this statement.
   a. The statement is true. You should administer the medication while holding the mouth closed with one hand.
   b. The statement is false. The medication should not be administered to a patient with an altered level of consciousness.
   c. The statement is true if the medication is administered by the oral route instead of the sublingual route.
   d. The statement is false. The patient must be unresponsive to pain before the medication can be administered.

3. Nitroglycerin is used for which of the following?
   a. Altered mental status
   b. Poisoning and overdose
   c. Chest pain
   d. Difficulty breathing

Note: Medication Reference Cards appear at the back of this workbook. There is a card for each of the following medications that EMTs are permitted to administer or assist with administering, with approval from medical direction: **activated charcoal, aspirin, epinephrine auto-injector, inhaled bronchodilator, nitroglycerin,** *and* **oral glucose.** *Each card includes information on medication names, indications, contraindications, form, dosage, administration, actions, side effects, and reassessment. Carry these cards with you for ready reference.*

Shock and Resuscitation

STANDARD

Shock and Resuscitation

COMPETENCY

Applies fundamental knowledge of the causes, pathophysiology, and management of shock, respiratory failure or arrest, cardiac failure or arrest, and post-resuscitation management.

OBJECTIVES

After reading this chapter, you should be able to:

15-1. Define key terms introduced in this chapter.
15-2. Explain the pathophysiology of shock (hypoperfusion), including the consequences of cellular hypoxia and death.
15-3. Describe the physiology of maintaining adequate perfusion.
15-4. Describe how inadequate vascular volume, inadequate heart function, and decreased peripheral vascular resistance can lead to shock.
15-5. Give examples of conditions that can lead to:
    a. Loss of vascular volume
    b. Inadequate heart function
    c. Decreased peripheral vascular resistance
15-6. Explain the mechanisms and pathophysiology of each of the following categories and types of shock:
    a. Hypovolemic (hemorrhagic and nonhemorrhagic)
    b. Distributive (anaphylactic, septic, neurogenic)
    c. Cardiogenic
    d. Obstructive
    e. Metabolic or respiratory
15-7. Explain how compensatory mechanisms to shock are maintained through:
    a. Direct nerve stimulation
    b. Release of hormones
15-8. Explain the body's compensatory responses to hypoperfusion and how they manifest in the early signs and symptoms of shock.

15-9. Differentiate between early (compensatory) and late (decompensatory/irreversible) signs of shock.

15-10. Describe the progression of shock through the compensatory, decompensatory (progressive), and irreversible stages.

15-11. Explain how to identify the patient who is in a shock state and demonstrate the assessment of patients to identify shock.

15-12. Explain the influence of age on the assessment and management of patients with shock.

15-13. Discuss the goals of prehospital management of patients with shock.

15-14. Describe the pathophysiology of cardiac arrest.

15-15. Differentiate between the electrical, circulatory, and metabolic phases of cardiac arrest.

15-16. Identify situations in which resuscitative attempts should be withheld.

15-17. Explain each of the links in the Chain of Survival of cardiac arrest for the adult and pediatric patient.

15-18. Explain the importance of early defibrillation in cardiac arrest.

15-19. Explain the rationale for the "push hard and push fast" approach to cardiopulmonary resuscitation (CPR).

15-20. Describe the features, functions, advantages, disadvantages, use, and precautions in the use of automated external defibrillators (AEDs).

15-21. Compare and contrast ventricular fibrillation, ventricular tachycardia, asystole, and pulseless electrical activity.

15-22. Given a series of cardiac arrest scenarios involving infants, children, and adults, demonstrate appropriate assessment and resuscitative techniques, including the integrated use of AEDs (automated and semiautomated), ventilation, and CPR, and explain the purpose and procedure for reassessment of the cardiac arrest patient.

15-23. Demonstrate assessment and management of a post-cardiac-arrest patient with return of spontaneous circulation.

15-24. Given a cardiac arrest scenario, make decisions regarding obtaining advanced cardiac life support (ACLS).

15-25. Describe the safety precautions to be taken to protect yourself, other EMS providers, the patient, and bystanders in resuscitation situations.

15-26. Explain the importance of AED maintenance, EMT training and skills maintenance, and medical direction in the Chain of Survival of cardiac arrest.

15-27. Discuss special considerations in the use of an AED in patients with cardiac pacemakers and automatic implanted cardioverter-defibrillators.

15-28. List the advantages and disadvantages of automated chest compression devices, impedance threshold devices, and other circulation-enhancing devices.

▌ KEY IDEAS

Shock is a condition that, if not managed effectively, will lead to patient death. This chapter describes different types of shock and the management for each. Resuscitation is the emergency care process that attempts to restore lost vital functions. This chapter additionally describes the causes, pathophysiology, and management of cardiac failure or arrest and post-resuscitation management.

■ Shock is a critical condition that results in the inadequate perfusion of cells, tissue, and organs. It carries a high morbidity and mortality if it is allowed to progress. Most of the emergency care of the patient in shock is geared toward maintaining or restoring oxygen and glucose delivery to the cells.

■ The three basic etiologies of shock are inadequate volume, inadequate pump function, and inadequate vessel tone.

■ The five major categories of shock are hypovolemic, distributive, cardiogenic, obstructive, and metabolic or respiratory shock.

■ The types of shock include hemorrhagic hypovolemic, nonhemorrhagic hypovolemic, burn, anaphylactic, septic, neurogenic, and cardiogenic shock.

- The compensatory mechanisms associated with shock are initiated and maintained through two major pathways: direct sympathetic nerve stimulation and the release of hormones.

- The three stages of shock are compensatory, decompensatory, and irreversible shock.

- The following are signs of poor perfusion: altered mental status; pale, cool, clammy skin; delayed capillary refill; decreased urine output; and weak or absent peripheral pulses.

- Successfully resuscitating an adult cardiac arrest patient is dependent upon the "adult Out of Hospital Cardiac Arrest (OHCA) Chain of Survival." This chain has five links: (1) immediate recognition and activation, (2) immediate high-quality CPR, (3) rapid defibrillation, (4) BLS care by EMT's to include high quality CPR and defibrillation, and (5) advanced life support and post arrest care. The provision of high-quality chest compressions and early defibrillation are two of the most critical factors.

- Successfully resuscitating a pediatric cardiac arrest patient is dependent upon the "pediatric Chain of Survival." This chain has five links: (1) prevention of arrest, (2) early, high-quality CPR, (3) rapid activation of EMS, (4) effective ACLS, (5) integrated post-cardiac-arrest care.

- There are two basic categories of external defibrillators: manual and automated. The automated external defibrillator (AED) is either fully automated or semiautomated.

- The rhythms for which automated external defibrillation is appropriate are ventricular fibrillation and pulseless ventricular tachycardia (patient is pulseless, apneic, or has agonal respirations).

- The AED is indicated for use on nontrauma cardiac arrest patients older than 1 year of age who are unresponsive, with no breathing and no pulse. For patients from 1 to 8 years of age, an adult AED with a dose attenuating system is preferred.

- Basic semiautomated (AED) adult sequence of two rescuers:
  - Take Standard Precautions.
  - Perform a brief assessment. If pulseless, apneic, or agonal respirations and no signs of life, start CPR using the chest compressions, airway, breathing (CAB) intervention sequence.
  - Continue chest compressions while AED is readied.
  - Turn on power to the AED.
  - Attach the defibrillation pads.
  - Begin analysis of the patient's cardiac rhythm.
  - If shock is indicated, press the shock or defibrillation button. If no shock is indicated, resume CPR.
  - After shock, immediately resume CPR, beginning with chest compressions.
  - After 2 minutes, the AED reanalyzes the rhythm. If a rhythm is indicated, check for pulse, responsiveness, and breathing
  - Repeat this sequence if the patient has no pulse, is unresponsive, or is apneic.
  - Follow local protocol regarding when to transport.

- The AED must be checked at the beginning of each shift to prevent device failure.

- AED operators should practice with the device every 90 days to refresh their skills.

▌MEDICAL TERMINOLOGY

Term	Prefix	Word Root Combining Form	Suffix	Definition
asystole (a-sis-TOL-le)	a (no, not, without)	systole (contraction)		The absence of electrical activity and pumping action in the heart
hypertension (high-per-TEN-shun)	hyper- (above, beyond, excessive)	tens (tension)	-ion (process)	A higher-than-normal blood pressure
hypoperfusion (high-poh-per-FYU-zhun)	hypo- (below, under, deficient)	perfusion (supplying an organ with nutrients and oxygen)		The insufficient supply of oxygen and other nutrients to some of the body cells that results from inadequate circulation of blood
hypovolemic (high-poh-vo-LEE-mik)	hypo- (below, under, deficient)	volem (volume)	-ic (pertaining to)	Diminished blood volume
systolic (sis-TOL-ik)		systole (contraction)	-ic (pertaining to)	The part of the heart cycle when the heart is contracting; pertaining to the top number of a blood pressure reading
vasoconstriction (VAYZ-oh-kon-STRIK-shun)	vas/o- (vessel)	constriction (narrowing)		The narrowing of a blood vessel's diameter
vasodilation (VAYZ-oh-dye-LAY-shun)	vas/o- (vessel)	dilation (widening)		The widening of a blood vessel's diameter

1. The medical term *hypertension* refers to a higher-than-normal blood pressure. The word root *tens* means
   a. the number 10.
   b. high, above.
   c. blood.
   d. tension.

2. The medical term *systolic* contains the word root *systole*, which means
   a. system.
   b. contraction.
   c. upper.
   d. pressure.

3. The medical term *vasoconstriction* contains the prefix *vas/o-*, which means
   a. heart.
   b. blood.
   c. cell.
   d. vessel.

4. In the term *asystole*, the prefix *a-* means
   a. with.
   b. some.
   c. other.
   d. without.

▍ TERMS AND CONCEPTS

1. Write the number of the correct term next to each definition.
   1. Anaphylactic shock
   2. Cardiac arrest
   3. Cardiogenic shock
   4. Decompensatory shock
   5. Defibrillation
   6. Distributive shock
   7. Downtime
   8. Hypovolemic shock
   9. Neurogenic shock
   10. Pulseless electrical activity (PEA)
   11. Septic shock
   12. Ventricular fibrillation (VF or V-Fib)
   13. Ventricular tachycardia (VT or V-Tach)

   _____ a. An advanced stage of shock in which the body's compensatory mechanisms are no longer able to maintain a blood pressure and perfusion of the vital organs. Also called *decompensated shock* or *progressive shock*.

   _____ b. Shock caused by the loss of blood or fluid from the intravascular space resulting in a low blood volume

   _____ c. A type of distributive shock that releases chemical mediators that cause massive and systemic vasodilation capillaries to become very permeable and to leak

   _____ d. A condition in which the heart generates a relatively normal electrical rhythm but fails to perfuse the body adequately because of a decreased or absent cardiac output from cardiac muscle failure or blood loss

   _____ e. The time from when the patient goes into cardiac arrest until CPR is effectively being performed

   _____ f. Electrical shock or current delivered to the heart through the patient's chest wall to help the heart restore a normal rhythm

   _____ g. The cessation of cardiac function with the patient displaying no pulse, no breathing, and unresponsiveness

   _____ h. A type of distributive shock caused by an infection that releases bacteria or toxins into the blood

_____ i. A very rapid heart rhythm that may or may not produce a pulse and is generally too fast to perfuse the body's organs adequately

_____ j. A type of distributive shock that results from massive vasodilation; also called *vasogenic shock*

_____ k. Poor perfusion resulting from an ineffective pump function of the heart

_____ l. Continuous, uncoordinated, chaotic rhythm that does not produce pulses

_____ m. A major category of shock that is associated with a decrease in intravascular volume caused by massive systemic vasodilation and an increase in the capillary permeability

▍CONTENT REVIEW

1. The three base etiologies of shock are inadequate volume, inadequate pump function, and
   a. increased volume.
   b. inadequate vessel tone.
   c. inadequate hemoglobin concentration.
   d. inadequate blood pressure.

2. BP = CO × _____.
   a. PBR
   b. SVR
   c. PP
   d. RR

3. This is a type of distributive shock that is caused by the release of chemical mediators that cause massive systemic vasodilation and cause the capillaries to become very permeable and to leak. What is the type of shock described?
   a. Nonhemorrhagic hypovolemic shock
   b. Hemorrhagic hypovolemic shock
   c. Anaphylactic shock
   d. Septic shock

4. The first stage of shock in which the body is able to maintain cardiac output is called
   a. compensated shock.
   b. systemic shock.
   c. baroreceptor reflex shock.
   d. early shock.

5. An elderly patient who takes multiple medications was struck in the abdomen. What signs may be the most profound indicators of shock in this patient?
   a. Altered mental status and tachypnea
   b. Pale skin and tachycardia
   c. Altered mental status and tachycardia
   d. Flushed skin and tachypnea

6. The compensatory mechanisms of shock are initiated and physiologically maintained through two major pathways. What are these two pathways?
   a. Direct sympathetic nerve stimulation and the release of hormones
   b. Direct parasympathetic nerve stimulation and the release of aldosterone
   c. Indirect parasympathetic nerve stimulation and the release of hormones
   d. Indirect and direct sympathetic nerve stimulation

7. Why is it not appropriate to hyperventilate the shock patient?
   a. It makes the blood viscous and decreases the off-loading of oxygen from the hemoglobin.
   b. It makes the blood alkalytic and decreases the off-loading of oxygen from the hemoglobin.
   c. It is appropriate to hyperventilate the shock patient to increase the oxyhemoglobin concentration.
   d. It makes the blood acidotic and increases the off-loading of oxygen from the hemoglobin.

8. Which of the following would you likely observe as a patient's blood volume depletes?
   a. The diastolic blood pressure increases, then the diastolic blood pressure drops, causing a widening pulse pressure.
   b. The systolic and diastolic blood pressures drop, causing the pulse pressure to widen.
   c. The systolic blood pressure maintains or increases as the diastolic blood pressure decreases, causing a narrowing pulse pressure.
   d. The systolic blood pressure drops and the diastolic blood pressure maintains or increases, creating a narrowing pulse pressure.

9. Certain medications, such as _____ or _____, can keep the heart rate from dramatically increasing, making it appear that the patient is not in a compensatory stage of shock.
   a. analgesics/antacids
   b. anticoagulants/antihistamines
   c. hormones/diuretics
   d. beta blockers/calcium channel blockers

10. In early distributive shock, the skin is typically
    a. white and cool.
    b. cyanotic and cool.
    c. flushed and warm.
    d. mottled and warm.

11. For children less than 10 years of age, a systolic blood pressure of _____ mmHg plus _____ times the age in years is a lower limit of normal.
    a. 50/0.5
    b. 60/1
    c. 70/2
    d. 80/3

12. Which of the following is a candidate for automated external defibrillation?
    a. An adult medical patient who is in cardiac arrest
    b. An unresponsive adult with a pulse
    c. An adult trauma patient who is in cardiac arrest
    d. A responsive adult who is having severe chest pain or discomfort

13. The American Heart Association describes a sequence of events called the *adult Out of hospital cardiac arrest (OHCA) chain of survival*. Choose two items that are components of the chain and are critical to adult patient survival of cardiac arrest.
    a. Immediate high-quality cardiac compressions and rapid defibrillation
    b. Access and ACLS
    c. Defibrillation and ACLS
    d. CPR and ACLS

14. The application of an electric shock to help the heart reorganize its electrical activity and restore its normal rhythm is known as which of the following?
    a. Vagal stimulation
    b. Shock therapy
    c. Defibrillation
    d. Cardiovascular therapy

15. Between 50 to 60% of cardiac arrest patients will be in what rhythm in the first eight minutes after becoming pulseless?
    a. asystole.
    b. PEA.
    c. VF.
    d. VT.

16. Which of the following is a characteristic of the fully automated external defibrillator but is not a characteristic of the semiautomated external defibrillator?
    a. It can deliver a first shock quickly, usually within the first minute.
    b. It allows for "hands-free" defibrillation through use of adhesive pads.
    c. The machine, not the operator, administers the defibrillation.
    d. The machine may be able to provide a record of its operation.

17. Pulse checks are not performed immediately after defibrillation because
    a. it takes several minutes for a perfusing rhythm to return.
    b. ventilations are required to oxygenate the patient's blood.
    c. the level of consciousness must be assessed, not the pulse.
    d. an airway must be inserted.

18. The AED
    a. is generally indicated for use in the traumatic cardiac arrest victim.
    b. is contraindicated for patients less than 1 year of age.
    c. is preferred for use in patients less than 1 year of age.
    d. dose attenuating system is preferred for the patient 1 year of age to puberty.

19. The AED prompts you to "check electrodes." Which action is most appropriate?
    a. Turn the unit off and allow it to reset.
    b. Use smaller electrode pads.
    c. Apply additional electrode jelly to the pad.
    d. Press down on the pad(s) or consider shaving the area.

20. The general sequence for AED use in a cardiac arrest is to
   a. quickly start CPR and proceed with the AED protocol as soon as the AED is ready.
   b. quickly start CPR and perform CPR for two minutes, then proceed with the AED protocol.
   c. proceed with the AED protocol first, and then perform CPR.
   d. proceed with the AED protocol, repeat the AED protocol twice, and then perform CPR.

21. When using the AED on a patient with an implanted cardioverter-defibrillator (ICD),
   a. place the AED pad directly over the ICD.
   b. the use of the AED on a patient with an ICD is contraindicated.
   c. avoid touching the ICD patient because the device may injure the EMT during discharge.
   d. place the electrodes 1 inch to the side of the ICD.

22. AED failure is most commonly attributed to which of the following?
   a. Operator error
   b. Cable failure
   c. Internal electronics failure
   d. Battery failure

23. It is recommended that all AED operators refresh or practice operational skills with the device every
   a. month.
   b. three months.
   c. six months.
   d. year.

24. Which of the following best describes an acceptable and safe use of an AED?
   a. Application of an AED on a patient who is lying in rainwater
   b. AED use on a patient who is on a metal catwalk
   c. AED use on a patient who is on ice or snow
   d. AED use on a patient who is on a dry tile floor

25. Which of the following is the first component of the pediatric Chain of Survival?
   a. Effective advanced life support
   b. Prevention of arrest
   c. Early, high-quality CPR
   d. Rapid activation of EMS

CASE STUDY 1

You have been dispatched to the scene of a cardiac arrest. Dispatch advises that an ALS unit is also responding to the incident. You arrive and observe a male patient who appears to be in his mid-60s supine on the floor. A family member is performing adequate CPR on the patient. You calculate the total downtime as about three minutes. You hear the siren of the approaching ALS vehicle.

1. Your next best action is to
   a. take over CPR, then stop and verify the absence of a pulse or breathing. Do nothing further until ALS arrives.
   b. stop CPR, perform a primary assessment, and verify the absence of pulse/breathing.
   c. obtain a detailed history of the event as the family member continues CPR, and then stop and verify the absence of pulse/breathing.
   d. quickly attach the AED and begin analysis of the rhythm.

2. Your partner took over CPR from the bystander. Which statement regarding CPR is correct?
   a. The EMT need not remove his hands from the patient's chest during rhythm analysis.
   b. The chest should be compressed at least 1½ inches in this patient.
   c. The EMT should minimize any interruptions in CPR during AED analysis and shock.
   d. If the patient's chest is hairy, it is critical to stop chest compressions and shave the chest.

3. The patient's rhythm is analyzed, and the AED shows that applying a shock will not benefit the patient ("no shock"). What is your next best action?
   a. Ventilate, then resume chest compressions.
   b. Reanalyze the rhythm, wait 30 seconds, then reanalyze the rhythm again.
   c. Resume with chest compressions and ventilations.
   d. Recheck the pulse. If there is no pulse, resume CPR for two minutes, and then reanalyze the rhythm.

CASE STUDY 2

You are working alone at a large convention complex as an EMT providing emergency medical coverage. You have been assigned to cover a concert for the evening. At the completion of the concert, you observe a 50-year-old male who collapsed in front of you. You have an AED with you. You quickly determine the patient is unresponsive, apneic, and pulseless.

1. What is your next best action?
   a. Verify the patient is unresponsive, with no pulse and breathing.
   b. Complete a rapid medical assessment.
   c. Attach the AED's external adhesive pads, turn the unit on, and initiate rhythm analysis.
   d. Use a pocket mask and attempt to give one ventilation to confirm an open airway.

2. You have delivered a shock and have resumed CPR. What is the next best action to take?
   a. Have a bystander request EMS.
   b. Reanalyze the rhythm and repeat two (or three) more shocks.
   c. Do nothing; resuscitation efforts are futile.
   d. Leave the patient to call for help from EMS dispatch.

3. Following two minutes of CPR, you reassess the patient's rhythm with the AED. The AED advises to check breathing and pulse. A pulse is present, but no ventilations. What should you do next?
   a. Check the SpO_2.
   b. Check the blood pressure.
   c. Ventilate the patient at 10–12 pm.
   d. Ventiilate the patient at 20–30 pm.

CHAPTER 15 SCENARIO 1: DOCUMENTATION EXERCISE

Read the following scenario and think about how you would document this call if you were the EMT who responded to the scene. Then answer the multiple-choice questions and fill in the sample prehospital care report, basing your documentation on information from the scenario.

It's 8:00 A.M. hours on a sultry Saturday morning. You and your partner, Mim, are performing your daily cleaning and inspection of your ambulance when a car pulls into the driveway. The frantic driver runs toward you screaming, "They stabbed my friend!" As you try to calm the driver to gain information, the station alerting system sounds. "Unit 1, EMS Battalion Chief, respond to 1600 14th Avenue for a patient stabbed. Law enforcement is on scene, and the scene is safe." The frantic man in your driveway has overheard the call. "That's my friend!" he interjects. Mim acknowledges the call, and you recognize the address as two blocks down from this street. You both apply gloves and eye protection before leaving the station.

As you approach the scene, you see many police cars and officers. One officer is pointing toward a particular police car. You advise dispatch that you are on scene. Upon exiting the ambulance, you see the patient lying on his left side next to the police car with an officer bending over him. You and Mim quickly pull the stretcher from the ambulance, making sure to bring your oxygen bag and trauma box.

As you and Mim approach the patient, you advise dispatch that you have made patient contact. The officer crouching by the patient says, "He got stabbed twice, once on the right side and once in the right inner-thigh area." The officer is holding direct pressure with a small bandage to the right lower lateral flank area and another to the right inner thigh. As you quickly open two large trauma dressings, you ask the officer to gently lift the bandages so you can inspect the wounds. You see two large puncture wounds. The wound to the right lower lateral flank area is bleeding freely with dark red blood. The wound to the inner thigh is spurting bright red blood. You quickly place the trauma dressings over the wounds and instruct the officer to apply firm, direct pressure over both wounds.

The patient is awake, alert, and talking to the officer. You ask if he was stabbed anywhere else on his body, and he says, "No, I don't think so." You ask him his name, and he replies, "Frank." You introduce yourself and Mim, explaining, "We will be your EMTs, and we're going to take good care of you."

Mim asks the patient if he has any medical history or takes any medication, and he replies, "No." She asks if he is allergic to anything, and he replies, "Not that I know of." Mim performs a quick initial assessment. There are no stridorous or crowing sounds with inhalation or exhalation. She indicates that Frank's breathing is normal at an approximate rate of 18 per minute. She also notes that his chest appears to be rising and falling, with adequate air flowing in and out of his mouth and nose and without use of accessory muscles. The patient's SpO_2 is 96%. Mim applies oxygen. She radios dispatch to notify the trauma center of a trauma alert and to launch the helicopter. She explains to Frank that he must go to a specialized trauma center in a neighboring town, and he will get there by helicopter. He states, "I trust you both. Please don't let me die." You recognize the wounds to be very serious. You ask the police officer if he has the knife or knows how long it was, and he replies, "The knife hasn't been located yet."

Mim feels for a radial pulse and finds a weak pulse at 90 beats per minute; the skin is warm and slightly diaphoretic; the capillary blanch is less than 2 seconds. She begins a rapid physical exam. The head reveals no deformities; the pupils are equal and react briskly to light. The nose, mouth, and ears are all clear of blood or fluid. The neck is soft without any obvious injuries or subcutaneous emphysema. The trachea is midline, and there is no deformity or pain to the posterior neck. She palpates the chest and notes equal chest rise and fall, finding no signs of trauma or use of accessory muscles. She carefully inspects the axillary area by lifting the arms and looking for hidden injuries. No trauma is noted.

Inspection of the abdomen reveals only the puncture wound located during the initial assessment. The abdomen is distended, with slight discoloration around the umbilicus and bilateral flank areas. Mim palpates the abdomen, and Frank responds with a grimaced face and remarks, "Ouch, that really hurts." Mim says she is sorry and that she is almost done. She notes that the pain is in all four quadrants and that the patient guards the area. She then turns to you and says, "The abdomen is distended and rigid with slight discoloration and pain on palpation." Mim quickly inspects the pelvis for deformity, contusions, abrasions, or penetrating injuries, and none are found. She rapidly assesses the extremities and finds no injuries other than the previously noted right-inner-thigh puncture wound. Frank indicates he can feel her touching each extremity, and he has good movement in all extremities. Mim remarks to you, "I can't find any distal pulses." She immediately feels for a femoral pulse, locates it, and reports that it is strong. She examines the posterior body and finds no trauma or sacral edema. She does note slight discoloration to the small of the back. The patient does not complain of any pain when the spine is palpated.

You position the cot next to the patient and, with Mim's assistance, you place the patient on the cot in a supine position. You both quickly wheel the cot to the ambulance while talking reassuringly to Frank. Your battalion chief arrives on scene and asks, "What do you have?" You briefly give him a size-up of Frank's condition. He asks, "How can I help you?" You inform him that you have a police officer assisting you and that you are in good shape right now. He informs you that he will set up the helicopter landing zone at a nearby park. You ask another police officer to drive your ambulance to the landing zone so you and Mim can both care for Frank in the patient compartment. You notify dispatch that you are en route to the landing zone area.

While en route to the landing zone, you assess the vital signs. You notice the patient's breathing rate has increased to 28 times a minute and is shallow, with use of accessory muscles. Frank appears more restless and anxious, and you reassure him.

You immediately insert a nasopharyngeal airway and provide positive pressure ventilation with the bag-valve mask (BVM) attached to oxygen. The carotid pulse is 130 beats per minute. The skin has become cool, sweaty, and pale. The blood pressure is 96/80 and difficult to auscultate. The SpO_2 is 93%. The capillary blanch is now delayed at 4 seconds.

As the police officer pulls the ambulance near the landing zone, you see that the helicopter is just touching down. Your battalion chief advises dispatch that the helicopter is on the ground. You hear a gentle knock on the rear door of the ambulance, and as it opens, you recognize flight medics Doug and Mike. Doug asks you what you have, and you give him a brief but thorough report. Mike notifies the pilot of the helicopter that they will be doing a "hot load." Frank is quickly loaded onto the helicopter. Less than a minute later, the helicopter lifts from the landing zone. The pilot advises the battalion chief that the patient will be at the trauma center in approximately 10 minutes.

You and Mim gather your thoughts while decontaminating your equipment and ambulance in preparation for the next call. Your battalion chief meets you at the ambulance and asks how you're doing. He coordinates a critique of the call for quality improvement purposes.

1. When Mim felt for distal pulses and could not locate any, she immediately felt for a femoral pulse and found it to be strong. What does this indicate?
   a. Blood is being pushed into the extremities.
   b. A severe state of shock exists.
   c. Respiratory effort has increased.
   d. The patient is in the early stages of shock.

2. You know that this patient has entered the late, decompensated stage of shock. Which of the following signs indicates that your patient has progressed into this stage?
   a. The patient developed bradycardia (abnormally slow heart rate).
   b. The patient developed bradypnea (abnormally slow respirations).
   c. The peripheral pulses became absent.
   d. The patient had a widening pulse pressure.

EMERGENCY TRIP SHEET

TRIP #	
MEDIC #	
BEGIN MILES	
~~ND~~ MILES	
~~DE~~___/___ PAGE___/___	
UNITS ON SCENE	

	BILLING USE ONLY
	DAY
	DATE
	RECEIVED
	DISPATCHED

NAME	SEX M F DOB ___/___/___
ADDRESS	RACE

CITY	STATE	ZIP

PHONE ( ) -	PCP DR.

RESPONDED FROM	CITY
TAKEN FROM	ZIP
DESTINATION	REASON

SSN - -	MEDICARE #	MEDICAID #

INSURANCE CO	INSURANCE #	GROUP #

RESPONSIBLE PARTY	ADDRESS

CITY	STATE	ZIP	PHONE ( ) -

EMPLOYER	

	EN-ROUTE		
ON SCENE		ON SCENE	
TO HOSPITAL			
AT HOSPITAL			
IN-SERVICE			

CREW	CERT	STATE #

IV THERAPY
SUCCESSFUL Y N # OF ATTEMPTS _____
ANGIO SIZE _____ga.
SITE _____
TOTAL FLUID INFUSED _____ cc
BLOOD DRAW Y N INITIALS

INTUBATION INFORMATION
SUCCESSFUL Y N # OF ATTEMPTS _____
TUBE SIZE _____ mm
TIME _____ INITIALS _____

TIME	ON SCENE (1)	ON SCENE (2)	ON SCENE (3)	EN-ROUTE (1)	EN-ROUTE (2)	AT DESTINATION
BP						
PULSE						
RESP						
SpO$_2$						
ETCO$_2$						
EKG						

MEDICAL HISTORY	

CONDITION CODES	

TREATMENTS

~~DICATIONS~~	

TIME	TREATMENT	DOSE	ROUTE	INIT

ALLERGIES

C/C

EVENTS LEADING TO C/C

ASSESSMENT

TREATMENT

GCS	E___ V___ M___ TOTAL =
GCS	E___ V___ M___ TOTAL =

HOSPITAL CONTACTED

CPR BEGUN BY B P TIME BEGUN	

EMS SIGNATURE

AED USED Y N BY:
RESUSCITATION TERMINATED - TIME

( ) OSHA REGULATIONS FOLLOWED

CHAPTER 15 SCENARIO 2: DOCUMENTATION EXERCISE

Read the following scenario and think about how you would document this call if you were the EMT who responded to the scene. Then answer the multiple-choice questions and fill in the sample prehospital care report, basing your documentation on information from the scenario.

It's a beautiful autumn day, and you and your partner, Tara, are the crew responsible for providing emergency medical care at a local football game. It's halftime, and the local team is winning 28 to 3. Both teams have left the field and are in the locker room. Suddenly, the portable radio squawks: "Unit 2, respond to the visitor's locker room for an elderly patient down; CPR is being administered; ALS Medic One is your backup." You mark or advise dispatch that you are en route to the locker room.

You and Tara quickly apply gloves and eye protection as you respond to the visiting team's locker room a short distance away. As you tell dispatch that you are at the locker room, Tara pulls the stretcher from the rear of the ambulance. You both place the necessary equipment, including the AED, on the stretcher and walk briskly toward the locker room. As you enter the locker room, you quickly scan the area, looking for any hazards. You notice that the room is filled to capacity with upset, screaming players and others. Tara solicits the help of a distressed but in-control adult standing in the room. She asks him to please help by moving all nonessential people out of the room.

As you approach the vicinity of the patient, you radio to dispatch that you have made patient contact and that this is a priority call. You recognize the patient as the coach from the visiting team. He is lying supine with a moribund look about him. Bystanders are administering highly effective CPR. An assistant coach states, "He was really giving it to the team, then his face turned red, and he fell to the floor. We immediately started CPR." Tara asks the bystanders to continue CPR while you perform a quick assessment. You see cyanosis around his lips and neck. You reassure the bystanders by saying what a good job they are doing and remind them to continue to push hard and fast.

Tara states she will ready the AED. As she exposes the patient's chest, you notice a large midchest scar extending from the suprasternal notch to the area just above the umbilicus. The assistant coach says, "The coach had a heart bypass two years ago." Tara attaches the defibrillation pads to the cables and then attaches them to the patient's bare chest.

After the pads are attached, she states in a loud, clear voice, "Stop CPR, and clear the patient so the AED can analyze the patient." Tara looks at the AED screen and recognizes the following rhythm.

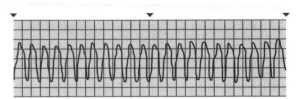

The AED indicates a "Shock advised and starts to charge the AED, CPR is continued until the AED advises "Press Shock" message. Tara quickly makes sure everyone is clear of the patient by looking from the patient's head to the feet. In a loud voice, she says, "I'm clear, you're clear, everyone is clear." She presses the shock button to deliver the shock. The patient's body convulses with a quick jerk and then relaxes. Tara and you quickly resume effective begin CPR and continue for two minutes, completing five sets of 30:2 compressions to ventilations. You reassess the patient's rhythm and the AED advises to "check pulse" and respirations. You feel for a carotid pulse and notice a strong pulse. The patient remains apneic. Tara quickly starts positive pressure ventilations with the BVM and supplemental oxygen. You hear on your portable radio that ALS Medic One has arrived on the scene.

Medic One's crew, Lieutenant Wilson and Paramedic Springer, approach you for a report on the patient's status. You report that the patient was a witnessed cardiac arrest, and prior to this event, the coach was visibly upset. You mention that you found him on the floor with highly effective CPR being performed. An estimated time of two minutes passed from the time the patient went into cardiac arrest until you arrived on scene. You relay that you immediately applied the AED and explain the rhythm that you found. You report that one shock was administered and that the patient just now has regained a pulse but remains apneic.

Tara continues to ventilate the patient with positive pressure ventilations. As Paramedic Springer positions the cot, you obtain a set of vital signs. The blood pressure is 138/64; the heart rate is 106 beats per minute, bounding but irregular. The skin is cool, pale, and clammy, but the color is improving. The SpO_2 is 94%. The pupils are dilated and very sluggish to respond to light. Lieutenant Wilson thanks you for a job well done. The patient is positioned on the cot and immediately loaded into Medic One and transported to the hospital eight minutes away.

The next morning, you and Tara receive a phone call at the station from the coach's wife, stating her gratitude for helping to save his life. You explain that you and Tara are but one link in the Out of Hospital Cardiac Arrest OHCA Chain of Survival and that there are others who deserve credit as well. You politely thank her for her comments and wish her and her husband well.

1. After Tara applied the AED, she found the patient in the following rhythm. You recognize this rhythm to be
   a. VF.
   b. VT.
   c. asystole.
   d. PEA.

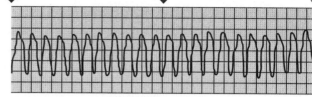

2. Tara asked everyone to stay clear of the patient when the AED entered the analyzing phase. Which of the following is a reason why it is important to ensure that everyone stays clear of the patient during this time?
   a. The AED may sense a bystander's heart rate and shut off.
   b. The AED defibrillation pads may become ineffective.
   c. The patient's body may deliver a residual (leftover) shock.
   d. The AED may sense movement and report inaccurately.

3. You explained to the coach's wife that your efforts were one of several in the adult out of hospital cardiac arrest (OHCA) Chain of Survival that helped save her husband's life.
   a. immediate recognition and activation, immediate high quality CPR, BLS and ALS and post arrest care.
   b. early notification, early CPR, early diagnosis, and early treatment.
   c. early diagnosis, early CPR, early hospitalization, and early rehabilitation.
   d. early CPR, early ALS, early defibrillation, and early hospitalization.

TRIP #	
MEDIC #	
BEGIN MILES	
END MILES	
CODE___/___ PAGE___/___	
UNITS ON SCENE	

EMERGENCY
TRIP SHEET

BILLING USE ONLY			
DAY			
DATE			
RECEIVED			
DISPATCHED			
EN-ROUTE			
ON SCENE			
TO HOSPITAL			
AT HOSPITAL			
IN-SERVICE			

NAME	SEX M F DOB ___/___/___	
ADDRESS	RACE	
CITY	STATE	ZIP
PHONE ( ) -	PCP DR.	
RESPONDED FROM	CITY	
TAKEN FROM	ZIP	
DESTINATION	REASON	
SSN - -	MEDICARE #	MEDICAID #
INSURANCE CO	INSURANCE #	GROUP #
RESPONSIBLE PARTY	ADDRESS	
CITY	STATE ZIP PHONE ( ) -	
EMPLOYER		

	CREW	CERT	STATE #

TIME	ON SCENE (1)	ON SCENE (2)	ON SCENE (3)	EN-ROUTE (1)	EN-ROUTE (2)	AT DESTINATION
BP						
PULSE						
RESP						
SpO$_2$						
ETCO$_2$						
EKG						

IV THERAPY
SUCCESSFUL   Y   N   # OF ATTEMPTS _____
ANGIO SIZE _____ga.
SITE _____
TOTAL FLUID INFUSED _____ cc
BLOOD DRAW   Y   N   INITIALS

INTUBATION INFORMATION
SUCCESSFUL   Y   N   # OF ATTEMPTS _____
TUBE SIZE _____ mm
TIME _____ INITIALS _____

MEDICAL HISTORY

MEDICATIONS

ALLERGIES

C/C

EVENTS LEADING TO C/C

ASSESSMENT

TREATMENT

CONDITION CODES				

TREATMENTS

TIME	TREATMENT	DOSE	ROUTE

GCS E___V___M___TOTAL =

GCS E___V___M___TOTAL =

HOSPITAL CONTACTED

CPR BEGUN BY   B   P   TIME BEGUN

AED USED   Y   N   BY:

RESUSCITATION TERMINATED - TIME

EMS SIGNATURE

(   ) OSHA REGULATIONS FOLLO

Respiratory Emergencies

▌ STANDARD

Medicine (Content Area: Respiratory)

▌ COMPETENCY

Applies fundamental knowledge to provide basic emergency care and transportation based on assessment findings for an acutely ill patient.

▌ OBJECTIVES

After reading this chapter, you should be able to:

16-1. Define key terms introduced in this chapter.

16-2. Explain the importance of being able to quickly recognize and treat patients with respiratory emergencies.

16-3. Describe the structure and function of the respiratory system, including:
   a. Upper airway
   b. Lower airway
   c. Gas exchange
   d. Inspiratory and expiratory centers in the medulla and pons

16-4. Demonstrate the assessment of breath sounds.

16-5. Describe the characteristics of abnormal breath sounds, including:
   a. Wheezing
   b. Rhonchi
   c. Crackles (rales)

16-6. Explain the relationship between dyspnea and hypoxia.

16-7. Differentiate respiratory distress, respiratory failure, and respiratory arrest.

16-8. Describe the pathophysiology by which each of the following conditions leads to inadequate oxygenation:
   a. Obstructive pulmonary diseases: emphysema, chronic bronchitis, and asthma
   b. Pneumonia
   c. Pulmonary embolism
   d. Pulmonary edema
   e. Spontaneous pneumothorax
   f. Hyperventilation syndrome

g. Epiglottitis

h. Pertussis

i. Cystic fibrosis

j. Poisonous exposures

k. Viral respiratory infections

16-9. As allowed by your scope of practice, demonstrate administering or assisting a patient with self-administration of bronchodilators by metered-dose inhaler and/or small-volume nebulizer.

16-10. Differentiate between short-acting beta$_2$ agonists appropriate for prehospital use and respiratory medications that are not intended for emergency use.

16-11. Describe special considerations in the assessment and management of pediatric and geriatric patients with respiratory emergencies, including:

a. Differences in anatomy and physiology

b. Causes of respiratory emergencies

c. Differences in management

16-12. Employ an assessment-based approach in order to recognize indications for the following interventions in patients with respiratory complaints/emergencies:

a. Establishing an airway

b. Administration of oxygen

c. Positive pressure ventilation

d. Administration/assistance with self-administration of an inhaled beta$_2$ agonist

e. Expedited transport

f. ALS backup

16-13. Given a list of patient medications, recognize medications that are associated with respiratory disease.

16-14. Use reassessment to identify responses to treatment and changes in the conditions of patients presenting with respiratory complaints and emergencies.

▌KEY IDEAS

This chapter describes respiratory distress and respiratory failure. Emphasis is placed on ensuring an open airway maintaining an SpO_2 reading of 94% or higher, providing continuous positive airway pressure (CPAP) or positive pressure ventilation, as needed, and not on trying to diagnose a specific underlying disease.

■ There is a wide variety of signs and symptoms of respiratory distress. They may include any of these: shortness of breath; restlessness; increased pulse rate or breathing rate; decreased breathing rate; skin color changes; noisy breathing; inability to speak; retractions; shallow, slow, or irregular breathing; abdominal breathing; coughing; patient in a tripod position; unusual anatomy (barrel chest); altered mental status; nasal flaring; tracheal tugging or deviations; paradoxical motion; and/or pursed-lip breathing.

■ Time is critical to the patient who is breathing inadequately. If signs of inadequate breathing are exhibited by the patient, you should immediately begin positive pressure ventilation with supplemental oxygen. If the breathing is adequate, supplemental oxygen should be administered. A nasal cannula at 2 to 4 lpm can be used to increase or maintain the SpO_2 reading at 94% or higher. Oxygen administration should be based on the patient's oxygenation status, measurement primarily guided by the pulse oximeter. The patient who presents with moderate to severe respiratory distress and who is awake and alert would benefit from CPAP. A patient presenting with a severely decreased SpO_2 reading and obvious signs of severe hypoxia may benefit from higher concentrations of oxygen delivered by a nonrebreather mask at 15 lpm. The SpO_2 of pregnant patients who present in respiratory distress should be maintained at a slightly higher level of $\geq 95\%$ to maintain adequate oxygenation of the fetus.

■ Metered-dose inhalers (MDIs) are used by some patients with chronic or recurring breathing problems. If the patient has a prescribed MDI, contact medical direction for an order to assist the patient with administering the medication. It may be necessary to coach the patient during the procedure to be sure the medication is taken by the patient in an effective manner.

- An increased work of breathing in the infant or child is an indication that he is compensating for inadequate oxygen and carbon dioxide exchange and may deteriorate into respiratory failure. You must recognize the wide range of symptoms and immediately provide oxygen if the infant or child is breathing adequately or provide positive pressure ventilation with supplemental oxygen if there are signs of inadequate breathing.

MEDICAL TERMINOLOGY

Term	Prefix	Word Root Combining Form	Suffix	Definition
apnea (AP-nee-ah)	a- (no, not, without, lack of)	pnea (to breathe or breathing)		Absence of breathing; respiratory arrest
bronchoconstriction (BRONG-koh-kun-STRIK-shun)		bronch/o (bronchi); constriction (narrowing an opening)		Constriction of the smooth muscles of the bronchi and bronchioles, causing a narrowing of the air passageways
bronchospasm (brong-koh-SPAZ-um)		bronch/o-(bronchi); spasm (constriction)		Spasm or constriction of the smooth muscles of the bronchi and bronchioles
dyspnea (DISP-nee-ah)	dys- (bad, difficult, painful)	pnea (to breathe or breathing)		Shortness of breath or perceived difficulty in breathing
diaphoresis (DYE-ah-for-EE-sis)	dia- (through, between)	phoresis (migration of ions)		Profuse sweating
hypotension (high-poh-TEN-shun)	hypo- (below, under, deficient)	tens (tension)	-ion (process)	Blood pressure lower than normal
tachycardia (tak-i-KAR-dee-ah)	tachy- (fast)	card (heart)	-ia (condition of)	Heart rate faster than normal
tachypnea (tak-ip-NEE-ah)	tachy- (fast)	pnea (to breathe or breathing)		Breathing rate faster than normal
syncope (SIN-koh-pee)	syn- (together, with)		-cope (strike, cut)	Fainting; transient loss of consciousness

1. The medical term *apnea* contains the word root *pnea*, which refers to
   a. heart.
   b. breathing.
   c. pain.
   d. lungs.

2. The prefix *tachy-*, used in the medical term *tachypnea*, means
   a. slow.
   b. irregular.
   c. regular.
   d. fast.

3. The prefix *a-* in the medical term *apnea* refers to
   a. no, not, without, lack of.
   b. bad, difficult, painful.
   c. out, away from.
   d. through, between.

4. The medical term *dyspnea* contains the prefix *dys-*, which means
   a. upon, over, above.
   b. below, under, deficient.
   c. out, away from.
   d. bad, difficult, painful.

5. Combining the prefix *a-* and the word root *pnea* creates a medical term that means
   a. inflammation of the cornea.
   b. absence of breathing; respiratory arrest.
   c. constriction of the bronchi.
   d. faster than the normal breathing rate.

TERMS AND CONCEPTS

1. Write the number of the correct term next to each definition.

   1. Apnea
   2. Bronchodilator
   3. Bronchospasm
   4. Dyspnea
   5. Grunting
   6. Metered-dose inhaler (MDI)
   7. Respiratory arrest
   8. Respiratory failure
   9. Spacer
   10. Tripod position

   _____ a. A drug that relaxes the smooth muscle of the bronchi and bronchioles

   _____ b. When breathing stops completely

   _____ c. Constriction of the smooth muscles of the bronchi and bronchioles

   _____ d. Device consisting of a plastic container and a canister used to inhale an aerosolized medication

   _____ e. A chamber that is connected to an MDI to collect medication until it is inhaled

   _____ f. A period with absence of breathing

   _____ g. A sound heard during exhalation in infants suffering from severe respiratory distress

   _____ h. Inadequate oxygenation of the blood and elimination of carbon dioxide

   _____ i. Shortness of breath or difficulty in breathing

   _____ j. Patient sits upright, leans slightly forward, and supports the body with arms in front and elbows locked

2. Which two of the terms listed in item 1 have essentially the same meaning? _____ and _____

CONTENT REVIEW

1. Your patient is experiencing difficulty breathing but has adequate tidal volume and respiratory rate. This patient is said to be _____ and your treatment should include _____.
   a. in respiratory failure/initiating immediate ventilation with a bag-valve mask (BVM)
   b. apneic/beginning aggressive ventilation at once
   c. experiencing dyspnea/administering oxygen at 6 lpm via nasal cannula
   d. in respiratory distress/administering oxygen to maintain SpO_2 at 94% or higher

2. You are treating your patient who complains of shortness of breath. The patient appears to be quite agitated and aggressive. This is likely due to
   a. hypercarbia.
   b. hyperventilation.
   c. hypoxia.
   d. hypotension.

3. While treating your patient who is experiencing respiratory distress, you find the skin to be pale, cool, and clammy (diaphoretic). This is likely a(n)
   a. late sign of hypoxia.
   b. early sign of hypoxia.
   c. late sign of hyperventilation.
   d. early sign of hyperventilation.

4. The tripod position is commonly indicative of which of the following?
   a. Severe respiratory distress
   b. Moderate respiratory distress
   c. Mild respiratory distress
   d. Apnea/respiratory arrest

5. Which of the following is a sign of severe respiratory distress?
   a. Speaking a couple of words between breaths
   b. Pink, warm skin
   c. Pulse oximeter reading of 97%
   d. Respiratory rate of 50 in infants

6. You are treating a patient complaining of respiratory distress. You know that a patient in a state of hypercarbia (high CO_2 levels) will present with which of the following?
   a. Patient will speak with stuttering speech.
   b. Lung sounds will become diminished.
   c. Pupils will become fixed and dilated.
   d. Patient will be confused and disoriented.

7. You are assessing your patient who complains of difficulty breathing. You hear crowing sounds with each breath; you suspect
   a. a partial airway obstruction.
   b. fluid in the lower lungs.
   c. an injured or ruptured diaphragm.
   d. inadequate blood flow to the lungs.

8. Your elderly patient is experiencing an acute onset of respiratory distress. The patient is obviously very agitated and aggressive toward your attempts to treat him. You suspect that the patient
   a. has had a reaction to medication.
   b. may be in an acute state of hypoxia.
   c. is hearing impaired and confused about your intentions.
   d. is an upset elderly person who is difficult to assess.

9. You are treating an unresponsive 3-year-old who is exhibiting signs of respiratory distress with decreased tidal volume. The respiratory rate is 14 per minute. Which of the following is correct?
   a. Immediately begin positive pressure ventilation.
   b. Begin positive pressure ventilation after the physical exam.
   c. Immediately apply oxygen by nonrebreather mask at 15 lpm.
   d. Apply oxygen by nasal cannula at 6 lpm after the physical exam.

10. You are treating an elderly man who complains of respiratory distress. He is breathing 18 times a minute with good chest rise and fall, and you feel a good volume of air at his nose and mouth upon exhalation. His SpO_2 is 92%. Which of the following is correct?
    a. Begin positive pressure ventilation.
    b. Apply oxygen by nasal cannula at 8 lpm.
    c. Apply oxygen and maintain the SpO_2 at 94% or greater.
    d. No ventilation or oxygen therapy is required.

11. Upon arrival on the scene, you make contact with a patient who is experiencing difficulty breathing. You observe that the patient's eyelids are beginning to droop and his head bobs with each respiration. Your immediate action should be to
    a. place the patient on a nonrebreather mask.
    b. interview the patient to determine the specific complaint.
    c. place the patient in the recovery position.
    d. administer positive pressure ventilations with the BVM.

12. The adult with respiratory distress and increased pulse rate and the infant or child with respiratory distress and slow pulse rate should both be transported immediately following the
    a. primary assessment.
    b. focused history.
    c. physical exam.
    d. reassessment.

13. Which of the following adult patients complaining of difficulty breathing should be administered oxygen to maintain an SpO_2 reading of greater than 94%?
    a. Respiratory rate of 20 with good air movement
    b. Respiratory rate of 18 with poor tidal volume
    c. Respiratory rate of 28 with adequate tidal volume
    d. Respiratory rate of 8 with little air movement

14. Suprasternal notch retractions indicate that the patient
    a. has a history of heart surgery.
    b. is experiencing substernal chest pain.
    c. is making an extreme effort to breathe.
    d. has a history that includes asthma.

15. Bradycardia in the adult, child, or infant is a sign of which of the following?
    a. Severe hypoglycemia
    b. Impending respiratory failure
    c. Possible myocardial infarction
    d. Imminent shock

16. When an area of the chest moves inward during inhalation and outward during exhalation, it is a common sign of chest injury leading to respiratory distress known as which of the following?
    a. Diaphragm breathing
    b. Accessory muscle use
    c. Paradoxical motion
    d. Intercostal retractions

17. If you are in doubt whether to ventilate with positive pressure or not, you should
    a. use a nonrebreather mask.
    b. contact medical direction for orders.
    c. provide positive pressure ventilation.
    d. wait for paramedic backup.

18. You have placed the pulse oximeter on your patient complaining of respiratory distress. The pulse oximeter reading is 88% while the patient is breathing room air. Which of the following statements best describes your findings?
    a. This is a normal reading for a patient breathing room air.
    b. This reading is an indication of severe hypoxia.
    c. This reading indicates a mild case of hypoxia.
    d. A reading below 90% is impossible; check the oximeter.

19. Number the following list in the proper order from 1 to 5 to provide emergency care for the patient with adequate breathing who is complaining of respiratory distress.

    _____ Complete the secondary assessment and physical exam.

    _____ Place the patient in a position of comfort and then transport.

    _____ Assess the vital signs.

    _____ Administer oxygen and maintain the SpO_2 at > 94%.

    _____ Determine if the patient has a prescribed MDI and contact medical direction for permission to administer it.

20. Your patient complains of shortness of breath. Following auscultation of the chest, you find decreased breath sounds on the right side; there is no evidence of trauma. You suspect
    a. spontaneous pneumothorax.
    b. bilateral hemothorax.
    c. pneumonia.
    d. flail segment.

21. To determine if your emergency medical care has decreased the patient's respiratory distress or if further intervention is necessary, you should
    a. perform a reassessment prior to transporting the patient.
    b. perform a reassessment while en route to the hospital.
    c. perform the secondary assessment while transporting.
    d. perform the secondary assessment before transporting.

22. For administering an MDI, which of the following procedures is correct?
    a. Coach the patient to breathe through the nose.
    b. Coach the patient to hold his breath as long as possible after inhalation of the medication.
    c. Depress the canister as the patient begins to exhale.
    d. Shake the canister for 10 seconds before removing the cap.

23. Which of the following is a sign of respiratory difficulty in children?
    a. Use of accessory muscles
    b. Hypertension and urticaria
    c. Sore or hoarse throat
    d. Respiratory rate of 15 to 30 breaths each minute

24. Which of the following is a sign of respiratory failure in infants and children?
    a. Seesaw or rocky breathing
    b. Increased muscle tone
    c. Bilateral breath sounds
    d. Rigid and painful abdomen

25. Your 4-year-old patient displays head bobbing and irregular breathing. You should
    a. administer oxygen; transport after completing the primary assessment.
    b. hold the nonrebreather mask next to the child's face; transport at once.
    c. immediately begin positive pressure ventilation; transport at once.
    d. immediately administer oxygen by nonrebreather mask; transport after completing the primary assessment.

26. A child experiencing respiratory distress should be placed in which position?
    a. Supine position
    b. Prone position
    c. Position of comfort
    d. Tripod position

27. Regarding epiglottitis in the infant or child, which of the following is true?
    a. Epiglottitis is usually self-rectifying and is seldom an emergency.
    b. The child usually sits straight up, juts the jaw forward, and drools.
    c. You should inspect the throat and mouth with a tongue depressor.
    d. You should perform foreign body airway obstruction maneuvers if respiratory distress is evident.

28. A cough that produces a sound like a barking seal is the hallmark sign of which of the following?
    a. Complete airway obstruction
    b. Partial airway obstruction
    c. Epiglottitis, swollen epiglottis
    d. Croup, swelling of the larynx

29. Which of the following conditions can lead to faster muscle fatigue and early respiratory failure in the patient complaining of respiratory distress?
    a. Difficulty breathing out (exhaling)
    b. Eupnea, relaxed breathing
    c. Increased lung sounds
    d. Increased tidal volume

30. You notice while assessing your patient who is having trouble breathing that his jugular veins are distended during inhalation and then return to normal during exhalation. You recognize this as
    a. paradoxical movement from a flail segment.
    b. an ominous sign of a traumatic brain injury with herniation.
    c. tachycardia, an increase in the heart rate above normal.
    d. Kussmaul sign, a severely increased pressure in the chest or around the heart.

31. You are treating your patient who has an extremely fast respiratory rate (tachypnea). This fast respiratory rate will likely result in
    a. adequate tissue perfusion due to the increased breathing rate.
    b. inadequate tidal volume due to inadequate filling of the lungs.
    c. inadequate blood pressure due to increased oxygenation of the cells.
    d. overinflation of the lungs leading to increased oxygenation of the tissue.

32. Your patient has signs of subcutaneous emphysema. Which of the following is correct pertaining to this condition?
    a. Subcutaneous emphysema is easily seen by visual inspection of the chest.
    b. Due to gravity, the air will settle to the lower chest in the seated patient.
    c. Subcutaneous emphysema is an indication of an air leak in the chest or neck.
    d. Subcutaneous emphysema cannot be felt; it must be auscultated with the stethoscope.

33. You are treating your patient who is breathing 36 times per minute with shallow tidal volume. The SpO_2 reading is 86% on room air. You should immediately
    a. ventilate with a BVM at 10 to 12 times per minute, imposing the ventilations over the patient's breathing rate.
    b. ventilate with a BVM at the patient's spontaneous respiratory rate.
    c. administer oxygen at 15 lpm due to the patient's ample spontaneous respiratory rate.
    d. place the patient on a nasal cannula at a low concentration due to the hyperventilation rate of the patient.

34. You are treating your patient suffering from bronchoconstriction with a $beta_2$ MDI. You note an increase in the heart rate following the administration of the MDI. What is likely the reason for this increase in heart rate?
    a. Decreasing the workload of the lungs increases the heart rate.
    b. Tachycardia is caused by the dilation of the smooth muscles.
    c. $Beta_4$ properties are a side effect to this type of MDI.
    d. $Beta_2$ MDI inhalers also have trace amounts of $beta_1$ properties.

35. Which of the following medical conditions is caused by an obstruction of blood flow in the pulmonary arteries due to an occlusion?
    a. Spontaneous pneumothorax
    b. Pulmonary embolism
    c. Pulmonary edema
    d. Tension pneumothorax

36. Choose the medical condition that describes a sudden rupture of a portion of the visceral lining of the lung, causing the lung to partially collapse.
    a. Spontaneous pneumothorax
    b. Pulmonary embolism
    c. Pulmonary edema
    d. Chronic emphysema

37. Your partner has just finished auscultation of the lungs on an elderly patient complaining of respiratory difficulty. She described the lung sounds as a high-pitched whistling heard primarily during exhalation. You recognize this to be
    a. wheezing.
    b. crackles.
    c. rhonchi.
    d. rales.

38. Choose the medical condition that is characterized by the destruction of the alveolar walls and distention of the alveolar sacs. It is more common in male patients, who may have a thin, barrel-chest appearance.
    a. Chronic bronchitis
    b. Emphysema
    c. Asthma
    d. Pulmonary embolism

39. You are treating a patient who is complaining of difficulty breathing. The patient has a history of congestive heart failure (CHF), and you suspect that the patient is suffering from acute cardiogenic pulmonary edema. Which of the following treatments is considered dangerous and may exacerbate the condition, causing the patient to become worse?
    a. If breathing is adequate, place the patient on a nonrebreather mask at 15 lpm.
    b. If breathing is inadequate, begin positive pressure ventilations immediately.
    c. Place the pulse oximeter probe on the patient's finger to obtain an SpO_2 value.
    d. Place the patient in the flat or supine position to decrease fluid buildup.

40. Which pulmonary disease is caused by changes in the mucus-secreting glands of the lungs? This disease is cited as one of the most common life-shortening genetic diseases and affects children.
    a. Emphysema
    b. Asthma
    c. Cystic fibrosis
    d. Chronic bronchitis

❙ CASE STUDY

It's 8:15 in the morning. You and your partner, Angie, have just received the report from the previous shift. With a cup of coffee in hand, you walk to the ambulance to inventory the supplies and equipment. The alerting system sounds: "Unit 105 respond to 155 Wick Avenue for an elderly patient complaining of difficulty breathing. Alert time 8:16 A.M." You and Angie get under way at once. En route, dispatch advises that they are on the phone with the son of the patient and that he is very apprehensive. You arrive at the scene and are met at the ambulance by the son. "Hurry! My mother is having trouble breathing." You quickly reassure him as he leads you to the patient. You find an elderly woman, Mrs. Frederick, sitting on the side of the bed, with slight use of accessory muscles. A quick survey of the house and room doesn't reveal indications of trauma. The patient's chest is rising and falling adequately. There is good air volume exchange. Auscultation of the lungs reveals breath sounds bilaterally, with a slight wheezy sound. The respiratory rate is 20 per minute and the SpO_2

is 93%. The patient responds appropriately and states, "I've been—(breath)—short of breath—(breath)—over an hour—(breath)—Hope—(breath)—you can—(breath)—help me."

1. From the information provided, what should your assessment and first emergency care step be?
   a. The patient is critical. Immediately begin positive pressure ventilation.
   b. Breathing is adequate. Apply oxygen and maintain the SpO_2 at 94% or greater.
   c. The patient is hyperventilating. Apply a nasal cannula at 6 lpm.
   d. The patient is hyperventilating. Place a paper bag over the nose and mouth.

2. Using the OPQRST questions to evaluate the history of the present illness, the question, "Does lying flat make the respiratory distress worse?" relates to which of the following?
   a. Provocation
   b. Quality
   c. Radiation
   d. Severity

During the secondary assessment, you learn that Mrs. Frederick has a history of asthma and has no known allergies. She does take albuterol when her breathing is difficult, but she has not taken any today. You inspect around the lips and mouth for cyanosis; none is found. Angie advises that the vitals are blood pressure 160/76, breathing rate 22 per minute, pulse 100 and regular.

3. Which of the following might cause the rapid breathing in this patient?
   a. Most asthmatics have rapid breathing continuously.
   b. The body attempts to make up for inadequate oxygenation.
   c. The elderly have higher respiratory rates.
   d. This is a common side effect of albuterol.

4. Which of the following is correct regarding albuterol?
   a. Alpha agonist bronchoconstrictor; constricts the smooth muscles; dilates the airway
   b. Alpha agonist bronchodilator; relaxes the smooth muscles; dilates the airway
   c. Beta agonist bronchodilator; relaxes the smooth muscles; dilates the airway
   d. Beta pacifist bronchoconstrictor; contracts the smooth muscles; constricts the airway

5. Before you and Angie assist in the administration of the patient's MDI, what three criteria must first be met (indications)?

6. After you administer an MDI, if there is little or no effect, you should
   a. check the expiration date, then readminister the dose.
   b. consult medical direction to consider readministering.
   c. shake the MDI for 15 seconds, then readminister the dose.
   d. have the patient begin deep breathing to increase the effect of the medication.

After administering the MDI, you perform a reassessment. Mrs. Frederick advises that her respiratory distress has decreased dramatically. The vitals are blood pressure 140/62, respiratory rate 14 per minute, SpO_2 of 96%, and pulse 74 and regular. After auscultating the lungs, you hear bilateral breath sounds without wheezing. Angie records and documents all the findings and readies the patient for transport.

7. In what position should you place this patient on the stretcher?
   a. Prone
   b. Lateral recumbent
   c. Supine
   d. Fowler or semi-Fowler's

Read the following scenario and think about how you would document this call if you were the EMT who responded to the scene. Then answer the multiple-choice questions and fill in the sample prehospital care report, basing your documentation on information from the scenario.

It's 6:00 P.M. in the evening; you and your partner, Captain Walls, have just sat down for a well-deserved dinner break. Suddenly, the alerting system sounds: "Unit 1, respond to grid 534, 55 Seaman Way for a 62-year-old female, short of breath." As you exit the dining area, Captain Walls acknowledges the call with dispatch. After a short emergency response, you arrive on the scene of a well-kept single-family residence. You apply gloves and eye protection as you exit the ambulance. You both quickly scan the scene, looking for any safety hazards. Not suspecting any potential hazards, you approach the house and ring the doorbell. There is no response, so you carefully open the front door and announce your presence. You hear a muffled voice state, "I—(breath)—am—(breath)—in—(breath)—the—(breath)—bed—(breath)—room." You cautiously proceed to the back bedroom, carefully assessing the scene.

As you and Captain Walls enter the bedroom, you find a patient who appears to be in her early 60s sitting on the edge of the bed in a tripod position. Captain Walls asks, "What seems to be the problem today?" She looks as if she is gasping for air, so Captain Walls quickly asks her if she is having trouble breathing. She nods her head indicating yes. You ask her name. She states very quickly with a gasp, "Mrs. Springer." Mrs. Springer seems very agitated, restless, and even somewhat confused by your presence. There are no stridorous or crowing sounds with inhalation or exhalation. Captain Walls indicates that the rate of Mrs. Springer's breathing is rapid at approximately 30 per minute. He also notes that her chest appears to be rising and falling, but little air is felt flowing from her mouth and nose, and she is using accessory muscles to breathe. You assess the radial pulse and find a strong, regular pulse. The skin is pale, cool, and clammy. A quick look at the patient's nail beds reveals a bluish gray color. You quickly apply the pulse oximeter, which provides an SpO_2 reading of 86% on room air. You place a nonrebreather mask on Mrs. Springer and set the liter flow to 15 lpm.

Captain Walls gives you a look that you recognize as meaning this is a priority call. He then calls for ALS backup. You reassess Mrs. Springer's mental status. She is now only responding to your verbal command to open her eyes with incomprehensible mumbling. Captain Walls sets up the cot as you proceed with the rapid secondary assessment. Her pupils are sluggish to respond to light and are slightly dilated. The area around her nose and mouth is cyanotic along with her oral mucosa. You find no jugular venous distention, tracheal tugging, or subcutaneous emphysema to the neck. You quickly inspect and palpate the chest and find no evidence of trauma or scars. Auscultation reveals a bubbly sound produced during inhalation in the lower lobes of the lungs, with decreased breath sounds bilaterally. Her abdomen is soft and not tender. Her lower extremities do not show any edema. Her distal pulses are present in all four extremities. She does not obey your commands to wiggle her toes or grasp your fingers. You pinch each extremity, which causes Mrs. Springer to moan slightly. You do not note any edema to the small of the back in the lower lumbar area.

As Captain Walls is positioning the cot, you obtain a set of baseline vital signs. The blood pressure is 190/86; the heart rate is 124 beats per minute and irregular; the respiratory rate is 30 per minute and labored; the skin is pale, cool, and clammy; and the pupils remain dilated and sluggish to respond to light. The SpO_2 reading is now at 87%. As you are positioning Mrs. Springer, you note that her chest is barely rising and falling. You quickly assess her breathing and find very little air movement. You immediately begin to ventilate her with a BVM device. You ask Captain Walls to connect the BVM device to oxygen at 15 lpm. You position the stretcher next to the bed and place the patient on the cot in a supine position as you continue to ventilate at 12 times per minute. With the patient continuously receiving positive pressure ventilation, you enlist the help of a First Responder at the scene to load the patient into the ambulance. As Captain Walls prepares for immediate transport to the medical facility, the ALS crew arrives. The paramedic climbs into the back of the unit and begins to provide ALS care.

A family member drives up to the scene and tells Captain Walls that she is Mrs. Springer's daughter. The daughter is placed in the front seat of the ambulance, and Captain Walls begins to collect a history from her. The daughter indicates that the patient is not under the care of a physician and takes no medications. She states that her mother has no known allergies. She notes that her mother called her earlier and stated she was cleaning the bathroom with a strong disinfectant cleaner. She said she didn't feel good and was going to lie down in bed. She called a little later and said that she was having trouble breathing while lying flat and that sitting upright on the edge of the bed made her breathing easier. The daughter denies that her mother complained of any other symptoms.

You conduct a reassessment and note the heart rate is 122 beats per minute and irregular. The breathing is 26 times a minute with better volume. The patient seems more relaxed and less aggravated.

She opens her eyes at your command. The pulse oximeter now indicates 98% SpO_2 with positive pressure ventilations. The blood pressure is 188/90, and the skin is warm and dry, without the bluish gray color.

The paramedic in the back of the ambulance indicates that she is ready for transport. Captain Walls pulls from the scene and heads toward the medical facility, which is three minutes away. You are beginning to perform another reassessment as Captain Walls indicates that you are at the emergency department.

1. Which of the following signs or symptoms did *not* contribute to the decision as to whether to provide positive pressure ventilation?
   a. SpO_2 of 86%
   b. Patient's age
   c. Agitation and restlessness
   d. Bluish gray color

2. The medical term used to describe the bluish gray color of the nail beds, which indicates severe hypoxia, is
   a. cyanosis.
   b. jaundice.
   c. flushed.
   d. urticaria.

3. The bubbly sound heard in the lower lung lobes with each inhalation while auscultating Mrs. Springer's chest is known as
   a. wheezing or stridor.
   b. rhonchi or sonorous.
   c. stridor or crowing.
   d. crackles or rales.

4. Captain Walls used the acronym OPQRST when questioning the patient's daughter. Mrs. Springer's daughter indicated that her mother's breathing became worse while lying flat. This is reported as which of the following?
   a. O—onset
   b. P—provocation
   c. Q—quality
   d. S—severity

EMERGENCY TRIP SHEET

TRIP #	
MEDIC #	
BEGIN MILES	
END MILES	
CODE___/___ PAGE___/___	
UNITS ON SCENE	

BILLING USE ONLY

DAY				
DATE				
RECEIVED				
DISPATCHED				
EN-ROUTE				
ON SCENE				
TO HOSPITAL				
AT HOSPITAL				
IN-SERVICE				

NAME _____ SEX M F DOB ___/___/___

ADDRESS _____ RACE

CITY _____ STATE _____ ZIP

PHONE ( )   -   PCP DR.

RESPONDED FROM _____ CITY

TAKEN FROM _____ ZIP

DESTINATION _____ REASON

SSN ___ - ___ - ___   MEDICARE # _____ MEDICAID #

INSURANCE CO ____ INSURANCE # ____ GROUP #

RESPONSIBLE PARTY ____ ADDRESS

CITY ____ STATE ____ ZIP ____ PHONE ( )   -

EMPLOYER

CREW	CERT	STATE #		

TIME	ON SCENE (1)	ON SCENE (2)	ON SCENE (3)	EN-ROUTE (1)	EN-ROUTE (2)	AT DESTINATION
BP						
PULSE						
RESP						
SpO$_2$						
ETCO$_2$						
EKG						

IV THERAPY

SUCCESSFUL Y N # OF ATTEMPTS _____
ANGIO SIZE _____ga.
SITE _____
TOTAL FLUID INFUSED _____ cc
BLOOD DRAW Y N INITIALS

INTUBATION INFORMATION

SUCCESSFUL Y N # OF ATTEMPTS _____
TUBE SIZE _____ mm
TIME _____ INITIALS _____

MEDICAL HISTORY

MEDICATIONS

ALLERGIES

C/C

EVENTS LEADING TO C/C

ASSESSMENT

TREATMENT

CONDITION CODES

TREATMENTS			
TIME	TREATMENT	DOSE	ROUTE

GCS E___ V___ M___ TOTAL =

GCS E___ V___ M___ TOTAL =

HOSPITAL CONTACTED

CPR BEGUN BY B P TIME BEGUN

AED USED Y N BY:

RESUSCITATION TERMINATED - TIME

EMS SIGNATURE

( ) OSHA REGULATIONS FOLLO

Cardiovascular Emergencies

CHAPTER

17

▌ STANDARD

Medicine (Content Area: Cardiovascular)

▌ COMPETENCY

Applies fundamental knowledge to provide basic emergency care and transportation based on assessment findings for an acutely ill patient.

▌ OBJECTIVES

After reading this chapter, you should be able to:

17-1. Define key terms introduced in this chapter.
17-2. Describe the relationship between chest pain or discomfort, heart disease, and cardiac arrest.
17-3. Describe the structure and function of the circulatory system, including:
   a. The cardiac conduction system
   b. Conductive tissue and conductivity
   c. Contractile tissue and contractility
   d. Automaticity
   e. Effects of the autonomic nervous system (sympathetic and parasympathetic) on the heart
   f. Gross anatomy of the heart
   g. Systemic and pulmonary circulation
   h. Coronary arteries
   i. Plasma and formed elements of the blood
17-4. Explain the relationship between electrical and mechanical events in the heart.
17-5. Describe the processes of depolarization and repolarization, and relate the waves and intervals of a normal electrocardiogram (ECG) to the physiological events they represent.
17-6. Discuss the relationship between hypoxia, damage to the cardiac conduction system, premature ventricular contractions, ventricular tachycardia, and ventricular fibrillation.
17-7. Describe the roles of the heart and blood vessels in maintaining normal blood pressure.
17-8. Explain the importance of early recognition of signs and symptoms and the early treatment of patients with cardiac emergencies.
17-9. Explain the pathophysiology and the appropriate assessment and management of the following conditions that may be classified as cardiac compromise or acute coronary syndrome:
   a. Angina pectoris
   b. Myocardial infarction

c. Aortic aneurysm or dissection
d. Congestive heart failure
e. Cardiogenic shock
f. Hypertensive emergencies
g. Cardiac arrest

17-10. Explain the typical presentation of myocardial ischemia or infarction in females.

17-11. Explain the indications, contraindications, forms, dosage, administration, actions, side effects, and reassessment for nitroglycerin.

17-12. Explain the special considerations in assessing and managing pediatric and geriatric patients with cardiac emergencies.

17-13. Explain the assessment-based approach to assessment and emergency medical care for cardiac compromise and acute coronary syndrome.

17-14. Discuss the indications and contraindications for percutaneous intervention (angioplasty) or fibrinolytic therapy in patients with cardiac emergencies.

17-15. Given a series of scenarios, demonstrate the assessment-based management of a variety of patients with cardiovascular emergencies including: Explain the indications, contraindications, forms, dosage, administration, actions, side effects, and reassessment for aspirin.

▌ KEY IDEAS

This chapter describes the assessment and emergency care of a patient suffering cardiovascular emergencies such as chest discomfort or pain and cardiac arrest.

■ Signs and symptoms of cardiac compromise and acute coronary syndromes may vary widely from patient to patient. However, chest discomfort or pain is the most common chief complaint and most important signal of patients suffering from an acute coronary syndrome.

■ All adult patients complaining of chest discomfort or pain should be treated as a cardiac emergency until proven otherwise.

■ Prehospital treatment by the EMT of the responsive patient suffering chest discomfort or pain should focus on airway and ventilation assessment and management application of the pulse oximiter and administration of oxygen to maintain a SpO_2 of 94% or greater, and transport—not on diagnosing the specific type of cardiac emergency that the patient is experiencing.

■ Not all patients experiencing chest discomfort or pain will go into cardiac arrest. If the patient does go into cardiac arrest, the EMT must be prepared to apply the automated external defibrillator (AED) and perform CPR rapidly.

■ The EMT can assist in fibrinolytic-therapy decision making by attaining answers to important questions that will determine if fibrinolytics are appropriate for the patient and promptly presenting the results to emergency department staff.

■ The female may present with different signs and symptoms from those of a male when experiencing a cardiac event.

■ The electrocardiogram (ECG or EKG) is a graphic representation of the heart's electrical activity and consists of the P wave, the QRS complex, and the T wave.

■ Conditions that are part of any acute coronary syndrome are *unstable angina* and *myocardial infarction* (heart attack).

■ Two types of life-threatening injuries that may occur to the aorta are an aortic aneurysm and aortic dissection. An aortic aneurysm occurs when a weakened section of the aortic wall, usually resulting from atherosclerosis, begins to dilate or balloon outward from the pressure exerted by the blood flowing through the vessel. An aortic dissection occurs when there is a tear in the inner lining of the aorta and blood enters the opening and causes separation of the layers of the aortic wall.

■ Heart failure can be categorized as *left ventricular failure* or *right ventricular failure*. The signs and symptoms of heart failure depend on the severity of the condition and whether it is an acute-onset or a long-term problem.

- A hypertensive emergency is defined as a severe, accelerated hypertension episode with a systolic pressure greater than 160 mmHg and/or a diastolic blood pressure greater than 94 mmHg.
- Cardiac arrest is the worst manifestation of cardiac compromise from an acute coronary event. It occurs when the heart, for any of a variety of reasons, is not pumping effectively or at all, and no pulses can be felt.

MEDICAL TERMINOLOGY

Term	Prefix	Word Root Combining Form	Suffix	Definition
angina pectoris (an-JYE-nah PEC-toris)		angina (to choke); pector (chest)		A symptom commonly associated with coronary artery disease
atherosclerosis (ath-ER-oh-skleh-roh-sis)		athero (fatty substance); sclera (hardening)	-osis (condition of)	Narrowing of arteries from fatty substances being deposited on the inner surface of the artery
atria (AY-tre-uh)		atri (atrium, entrance room)		The two upper chambers of the heart
arteriole (ar-TEER-e-ol)		arter (artery, road, channel)	-ole (small)	Smallest artery, leading to a capillary
arteriosclerosis (ar-TEER-e-oh-skleh-roh-sis)		arter (artery, road, channel); sclera (hardening)	-osis (condition of)	A condition that causes the arteries to become stiff and less elastic
artery (AR-tuh-re)		arter (artery, road, channel)		Blood vessel that carries blood away from the heart
capillary (KAP-uh-lair-e)		capillaries (hairlike)		Tiny blood vessel connecting to venules; site for gas and nutrient exchange
dysrhythmia (dis-RYTH-me-ah)	dys (bad, difficult, painful)	rhyth (rhythm)	-ia (condition of)	An abnormal rhythm of the heart
myocardial infarction (my-oh-CAR-dee-al in-FARC-shun)		myo (muscle); card (heart); infarct (necrosis of an area)	-ion (process)	Occurs when a portion of the heart muscle dies because of the lack of an adequate supply of oxygenated blood
perfusion (per-FU-zhun)	per- (through)	fus (pour)	-ion (process)	Delivery of oxygen and nutrients to the body cells and removal of wastes by blood flowing through the capillaries
pulmonary artery (PUL-mun-air-e AR-tuh-re)		pulmo (lung); artery	-ary (pertaining to)	Vessel carrying oxygen-depleted blood from the heart's right ventricle to the lungs
pulmonary vein (PUL-mun-air-e vane)		pulmo (lung); vein	-ary (pertaining to)	Vessel carrying oxygen-rich blood from the lungs to the left atrium of the heart
vein (vane)		ven (vein)		Vessel that carries blood toward the heart
ventricles (VEN-trik-ulz)		ventriculus (little belly, small cavity)		The two lower chambers of the heart

1. In each space, write the word form that matches the given definition. Not all terms will be used.

arter   card   ion   pulmo

ary   fus   myo   ven

atri   infarct   per   ventriculus

_____ a. Through

_____ b. Atrium

_____ c. Pour

_____ d. Artery

_____ e. Process

_____ f. Pertaining to

_____ g. Vein

_____ h. Small cavity

_____ i. Necrosis of an area

_____ j. Muscle

_____ k. Heart

TERMS AND CONCEPTS

1. Write the number of the correct term next to each definition. Not all terms will be used.

1. Arteriole
2. Atria
3. Capillary
4. Cardiac conduction system
5. Coronary arteries
6. Pulmonary vein
7. Valves
8. Venae cavae
9. Ventricles
10. Venule

_____ a. The two upper chambers of the heart

_____ b. Membranes located within the heart to prevent backflow of blood

_____ c. Two lower chambers of the heart

_____ d. Vessel carrying oxygen-rich blood from the lungs to the left atrium of the heart

_____ e. The smallest vein

_____ f. The two major veins that carry oxygen-depleted blood back to the heart

_____ g. Specialized contractile and conductive tissue of the heart that generates electrical impulses and causes the heart to beat

_____ h. Network of arteries that supply the heart with blood

_____ i. The smallest artery

CONTENT REVIEW

1. On the appropriate line, identify each structure of the circulatory system.

   Alveoli   Lung capillaries

   Arteries   Pulmonary artery

   Arterioles   Pulmonary vein

   Body capillaries   Veins

   Bronchi   Venules

   A. _____

   B. _____

   C. _____

   D. _____

   E. _____

   F. _____

   G. _____

   H. _____

   I. _____

   J. _____

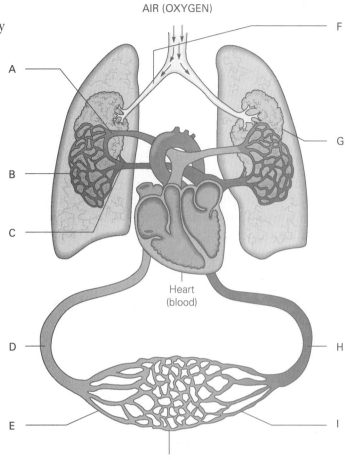

2. The three components of the circulatory system are the
   a. liver, kidneys, and blood.
   b. heart, blood vessels, and blood.
   c. heart, lungs, and blood.
   d. liver, lungs, and heart.

3. Hypoperfusion resulting from nervous system interference
   a. creates a vascular system that is too small for the amount of available blood.
   b. is only a theoretical consideration and never occurs in a clinical situation.
   c. creates a vascular system that is too large for the amount of available blood.
   d. directly affects the normal pumping action of the heart.

4. Which is the proper sequence for the primary assessment of the responsive cardiac patient who is suffering chest discomfort or pain?
   a. Assess circulation, breathing, airway, skin, and oxygenation.
   b. Assess airway, breathing, oxygenation, circulation, and skin.
   c. Assess breathing, circulation, airway, oxygenation, and skin.
   d. Assess oxygenation, skin, airway, breathing, and circulation.

5. Oxygen administration to a patient with acute coronary syndrome
   a. should be administered in high concentrations via a nonrebreathing face mask.
   b. should be administered in high concentrations via a nasal cannula.
   c. can be detrimental if administered in high concentrations.
   d. reduces the effects of reperfusion syndrome.

6. Using the OPQRST questions to evaluate the history of the present illness, the question "On a scale of 1 to 10, how would you rate your discomfort or pain?" is an example of which of the following?
   a. Onset
   b. Quality
   c. Severity
   d. Provocation

7. Some acute coronary syndrome patients, such as those suffering a heart attack, may not follow a typical pattern of signs and symptoms. This atypical pattern is known as
   a. a suspicious heart attack.
   b. an unconfirmed heart attack.
   c. an invalid heart attack.
   d. a silent heart attack.

8. Nitroglycerin in spray or tablet form is administered by what route?
   a. Sublingual
   b. Topical
   c. Intravenous
   d. Intramuscular

9. Which statement is a contraindication for the administration of nitroglycerin?
   a. The patient has signs and symptoms of chest discomfort.
   b. The patient's systolic blood pressure is below 100 mmHg.
   c. The patient's systolic blood pressure is 10 mmHg lower than the baseline reading.
   d. The patient has extreme bradycardia.

10. Which is correct regarding managing a patient with acute myocardial infarction (AMI) or a patient with heart failure?
    a. The EMT must be able to diagnose what condition is causing the signs/symptoms.
    b. The EMT's assessment and care will be the same regardless of the cause of the patient's signs/symptoms.
    c. The EMT will administer nitroglycerin only to patients known to be suffering from angina pectoris.
    d. The EMT needs to know which condition is likely to deteriorate into cardiac arrest.

11. While preparing to administer nitroglycerin spray to your patient experiencing chest pain, he states that he takes Viagra. What should you do?
    a. Do not administer nitroglycerin, and contact medical direction for orders.
    b. Administer the first nitroglycerin spray and reevaluate the patient.
    c. Double the dose of nitroglycerin, then contact medical direction.
    d. Reduce the nitroglycerin dose by half and reevaluate the patient.

12. The primary contributing factor to coronary artery disease is
    a. aortic dissection.
    b. lactic acid formation.
    c. peripheral vasodilation.
    d. atherosclerosis.

13. Which of the following most accurately states the factors that affect the signs, symptoms, and severity of acute coronary syndrome?
    a. The patient's resting pulse rate, the artery occluded, how much blood the coronary artery supplies to the heart, and the size or portion of the heart muscle not being supplied with oxygenated blood
    b. The site of the occlusion, the artery occluded, how much blood the occluded coronary artery supplies to the heart, the size or portion of the heart muscle not being supplied with oxygenated blood, and the length of time the artery has been occluded
    c. The patient's resting pulse rate, the patient's resting blood pressure, the artery occluded, how much blood the coronary artery supplies to the heart, and the size or portion of the heart muscle not being supplied with oxygenated blood
    d. The patient's resting pulse rate, the patient's resting blood pressure, the size or portion of the heart muscle not being supplied with oxygenated blood, and the length of time the artery has been occluded

14. Which statement is correct relating to cardiac compromise?
    a. Time is not an important consideration.
    b. Early recognition is not an important factor relating to patient survival.
    c. Heart muscle cell death is reversible.
    d. Some patients may be eligible for drugs or mechanical therapy that will restore blood flow.

15. Angina pectoris
    a. is infrequently associated with coronary artery disease.
    b. typically occurs when a decreased workload is placed on the heart.
    c. most commonly will last from two to five minutes.
    d. is a symptom of inadequate blood supply to the heart muscle.

16. The signs and symptoms of angina pectoris may include
    a. steady discomfort in the lower abdomen.
    b. chest pain or discomfort that lasts longer than 20 minutes.
    c. nausea and/or vomiting.
    d. numbness or tingling of the lips.

17. Appropriate emergency medical care for angina pectoris includes
    a. administering a patient's prescribed nitroglycerin.
    b. establishing an open airway and administering aspirin at 650 mg.
    c. applying the pulse oximeter when en route to the hospital.
    d. administering a patient's prescribed metered-dose inhaler.

18. An AMI
    a. most frequently is the result of a coronary artery spasm.
    b. occurs when a portion of the heart muscle dies.
    c. is commonly known as Graves' disease.
    d. will cause heart muscle death within two to five minutes.

19. In the patient suffering from AMI,
    a. ventricular fibrillation infrequently results in cardiac arrest.
    b. ventricular fibrillation usually occurs within the first four hours.
    c. thrombolytic drugs will reverse heart muscle damage.
    d. ischemic heart tissue can cause dysrhythmias.

20. Complete the chart by indicating if the sign or symptom is most likely associated with angina pectoris, AMI, or heart failure. Indicate with a check mark if the item is a common sign or symptom. One, two, or three check marks may be used for each sign or symptom.

Signs/Symptoms	Angina Pectoris	AMI	Heart Failure
Steady discomfort usually located in the center of the chest, but may be more diffuse throughout the front of the chest			
Chest discomfort radiating to the jaw, arms, shoulders, or back			
Nausea or vomiting			
Severe dyspnea			
Cyanosis			
Anxiety			
Dyspnea			
Signs and symptoms of pulmonary edema			
Complaint of indigestion pain			
Distended neck veins—jugular vein distention (JVD) (late sign)			
Sense of impending doom			
Distended and soft, spongy abdomen			
Tachypnea			
Diaphoresis			
Discomfort usually described as pressure, tightness, or an aching, crushing, or heavy feeling			
Edema in the ankles, feet, and hands			
Light-headedness or dizziness			
Fatigue on any exertion			
Crackles and possibly wheezes on auscultation of the chest			
Tachycardia			
Weakness			
Upright position with legs, feet, arms, and hands dangling			
Decreased SpO_2 (oxygen saturation) reading			

21. Heart failure
    a. can be categorized as upper-chamber or lower-chamber failure.
    b. may be caused by hypoperfusion, kidney failure, or liver failure.
    c. seldom results in peripheral edema, or swelling of the extremities.
    d. results when blood is not adequately ejected from the ventricle.

22. Management of the heart failure patient with pulmonary edema
    a. is vastly different from treatment of the patient with an AMI.
    b. commonly results in a pneumothorax from positive pressure ventilation treatment.
    c. becomes more complicated if the patient is taking a "water pill."
    d. can result in drastic improvement following positive pressure ventilation.

23. The stage in which electrical charges of the heart muscle change from positive to negative and cause the heart muscle to contract is known as
    a. repolarization.
    b. depolarization.
    c. automaticity.
    d. conduction.

24. A normal ECG has stages that represent different activities in the normal heart cycle. Which of the following represents the second waveform, which signifies depolarization (contraction) of the ventricles of the heart?
    a. P wave
    b. PR interval
    c. QRS complex
    d. T wave

25. The T wave in a normal ECG represents which of the following?
    a. Repolarization, or relaxation, of the ventricles
    b. Depolarization, or contraction, of the atria
    c. Depolarization, or contraction, of the ventricles
    d. Repolarization, or relaxation, of the atria

26. From the following, choose the ECG interval that represents the time that it takes the heart's electrical impulses to travel from the atria to the ventricles.
    a. RR interval
    b. PR interval
    c. PP interval
    d. PS interval

27. The heart's primary pacemaker site that is located in the upper portion of the right atrium and is responsible for the generating impulses that trigger the rest of the heart to contract is known as the
    a. sinoatrial (SA) node.
    b. atrioventricular (AV) node.
    c. Purkinje fibers.
    d. aortic arch fibers.

28. The clinical state in which the left or right ventricle fails to pump enough blood to meet the demands of the body is
    a. cardiogenic shock.
    b. angina pectoris.
    c. AMI.
    d. acute coronary syndrome.

29. Which of the following is a contraindication to the administration of any additional nitroglycerin?
    a. A systolic blood pressure of 100 mmHg, or 20 mmHg less than the patient's baseline systolic blood pressure
    b. A diastolic blood pressure of 90 mmHg, or 10 mmHg greater than the patient's baseline diastolic blood pressure
    c. A systolic blood pressure of 90 mmHg, or 30 mmHg less than the patient's baseline systolic blood pressure
    d. A diastolic blood pressure of 90 mmHg, or 40 mmHg greater than the patient's baseline diastolic blood pressure

30. Which of the following is NOT an absolute contraindication for fibrinolytic therapy?
    a. Closed head trauma
    b. Prolonged history of arthritis
    c. Prior history of intracranial hemorrhage
    d. Suspected aortic dissection

❙ CASE STUDY

You and your partner, Sprenger, are dispatched to 86 North Broadway Street, a residence where there is a report of an elderly man having a heart attack. You are met at the door by the patient's wife, and she thanks you for your prompt response. She leads you to the back porch, where you find her husband sitting, clutching his chest. You introduce yourselves, and the patient says his name is Devin Harley. A quick visual assessment reveals that the patient is pale, moderately short of breath, and very anxious.

1. You instruct Sprenger to place Mr. Harley on oxygen. Which is the most appropriate means of delivering the oxygen?
    a. The patient's own home oxygen apparatus
    b. Administer via nasal cannula to maintain an SpO_2 of 94%
    c. Nonrebreather mask at 15 lpm
    d. Positive pressure ventilation with supplemental oxygen

As you perform the primary assessment, you note that Mr. Harley's radial pulse is very weak and irregular. You compare his radial pulse with the carotid pulse and find that the carotid is strong, but both are irregular.

2. On the basis of the information you gathered on arrival plus this additional information, you determine that
    a. Mr. Harley is experiencing cardiac compromise; however, early transport is not necessary.
    b. Mr. Harley is experiencing cardiac compromise, and early transport is necessary.
    c. Mr. Harley is not experiencing cardiac compromise; however, early transport is necessary.
    d. Mr. Harley is not experiencing cardiac compromise, and early transport is not necessary.

Mr. Harley states the only medicine that his physician prescribes for him is an aspirin a day and nitroglycerin for chest pain. You ask Mr. Harley if he took any nitroglycerin with this episode of chest discomfort. He states, "One about five minutes before you arrived, but the pain is getting worse." You reassure Mr. Harley as you quickly obtain the vital signs, which are pulse 70 per minute, weak and irregular; respirations 24 per minute; BP 152/74; SpO_2 of 94%. His skin is slightly pale and sweaty. Pupils are normal. You call medical direction for permission to administer additional nitroglycerin. Permission is granted by Dr. Heltman for a total of three doses, including the dose Mr. Harley has already taken, so long as the patient's blood pressure is stable.

3. Shortly after you administer sublingual nitroglycerin spray, Mr. Harley complains of a headache. You should
   a. reassure him that this is a common side effect and the pain should pass.
   b. immediately remove the tablet; the headache indicates an allergic response.
   c. have him swallow the tablet; this will speed its absorption.
   d. reestablish contact with medical direction to ask for direction.

4. Mr. Harley's chest discomfort has improved dramatically. Since the crisis appears to be over, you should
   a. relax and complete the medical report.
   b. continue to evaluate him en route to the emergency department and update the receiving emergency department of any changes.
   c. administer the third nitroglycerin tablet to increase the therapeutic level.
   d. contact medical direction for permission to administer an aspirin to reduce the chest discomfort.

CHAPTER 17 SCENARIO: DOCUMENTATION EXERCISE

Read the following scenario and think about how you would document this call if you were the EMT who responded to the scene. Then answer the multiple-choice questions and fill in the sample prehospital care report, basing your documentation on information from the scenario.

It is 6:00 P.M. on a Saturday afternoon. You and your partner, Nancy, are on the way to a local grocery store to pick up some items for supper when dispatch calls: "Squad 1220, respond to 1061 Black Key Road, cross street Chulahoma Avenue, for a 65-year-old male patient with chest discomfort." You advise dispatch that you are responding to the call.

In about five minutes, you arrive on the scene. It is a residential area of small apartments and mobile homes. You ring the doorbell of a small but tidy mobile home and wait for an answer. A woman who appears to be in her mid-60s answers the door. With Standard Precautions taken, you and Nancy enter. You introduce yourself and your partner, and ask, "What's the problem today?" As you are walking toward a back bedroom, she tells you that her husband, Mr. Auerbach, has been complaining of severe indigestion.

You enter the room and observe Mr. Auerbach sitting up in bed with a balled fist against the center of his chest. His opposite hand clasps his fist. His eyes are open and he glances at you as you enter the room. His skin looks blue, and you notice copious amounts of sweat on his forehead. He seems to be restless as he rocks back and forth in bed. He is breathing adequately, with no audible, abnormal respiratory sounds.

You begin your assessment by introducing yourselves and saying, "We're EMTs and we're here to help you. What's the problem today?" Mr. Auerbach replies, "My chest hurts!" You place the AED next to the patient. You have a nasal cannula and oxygen prepared, and you place it on Mr. Auerbach. You adjust the flow rate to 2 lpm. You assess the radial pulse. It appears to be rapid at a rate of approximately 120 beats per minute, and Mr. Auerbach's skin is cool and clammy.

Nancy quickly begins to take the vital signs as you begin a secondary assessment and physical exam. You ask, "When did the pain start? What were you doing when it started? Did it start all of a sudden?" Mr. Auerbach replies, "I was sitting here reading the newspaper, and it started all of a sudden. It was about an hour ago when it started. You guys gotta help me. It really hurts!" You quickly say, "We're doing everything we can for you, and to help you, we need to ask you some additional questions." Nancy finishes taking Mr. Auerbach's pulse. She tells you it is 120, regular and strong. His skin is cool, clammy, and cyanotic. Nancy places the pulse oximeter, and you note that his SpO$_2$ is 94%.

Given the information you have gained, ALS backup is required, and you quickly advise dispatch of the need. Nancy continues with the vital signs while you continue with the secondary assessment and physical exam. You ask Mr. Auerbach, "Does anything make the discomfort better or worse?" He says, "No, it just hurts. I can't make it go away! Nothing seems to help it!" You ask him, "Can you describe the discomfort you are having? Is it sharp

© 2014 by Pearson Education, Inc.

CHAPTER 17 Cardiovascular Emergencies **169**

or dull, pressing or squeezing? What does it feel like?" He says, "It feels like someone is sitting on my chest. I don't really know how else to describe it." Nancy states that the patient's respirations are 18 per minute, full and regular, and that the breath sounds are clear and equal bilaterally. You continue your assessment by inquiring, "Does this discomfort you are experiencing move or radiate to any other part of your body?" He replies, "You know . . . now that you said that, it does. It hurts in my shoulder and left arm—the inside part of my left arm." You ask Mr. Auerbach if the oxygen is helping him. "Well, yes, it does seem to be helping me," he replies.

Mrs. Auerbach is standing in the corner and appears to be disturbed by the activities taking place in her bedroom. You place your hand on her shoulder and speak to her softly. "Mrs. Auerbach, we are doing everything we can right now. Could you please help us by getting any medications together that Mr. Auerbach is currently taking and bring them to me?" She says, "Yes, yes. I am so worried about him. You know he is all I have. I'll get the medications together for you." Mrs. Auerbach heads toward the bathroom.

Nancy tells you the blood pressure is 180/90, and the pupils are equal and reactive. You look at Mr. Auerbach's neck veins, and they appear flat. His abdomen is distended and nontender, and you note no palpable masses. You don't see any swelling in his lower extremities or back region. Nancy finishes the vital signs. You ask her to bring the cot into the house as you continue your secondary assessment and physical exam. "Mr. Auerbach, have you ever had any discomfort like this before?" You wait for his response. "No, I don't think I have," he states. "On a scale of 1–10, with 10 being the worst discomfort you have ever had, how would you rate your current discomfort?" you ask. He replies, "It's at least a 9 or a 10. It really hurts." Next, you ask, "Mr. Auerbach, when did this start? I know you told me about an hour ago. It's 6:05 P.M. now so it started about 5:00 P.M., right?" He responds by saying, "No, it really started about 4:30 this afternoon."

Mrs. Auerbach returns to the room with her husband's medications. The only medication he is taking is an over-the-counter medication for arthritis. You ask Mr. Auerbach if he is allergic to any medications, and he shakes his head no. You ask if he is allergic to aspirin. He shakes his head no again. You ask him to chew a baby aspirin and then swallow a second 160-mg tablet.

A knock on the door is followed by the voice of Paramedic Carney. She enters the room. You introduce Mr. Auerbach to Paramedic Carney and provide a brief report. You help Paramedic Carney and her partner move Mr. Auerbach to the front of the mobile home and into the ALS vehicle.

1. Mr. Auerbach is most likely suffering from
   a. angina pectoris.
   b. AMI.
   c. congestive heart failure.
   d. acute hypertension.

2. What physical findings or information suggests that Mr. Auerbach's condition is critical and requires ALS assistance?
   a. His abdominal distention
   b. His respiratory rate of 18 per minute
   c. The timing of his chest discomfort
   d. His mental status

3. Mr. Auerbach's clenched fist positioned over the center of his chest is called _____ sign.
   a. Wilson's
   b. Orchid's
   c. Levine's
   d. Cardiac's

4. The use of the AED on Mr. Auerbach is
   a. appropriate and should have been placed during the primary assessment.
   b. appropriate and should have been placed following obtaining the vital signs.
   c. inappropriate unless he becomes unresponsive.
   d. inappropriate; the AED should not have been taken from the vehicle.

5. The method used for assessing the patient's chest discomfort is referred to as the _____ method.
   a. cardiac history
   b. referral
   c. OPQRST
   d. summary

EMERGENCY TRIP SHEET

TRIP #	
MEDIC #	
BEGIN MILES	
END MILES	
CODE___/___ PAGE___/___	
UNITS ON SCENE	

BILLING USE ONLY				
DAY				
DATE				
RECEIVED				
DISPATCHED				
EN-ROUTE				
ON SCENE				
TO HOSPITAL				
AT HOSPITAL				
IN-SERVICE				

NAME   SEX   M   F   DOB ___/___/___

ADDRESS   RACE

CITY   STATE   ZIP

PHONE ( )   -   PCP DR.

RESPONDED FROM   CITY

TAKEN FROM   ZIP

DESTINATION   REASON

SSN   -   -   MEDICARE #   MEDICAID #

INSURANCE CO   INSURANCE #   GROUP #

RESPONSIBLE PARTY   ADDRESS

CITY   STATE   ZIP   PHONE ( )   -

EMPLOYER

CREW	CERT	STATE #

TIME	ON SCENE (1)	ON SCENE (2)	ON SCENE (3)	EN-ROUTE (1)	EN-ROUTE (2)	AT DESTINATION
BP						
PULSE						
RESP						
SpO_2						
$ETCO_2$						
EKG						

IV THERAPY
SUCCESSFUL   Y   N   # OF ATTEMPTS _____
ANGIO SIZE _____ ga.
SITE _____
TOTAL FLUID INFUSED _____ cc
BLOOD DRAW   Y   N   INITIALS

INTUBATION INFORMATION
SUCCESSFUL   Y   N   # OF ATTEMPTS _____
TUBE SIZE _____ mm
TIME _____ INITIALS _____

MEDICAL HISTORY

CONDITION CODES

TREATMENTS

MEDICATIONS

TIME	TREATMENT	DOSE	ROUTE	INIT

ALLERGIES

C/C

EVENTS LEADING TO C/C

ASSESSMENT

TREATMENT

GCS   E___ V___ M___ TOTAL =

GCS   E___ V___ M___ TOTAL =

HOSPITAL CONTACTED

CPR BEGUN BY   B   P   TIME BEGUN

EMS SIGNATURE

AED USED   Y   N   BY:

RESUSCITATION TERMINATED - TIME

( ) OSHA REGULATIONS FOLLOWED

Altered Mental Status, Stroke, and Headache

STANDARD

Medicine (Content Area: Neurology)

COMPETENCY

Applies fundamental knowledge to provide basic emergency care and transportation based on assessment findings for an acutely ill patient.

OBJECTIVES

After reading this chapter, you should be able to:

18-1. Define key terms introduced in this chapter.

18-2. List possible structural, toxic-metabolic, and other causes of altered mental status.

18-3. Describe an assessment-based approach to altered mental status. Obtain information.

18-4. Explain the reason for paying particular attention to airway assessment and management in patients with altered mental status.

18-5. List signs and symptoms of altered mental status commonly associated with:
   a. Trauma
   b. Nontraumatic or medical conditions

18-6. Determine the need for the following interventions in patients with altered mental status:
   a. Manual spinal stabilization
   b. Opening and maintaining the airway
   c. Oxygenation
   d. Ventilation
   e. Positioning
   f. Transport

18-7. Explain the responsibilities of the general public and EMS in the care for a stroke patient that are identified by the American Heart Association as "Detection," "Dispatch," and "Delivery."

18-8. Describe the pathophysiology of stroke and distinguish between ischemic strokes and hemorrhagic strokes.

18-9. Describe the relationship between stroke and transient ischemic attack.

18-10. Describe an assessment-based approach to stroke and transient ischemic attack.

18-11. Discuss the use of the Cincinnati Prehospital Stroke Scale and the Los Angeles Prehospital Stroke Screen.

18-12. Discuss the role of blood glucose determination in the assessment of patients with altered mental status and neurological deficits.

18-13. Describe ways of communicating with patients who have difficulty speaking.

18-14. Recognize indications that a headache may have a potentially life-threatening underlying cause, such as toxic exposure, hypertension, infectious disease, or hemorrhagic stroke.

18-15. Describe the appropriate emergency medical care for a patient suffering from headache.

▌ KEY IDEAS

An altered mental status may sometimes be accompanied by a loss of speech, sensory, or motor function. This chapter focuses on the assessment and management of patients with these signs.

■ An altered mental status with loss of function may be caused by external trauma or by a nontraumatic brain injury, such as that caused by stroke.

■ It is important to monitor and manage closely the airway and breathing of the patient who is suffering an altered mental status with loss of speech, sensory, and motor function.

▌ MEDICAL TERMINOLOGY

Term	Prefix	Word Root Combining Form	Suffix	Definition
aphagia (ah-FAY-juh)	a- (lack of)	phag (to eat, engulf)	-ia (condition of)	Lack of the ability to eat or swallow
aphasia (ah-FAY-zhuh)	a- (no, not, without, lack of)	phas (to speak)	-ia (condition of)	Lack of the ability to speak
atherosclerosis (ath-uh-roh-skluh-RO-sis)		ather/o (fatty substance, porridge); scler (hardening)	-osis (condition of)	Condition of hardening of the arteries caused by fatty deposits that progress to calcified plaque
dysphagia (dis-FAY-juh)	dys- (bad, difficult, painful)	phag (to eat, engulf)	-ia (condition of)	Difficulty in eating or swallowing
dysphasia (dis-FAY-zhuh)	dys- (bad, difficult, painful)	phas (to speak)	-ia (condition of)	Difficulty in speaking
embolism (EM-boh-lizm)		embol (to cast, to throw)	-ism (condition of)	Condition in which a blood clot obstructs a blood vessel
hemiparesis (hem-ee-puh-REE-sis)	hemi- (half)		-paresis (weakness)	Slight paralysis or weakness that affects one side of the body
hemiplegia (hem-ee-PLEE-juh)	hemi- (half)		-plegia (paralysis, stroke)	Paralysis that affects half of the body
monoplegia (mon-oh-PLEE-juh)	mono- (one)		-plegia (paralysis, stroke)	Paralysis that affects only one extremity

paraplegia (pair-uh-PLEE-juh)	para- (beside, alongside, abnormal)		-plegia (paralysis, stroke)	Paralysis of both legs or the lower portion of the body
quadriplegia (kwahd-ruh-PLEE-juh)	quadri- (four)		-plegia (paralysis, stroke)	Paralysis in all four extremities
subarachnoid (sub-ah-RAK-noyd)	sub- (below, under, beneath)	arachn/e (spider)	-oid (resemble, form)	Below the arachnoid membrane; between the arachnoid membrane and the pia mater
thrombosis (throm-BOH-sis)		thromb (clot of blood)	-osis (condition of)	Condition in which there is a blood clot within the vascular system

1. The medical term *aphasia* contains the word root *phas*, which means
   a. without.
   b. paralysis.
   c. to eat, hunger.
   d. to speak.

2. *Dysphagia*, a medical term, contains the prefix *dys-*, which means
   a. down, away from.
   b. bad, difficult, painful.
   c. through, between.
   d. apart, separate.

3. The medical term *atherosclerosis* includes the word root *scler*, which means
   a. spine.
   b. narrowing.
   c. shoulder.
   d. hardening.

4. Your patient has a history of hemiparesis. The prefix *hemi-* means
   a. half.
   b. water.
   c. different.
   d. below, under.

5. The medical term *quadriplegia* includes the suffix *-plegia*, which refers to
   a. weakness.
   b. paralysis, stroke.
   c. surgical repair.
   d. formation.

TERMS AND CONCEPTS

1. Write the number of the correct term next to each definition.

   1. Neurological deficit
   2. Nontraumatic brain injury
   3. Stroke
   4. Transient ischemic attacks (TIAs)

   _____ a. Brief, intermittent episodes with strokelike symptoms that typically disappear within 10 to 15 minutes and resolve within 24 hours

   _____ b. A medical injury to the brain, such as a stroke, that is not caused by an external injury

   _____ c. Any deficiency in the brain's functioning

   _____ d. A sudden disruption in blood flow to the brain that results in brain cell damage

CONTENT REVIEW

1. Which of the following is a sign or symptom of neurological deficit?
   a. Slurred speech
   b. Substernal chest pain
   c. Hypoglycemia
   d. Hypotension

2. One kind of nontraumatic (medical) brain injury is a stroke. Using the illustrations as your guide, choose possible causes of a stroke from the following list.
   1. Rupture of a blood vessel in the brain
   2. Blockage of a blood vessel in the brain
   3. Laceration of the carotid artery
   4. Dilation of the blood vessels in the brain

   a. 1 and 2
   b. 3 and 4
   c. 2 and 3
   d. 1 and 4

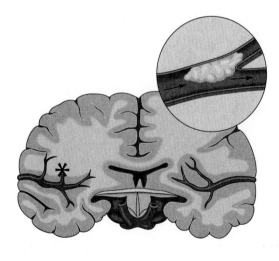 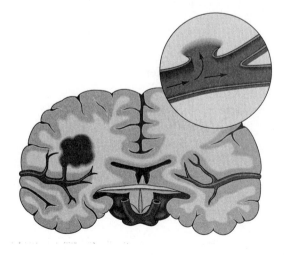

3. Which of the following is a common risk factor of hemorrhagic strokes?
   a. Hypoglycemia
   b. Chronic hypertension
   c. Alcoholism
   d. Chronic asthma

4. An ischemic stroke is one in which an inadequate amount of blood is being delivered to a portion of the brain due to a blood clot. The ischemic stroke is also known as a
   a. brain bleed.
   b. brain attack.
   c. brain accident.
   d. brain incident.

5. Which of the following signs and symptoms is a rare finding in the stroke patient?
   a. Hypertension
   b. Hemiplegia
   c. Hypotension
   d. Hemiparesis

6. A stroke that results from a piece of plaque or other substance that breaks off from inside a vessel or the heart and travels into the brain, becoming lodged in a cerebral vessel and cutting off circulation to the brain tissue, is known as
   a. acute stroke.
   b. embolic stroke.
   c. hemorrhagic stroke.
   d. systemic stroke.

7. Which of the following is a likely sign or symptom of stroke?
   a. Hemiparesis of the right arm and foot
   b. Paralysis to both right and left legs
   c. Bilateral paralysis of right and left arms
   d. Substernal nonradiating chest pain

8. You are treating an alert patient who you suspect suffered a stroke. The patient's breathing has become faster than normal with a decreased tidal volume; the SpO_2 is 93%. You should
   a. administer positive pressure ventilation with supplemental oxygen.
   b. administer oxygen via nonrebreather mask at 6 lpm.
   c. administer oxygen via nasal cannula 2 lpm to maintain an SpO_2 of 94% or greater.
   d. administer oxygen via a Venturi mask 6–12 lpm.

9. You are treating a patient with signs and symptoms of a stroke who is unresponsive. In which position is it most appropriate to place this patient?
   a. Supine position; legs elevated
   b. Supine position; head and chest elevated
   c. Lateral recumbent position
   d. Prone position with knees to the side

10. When using the Cincinnati Prehospital Stroke Scale to evaluate your patient, you know that an abnormal arm drift is defined as when, after the patient extends both arms with eyes closed,
    a. both arms drift downward together.
    b. both arms drift upward together.
    c. one arm drifts upward.
    d. one arm drifts downward.

11. Because the patient with a nontraumatic brain injury may deteriorate rapidly, you should frequently perform which of the following?
    a. A rapid physical assessment
    b. A focused trauma assessment
    c. A detailed physical exam
    d. A reassessment

12. Strokes most often affect elderly patients with certain kinds of medical history. Which of the following contributes to strokes?
    a. A history of heart disease
    b. A history of osteoporosis
    c. A history of diabetes
    d. A history of emphysema

13. Your patient has experienced the signs and symptoms of a TIA. However, he is feeling better and is refusing treatment. You must encourage the patient to be treated because
    a. approximately one-third of those who suffer a TIA will have a stroke.
    b. approximately one-half of those who suffer a TIA will have a heart attack.
    c. nearly all of the patients who suffer a TIA sustain permanent neurological deficit.
    d. nearly all of the patients who suffer a TIA experience electrolyte imbalances.

14. It is extremely important to recognize the signs and symptoms of a stroke early. Which of the following strongly suggests that your patient may be suffering from a stroke?
    a. The patient has dilated pupils that constrict equally when a light source is applied.
    b. The patient uses wrong words when repeating, "You can't teach an old dog new tricks."
    c. The patient presents with an elevated blood glucose level and pale, cool, diaphoretic skin.
    d. The patient experiences sudden and complete paralysis to the lower extremities.

15. You are assessing an elderly patient who appears to have suffered a stroke. Why is it important to determine if there is a history of diabetes?
    a. An elderly diabetic patient should not be given oxygen.
    b. An elderly stroke patient is likely to develop diabetes.
    c. Elderly hyperglycemic diabetics suffer more strokes than elderly nondiabetics.
    d. An elderly diabetic patient who is hypoglycemic may present with signs and symptoms similar to a stroke.

16. You suspect your patient is suffering from a stroke. What information is crucial to obtain from family or bystanders that will aid in proper treatment?
    a. When was the last meal consumed?
    b. Has the patient experienced a loss of time?
    c. Does the patient seem more agitated than normal?
    d. What was the time of onset of the symptoms?

17. Rapid transport of the stroke patient is critical because
    a. hyperventilation with a bag-valve mask (BVM) may be necessary.
    b. increased secretions may compromise the airway.
    c. the emergency department may be able to administer clot-dissolving drugs.
    d. the patient will likely become unresponsive to voice commands.

18. The type of stroke that occurs when the cerebral artery is blocked by a clot or other foreign matter is known as a(n)
    a. hemorrhagic stroke.
    b. ischemic stroke.
    c. hyperglycemic stroke.
    d. compression stroke.

19. The type of stroke that occurs from bleeding within the brain from a ruptured cerebral artery is known as a(n)
    a. hemorrhagic stroke.
    b. ischemic stroke.
    c. hyperglycemic stroke.
    d. compression stroke.

20. Which sign or symptom would you associate with the patient suffering from a hemorrhagic stroke?
    a. Gradual onset
    b. Rapidly improving mental status
    c. History of low blood pressure
    d. Severe headache

21. Which of the following statements best describes the thrombotic-type stroke?
    a. Usually presents with a severe headache
    b. Caused by narrowed arteries through a process called atherosclerosis
    c. Comes on suddenly and is the rarest of the stroke types
    d. Occurs after a blood clot lodges in the small arteries of the brain

22. Which of the following types of headaches usually presents with pain found only on one side of the head or face? The patient may also complain of excessive tear production on the side of the pain, nasal congestion, or a runny nose (rhinorrhea).
    a. Vascular headaches
    b. Cluster headaches
    c. Tension headaches
    d. Inflammatory headaches

23. Which type of headache is usually described as being "tight" or "viselike"? The pain usually occurs on both sides of the head and is described as throbbing, aching, squeezing, or forceful pressure.
    a. Vascular headache
    b. Cluster headache
    c. Inflammatory headache
    d. Tension headache

▍CASE STUDY

You and your partner, Lynn, are dispatched to an unknown medical problem in a high-rise apartment. You are met in the parking lot by a security guard, who directs you to the elevator. He says, "José, the other guard, is with the patient, Mrs. Peters, and he will meet you up there." José directs you to the bedroom, where you find an elderly female lying in bed. As you introduce yourself, the patient looks at you with a terrified glare. You reassure her and ask if she can understand you. She nods her head to indicate yes. The patient tries to communicate, but her speech is incomprehensible. Her feelings of frustration are obvious. You explain that you will ask "yes" or "no" questions, and she can reply by shaking or nodding her head.

1. Mrs. Peters's breathing is approximately 14 per minute, with good tidal volume. There are no signs of hypoxia, and the SpO_2 is 96% on room air. Which is most appropriate?
   a. Place her on oxygen at 15 lpm via a nonrebreather mask.
   b. Mrs. Peters's breathing is adequate, so there is no need for oxygen.
   c. Place her on oxygen at 2 to 4 lpm via nasal cannula.
   d. Administer positive pressure ventilation with supplemental oxygen.

Further interviewing reveals that Mrs. Peters's only medical history is hypertension. You notice significant facial drooping and paralysis to the right side of her body. Lynn suggests that the portable suction unit be set up and ready for immediate use. You agree. You prepare Mrs. Peters for transport, carefully protecting her paralyzed extremities so as not to injure them.

2. Briefly explain why the suction unit may be needed even though Mrs. Peters's airway is adequate.

As you and Lynn are transporting Mrs. Peters in the elevator, the patient grabs her head with her left hand. You ask her if she has a terrible headache. She nods yes, and then becomes unresponsive, and her breathing becomes inadequate at 8 breaths per minute.

3. With this change in the patient's status, which of the following is now most appropriate?
   a. Administer oxygen at 15 lpm via a nonrebreather mask.
   b. Administer positive pressure ventilation at 10 to 12 ventilations per minute with supplemental oxygen.
   c. Administer positive pressure ventilation at 20 ventilations per minute with supplemental oxygen.
   d. Administer positive pressure ventilation at greater than 24 ventilations per minute with supplemental oxygen.

▍CHAPTER 18 SCENARIO: DOCUMENTATION EXERCISE

Read the following scenario and think about how you would document this call if you were the EMT who responded to the scene. Then answer the multiple-choice questions and fill in the sample prehospital care report, basing your documentation on information from the scenario.

You and your partner, Cory, are attending an on-duty continuing education class when your portable radio sounds: "Unit 3 respond to 428 45th Street for a man in his 50s acting inappropriately." You and Cory walk briskly to the ambulance. You both check the map book to confirm the location, and then mark en route. After a short emergency response, you arrive on the scene of a modest single-family residence. You both put on protective gloves and eyewear and scan the area for any obvious hazards. As you are placing the equipment on your cot, a frantic woman meets you at the rear of the ambulance. She cries,

"Hurry! It's my husband, Brian. I think he's had a stroke." As you approach and enter the home, you again scan the area for possible hazards and note the best access and egress of the house.

As you and Cory enter the living room, you find an approximately 50-year-old man sitting on the floor leaning against the sofa. Cory asks, "What seems to be the problem today?" The patient responds in a muffled voice, "I don't know." You ask him his name and if he hurts anywhere. He responds with slurred speech, "My name is Brian, and I have a headache." You notice the airway is intact, with good air exchange at a rate of approximately 14 breaths per minute. Brian's face seems drawn down on the right side. His chest is rising and falling, with adequate air moving in and out of the mouth and nose and no use of accessory muscles. Cory quickly assesses the radial pulse and finds it strong and regular. The skin is warm and dry with no cyanosis noted. The pulse oximeter reveals a reading of 98% on room air.

You notify dispatch that this is a priority call and to send ALS backup immediately and notify the hospital emergency department of a possible stroke alert. You look at the patient and his wife and explain that you suspect a possible stroke. As you and Cory lift the patient from the floor and place him on the stretcher, you notice the patient is supporting his right arm by holding it with his left. You ask Cory to prepare the suction and BVM and place them nearby, ready for use if needed, while you begin to administer the Cincinnati Prehospital Stroke Scale. You ask Brian to look straight at you and smile, then show his teeth. The right side of his face droops downward. Next, you have the patient lift both arms outward and close his eyes and ask him to hold this position for 10 seconds. You notice his right arm drifts downward while the left remains in the outward position. Last, you ask Brian to repeat, "You can't teach an old dog new tricks." Brian repeats with a puzzled look on his face, "You train old sticks with new dogs." You can see that Brian is becoming frustrated.

While you are completing the Cincinnati Prehospital Stroke Scale, Cory positions the patient and proceeds with a rapid medical exam. You obtain a blood glucose level of 126 mg/dL with the glucometer. Cory shines a pocket penlight into Brian's eyes and remarks, "The left is midposition and reacts to light. The right is dilated and unreactive." He states, "Other than the facial droop, the face is unremarkable." There is no jugular vein distention (JVD), tracheal

tugging, or subcutaneous emphysema to the neck. He quickly exposes and palpates the chest and finds no evidence of trauma or scars. Auscultation reveals lung sounds that are clear bilaterally. The abdomen is soft and not tender. The lower extremities do not show edema, and distal pulses are felt in all four extremities. Cory notes that the right arm and leg both have no sensation to pain or movement, while the left arm and leg are both normal. There is no noted edema to the small of the back in the lumbar area.

You obtain a set of baseline vital signs. The blood pressure is 230/124; the heart rate is 88 beats per minute and regular; the respiratory rate is 16 per minute; the skin is pink, warm, and dry; and the pupils remain the same. The SpO_2 reading is 98%.

You advise Brian's wife that you will be transporting soon and will meet the ALS unit en route. Cory helps to load the patient into the ambulance and then seats Brian's wife in the front seat, ensuring that her seat belt is fastened. You quickly interview the wife to gain valuable information. You discover that Brian is 52 years of age, has a history of hypertension, and takes a multivitamin and high-blood-pressure medicine every day. He has no known drug allergies. She states he was watching his favorite team lose in the finals on television when he suddenly stood up from the couch and said he had a terrible headache. Shortly after, she noticed his speech was slurred and his face had drooped. You ask her exactly what time this was. She indicates it was 10 minutes before she called you. You contact dispatch to ascertain what time the call came in to dispatch. You add 10 minutes to the call time and document it, so as not to forget.

En route to the hospital, you meet ALS Medic Four. The paramedic steps into the rear of your ambulance, carrying her equipment. You recognize her as Lieutenant Meads. She introduces herself to the patient and his wife. As she gathers the report and prepares to provide advanced life support, you begin to perform a reassessment of the patient. You obtain the following vital signs: blood pressure 226/120, heart rate 80 beats per minute and regular, respiratory rate 16 per minute. The skin remains pink, warm, and dry. The pupils are unchanged. You ask the patient to describe the pain in his head, and he states, "It's the worst pain I've ever had, and it's all over my head." The patient remarks that his vision seems blurred. A few minutes later, Cory advises you that you have arrived at the emergency department.

1. What is the significance of the patient replying, "You train old sticks with new dogs"?
   a. This is a response that indicates a possible underlying diabetic condition.
   b. This response was normal. Many patients, under stress, confuse these words.
   c. This was a normal response according to the Los Angeles Prehospital Stroke Screen.
   d. This was an abnormal response according to the Cincinnati Prehospital Stroke Scale.

2. Why is it important to obtain a blood glucose level with the glucometer in a patient who you suspect is having a stroke?
   a. Symptoms of a diabetic emergency can mimic those of the stroke patient.
   b. Blood glucose levels in stroke patients can rapidly rise to dangerous levels.
   c. Ischemic strokes can be positively diagnosed by determining blood glucose level.
   d. The Cincinnati Prehospital Stroke Scale requires the collection of these data.

3. Proper positioning is very important when treating the stroke patient. You have determined that this patient can protect his own airway. In what position should you place this patient?
   a. Supine, with the head and chest elevated no more than 30 degrees
   b. Right lateral recumbent, with the head elevated 10 degrees
   c. Supine, with head lower than body 20 degrees
   d. Left lateral recumbent, with the head lower than the chest

4. This patient complained of a severe headache that came on suddenly. The signs and symptoms of stroke also developed rapidly. He has a history of hypertension treated with medication. All of these would lead you to believe that your patient is suffering from which of the following?
   a. Ischemic stroke
   b. Hemorrhagic stroke
   c. Transient ischemic stroke
   d. Progressive stroke

5. Why was it important to determine the exact time that the symptoms were first noticed?
   a. Onset time is important to determine if the patient is a candidate for surgery.
   b. The time elapsed from first symptoms corresponds to probable recovery time.
   c. Time of onset is crucial in determining if clot-dissolving drugs can be administered.
   d. Onset-to-treatment time helps hospital personnel determine how symptoms will progress.

EMERGENCY TRIP SHEET

TRIP #		BILLING USE ONLY			
MEDIC #		DAY			
BEGIN MILES		DATE			
MILES		RECEIVED			
CODE __/__	PAGE __/__	DISPATCHED			
UNITS ON SCENE					

NAME	SEX M F DOB __/__/__	EN-ROUTE
ADDRESS	RACE	ON SCENE
CITY	STATE	ZIP	TO HOSPITAL
PHONE ( ) -	PCP DR.	AT HOSPITAL
RESPONDED FROM	CITY	IN-SERVICE

TAKEN FROM	ZIP	CREW	CERT	STATE #
DESTINATION	REASON			
SSN - -	MEDICARE #	MEDICAID #		
INSURANCE CO	INSURANCE #	GROUP #		
RESPONSIBLE PARTY	ADDRESS			
CITY	STATE	ZIP	PHONE ( ) -	
EMPLOYER				

IV THERAPY
SUCCESSFUL Y N # OF ATTEMPTS _____
ANGIO SIZE _____ ga.
SITE _____
TOTAL FLUID INFUSED _____ cc
BLOOD DRAW Y N INITIALS

TIME	ON SCENE (1)	ON SCENE (2)	ON SCENE (3)	EN-ROUTE (1)	EN-ROUTE (2)	AT DESTINATION
BP						
PULSE						
RESP						
SpO$_2$						
ETCO$_2$						
EKG						

INTUBATION INFORMATION
SUCCESSFUL Y N # OF ATTEMPTS _____
TUBE SIZE _____ mm
TIME _____ INITIALS _____

MEDICAL HISTORY

CONDITION CODES

TREATMENTS

TIME	TREATMENT	DOSE	ROUTE	INIT

MEDICATIONS

ALLERGIES

C/C

EVENTS LEADING TO C/C

ASSESSMENT

TREATMENT

GCS E__ V__ M__ TOTAL =

GCS E__ V__ M__ TOTAL =

HOSPITAL CONTACTED

CPR BEGUN BY B P TIME BEGUN

EMS SIGNATURE

AED USED Y N BY:

RESUSCITATION TERMINATED - TIME

( ) OSHA REGULATIONS FOLLOWED

Seizures and Syncope

CHAPTER

19

▌ STANDARD

Medicine (Content Area: Neurology)

▌ COMPETENCY

Applies fundamental knowledge to provide basic emergency care and transportation based on assessment findings for an acutely ill patient.

▌ OBJECTIVES

After reading this chapter, you should be able to:

19-1. Define key terms introduced in this chapter.

19-2. Describe the various ways that seizures can present.

19-3. Discuss the pathophysiology of seizures.

19-4. Explain the concerns associated with prolonged or successive seizures.

19-5. Describe the assessment and emergency medical care of patients with tonic-clonic, simple partial, complex partial, absence, and febrile seizures.

19-6. Anticipate bystander reactions to patients having seizures and take measures to stop unnecessary or inappropriate interventions.

19-7. Describe the assessment and emergency medical care of patients in a postictal state.

19-8. Describe the assessment and emergency medical care of patients who are unresponsive, actively seizing, or in status epilepticus.

19-9. Recognize situations in which the patient who is having or has had a seizure must be a higher priority for transport.

19-10. Discuss the role of blood glucose determination in patients who have had a seizure.

19-11. Discuss relevant questions to ask while gathering a history of the seizure activity.

19-12. Describe common causes of syncope.

19-13. Describe the scene size-up, assessment, and emergency medical care of patients with syncope, including differentiating syncope from seizure.

KEY IDEAS

This chapter focuses on seizures, their causes and characteristics, and their management in the prehospital setting. Syncope, or fainting, is also discussed.

- A common cause of seizures is epilepsy, but seizures are caused by a variety of conditions.
- The most common type of epileptic seizure is the generalized tonic-clonic seizure.
- It is important to protect the airway in the seizing and postseizure patient.
- Oxygen is administered to maintain a SpO_2 level of > 94% to the seizure patient. If breathing is inadequate, it may be necessary to assist it.
- It is important to prevent injury to the seizing patient.
- *Syncope* is a temporary loss of responsiveness and may be confused with a seizure. Among other distinctions between a seizure and syncope, the patient who has fainted usually becomes responsive and recovers almost immediately.

TERMS AND CONCEPTS

1. Write the number of the correct term next to each definition.
   1. Aura
   2. Epilepsy
   3. Generalized tonic-clonic seizure
   4. Postictal state
   5. Seizure
   6. Status epilepticus
   7. Syncope

   _____ a. An unusual sensory sensation that may precede a seizure episode

   _____ b. A sudden and temporary alteration in the mental status caused by massive electrical discharge in a group of nerve cells in the brain

   _____ c. Recovery period that follows the clonic phase of a generalized seizure

   _____ d. A medical disorder characterized by recurrent seizures

   _____ e. A seizure lasting longer than 10 minutes, or seizures that occur consecutively without a period of responsiveness between them

   _____ f. A brief period of unresponsiveness due to a lack of blood flow to the brain

   _____ g. A common type of seizure that produces unresponsiveness and a generalized jerking muscle activity; a generalized tonic-clonic seizure

CONTENT REVIEW

1. A seizure is a sign of an underlying defect. Which of the following may be a cause of seizures?
   a. Head injury
   b. Abdominal aortic aneurysm
   c. Hypothermia
   d. Asthma

2. Select, in order, the six stages of a typical generalized tonic-clonic seizure.
   a. Aura, loss of consciousness, tonic, hypertonic, clonic, postictal
   b. Hypertonic, aura, loss of consciousness, postictal, clonic, tonic
   c. Aura, clonic, hyperlactic, tonic, hypertonic, postictal
   d. Postictal, hyperlactic, clonic, hypertonic, tonic, aura

3. You arrive on the scene of a seizure patient. In what state will you most often encounter the seizure patient?
   a. Aura phase
   b. Tonic phase
   c. Clonic phase
   d. Postictal phase

4. Since hypoglycemia is one possible cause of seizure, you should assess the blood glucose level in a seizure patient using a glucose meter. You should suspect that the seizure is due to hypoglycemia if the blood glucose level is
   a. below 60 mg/dL.
   b. below 70 mg/dL.
   c. between 80 and 120 mg/dL.
   d. above 120 mg/dL.

5. When you encounter a patient seizing with jerky body movements, to help prevent further injury, you should
   a. place a spoon in the mouth to stop the patient from swallowing his tongue.
   b. move objects away from the patient's area and guide his movements.
   c. physically restrain the patient's body movements until he becomes postictal.
   d. restrain the patient by securing him on a long spine board.

6. Following a generalized seizure, paralysis that affects one area or one side of the body that may indicate a space-occupying problem in the brain is known as
   a. Jackson paralysis.
   b. simple paralysis.
   c. Todd paralysis.
   d. grand mal paralysis.

7. Which of the following is the most appropriate treatment for a patient suffering status epilepticus?
   a. Positive pressure ventilation, transport after secondary assessment, and physical exam
   b. Positive pressure ventilation and immediate transport to a medical facility
   c. Oxygen at 15 lpm via a nonrebreather mask and transport after primary assessment and secondary assessment
   d. Oxygen at 6 lpm via a nasal cannula and immediate transport to a medical facility

8. You are responding to a report of a child seizing. Which of the following is a common cause of seizures in infants and young children?
   a. Head injury
   b. Diabetes
   c. High fever
   d. Epilepsy

9. It is important to recognize when the seizure patient needs immediate transport. Which of the following patients is more stable, meaning that transport can be delayed more than the other situations?

   a. The seizing patient who is pregnant, has a history of diabetes, or is injured
   b. The patient whose seizure has occurred in the water, such as a swimming pool or lake
   c. The patient who has suffered a seizure, regained responsiveness, then suffered another seizure an hour later
   d. The patient who remains unresponsive following the seizure activity

10. You are treating a 4-year-old child who experienced a generalized seizure that lasted approximately 30 seconds. His mother states that the patient has been sick with a high fever all day. From this information, which of the following seizures is this child likely experiencing?

    a. Generalized tonic-clonic seizure
    b. Grand mal seizure
    c. Absence (petit mal) seizure
    d. Febrile seizure

11. You are preparing to ventilate your patient, who is experiencing a generalized tonic-clonic seizure. Which of the following is the best way to ventilate this patient?

    a. Use the head-tilt, chin-lift maneuver and ventilate with a bag-valve mask (BVM).
    b. Restrain the patient's head and ventilate with a BVM.
    c. Insert an oropharyngeal airway and ventilate with a BVM.
    d. Insert a nasopharyngeal airway and ventilate with a BVM.

12. The postictal patient with no suspected spinal injury should be placed in which position?

    a. Semi-Fowler's
    b. Lateral recumbent
    c. Supine
    d. Prone

13. A generalized seizure typically involves both cerebral hemispheres (large lobes) of the brain and another system, also known as the *wake/sleep system*. The wake/sleep system is known as the

    a. left cerebral hemisphere (LCH).
    b. mid medulla oblongata (MMO).
    c. reticular activating system (RAS).
    d. right cerebral hemisphere (RCH).

14. You know that primary seizures are categorized as generalized or partial. Which of the following best describes the generalized seizure?

    a. Related to abnormal activity in one hemisphere; the patient usually remains conscious
    b. Related to abnormal activity in both hemispheres; the patient usually remains conscious
    c. Related to abnormal activity in one cerebral hemisphere; usually renders the patient unconscious
    d. Related to abnormal activity in both hemispheres; usually renders the patient unconscious

15. Which type of seizure generally produces jerky muscle activity in one area of the body, arm, leg, or face? These patients cannot control the jerky movement but remain awake and aware of the seizure activity.
    a. Simple partial seizure
    b. Complex partial seizure
    c. Absence or (petit mal) seizure
    d. Febrile seizure

16. Which of the following signs and symptoms usually precedes the typical syncopal episode?
    a. Chest pain, breathing difficulty
    b. Yawning, diaphoresis, nausea
    c. Stuttering, hypertension, numbness
    d. Blurred vision, belching

17. Which of the following is unlikely to be associated with a syncopal episode?
    a. The brain is briefly deprived of oxygen.
    b. The skin is usually warm, pale, and dry.
    c. The patient usually remembers feeling faint.
    d. The event usually begins in a standing position.

18. You are treating a patient that you suspect experienced a vasovagal faint. This type of syncopal episode is caused by which of the following?
    a. The parasympathetic nervous system causes the vessels to dilate throughout the body.
    b. The sympathetic nervous system constricts the vessels through stimulation of the vagus nerve.
    c. The parasympathetic nerves constrict blood vessels, causing the blood pressure to increase.
    d. The sympathetic nervous system causes hyperperfusion of the brain through vasoconstriction.

CASE STUDY

You and your partner, Gruwell, are at a local supermarket picking up groceries for dinner when an elderly woman screams for help: "There's a man over here dying!" You ask Gruwell to bring the ambulance closer to the building and bring the equipment and stretcher. You reach into your pocket for your extra pair of gloves and eye protection and put them on as you hurry to the patient's side. You find an elderly man on the ground, shaking uncontrollably. A closer look reveals the identity of the patient. You recognize him as Karl Louis, a local homeless man with a history of epilepsy and chronic alcoholism. The bystander states, "I found him lying on the ground shaking. I don't know how long he was like that, but he's been shaking for three or four minutes just since I found him!"

1. While you are waiting for Gruwell to bring the equipment, you should
   a. guide the body movements and move obstacles.
   b. restrict the patient to limit movement.
   c. place the patient in a Fowler position.
   d. place your finger into the mouth to position the tongue.

Gruwell approaches with the stretcher and equipment. You advise him that it's a known patient, Karl Louis, and that you have never seen him this bad. The seizure stops, and you try to arouse Karl, but he remains unresponsive. As you are assessing his breathing, he begins to seize again, violently. You notice blood flowing from his mouth.

2. Which of the following is the most appropriate emergency care?
   a. Administer oxygen via a nonrebreather mask at 15 lpm, wait for the seizure to end, and suction.
   b. Suction, administer oxygen via a nonrebreather mask at 15 lpm, and transport immediately.
   c. Suction, begin positive pressure ventilation with an oropharyngeal airway in place, and use rapid transport.
   d. Suction, begin positive pressure ventilation with a nasopharyngeal airway in place, and use rapid transport.

3. Briefly explain why you might see blood coming from the mouth of a seizure patient and how you would treat this problem.

En route to the medical facility, Karl stops seizing. While you are reassessing Karl's mental status, you ask Gruwell to obtain baseline vital signs. Karl responds to a painful stimulus by pulling away. Then he opens his eyes sluggishly and asks you to stop. He looks exhausted. Your physical exam reveals no injuries. The vital signs include heart rate 118 beats per minute, blood pressure 164/68, and breathing adequate at 20 per minute. The pulse oximeter displays an SpO_2 of 98% with the BVM.

4. Now that Karl is responsive, you recognize that he is in which phase?
   a. Aura phase
   b. Clonic phase
   c. Postictal phase
   d. Tonic phase

5. What should you now do for Karl?
   a. Place Karl in a supine position, and administer positive pressure ventilation with supplemental oxygen.
   b. Place Karl in a semi-sitting position, administer oxygen by BVM, and hyperventilate him at greater than 24 ventilations per minute.
   c. Place Karl in a full sitting position, and administer oxygen by a nonrebreather mask at 15 lpm.
   d. Place Karl in a lateral recumbent position, and maintain his SpO_2 at > 94%.

You arrive at the medical facility. Karl is feeling much better, although still somewhat confused and disoriented. You reassure him and give your report to the emergency nurse.

CHAPTER 19 SCENARIO: DOCUMENTATION EXERCISE

Read the following scenario and think about how you would document this call if you were the EMT who responded to the scene. Then answer the multiple-choice questions and fill in the sample prehospital care report, basing your documentation on information from the scenario.

While you and your partner, Jill, are cleaning the station, the alerting system sounds: "Unit 1 respond to 5555 Twentieth Street for a patient possibly having a seizure. Your ALS backup will be Medic Two." You acknowledge the call while Jill checks the location on the wall map. After a short emergency response, you arrive at a large retail store. You both quickly put on your gloves and eye protection. The store's manager meets you at the entrance and asks you to hurry—the patient is in the checkout area and is still seizing.

As you follow the manager to where the patient is located, you quickly scan the area for hazards and the best way to gain access to the patient. As you and Jill enter the checkout area, you find an approximately 30-year-old male lying supine on the floor. The patient's whole body is shaking with tonic-clonic movement. You radio your dispatch to advise that this is a priority call. The patient's body is up against shopping carts, and you ask the manager to move the carts carefully as you hold the patient's head and guide the patient's movements. Jill asks if anyone witnessed what happened. A checkout clerk says, "The man said he had a funny taste in his mouth, and then he sat down on the floor and went into a seizure."

Suddenly, the tonic-clonic movement ceases. You quickly assess the patient. You gently shake his shoulder and ask if he can hear you. There is no response. You assess the airway and note the patient is breathing approximately 20 times a minute with good air movement in and out of the lungs. There are no stridorous or crowing sounds with inhalation or exhalation. You check a radial pulse and find it to be strong at a rate of approximately 100 beats each minute and regular. The patient's general appearance is face flushed, with slight cyanosis around the lips and nail beds. The skin is warm and diaphoretic. Jill notices a medical alert bracelet on the patient's wrist. It reads that the patient has a history of epilepsy and takes Dilantin, which you know to be a seizure medication. You ask if there are any family or friends with the patient, and the checkout clerk states that she thought the patient was alone. You quickly apply the pulse oximeter, which indicates 98% while on oxygen.

Before the patient becomes responsive, he slips back into a full-body seizure. Again, the body convulses with tonic-clonic movement. You and Jill quickly place the patient onto the stretcher and make your way toward the ambulance, which is close by. After placing the patient into the ambulance, you perform a rapid assessment and note the patient's breathing has decreased to approximately six times each minute with poor tidal volume. You open the airway using the head-tilt, chin-lift maneuver. You ask Jill to insert a nasopharyngeal airway and provide positive pressure ventilations with the BVM with supplemental oxygen. The patient actively seizes for approximately two minutes before the activity once again subsides. Again the patient looks exhausted, with slight cyanosis of the lips. You instruct Jill to continue to support the ventilations with the BVM. Jill notices a small amount of saliva and blood dripping from the patient's mouth, and she immediately suctions the secretions with the portable suction unit.

The patient responds with purposeful movement by trying to push the BVM from his face. Despite his efforts to remove the BVM, you continue to provide positive pressure ventilations and reassure him. The patient now appears extremely sleepy, weak, and disoriented. You reassess his mental status. You ask him his name and he responds with a tired sigh, "Tyler, my name is Tyler." Jill proceeds with a medical exam. His pupils are equal and react briskly to light. The areas around his mouth and nail beds are now pink. You find no jugular venous distention, tracheal tugging, or subcutaneous emphysema to the neck. You quickly inspect and palpate the chest and find no evidence of trauma or scars. Auscultation reveals normal lung sounds with good tidal volume. Tyler's abdomen is soft and not tender. His lower extremities do not show any edema. Distal pulses are present in all four extremities. He obeys your commands to wiggle his toes and grasp your fingers. He states he can feel you touching his hands and feet. You do not note any edema to the small of the back in the lower lumbar area. Jill obtains vital signs. The blood pressure is 132/78; pulse is 100 beats each minute and regular. The patient is breathing 20 times a minute with good tidal volume. The pulse oximeter reading remains at 98%.

You hear on the radio that Medic Two is now on scene. As the paramedic lieutenant Logsdon enters the rear of your ambulance, you begin to give him a report while Jill, using the glucometer, obtains a blood glucose level of 110 mg/dL. You instruct Jill to drive the ambulance, responding in the emergency mode so as to not delay transport. The patient becomes more awake and alert, and he tells you that he has not experienced a seizure for over a year. He thought his seizures were cured, so he stopped taking his Dilantin. You ask him if he has any drug allergies, and he states, "None that I know of." Paramedic Logsdon starts an intravenous line in preparation for drug therapy. You obtain repeat vital signs, which are blood pressure 130/74, pulse 90 beats per minute, and respirations 16 each minute with good tidal volume. As you perform a reassessment, Jill advises that you have arrived at the emergency department.

1. The kind of seizure this patient was experiencing, with the whole body shaking with tonic-clonic movement, is most likely which type of seizure?
   a. Simple partial seizure
   b. Generalized tonic-clonic seizure
   c. Febrile seizure
   d. Focal motor seizure

2. The checkout clerk said that before the man went into a seizure, he said he had a funny taste in his mouth. The odd taste was likely a(n)
   a. postictal.
   b. aura.
   c. epilepticus.
   d. aspiration.

3. The patient had been seizing for several minutes before you arrived on scene and then had a second seizure without a period of responsiveness between seizures. Therefore, you recognized his condition as
   a. focal.
   b. syncopal.
   c. status epilepticus.
   d. postictal.

4. When the patient responded with purposeful movement and a sleepy, weak, disoriented appearance, he was likely in the
   a. postictal state.
   b. aura state.
   c. clonic state.
   d. tonic state.

5. Why did Jill obtain a blood glucose level on this patient?
   a. The seizures may have been caused by hypoxia.
   b. The seizures may have been caused by an allergic reaction.
   c. The seizures may have been caused by hypoglycemia or hyperglycemia.
   d. The seizures may have been caused by eclampsia.

EMERGENCY TRIP SHEET

TRIP #	
MEDIC #	
BEGIN MILES	
END MILES	
CODE___/___	PAGE___/___
UNITS ON SCENE	

BILLING USE ONLY

DAY	
DATE	
RECEIVED	
DISPATCHED	
EN-ROUTE	
ON SCENE	
TO HOSPITAL	
AT HOSPITAL	
IN-SERVICE	

NAME	SEX M F DOB ___/___/___
ADDRESS	RACE
CITY	STATE	ZIP
PHONE ( ) -	PCP DR.
RESPONDED FROM	CITY
TAKEN FROM	ZIP
DESTINATION	REASON
SSN - -	MEDICARE #	MEDICAID #
INSURANCE CO	INSURANCE #	GROUP #
RESPONSIBLE PARTY	ADDRESS
CITY	STATE	ZIP	PHONE ( ) -
EMPLOYER	

CREW	CERT	STATE #

TIME	ON SCENE (1)	ON SCENE (2)	ON SCENE (3)	EN-ROUTE (1)	EN-ROUTE (2)	AT DESTINATION
BP						
PULSE						
RESP						
SpO_2						
$ETCO_2$						
EKG						

IV THERAPY
SUCCESSFUL Y N # OF ATTEMPTS _____
ANGIO SIZE _____ ga.
SITE _____
TOTAL FLUID INFUSED _____ cc
BLOOD DRAW Y N INITIALS _____

INTUBATION INFORMATION
SUCCESSFUL Y N # OF ATTEMPTS _____
TUBE SIZE _____ mm
TIME _____ INITIALS _____

MEDICAL HISTORY

MEDICATIONS

ALLERGIES

C/C

EVENTS LEADING TO C/C

ASSESSMENT

TREATMENT

CONDITION CODES				

TREATMENTS

TIME	TREATMENT	DOSE	ROUTE	

GCS E___ V___ M___ TOTAL =
GCS E___ V___ M___ TOTAL =

HOSPITAL CONTACTED

CPR BEGUN BY B P TIME BEGUN

AED USED Y N BY:

RESUSCITATION TERMINATED - TIME

EMS SIGNATURE

(   ) OSHA REGULATIONS FOLLOWED

Acute Diabetic Emergencies

CHAPTER

20

STANDARD

Medicine (Content Area: Endocrine Disorders)

COMPETENCY

Applies fundamental knowledge to provide basic emergency care and transportation based on assessment findings for an acutely ill patient.

OBJECTIVES

After reading this chapter, you should be able to:

20-1. Define key terms introduced in this chapter.
20-2. Describe the following regarding glucose:
    a. The function of glucose in the body
    b. Response of brain cells and other body cells to insufficient glucose levels
    c. Relationships of glucose and water
20-3. Describe how insulin and glucagon function to control blood glucose levels.
20-4. Describe how glucose levels are regulated in normal metabolism.
20-5. Explain the purposes and process of checking blood glucose levels.
20-6. Discuss the pathophysiology of diabetes mellitus (DM) and contrast type 1 insulin-dependent diabetes mellitus (IDDM) with type 2 non-insulin-dependent diabetes mellitus (NIDDM).
20-7. Discuss the pathophysiology, assessment, and emergency medical care of a hypoglycemic emergency.
20-8. Identify indications and contraindications to the administration of oral glucose.
20-9. Discuss the pathophysiology, assessment, and emergency medical care of diabetic ketoacidosis (DKA).
20-10. Compare and contrast the speed of onset and the signs and symptoms of hypoglycemia and hyperglycemia.
20-11. Describe the primary differences between DKA and hyperglycemic hyperosmolar nonketotic syndrome (HHNS).
20-12. Discuss the pathophysiology, assessment, and emergency medical care of HHNS.
20-13. Discuss the assessment-based approach to a patient with an altered mental status in a diabetic emergency.

KEY IDEAS

This chapter focuses on the patient with an acute diabetic emergency. Emphasis is placed on assessing the patient's mental status, determining if the patient has a history of diabetes controlled by medication, and determining if the patient is alert enough to swallow before administering oral glucose with permission from medical direction.

■ It is important to distinguish between the patient with an altered mental status who has a history of diabetes controlled by medication and the patient with an altered mental status who does not have a known history of diabetes.

■ Airway management is a major concern in the patient suffering from an acute diabetic emergency.

■ With on-line or off-line approval from medical direction, oral glucose may be administered to the patient with an altered mental status and a history of diabetes controlled by medication who is alert enough to swallow.

MEDICAL TERMINOLOGY

Term	Prefix	Word Root Combining Form	Suffix	Definition
hypoglycemia (HY-po-gly-SEE-mee-uh)	hypo- (below, under, deficient)	glyc (glucose, sweet, sugar)	-emia (blood condition)	Low blood sugar
hyperglycemia (HY-per-gly-SEE-mee-uh)	hyper- (above, beyond, excessive)	glyc (glucose, sweet, sugar)	-emia (blood condition)	High blood sugar
polyuria (POL-ee-YOO-ree-uh)	poly- (many, much, excessive)	ur (urine)	-ia (condition of)	Excessive urination
polyphagia (POL-ee-FAY-juh)	poly- (many, much, excessive)	phag (to eat, engulf)	-ia (condition of)	Excessive hunger
polydipsia (POL-ee-DIP-see-uh)	poly- (many, much, excessive)	dips (thirst, to drink)	-ia (condition of)	Excessive thirst

1. The medical term *hypoglycemia* contains the word root *glyc*, which refers to
   a. protein.
   b. globe.
   c. glomerulus.
   d. sugar.

2. The suffix *-emia* in such medical terms as *hyperglycemia* means
   a. blood condition.
   b. pertaining to.
   c. surgical repair.
   d. diabetic condition.

3. The prefix *poly-* in such medical terms as *polyuria* means
   a. many, much, excessive.
   b. similar, same, likeness.
   c. cut, away, from.
   d. below, under, deficient.

4. The medical term *polyuria* contains the word root *ur,* which means
   a. uterus.
   b. urine.
   c. uvea.
   d. ureter.

5. The medical term *polyphagia* contains the word root *phag,* which refers to
   a. sweating, perspiration.
   b. thirst, to drink.
   c. to eat, engulf.
   d. drum membrane.

TERMS AND CONCEPTS

1. Write the number of the correct term next to each definition.
   1. Altered mental status
   2. Diabetes mellitus
   3. Glucose
   4. Hyperglycemia
   5. Hypoglycemia
   6. Insulin

   _____ a. High blood glucose

   _____ b. Hormone secreted by the pancreas that promotes the movement of glucose into the sugar-storing cells

   _____ c. Disease characterized by the body's inability to produce insulin

   _____ d. Condition in which the patient displays a change ranging from disorientation to complete unresponsiveness

   _____ e. Low blood glucose

   _____ f. Form of sugar that is the body's basic source of energy

CONTENT REVIEW

1. You are treating your diabetic patient with an altered mental status. You know the altered mental status indicates that the
   a. plantar nervous system has been affected.
   b. brachial nervous system has been affected.
   c. peripheral nervous system has been affected.
   d. central nervous system has been affected.

2. Which of the following is the primary energy source for cells?
   a. Carbohydrates
   b. Fats
   c. Adipose
   d. Proteins

3. Your EMS medical director has approved orders to obtain patient blood glucose levels through the use of a blood glucose meter (glucometer). Which statement is true pertaining to the use of glucometers?
   a. The glucometer analyzes glucose in the blood by obtaining a drop of arterial blood.
   b. Glucometers measure blood glucose levels in grams per liter (g/L).
   c. Glucometers are complex diagnostic equipment that require extensive special training.
   d. The glucometer analyzes glucose in the blood by obtaining a drop of capillary blood.

4. The blood glucose level in a nondiabetic patient following a meal will typically rise to _____ mg/dL.
   a. 70–90
   b. 100–110
   c. 120–140
   d. 140–160

5. Glucometers measure the glucose in the blood in milligrams per deciliter (mg/dL). Which of the following blood glucose levels would indicate hyperglycemia?
   a. 50 mg/dL
   b. 80 mg/dL
   c. 120 mg/dL
   d. 150 mg/dL

6. When assessing the patient's blood glucose with a glucometer, you should
   a. ask the patient about allergies to latex.
   b. apply a venous restricting band before obtaining the blood sample.
   c. determine when the patient last had something to eat or drink.
   d. encourage the patient to sip water before taking a blood sample.

7. Your patient has experienced a rapid onset of altered mental status and has cool, moist skin, an elevated heart rate, and other signs indicating that he is experiencing a diabetic emergency. He has no medical ID tag or medications on his person, and you are unable to confirm that he has a history of diabetes controlled by medication. However, he is clearly still able to swallow. Which of the following emergency care measures should you first provide?
   a. Ensure an open airway.
   b. Provide oxygen by a nasal cannula at 4 lpm.
   c. Administer oral glucose.
   d. Position the patient in a supine position.

8. Which of the following best describes type 2 diabetes?
   a. The blood glucose level is usually controlled by diet.
   b. No insulin is produced by the body.
   c. It is commonly acquired during the childhood years.
   d. Insulin must be injected daily.

9. You are assessing a patient who has a history of diabetes mellitus. The patient presents with tachycardia, diaphoresis, and pale, cool skin typically seen in the hypoglycemic patient. Which of the following is responsible for these signs?
   a. Release of epinephrine (adrenaline)
   b. Increasing blood pressure (hypertension)
   c. Narrowing of blood vessels (vasoconstriction)
   d. Inflammation of the renal glomeruli (glomerulitis)

10. You are assessing your patient who has a history of diabetes. Which of the following questions will not aid you in your assessment of this patient?
    a. Did you take your medication today?
    b. Have you eaten (or skipped any) regular meals today?
    c. Did you do any unusual exercise or physical activity today?
    d. Does a history of cancer run in your family?

11. Signs and symptoms that mimic a stroke, such as weakness or paralysis on one side of the body, may occur more frequently in the diabetic patient who is
    a. young.
    b. hyperglycemic.
    c. elderly.
    d. on cardiac medications.

12. Which of the following indicates that a patient has a history of diabetes that is controlled by medication?
    a. Medical identification device (medical alert bracelet, tag, or tattoo)
    b. Unequal pupils
    c. Pale, cool, diaphoretic skin
    d. 1-cc syringes are found

13. You are treating a patient who is experiencing an acute diabetic emergency with an altered mental status. After establishing and maintaining the airway, you should next
    a. administer oral glucose per protocol.
    b. determine if the patient can swallow.
    c. reassess airway, breathing, and circulation.
    d. perform a reassessment of the patient's condition.

14. Select the correct statement regarding reassessment following administration of oral glucose.
    a. Reassess the patient's mental status, expecting an improvement in 3 minutes or less.
    b. Reassess the patient's mental status, understanding that improvement may not be apparent for 20 minutes or more.
    c. Assume that the patient's mental status will not deteriorate once oral glucose has been administered.
    d. If the patient loses responsiveness or seizes, insert a tongue depressor to prevent the patient from biting his tongue.

15. While attending a continuing education class on diabetes mellitus, you are asked which of the following best describes glucagon.
    a. It contains sugars to control the blood levels.
    b. It is a hormone that stimulates the breakdown of glycogen.
    c. It transports simple sugars into the cells from the bloodstream.
    d. It prevents the free movement of glucose across the blood-brain barrier.

16. You are assessing a 42-year-old patient who presents with a furrowed tongue, sunken eyes, and poor skin turgor (tenting). You suspect the patient is dehydrated. You should
    a. place the patient in a prone position.
    b. apply cold packs to the external neck great veins.
    c. immediately palpate the abdomen for abnormalities.
    d. check the patient's blood glucose level (BGL).

17. You are treating a patient that you suspect is suffering from diabetic ketoacidosis (DKA). You know that the DKA patient's altered mental status is caused by
    a. dehydration and acidosis affecting the brain.
    b. a lack of glucose affecting the brain.
    c. rapid onset of hypoglycemia affecting the brain.
    d. decrease in blood from hypotension affecting the brain.

18. If insulin is not available to help glucose enter the cell, glucose will move into the cell up to how many times slower than with insulin?
    a. 10 times
    b. 20 times
    c. 30 times
    d. 50 times

19. You are treating your patient who is experiencing an acute diabetic emergency. You know the normal blood glucose range is
    a. 40–60 mg/dL.
    b. 50–70 mg/dL.
    c. 80–120 mg/dL.
    d. 150–200 mg/dL.

20. You are assessing a patient who you suspect is experiencing an acute diabetic emergency. Which of the following medications can hide the signs and symptoms of hypoglycemia?
    a. Bronchodilators
    b. Alpha enhancers
    c. Analgesics
    d. Beta blockers

UNDERSTANDING DIABETES MELLITUS

1. Insulin is secreted when the blood glucose level is elevated. Insulin has three main functions. Which of the following is a function of the hormone glucagon rather than insulin?
    a. Increases the movement of glucose out of the blood and into the cells
    b. Converts noncarbohydrate substances into glucose
    c. Causes the liver to take glucose out of the blood and convert it to glycogen
    d. Decreases blood glucose levels

2. The hormone glucagon is secreted by the pancreas. Its major role in the body is to
    a. raise and maintain the blood glucose level.
    b. facilitate the movement of glucose out of the blood.
    c. increase insulin levels in the blood and brain.
    d. slow the secretion of glycogen, which lowers glucose levels.

3. Diabetes mellitus patients suffering from the lack of insulin will typically complain of frequent thirst (polydipsia), frequent urination (polyuria), and hunger (polyphagia). This is referred to as the "three Ps." Which best describes the reason that these patients often complain of the three Ps?
   a. The liver collects the hormone insulin, which helps to regulate water absorption.
   b. The kidneys spill glucose into the urine; the large molecule of glucose draws water.
   c. The glycogen molecule is very small, which draws water from the kidneys into the cells.
   d. The pancreas overproduces the hormone insulin, which draws water from the cells.

4. Type 1 and type 2 diabetes mellitus each have specific characteristics. Which characteristic best describes type 1 diabetes mellitus?
   a. Most often, the pancreas will not produce and secrete any insulin.
   b. Typically it is diagnosed in patients older than 50 years of age.
   c. It is characteristically found in the heavy or obese patient.
   d. Rarely will these patients suffer from DKA or hypoglycemia.

5. Which of the following is typical of the patient suffering from DKA?
   a. Blood glucose levels are drastically low, usually below 40 mg/dL.
   b. Signs and symptoms of DKA occur immediately following the onset of hypoglycemia.
   c. The electrolytes in the body become balanced to form a homeostatic state.
   d. The cells begin to burn fat for energy as glucose collects in the blood.

6. Most often the signs and symptoms of DKA are produced by dehydration and acid buildup. Which of the following is a very late sign of DKA?
   a. Acetone breath
   b. Polyuria
   c. Coma
   d. Kussmaul respirations

7. In the absence of glucose, some cells of the body are able to use fats and proteins as an energy source. Which of the following organ cells can use only glucose as a source of fuel and will dysfunction, shut down, and eventually begin to die without it?
   a. Cardiac muscle cells
   b. Skeletal muscle cells
   c. Brain tissue cells
   d. Liver cells

CASE STUDY

You and your partner, Emil, are dispatched to a local park, where there is a report of a young female acting strangely. You approach the scene and find an approximately 30-year-old female in a jogging outfit sitting on a bench. It appears that she is anxious and speaking with inappropriate words. You notice a medical identification bracelet informing you that she is an insulin-dependent diabetic. The patient's airway is patent and her breathing appears adequate; however, the SpO$_2$ on the pulse oximeter registers at 92%. You place her on oxygen. The patient does not answer any of your questions appropriately, and none of the bystanders who have gathered know her. Her vital signs include heart rate 104 per minute, blood pressure 100/64, and respirations 20 per minute. The skin is cool and moist. You and Emil both suspect a diabetic emergency and decide that she is alert enough to swallow. You ask Emil to prepare to administer oral glucose following the protocol established off-line by your medical direction.

1. From the information provided in this case, list the signs that support your suspicion that the patient is suffering from a diabetic emergency.

2. You place the patient on oxygen. Which of the following is most appropriate for this patient?
   a. Nasal cannula at 2 lpm
   b. Nonrebreather mask at 15 lpm
   c. Simple face mask at 15 lpm
   d. Positive pressure ventilation

3. You and your partner determine that the patient has met the three criteria for administration of oral glucose. Which of the following criteria would *not* aid you in your decision?
   a. The patient's blood pressure must be within the normal range.
   b. The patient must have an altered mental status.
   c. The patient must have a history of diabetes controlled by medication.
   d. The patient must be able to swallow.

4. Approval to administer oral glucose was given off-line in this scenario. In some jurisdictions, approval to administer oral glucose must be given on-line. Which of the following best describes "on-line" medical direction?
   a. Approval given by radio or phone
   b. Approval given by standing orders
   c. Approval given by prearranged written protocol
   d. Approval given by the EMS supervisor

After you administer the oral glucose, the patient begins feeling much better. En route to the hospital, she is able to converse normally. She informs you that her name is Pat, she lives on Third Avenue, and she knows that it is Tuesday. She took her insulin this morning but went for a jog and forgot to eat lunch. You continue to assess her during transport to the hospital.

❙ CHAPTER 20 SCENARIO: DOCUMENTATION EXERCISE

Read the following scenario and think about how you would document this call if you were the EMT who responded to the scene. Then answer the multiple-choice questions and fill in the sample prehospital care report, basing your documentation on information from the scenario.

You and your partner, Lieutenant Graves, are returning to the station from the hospital after completing a call. The radio sounds with an emergency tone: "Squad 11 respond to 1729 17th Avenue for an elderly male that is confused. Time out 1634 hours." Lieutenant Graves acknowledges the call, "Squad 11 en route." After a short emergency response, your unit arrives at the scene of an older, run-down single-family residence. You both put on gloves and eye protection as you scan the area for possible safety hazards. Seeing no obvious or potential hazards, you approach the house and knock on the front door.

A well-dressed, middle-aged woman answers. She introduces herself and says she is the patient's younger sister, who lives across town. She states she tried to call her brother on the phone for the past few hours and then became worried, so she drove over to check on him. As you enter the house, you quickly scan the area, looking for any hazards or obstacles that may inhibit moving the patient. She leads you to the living room, where you find a man you estimate to be about 60 years old sitting on the couch rocking back and forth while repeating words that don't make sense. The patient seems agitated, perhaps even aggressive. He speaks in loud shouts, but without slurred speech.

Lieutenant Graves begins the primary assessment. He touches the patient gently on the shoulder and asks him, "What seems to be the problem today?" The patient responds with an inappropriate statement but follows you with his eyes. His sister says, "He has diabetes and sometimes will have episodes like this. We've had the ambulance out here before." Your general impression is that the patient is weak, pale, and sweating profusely. Lieutenant Graves asks the patient his name. He responds with a sluggish, mumbled "Dale." "Did you eat lunch today?" Lieutenant Graves asks. Dale responds with a delayed "No." You ask him if he took his insulin today. He responds "Yes." You observe that the patient has an adequate airway with respirations approximately 20 per minute; however, the SpO_2 on the pulse oximeter is 92%. You place a nasal cannula on the patient at 2 lpm. You then assess the radial pulse and find it to be around 80 beats per minute and regular. The skin is very diaphoretic and cool. There is no noted cyanosis. Lieutenant Graves calls for ALS backup and positions the cot next to the patient.

You begin a rapid medical exam. Dale's pupils respond normally to light. You do not notice any acetone smell from the mouth; however, the patient is drooling copious amounts of saliva. There is no noted unilateral facial droop. You find no jugular vein distention or tracheal tugging. You quickly inspect and palpate the chest and find no evidence of trauma or scars. Auscultation of the lungs reveals that they are clear in all fields with a normal tidal volume. His abdomen is soft and not tender. The lower extremities do not show any edema. The upper extremities are unremarkable, and good distal pulses are found in all extremities. Dale does not respond to your request to wiggle his fingers and toes but responds with a loud "Ouch" when you pinch each extremity. There is no edema to the lower lumbar area of the back.

Lieutenant Graves asks Dale's sister if she can provide answers to some medical questions. She responds, "I hope I can remember everything." He reassures her. She states that Dale has no known allergies; he takes an injection of insulin in the morning and one right before dinner every day; he takes no other medications except for over-the-counter vitamins. She adds, "He always eats a good breakfast every morning, but he must have missed his lunch today."

Lieutenant Graves obtains a set of baseline vital signs. The blood pressure is 162/84; the heart rate is 86 beats per minute and regular; the respiratory rate is 18 per minute and nonlabored; the skin is pale, cool, and very diaphoretic; the pupils respond appropriately to light; the SpO_2 reading on the pulse oximeter is 95% with the oxygen. You prepare to obtain a blood glucose level as per your offline protocol. You let Dale's arm and hand dangle from the edge of the couch and briefly warm the fingers by placing them in your hands. Lieutenant Graves prepares the glucometer and test strip for the application of capillary blood. You grasp a finger close to the distal end and clean it with alcohol prep. The finger is pricked, and you gently squeeze a drop of blood onto the test strip. Lieutenant Graves takes the glucometer while you place a bandage on the pricked site, and Lieutenant Graves remarks, "The BGL is 42 mg/dL."

You determine that Dale is alert enough to swallow and prepare for the administration of oral glucose. You administer small amounts of oral glucose between his cheek and gum, making sure not to compromise his airway. You and Lieutenant Graves position Dale on the cot and prepare him for transport. As you move him to the ambulance, the ALS backup, Medic Six, arrives on the scene. You reassess the patient and find that Dale is becoming more alert and aware of his surroundings. His vital signs are blood pressure 158/80, heart rate 80 beats per minute and regular, and respiratory rate 20 per minute and nonlabored. His skin is less diaphoretic but still pale. The SpO_2 reading on the pulse oximeter remains 95% with the oxygen. Dale remarks, "Oh, I must have been out for awhile. I should have eaten lunch." You assist the crew of Medic Six and transport Dale to the emergency department located approximately 10 minutes away.

1. Why is it significant for Lieutenant Graves to ask if the patient has eaten or taken his insulin today?
   a. If the patient ate without taking insulin, this is a critical mistake, which could lead to death.
   b. Administering insulin and then not eating signifies the patient is a danger to himself.
   c. Taking insulin injections and then not eating will likely lead to a high blood glucose level.
   d. If the patient took his insulin but did not eat, you would suspect hypoglycemia.

2. How would the smell of acetone on the patient's breath be of value in your assessment of the diabetic patient?
   a. Acetone breath may indicate a buildup of ketones, a sign of DKA.
   b. This smell is evidence that the patient has consumed alcohol and may be intoxicated.
   c. Acetone breath indicates the need for immediate administration of ipecac syrup.
   d. The fruity acetone breath is an indication of impending unresponsiveness.

3. Why is it important to let the patient's hand dangle and to warm the patient's fingertips when obtaining a blood glucose level?
   a. Bleeding is better controlled when the hand is lowered and warmed.
   b. Lowering the hand lessens the likelihood of developing complications like thrombus.
   c. This allows better blood flow to the fingers and provides a better sample.
   d. Lowering the hand will keep the blood from coagulating and ruining the sample.

4. This patient's BGL was 42 mg/dL. Which of the following statements best describes this finding?
   a. The BGL is above the normal range. This patient shows signs of hyperglycemia.
   b. The BGL is within the normal range. However, the patient exhibits abnormal behavior.
   c. The BGL is below normal, but the patient is responsive. This is a normal response.
   d. The BGL is below normal with signs and symptoms. This patient is hypoglycemic.

5. What criteria did this patient have to meet before you were able to treat him with oral glucose? The patient must
   a. be over 30 years of age, have a history of diabetes controlled by diet, and have an intact gag reflex.
   b. have an altered mental status, have a history of diabetes controlled by medication, and have the ability to swallow.
   c. be responsive to tactile stimulation, have a history of diabetes controlled by diet, and have an intact gag reflex.
   d. have an altered mental status, have a history of diabetes controlled by diet or medication, and be able to respond to commands.

TRIP #		**EMERGENCY**	BILLING USE ONLY

			BILLING USE ONLY
TRIP #		**EMERGENCY**	
MEDIC #		**TRIP SHEET**	DAY
BEGIN MILES			DATE
MILES			RECEIVED
CODE___/___ PAGE___/___			DISPATCHED
UNITS ON SCENE			

NAME	SEX M F DOB ___/___/___	EN-ROUTE
ADDRESS	RACE	ON SCENE
CITY STATE	ZIP	TO HOSPITAL
PHONE ( ) - PCP DR.		AT HOSPITAL
RESPONDED FROM	CITY	IN-SERVICE

TAKEN FROM	ZIP	CREW	CERT	STATE #
DESTINATION	REASON			
SSN - - MEDICARE #	MEDICAID #			
INSURANCE CO INSURANCE #	GROUP #			
RESPONSIBLE PARTY ADDRESS				
CITY STATE ZIP PHONE ( ) -				
EMPLOYER				

IV THERAPY
SUCCESSFUL Y N # OF ATTEMPTS _____
ANGIO SIZE _____ ga.
SITE _____
TOTAL FLUID INFUSED _____ cc
BLOOD DRAW Y N INITIALS _____

TIME	ON SCENE (1)	ON SCENE (2)	ON SCENE (3)	EN-ROUTE (1)	EN-ROUTE (2)	AT DESTINATION
BP						
PULSE						
RESP						
SpO$_2$						
ETCO$_2$						
EKG						

INTUBATION INFORMATION
SUCCESSFUL Y N # OF ATTEMPTS _____
TUBE SIZE _____ mm
TIME _____ INITIALS _____

MEDICAL HISTORY	CONDITION CODES

TREATMENTS

MEDICATIONS	TIME	TREATMENT	DOSE	ROUTE	INIT

ALLERGIES

C/C

EVENTS LEADING TO C/C

ASSESSMENT

TREATMENT

GCS E___ V___ M___ TOTAL =

GCS E___ V___ M___ TOTAL =

HOSPITAL CONTACTED

CPR BEGUN BY B P TIME BEGUN

EMS SIGNATURE

AED USED Y N BY:

RESUSCITATION TERMINATED - TIME

(   ) OSHA REGULATIONS FOLLOWED

Anaphylactic Reactions

STANDARD

Medicine (Content Area: Immunology)

COMPETENCY

Applies fundamental knowledge to provide basic emergency care and transportation based on assessment findings for an acutely ill patient.

OBJECTIVES

After reading this chapter, you should be able to:

21-1. Define key terms introduced in this chapter.
21-2. Explain the importance of being able to recognize and treat anaphylactic reactions.
21-3. Describe the pathophysiological process by which exposure to an antigen results in anaphylaxis.
21-4. Explain the life-threatening mechanisms of anaphylaxis, including airway compromise, impaired ventilation and oxygenation, and impaired perfusion.
21-5. Describe the difference between an anaphylactic and an anaphylactoid reaction.
21-6. Discuss the ways that an antigen can be introduced into the body and substances that commonly cause anaphylactic or anaphylactoid reactions.
21-7. Explain an assessment-based approach to anaphylactic reaction including scene size-up, primary and secondary assessments, and reassessment.
21-8. Recognize the signs and symptoms of anaphylactic reaction.
21-9. List the two key categories of signs and symptoms that specifically indicate a severe anaphylactic reaction.
21-10. Develop a treatment plan for the patient with an anaphylactic reaction.
21-11. Describe the role of epinephrine in the treatment of anaphylaxis and the criteria and procedure administration of epinephrine.

KEY IDEAS

An anaphylactic reaction can quickly be life threatening. It is important for the EMT to rapidly assess and manage patients suffering an anaphylactic reaction. Appropriate assessment and management techniques for anaphylactic reactions are the focus of this chapter.

- An anaphylactic reaction is a misdirected or excessive response by the immune system to a foreign substance or allergen. An allergen can enter the body by injection, ingestion, inhalation, or contact.

- Causes of anaphylactic reactions include venom from bites or stings, foods, pollen, and medications. Medications taken orally or injected are the most common cause.
- Hives and itching are hallmark signs and symptoms of an anaphylactic reaction.
- Most anaphylactic reactions are mild. A severe form of anaphylactic reaction is anaphylaxis, or anaphylactic shock.
- In anaphylactic shock, the entire body is affected by the release of histamine by the immune system. There is swelling in the upper airway and bronchoconstriction and swelling in the lower airways. Blood vessels dilate and decrease the blood pressure. Anaphylaxis is a life-threatening condition that, without proper treatment, leads to death.
- The two key categories of signs and symptoms that specifically indicate anaphylaxis are respiratory compromise and shock (hypoperfusion).
- Emergency medical care for anaphylaxis includes maintaining a patent airway, oxygen therapy, administering epinephrine by prescribed auto-injector, calling for advanced life support, and early transport. It may be necessary to provide positive pressure ventilation to force air past the swollen upper airway.

TERMS AND CONCEPTS

1. Write the number of the correct term next to each definition.

1. Allergen
2. Allergic reaction
3. Anaphylactoid reaction
4. Anaphylactic shock
5. Antibodies
6. Histamine
7. Hives
8. Immune system
9. Malaise
10. Sensitization

_____ a. The process by which antibodies are produced after exposure to an antigen

_____ b. Misdirected and excessive response by the immune system to a foreign substance or an allergen

_____ c. Raised, red blotches associated with some anaphylactic reactions

_____ d. Special proteins produced by the immune system that search out antigens, combine with them, and destroy them

_____ e. The body's defense mechanism against invasion by foreign substances

_____ f. A state of hypoperfusion that results from dilated and leaking blood vessels related to severe anaphylactic reaction

_____ g. A substance that enters the body by ingestion, injection, inhalation, or contact and triggers an anaphylactic reaction

_____ h. A general feeling of weakness or discomfort

_____ i. Primary chemical mediator released from mast cells and basophils

_____ j. A reaction that requires no previous sensitization

CONTENT REVIEW

1. For each sign or symptom of an anaphylactic reaction in the following list, indicate if it is a sign or symptom of a mild (M) reaction or a severe (S) reaction.

   _____ a. Localized flushed skin

   _____ b. Cyanosis

   _____ c. Altered mental status

   _____ d. Watery eyes

   _____ e. Wheezing in all lung fields

   _____ f. Severe respiratory distress

2. The *most* common cause of anaphylaxis is
   a. glue and adhesives.
   b. pollen from ragweed.
   c. medications.
   d. mosquito bites.

3. Which of the following is a route by which an allergen may enter the body?
   a. Ulnar
   b. Excretion
   c. Contact
   d. Vagus

4. In an anaphylactoid reaction
   a. the second time an antigen is introduced into the body, chemical mediators are released.
   b. bronchoconstriction, decreased capillary membrane permeability, and vasoconstriction occur.
   c. the treatment is significantly different from anaphylaxis.
   d. the patient will not have experienced a previous exposure to an antigen.

5. When assessing respiratory sounds, stridor or crowing indicates
   a. significant swelling to the upper airway, requiring positive pressure ventilation.
   b. significant swelling to the upper airway, requiring insertion of an airway adjunct.
   c. significant swelling to the bronchioles, requiring oxygen at 15 lpm by a nonrebreather mask.
   d. possible collapse of the alveoli of the lungs, requiring endotracheal intubation.

6. You are providing positive pressure ventilation to an anaphylaxis patient who is experiencing respiratory difficulty. The bag-valve-mask (BVM) device's pop-off valve releases air with each squeeze of the bag. What is the *best* action to take?
   a. Deactivate the valve or place your thumb over it and continue with ventilations.
   b. Continue ventilating the patient and increase the rate of ventilations.
   c. Continue until advanced life support (ALS) arrives and report your finding to the crew.
   d. Reduce the pressure that you are using to squeeze the bag to prevent the valve from opening.

7. Hives may be present all over the skin in a patient experiencing an anaphylactic reaction. Hives are usually accompanied by
   a. severe coughing.
   b. severe stuffy nose.
   c. severe itching.
   d. severe headache.

8. Most anaphylactic reactions are apparent within _____ minute(s) after exposure.
   a. 1
   b. 5
   c. 10
   d. 20

9. The two key categories of signs and symptoms that specifically indicate anaphylaxis are
   a. gastrointestinal compromise and shock.
   b. respiratory compromise and shock.
   c. central nervous system compromise and shock.
   d. respiratory compromise and gastrointestinal complaints.

10. Anaphylaxis can be mistaken for other conditions with similar signs and symptoms, such as
    a. an anxiety attack.
    b. a stroke.
    c. meningitis.
    d. epilepsy.

11. A common substance that causes an anaphylactoid reaction is
    a. pollen.
    b. a nonsteroidal anti-inflammatory drug (NSAID).
    c. food additives.
    d. eggs.

12. Histamine release causes
    a. bronchodilation, vasodilation, and decreased capillary membrane permeability.
    b. bronchoconstriction, vasodilation, and increased capillary membrane permeability.
    c. bronchoconstriction, vasoconstriction, and decreased capillary membrane permeability.
    d. bronchodilation, vasodilation, and decreased capillary membrane permeability.

13. Anaphylaxis is a condition that
    a. is a minor medical problem with a low mortality rate.
    b. causes pulmonary hypertension and pulmonary emboli.
    c. causes blood vessels to constrict, increasing the blood pressure to dangerous levels.
    d. may make positive pressure ventilation of the patient difficult.

14. The criteria that must be met before an EMT can administer epinephrine by auto-injector to a patient are (1) _____, (2) the medication has been prescribed to the patient, and (3) the EMT has received an order from medical direction.
    a. abdominal cramping and bloating
    b. headache and blurred vision
    c. respiratory distress and/or hypotension
    d. flushed, red skin and/or itching

15. You respond to a call for a patient who was stung by a bee. The patient's family reports that the patient is allergic to bee stings. As you approach the patient, you note that the face, neck, tongue, and lips are swollen. Given this information, you know that it is most likely that
    a. the patient will complain of yellow vision.
    b. the patient will have peripheral edema.
    c. the patient is stable and will require limited care.
    d. the upper airway is also likely to be swollen.

16. The type of antibodies produced specific to anaphylaxis is called
    a. anaphylaxis antibody 7 and is abbreviated Aa7.
    b. immunoglobin E and is abbreviated as IgE.
    c. urticaria antibody C and is abbreviated UaC.
    d. allergen property A and is abbreviated ApA.

17. Which of the following is the most common early physical assessment finding in your patient experiencing anaphylaxis?
    a. Rhinitis (stuffy, runny, itchy nose)
    b. Urticaria (hives)
    c. Anisocoria (unequal pupil size)
    d. Pneumonitis (inflammation of lung tissue)

❙ CASE STUDY

You have responded to a call for a child who has been stung by a bee. The scene appears safe as you arrive at a small home. A frantic-looking woman meets you at the front of the house and cries out to you, "Please hurry up!" As you follow her to the backyard, you introduce yourself and your partner and ask, "Why did you call the ambulance today?" She replies, "My daughter was just stung by a bee!"

The patient appears to be about 10 years old. She is sitting in a chair and looks up at you as you approach. Your general impression is that she looks well. Her skin color is red. She responds to your questions appropriately. She says her name is Caitlin. She tells you that she was stung by a bee about five minutes ago. She doesn't appear to have any difficulty breathing. She complains of a "lump" in her throat and her stomach feels "upset." Her pulse is strong and regular. There is no sign of trauma, and no bleeding is present.

You complete the OPQRST and history. You find out that she had an anaphylactic reaction to a yellow jacket sting one year ago. She has a prescription for an EpiPen Jr. During the physical exam, you observe the small, red sting site on her arm but make no other findings.

1. Which of the following is true about this patient?
    a. She is not showing signs of an anaphylactic reaction. Caitlin does not require transport or additional treatment.
    b. She is not showing signs of an anaphylactic reaction. Caitlin should be transported by her mother for additional evaluation at a local hospital.
    c. She is showing late signs of anaphylaxis. Place Caitlin on oxygen and closely evaluate while you wait for ALS backup.
    d. She is showing early signs of an anaphylactic reaction. Provide supplemental oxygen, maintain an SpO_2 reading at or above 94%, call for ALS backup, prepare for suction and to assist ventilations, and initiate early transport.

2. You should carefully monitor Caitlin for which of the following?
    a. Signs of developing hives and itching
    b. Signs of abdominal cramping
    c. Loss of bowel control
    d. Airway and respiratory compromise and poor perfusion

3. En route to the hospital, Caitlin develops respirations that sound noisy, with a rattling sound on inspiration and exhalation. These sounds are probably caused by
    a. swelling of the tongue.
    b. severe bronchoconstriction.
    c. excessive mucus in the upper airways.
    d. excessive mucus in the lower airways.

4. What additional signs and symptoms might you expect Caitlin to develop?
  a. Constipation
  b. Coughing and hoarseness
  c. Pinpoint pupils
  d. Hypertension

CHAPTER 21 SCENARIO: DOCUMENTATION EXERCISE

Read the following scenario and think about how you would document this call if you were the EMT who responded to the scene. Then answer the multiple-choice questions and fill in the sample prehospital care report, basing your documentation on information from the scenario.

It is 11:00 A.M. on a bright summer day. You and your partner, Nancy Ann, have just completed a call for an elderly man who fell. You are returning to the station when dispatch calls: "Unit 2, respond to 1220 Little Wing Road, cross street Moulin Avenue, for difficulty breathing. Time out 1100 hours." Nancy advises dispatch that you are responding to the incident. You arrive on scene in about three minutes.

When you arrive, you notice a small crowd of people standing and squatting next to a man on the ground. He is located in a grassy area next to a lake filled with ducks and swans. You observe a city Parks Department truck parked near the man. You park in a safe area and exit the emergency vehicle. Having taken Standard Precautions, you and Nancy walk toward the crowd and note that the man appears to be in his mid-30s. He is on his knees, leaning forward, and struggling to breathe. He is in obvious respiratory distress. Even as you approach, you can hear wheezing, and stridor is present on inspiration. He leans forward on his hands to breathe, his nostrils flare with each breath, and his respirations are rapid. His brow is covered with sweat. His color is flushed red, and there are hives on both arms, as well as his neck and face. He begins scratching his arms and neck aggressively.

You quickly introduce yourself and your partner, and say to the patient and bystanders, "We are EMTs, and we're here to help you. Does anyone know what happened today?" Nancy begins the primary assessment while you set up the oxygen equipment. A bystander states that the patient's name is Kyle Patrick and that he is a coworker with the Parks Department. He tells you that he and Kyle were capturing swans to take for an annual veterinarian visit when a bee stung Kyle on the forearm. He goes on to say that Kyle has a history of similar episodes and that he has some kind of medication that he is supposed to take.

You quickly request paramedic backup. Dispatch confirms your request and tells you that paramedics are about 10 minutes out. The patient appears to be in severe respiratory distress. The SpO_2 on room air is 78% as you set the oxygen flow rate to 15 lpm and attempt to place the nonrebreather mask on him. You ask the patient's coworker to locate the patient's medication and bring it to you as quickly as possible. The patient refuses to allow you to place the nonrebreather face mask, so you hold the oxygen mask close to his nose and mouth. Nancy utters softly, "The patient's pulse is 160 per minute, regular, and bounding; the skin is cool, clammy, and flushed; respirations are 30 per minute, shallow, and labored. He responds to verbal stimuli appropriately. Pupils are equal and reactive. The SpO_2 is 80%, and his blood pressure is 90 by palpation."

The coworker returns with a prescribed epinephrine auto-injector and hands it to you. The label identifies the medication as the patient's, and the medication is not expired. You quickly expose the patient's thigh by cutting away the pants, administer the medication, and hold it in place for 10 seconds. You continue to administer oxygen and comfort the patient while the epinephrine takes effect. In about two minutes, the patient's respiratory status has improved dramatically, and he is able to answer questions. He shows you the spot on his arm where the bee stung him. Nancy had earlier removed the stinger while she was taking the patient's blood pressure. The patient states that he feels sick to his stomach and has a horrible headache.

You hear a siren in the distance and know that the paramedic unit will arrive soon. You complete a reassessment and have the following findings: The patient is alert and oriented and is breathing adequately; the pulse is 120 per minute, strong, and regular; the skin is cool, moist, and slightly flushed; respirations are 22 per minute and normal; pupils are equal and reactive. The blood pressure is 100/76 by auscultation. The SpO_2 is 97%, Nancy switched the oxygen to a nasal cannula at 2 lpm. You ask Kyle Patrick if he has any allergies, and he advises that he is only allergic to bee stings. You go on to ask if he takes any additional medications, and he says only the epinephrine auto-injector. You ask, "Do you have any other medical conditions or problems?" Kyle replies, "No, only the allergy to bee stings." You ask, "When was the last time you ate or drank anything?" He tells you, "It was about three hours ago. I ate a normal breakfast of Frosted Flakes and toast." You try to clarify the information presented to you by saying, "OK, Kyle, let me make sure I understand what happened to you this morning. You were working here capturing swans to take to the veterinarian when a bee stung you on the arm. Is that correct?" "Yes," he says with a slight grin.

You hear the door of the ALS vehicle close and look up to see Paramedic Logsdon walking toward you. You introduce Kyle Patrick to Lieutenant Paramedic Logsdon and provide a brief report of the patient's condition. You help place Kyle on the cot and then into the ALS ambulance. You and Nancy Ann return your equipment to the vehicle and prepare the unit to respond to another call. You report to dispatch that you are available.

1. What sign(s) that Kyle Patrick presented would be considered the hallmark sign(s) of an anaphylactic reaction?
   a. Hives and severe itching
   b. Blood pressure of 90 mmHg
   c. Respiratory distress
   d. SpO_2 of 78%

2. Kyle Patrick was in respiratory distress and had an SpO_2 of only 78%. What mechanism was the most likely cause of these signs and symptoms?
   a. Bronchoconstriction
   b. Blood vessel dilation and leaking
   c. Psychogenic reaction
   d. Hypertension

3. When administering the epinephrine auto-injector, where is the preferred location to inject the contents?
   a. Proximal end of the medial thigh
   b. Distal end of the medial thigh
   c. Midpoint of the lateral thigh
   d. Distal end of the lateral thigh

4. Kyle Patrick complains of a severe headache and nausea. This finding is most likely to indicate
   a. recurrence of the anaphylactic reaction.
   b. normal side effect of the epinephrine.
   c. hypoperfusion.
   d. nothing of significance.

5. Instead of cutting Kyle Patrick's pants to administer the epinephrine, the EMT could have administered the epinephrine into
   a. the lateral aspect of his upper arm muscle.
   b. the medial aspect of his upper arm muscle.
   c. his lower leg with pant leg raised.
   d. his thigh through his pants.

EMERGENCY TRIP SHEET

TRIP #	
MEDIC #	
BEGIN MILES	
END MILES	
CODE ___/___	PAGE ___/___
UNITS ON SCENE	

NAME	SEX M F DOB ___/___/___
ADDRESS	RACE
CITY STATE	ZIP
PHONE ( ) - PCP DR.	
RESPONDED FROM	CITY
TAKEN FROM	ZIP
DESTINATION	REASON
SSN - - MEDICARE #	MEDICAID #
INSURANCE CO INSURANCE #	GROUP #
RESPONSIBLE PARTY ADDRESS	
CITY STATE ZIP PHONE ( ) -	
EMPLOYER	

BILLING USE ONLY

DAY		
DATE		
RECEIVED		
DISPATCHED		
EN-ROUTE		
ON SCENE		
TO HOSPITAL		
AT HOSPITAL		
IN-SERVICE		

CREW	CERT	STATE #

TIME	ON SCENE (1)	ON SCENE (2)	ON SCENE (3)	EN-ROUTE (1)	EN-ROUTE (2)	AT DESTINATION
BP						
PULSE						
RESP						
SpO2						
ETCO2						
EKG						

IV THERAPY
SUCCESSFUL Y N # OF ATTEMPTS _____
ANGIO SIZE _____ ga.
SITE _____
TOTAL FLUID INFUSED _____ cc
BLOOD DRAW Y N INITIALS

INTUBATION INFORMATION
SUCCESSFUL Y N # OF ATTEMPTS _____
TUBE SIZE _____ mm
TIME _____ INITIALS _____

MEDICAL HISTORY

MEDICATIONS

ALLERGIES

C/C

EVENTS LEADING TO C/C

ASSESSMENT

TREATMENT

CONDITION CODES				

TREATMENTS

TIME	TREATMENT	DOSE	ROUTE	INIT

GCS E___ V___ M___ TOTAL =
GCS E___ V___ M___ TOTAL =

HOSPITAL CONTACTED

CPR BEGUN BY   B   P   TIME BEGUN

AED USED   Y   N   BY:

RESUSCITATION TERMINATED - TIME

EMS SIGNATURE

( ) OSHA REGULATIONS FOLLOWED

Toxicologic Emergencies

STANDARD

Medicine (Content Area: Toxicology)

COMPETENCY

Applies fundamental knowledge to provide basic emergency care and transportation based on assessment findings for an acutely ill patient.

OBJECTIVES

After reading this chapter, you should be able to:

22-1. Define key terms introduced in this chapter.

22-2. List the primary concerns of the EMT in managing drug and alcohol emergencies.

22-3. Describe each of the four routes by which a poison can enter the body:
  a. Ingestion
  b. Inhalation
  c. Injection
  d. Absorption

22-4. Describe the important steps in managing a poisoning patient, regardless of the specific poison or route of exposure.

22-5. Explain the limited role of specific antidotes in toxicologic emergencies.

22-6. Given a scenario involving a patient who has ingested a poison, describe the steps of assessment-based management.

22-7. Describe the indications, contraindications, mechanism of action, side effects, dosage, and administration of activated charcoal.

22-8. Given a scenario involving a patient who has inhaled a poison, describe the steps of assessment-based management.

22-9. Given a scenario involving a patient who has been exposed to an injected poison, describe the steps of assessment-based management.

22-10. Given a scenario involving a patient who has absorbed a poison, describe the steps of assessment-based management.

22-11. Describe special considerations in assessing and managing patients with each of the following:
  a. Food poisoning
  b. Carbon monoxide poisoning
  c. Cyanide poisoning

      d. Exposure to acid or alkali substances

      e. Exposure to hydrocarbons

      f. Methanol ingestion

      g. Isopropanol ingestion

      h. Ethylene glycol ingestion

      i. Exposure to poisonous plants

22-12. Explain the importance of contacting the poison control center with as complete a patient history as possible, and list specific types of information you should include.

22-13. Given a scenario involving a patient experiencing a drug or alcohol emergency, describe the steps of assessment-based management.

22-14. Describe special considerations in managing violent drug or alcohol abuse patients.

22-15. Describe special considerations in assessing and managing patients experiencing emergencies associated with each of the following:

      a. Drug withdrawal

      b. Alcoholic syndrome

      c. Withdrawal syndrome, including delirium tremens

      d. PCP use

      e. Cocaine use

      f. Amphetamines and methamphetamines

      g. Medication overdose

      h. Huffing

❙ KEY IDEAS

This chapter focuses on the assessment and management of toxicologic emergencies, including poisoning and drug and alcohol abuse. Thousands of people become seriously ill or die each year due to accidental or intentional poisonings. Drugs and alcohol are abused by a number of people in a variety of ways. You may encounter such patients in virtually any setting. In addition to the medical emergency created by drug or alcohol ingestion or withdrawal, these individuals are often trauma patients and may exhibit aggressive or violent behavior toward the EMS crew. It is important that you have a good understanding of the assessment and emergency care needed to manage these patients effectively. Key concepts include the following:

- A poison is any substance (liquid, solid, or gas) that impairs health or can cause death by its chemical effect when it enters the body or comes in contact with the skin.

- Poisons may enter the body via absorption, ingestion, inhalation, or injection.

- Children are the most frequent victims of accidental poisoning by ingestion of prescription or illicit drugs, cleaning agents, or cosmetics.

- The scene size-up must be carefully conducted to prevent the exposure of emergency response personnel to hazardous substances that may be present on the emergency scene.

- The first priority of care in the management of poisoning emergencies is to ensure that any life-threatening findings to the airway, breathing, oxygenation, or circulation are immediately managed when discovered.

- Continually monitor the airway, breathing, oxygenation, circulation, and mental status of the poisoned patient because rapid deterioration could occur. A sudden decrease in the mental status may indicate rapid patient deterioration.

- Safety must be a primary concern for the EMT at the scene of drug or alcohol emergencies, since these patients may exhibit aggressive or violent behavior and are also often infected with blood-borne or airborne diseases.

- Overdose and withdrawal are potentially life-threatening emergencies.

- The signs and symptoms of high-priority drug and alcohol patients include unresponsiveness or an altered mental status, inadequate breathing, fever, abnormal pulse rates, vomiting, and seizures.

- Management of drug and alcohol emergencies requires careful attention to the maintenance of airway, breathing, assessment of oxygenation, and circulation status as well as to controlling potentially volatile situations with unpredictable patients.

TERMS AND CONCEPTS

1. Write the number of the correct term next to each definition.
    1. Absorption
    2. Ingestion
    3. Inhalation
    4. Injection
    5. Poison
    6. Toxin
    7. Drug abuse
    8. Huffing
    9. Overdose
    10. Pharming
    11. Withdrawal

    _____ a. Substance that can impair health or cause death

    _____ b. Exposure that results from breathing a substance

    _____ c. Passage of a substance through the skin surface upon contact

    _____ d. Exposure that results from swallowing a substance

    _____ e. A poison of animal, plant, or bacterial origin

    _____ f. Forceful introduction of a substance through the penetration of the skin surface

    _____ g. Physical syndrome that occurs after a period of abstinence from a substance to which a person's body has become accustomed

    _____ h. Self-administration of legal or illicit substances in a manner that is not in accord with approved medical or social patterns

    _____ i. An emergency that involves poisoning or toxicity caused by drugs or alcohol

    _____ j. Raiding parents' or friends' medicine cabinets for prescription medications

    _____ k. Inhaling paints or propellants in order to "get high"

CONTENT REVIEW

1. Which statement is most correct with regard to poisoning emergencies?
    a. Approximately 1,000 poisonings occur each year in the United States.
    b. Most poisonings are intentional and result from homicide or suicide.
    c. Toxicology is the study of beneficial drugs and their effects on the body.
    d. Poisoning is commonly defined as exposure to a substance other than a drug or medication.

2. Poisoning by inhalation
    a. produces a more delayed effect than by ingestion.
    b. results in only respiratory signs and symptoms.
    c. may cause lung tissue damage that may lead to pulmonary edema.
    d. rarely has direct effects on the pulmonary system.

3. During the physical exam of a 16-year-old male patient who is unresponsive, you observe a yellow substance on the patient's lips and around his nose. The same substance is observed on the patient's nose hairs. The patient most likely
   a. used "free-based" crack cocaine.
   b. has ingested psychoactive "bath salts" (PABS).
   c. smoked "ice" or "crystal."
   d. intentionally inhaled paint or some other substance.

4. At the scene of a poisoning emergency, your medical priority is to
   a. identify the poisonous substance.
   b. contact the regional poison control center.
   c. maintain the patient's airway.
   d. verify the type of exposure.

5. Inhaled poisons may cause airway and breathing compromise as a result of which three factors?
   a. Enhanced airway reactivity, respiratory depression, and direct damage to airway tissues
   b. Diminished bronchial cleansing, enhanced airway reactivity, and direct damage to airway tissues
   c. Alteration of mental status, respiratory depression, and direct damage to airway tissues
   d. Alteration of mental status, diminished bronchial cleansing, and direct damage to airway tissues

6. Inhaled poisonings
   a. cause millions of deaths each year in the United States.
   b. most frequently occur as a result of chemical spills in industrial settings.
   c. are frequently successfully resuscitated, even with long exposure times.
   d. that are most common include carbon monoxide and carbon dioxide.

7. From the following list, indicate the items that typically suggest the signs and symptoms associated with poisoning by inhalation (INH), ingestion (ING), injection (INJ), or absorption (ABS).

   _____ Abdominal pain, tenderness, and cramping

   _____ Pupillary changes

   _____ Hoarseness

   _____ Body or breath odor

   _____ Difficulty breathing

   _____ Liquid or powder on skin

   _____ Diarrhea

   _____ Copious secretions

   _____ Itching and burning

   _____ Pain, redness, and swelling at injection site

   _____ Singed nasal hairs

   _____ Fever and chills

   _____ Redness or swelling

8. From the following list, select the items that may indicate poisoning. Indicate yes (Y) if it is a possible indicator or no (N) if it is not a possible indicator.

   _____ a. Behavior changes (clumsiness, drowsiness, altered mental status)

   _____ b. Crackles on auscultation of the chest

   _____ c. Pupils normal in size and reaction

_____ d. Excessive salivation

_____ e. Normal skin and mucosa findings

_____ f. No paralysis

9. Timmy is a 2-year-old who has ingested a corrosive acid. In addition to maintaining his airway and oxygenation, you should
   a. dilute the substance by giving him large amounts of milk or water.
   b. prevent further injury by rinsing the substance from his mouth and lips.
   c. administer activated charcoal per local protocol or medical direction.
   d. talk seriously with his mother about child safety issues.

10. Activated charcoal
    a. is a commonly used antidote to most ingested poisons.
    b. neutralizes caustic and corrosive poisonous substances.
    c. is rarely used in the emergency medical care of ingested poisonings.
    d. reverses the toxic effects of drugs and alcohol.

11. When ordered by medical direction or the poison control center, activated charcoal is indicated for the patient who has
    a. recently ingested poisons by mouth.
    b. inhaled toxic chemical substances.
    c. made skin contact with corrosive powders.
    d. been bitten by a poisonous snake.

12. Medical direction may order the administration of activated charcoal if it can be immediately administered shortly after ingestion of which of the following medication types?
    a. Nonsteroidal anti-inflammatory drugs (NSAIDs)
    b. Anticoagulants
    c. Antioxidants
    d. Opioids

13. The usual adult dosage of activated charcoal is
    a. 10 grams.
    b. 12–20 grams.
    c. 30–100 grams.
    d. 150 grams.

14. Activated charcoal is also known by the brand name
    a. CharAway.
    b. GoChar.
    c. Actidose.
    d. Toxi-aid.

15. Which patient is the most likely candidate for the use of activated charcoal?
    a. A patient who responds to verbal stimuli and has ingested ethanol
    b. A patient who is alert and oriented and recently ingested an anticholinergic drug
    c. A patient who is alert and oriented and ingested ammonia
    d. A patient who is confused and is unable to swallow

16. A common side effect seen with administration of activated charcoal is
    a. blackened stool.
    b. headache.
    c. rapid pulse.
    d. seizures.

17. The majority of toxic inhalations occur as a result of
    a. recreational use of inhalants.
    b. industrial accidents.
    c. fire-related incidents.
    d. hazardous materials incidents.

18. The primary symptom associated with toxic inhalation that is most likely to occur first is
    a. an altered mental status.
    b. respiratory symptoms.
    c. increased tearing from the eyes.
    d. nausea.

19. An appropriate action in the management of a toxic inhalation is to
    a. perform the assessment where the patient is found.
    b. have the patient removed to fresh air as soon as possible.
    c. administer activated charcoal to minimize absorption.
    d. avoid positive pressure ventilation of the patient.

20. As an EMT, when managing poisons due to absorption, one thing you should pay particular attention to is
    a. preventing the substance from contacting your own skin.
    b. avoiding irrigation of chemical burns to the patient's eyes.
    c. keeping the patient's clothing and jewelry intact and on the patient.
    d. flushing dry powder from the skin with copious amounts of water.

21. Food poisoning
    a. commonly results in death.
    b. is decreasing in incidence from prior years in the United States.
    c. is often caused by tainted vegetables but seldom by tainted fish.
    d. is difficult to detect because the signs and symptoms vary greatly.

22. Carbon monoxide
    a. is generally easy to detect because of its foul smell.
    b. increases the amount of oxygen carried on the hemoglobin.
    c. inhibits the ability of body cells to utilize oxygen.
    d. is only rarely a cause of death in the United States.

23. Carbon monoxide poisoning should be suspected if
    a. the patient has a fever and a slower-than-normal respiratory rate.
    b. flulike symptoms are shared by people in the same environment.
    c. the patient's pupils are unequal in size and reactivity.
    d. chest pain and choking are experienced by people in the same environment.

24. This poison can enter the body through inhalation, absorption, injection, or ingestion. It is found in many household products, including rodent poisons and silver polish, and in cherry and apricot pits. Inhalation of this poison can occur in fires where plastics, silk, and synthetic carpets may be burning. The poison is
    a. carbon monoxide.
    b. carbon dioxide.
    c. chlorine.
    d. cyanide.

25. The smell of bitter almonds is most closely associated with _____ poisoning.
    a. carbon monoxide
    b. carbon dioxide
    c. chlorine
    d. cyanide

26. Strong acids
    a. have an extremely high pH.
    b. will cause the most severe burns in the esophagus if ingested.
    c. will typically burn for only 1–2 minutes.
    d. cause little if any abdominal pain if ingested.

27. Alkalis
    a. will produce burns that are not as deep as acid burns.
    b. will typically burn for only 1–2 minutes.
    c. will likely injure the stomach tissue if ingested.
    d. have an extremely low pH.

28. Hydrocarbon
    a. poisoning frequently involves elderly patients.
    b. toxicity is somewhat dependent upon the viscosity of the substance.
    c. poisoning can be safely treated with activated charcoal.
    d. products include most commercial drain cleaners.

29. Methanol
    a. is also known as domestic alcohol.
    b. is found in most alcoholic beverages.
    c. poisoning occurs only through ingestion.
    d. ingestion will produce large amounts of acid in the body.

30. Isopropanol
    a. acts as a cardiac depressant, causing bradycardia.
    b. is also known as isopropyl alcohol or rubbing alcohol.
    c. poisoning occurs most frequently by inhalation.
    d. is frequently found in antifreeze.

31. Ethylene glycol
    a. is found in detergents, radiator antifreeze, and windshield deicers.
    b. poisoning occurs infrequently in children due to its bitter taste.
    c. poisoning occurs in two distinct stages.
    d. poisoning is unresponsive to drinking ethanol (drinking alcohol).

32. Which statement related to poisonous plants is most correct?
  a. About 5 percent of all Americans are allergic to urushiol.
  b. For a reaction to poison ivy to occur, direct contact is necessary.
  c. Poison sumac is found mostly in the Northeast and Southeast of the United States.
  d. Stinging nettle, crown of thorns, and buttercup can cause mild to severe dermatitis.

33. Poison control centers
  a. are staffed and available for service from 8:00 A.M. to 5:00 P.M. EST seven days a week.
  b. are able to provide information on only a small number of poisons.
  c. provide follow-up via telephone calls to monitor the patient's progress.
  d. should not be consulted by EMTs on a routine basis.

34. Which of the following are the goals at the scene of a drug or an alcohol emergency?
  a. Identify and reverse the effects of the abused substance.
  b. Identify and treat the loss of vital functions caused by the drug.
  c. Notify police of illegal drug use.
  d. Identify the abused substance and control the behavior of the patient.

35. What are three common potential dangers at the scene of a drug or an alcohol emergency?
  a. Communicable disease, violent behavior, and weapons
  b. Violent behavior, weapons, and hazardous substances
  c. Infectious disease, violent behavior, and traffic
  d. Hazardous substances, weapons, and infectious disease

36. Your patient is found unresponsive on the living room floor, surrounded by nearly a dozen empty and partially filled pill bottles. What should be done with the bottles?
  a. Do nothing with the pill bottles. They are of little importance.
  b. Keep the pill bottles with the patient as a source of information.
  c. Turn the pill bottles over to the police. They may be a source of evidence.
  d. Return the pill bottles to the patient's family so they may be refilled.

37. In drug or alcohol emergencies, expect
  a. signs and symptoms that mimic only one or two medical disorders.
  b. to identify and treat the loss of vital functions caused by the drug or alcohol.
  c. scenes that seldom involve violent acts or physical abuse.
  d. scenes that do not require the use of Standard Precautions.

38. Upon completion of your assessment, you suspect that your unresponsive patient's condition may be due to drugs or alcohol. Which action is most appropriate to take next?
  a. Move the patient to the ambulance and transport immediately.
  b. Contact medical direction and seek additional guidance.
  c. With a gloved hand, check the mouth for signs of pills or tablets.
  d. Ask bystanders for information about precipitating events.

39. From the following list, select those signs and symptoms that indicate a life-threatening drug or alcohol emergency. Mark those that indicate a life threat with a Y for yes and those that do not with an N for no.

  _____ a. Normal level of responsiveness

  _____ b. Respiratory difficulty

  _____ c. Vomiting, with a normal level of responsiveness

_____ d. Fever

_____ e. Slow pulse rate

_____ f. Seizures

_____ g. Right-lower-quadrant abdominal pain

_____ h. Lower back discomfort

40. The most reliable indicators of a drug or alcohol emergency are likely to come from which two of the following phases of the patient assessment?
a. Physical exam and vital signs
b. Vital signs and patient history
c. Scene size-up and patient history
d. Physical exam and reassessment

41. You are on scene with a disoriented patient who reports taking an overdose of pain medication. Number the following list in the proper order from 1 to 5 to show the emergency care steps for this patient.

_____ Administer oxygen at 15 lpm by a nonrebreather mask if signs of severe hypoxia are present.

_____ Transport the patient to the hospital.

_____ Take measures to maintain body temperature and prevent shock.

_____ Establish and maintain a patent airway.

_____ If local protocol permits, assess the blood glucose level.

42. Hallucinogenic substances
a. such as phencyclidine (PCP) can cause extreme agitation or excitation.
b. are also known as "imbecilic drugs."
c. are commonly derived from opiates and opioids.
d. cause central nervous system (CNS) depression and drowsiness.

43. The EMT pictured here is talking with a patient who is experiencing an alcohol emergency. Which of the following is the most correct comment about the technique being demonstrated?
a. Touch can be comforting; always touch the alcohol emergency patient.
b. Touch can be comforting; however, never touch the patient without his permission.
c. Pat the patient on the back to help clear his airway.
d. Grasp the shoulder and forearm to initiate restraint.

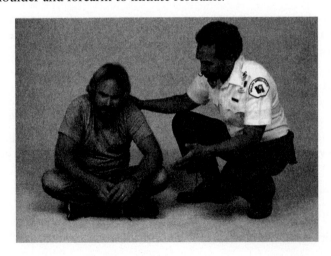

44. You are attempting to treat a drug abuse patient experiencing a "bad trip." Which of the following is *not* an element of the "talk-down technique"?

    a. Transport the patient immediately and attempt to calm while en route to the hospital.

    b. Help the patient verbalize what is happening to him.

    c. Make simple statements to help orient the patient to time and place.

    d. Reassure the patient that his condition is caused by the drug.

45. CNS stimulant drugs typically cause

    a. constricted pupils.

    b. dilated pupils.

    c. no effect on the patient's pupils.

    d. unequal pupils.

46. Bradycardia, hypotension, inadequate breathing rates and volume, cool and clammy skin, constricted pupils, and nausea are most commonly associated with

    a. CNS stimulants.

    b. CNS depressants.

    c. CNS depressants derived from narcotics.

    d. hallucinogens.

47. The physically dependent drug user

    a. deals normally with problems and seldom thinks about using the drug.

    b. undergoes physiological changes within the body that require the drug to be present.

    c. has no physiological consequences from drug withdrawal.

    d. may develop tolerance to a drug, in which case smaller doses are needed.

48. Common signs and symptoms of drug withdrawal

    a. typically peak at 12–24 hours.

    b. include urinary retention, lower leg cramps, and dilated pupils.

    c. include excessive thirst, lower leg cramps, and indigestion.

    d. include nausea, abdominal cramping, and tremors.

49. A chronic brain syndrome resulting from the toxic effects of alcohol on the CNS combined with malnutrition is called

    a. Jackson-Pierce disease.

    b. Wernicke-Korsakoff syndrome.

    c. Alcoholic nutritional syndrome.

    d. Perkins-Brower syndrome.

50. Which is the correct term for a combination of problem drinking (to relieve tension) and true addiction to alcohol (in which abstinence causes physical withdrawal symptoms)?

    a. Addiction syndrome

    b. Withdrawal syndrome

    c. Alcoholic syndrome

    d. Intoxication syndrome

51. Which is the correct term for the syndrome that occurs when the alcoholic's alcohol level falls below the amount usually ingested?

    a. Abstinence syndrome

    b. Hypoalcohol syndrome

    c. Addiction syndrome

    d. Withdrawal syndrome

52. Stage 1 of alcohol withdrawal occurs within about _____ and is characterized by nausea, insomnia, sweating, and tremors.
    a. 2 hours
    b. 4 hours
    c. 6 hours
    d. 8 hours

53. The last stage of alcohol withdrawal is a life-threatening condition with a mortality rate between 5 and 15 percent. This stage is called
    a. alcohol poisoning.
    b. delirium tremens.
    c. Jackson-Pierce syndrome.
    d. terminal alcohol toxicity.

54. Which of the following is a drug that is cheap to make and produces horrible psychological effects that can last for years? It is known by multiple names, such as angel dust, killer weed, supergrass, crystal cyclone, and many others.
    a. AGN
    b. PCP
    c. Amnioglycoside
    d. DHT

55. Cocaine
    a. is mildly addictive.
    b. is taken only by inhalation through the nose.
    c. requires treatment that is very different from that for PCP.
    d. is also known as crack and may be inhaled (free-based).

56. The first priority of care for a patient under the influence of PCP is to
    a. begin the talk-down technique to manage the patient.
    b. quickly check for injuries that require attention.
    c. protect the safety of yourself and your response crew.
    d. monitor the vital signs and transport quickly.

57. Intentionally inhaled poisons commonly
    a. contain the chemical agent oban.
    b. improve oxygen movement across the alveolar membrane.
    c. have a more delayed onset of symptoms than injected poisons.
    d. accumulate in the regions of the brain responsible for feelings of pleasure.

58. Methamphetamine
    a. is a type of depressant drug.
    b. use calms and relaxes the patient.
    c. is commonly called "crank" or "go."
    d. can only be used by injection.

59. You arrive on the scene, where it appears that the patient may have applied the use of a suicide bag. Your first and most important action is to
    a. quickly cut or remove the tie and bag from around the neck and head of the patient.
    b. secure the bag in place until the police can take control of the scene.
    c. immediately exit the room to fresh air and await for the arrival of the fire department.
    d. expose the patient; administer ventilation breaths by bag-valve-mask (BVM) with supplemental oxygen.

60. You are assessing a patient that you suspect has ingested PABS. Which of the following would you likely expect to encounter with this type of drug?

a. Hypertension

b. Bradycardia

c. Hypothermia

d. Unequal pupils

▌CASE STUDY 1

You have just returned the emergency unit to service following a minor traffic accident call when you are dispatched to 1980 Brandywine Ski Road for "a male that is unconscious." You note no obvious hazards as you approach the house. A neighbor with a house key lets you in. The neighbor reports that the occupant's wife called her from work and asked her to please check on her husband, Mr. Johnson. The neighbor tried to enter the basement but was unable to do so because of a strong odor. She thinks 50-year-old Mr. Johnson is lying on the floor of his basement workshop. You are aware of an overwhelmingly pungent chemical odor that burns your nose and eyes as you attempt to descend the stairs.

1. What action should you take?

a. Retreat to a safe area and call for personnel with self-contained breathing apparatus.

b. Continue down the stairs until you can determine the source of the hazard.

c. Proceed down the stairs and quickly remove Mr. Johnson from the basement.

d. Hold your breath as you quickly remove Mr. Johnson from the basement.

2. Following the removal of Mr. Johnson from the basement, which of the following best describes the care that should be provided before transport?

a. Maintain spinal immobilization, ensure a patent airway, check for breathing, provide positive pressure ventilation if required, and loosen tight clothing.

b. Apply a nonrebreather mask with oxygen flowing at 15 lpm, place Mr. Johnson in a lateral recumbent position, and be prepared to suction.

c. Maintain spinal immobilization, administer oxygen by a nonrebreather mask at 15 lpm, and place the patient on a plastic-lined sheet.

d. No care should be provided to Mr. Johnson until he is properly decontaminated.

You find Mr. Johnson to be unresponsive, with rapid, shallow, labored breathing. His pulse is rapid. His skin is pale, cool, and sweaty. There are no signs of trauma.

3. From the following list of treatment descriptions, indicate yes (Y) if it is an appropriate treatment or no (N) if it is not an appropriate treatment for Mr. Johnson.

_____ a. Inspect Mr. Johnson for any poison that may still be on his body or clothes.

b. Perform a rapid physical exam.

_____ c. Have someone wearing self-contained breathing apparatus retrieve any containers that Mr. Johnson might have been using.

_____ d. Give careful attention to Mr. Johnson's airway and breathing.

The neighbor reports that Mr. Johnson has "never been sick a day in his life." He takes no medications and has no known allergies. She says she does not know when he last ate. She knows that Mr. Johnson enjoys refinishing furniture.

4. How often does Mr. Johnson require reassessment en route to the hospital?
   a. Every 5 minutes
   b. Every 10 minutes
   c. Every 15 minutes
   d. Every 20 minutes

CASE STUDY 2

You have just finished cleaning up the station kitchen following a great dinner prepared by your partner when the alarm sounds. You are dispatched to a call for an unresponsive patient. You arrive on scene and find a 17-year-old female who was found unresponsive on the floor of her bedroom by her mother. She was last seen about four hours ago. Your initial assessment finds her unresponsive, with snoring respirations of approximately 8 per minute. There is vomitus on the floor near her head. Her pulse is slow and irregular. Her skin is pale, cool, and dry.

1. What is your first priority in managing this patient?
   a. Cover the patient to maintain body temperature.
   b. Ensure that the airway is clear of vomitus.
   c. Quickly begin positive pressure ventilation.
   d. Immobilize on a long spine board.

   The mother reports that her daughter has been depressed since the death of her boyfriend in a car crash last month, but she has no medical problems or allergies. Your partner finds four empty pill bottles and a partially full wine bottle in the adjacent bathroom.

2. Your partner read in a journal about the usefulness of activated charcoal for one of the drugs the patient ingested. He suggests that you should administer activated charcoal. Should this patient be administered activated charcoal?
   a. Yes, at a dose of 3 g/kg.
   b. Yes, at a dose of 1 g/kg.
   c. No, because the patient has an altered level of consciousness.
   d. No, because the patient has ingested alcohol.

3. Which statement best describes the management of this patient?
   a. This is a life-threatening situation. The patient is a high priority for transport. Give the pill bottles and wine bottle to the police. Complete the physical exam and the baseline vital signs. Perform a reassessment every 5 minutes during transport and closely monitor the airway and breathing.
   b. This is a life-threatening situation. The patient is a high priority for transport. Transport the pill bottles, wine bottle, and a sample of the vomitus to the emergency department. Complete the physical exam and the vital signs. Perform a reassessment every 5 minutes during transport and closely monitor the airway and breathing.
   c. This is a non-life-threatening situation. The patient is a low priority for transport. Complete the physical exam and the baseline vital signs. Perform a reassessment every 15 minutes during transport.
   d. This is a non-life-threatening situation. The patient is a low priority for transport. Transport the pill bottles and wine bottle and a sample of the vomitus to the emergency department. Perform an ongoing assessment every 15 minutes during transport.

CHAPTER 22 SCENARIO 1: DOCUMENTATION EXERCISE

Read the following scenario and think about how you would document this call if you were the EMT who responded to the scene. Then answer the multiple-choice questions and fill in the sample prehospital care report, basing your documentation on information from the scenario.

It is 8:30 A.M. on an overcast Saturday. You are working with your partner, Laci Richard, when the alarm sounds: "Unit 1 respond to an unknown medical at 1621 Lake Hollingsworth Road, cross street Ingraham. Time out 0830 hours." Dispatch advises that the caller is hysterical and is unable to provide any information related to the patient.

You arrive on the scene in about 5 minutes. The home is located in a neighborhood of expensive homes in an exclusive area of town. You pull up in the driveway of a three-story home and park next to several bikes that are scattered across the driveway. As you are walking toward the door with your Standard Precautions on, a boy of about 10 or 12 years of age comes running out of the house. He tells you that his younger brother ate some medicine and that his mom was "really upset." You introduce yourself and your partner and find out that his name is Jake and that his younger brother's name is Jimmy. Jimmy is about 2 years of age. You enter the house and proceed to a bathroom at the back, where a small boy is sitting on the floor on which some medicine containers are scattered. The mother grabs Laci and loudly screams, "You've got to do something for my son, NOW!"

Jimmy appears to be in minor distress. He looks at you as you enter. His skin color looks normal, with no abnormal respiratory sounds present, and he appears to be breathing normally. No signs of trauma are present. You reach down to check his pulse. His skin is warm and dry, and his pulse is rapid and strong. You introduce yourself and Laci to the mother and say, "We are EMTs, and we are here to help your son. Can you tell us what happened today?" Laci begins a primary assessment and tells you she will obtain the vitals. Meanwhile, the crying mother says, "I don't know how it happened. I was talking to my sister on the phone, and I thought Jimmy was next to me, but he got into the bathroom, and I guess he crawled up on the sink and got into the medicine cabinet. By the time I found him, he had all these bottles open, and I don't know what he swallowed." You ask, "What's your name, ma'am?" She says, "It's Mrs. Wilson."

You continue by saying, "Mrs. Wilson, we are going to do all we can to help Jimmy. How much does he weigh, and when did he get into the medicines?" She tells you, "He weighs about 28 pounds, and this happened about 10 or 15 minutes ago." You ask, "Has he complained of anything?" "No," she replies. "He doesn't know why I'm so upset." You ask, "Was your son sick to his stomach before we arrived?" "No," she says. You ask, "Does your son have any allergies?" The mother says, "No, he is not allergic to anything." You next ask, "Is your son taking any medications?" "No," she replies. You continue the assessment. "Has your son ever been sick before or hospitalized?" "No," she quickly states. You then ask, "When was the last time your son ate, and how much did he eat?" She says, "He ate a bowl of cereal about an hour ago . . . and some toast, too. I don't see what this all has to do with helping my son. Please do something!"

You ask the mother to please gather up all the containers of medication that she thinks Jimmy could possibly have gotten into and bring them along to the hospital. Laci has established a good rapport with Jimmy by allowing him to participate in the evaluation. She advises that his respirations are normal at 28 per minute; pulse is strong and regular at 110; skin color is normal, warm, and dry; and pupils are equal, reactive, and respond briskly to light. Perfusion appears adequate; the SpO_2 is 99%. There is no abdominal tenderness. You quickly jot down the vitals and say that you are going to contact poison control. You explain to Mrs. Wilson that poison control will advise you of the very best and most up-to-date treatment for Jimmy.

You call poison control and advise the registered nurse (RN) of the situation. You tell him Jimmy's age and weight, and you quickly summarize his general condition. You provide his vital signs and say that he may have ingested an undetermined number of pills and capsules from at least three different medications. The three medications are Prilosec (omeprazole SA) 20 mg, Lipitor (atorvastatin) 10 mg, and Norvasc (amlodipine besylate) 10 mg. You tell him the child ate a bowl of cereal and some toast about an hour ago. The RN advises that he is most concerned about the possibility that Jimmy may have ingested the Norvasc. You ask Mrs. Johnson who is taking the Norvasc. She tells you that it is her father, who was visiting a few months ago and left it in the medicine cabinet. You relay this information to the RN and he advises you that he will contact the receiving emergency department with additional instructions. He tells you to monitor Jimmy closely and transport. You complete your assessment and transport Jimmy and his mother and brother and a paper bag containing all the medications from the bathroom to the local emergency department.

1. When Laci assessed Jimmy's vital signs
   a. she should have assessed the blood pressure early.
   b. she should have assessed the blood pressure by palpation.
   c. she was correct in not assessing the blood pressure, which is generally not assessed in children less than 3 years of age.
   d. she was correct in not assessing the blood pressure, which is generally not assessed in children less than 5 years of age.

2. Your treatment of Jimmy is primarily focused on
   a. watching closely for life threats and providing information to poison control.
   b. providing an antidote to the medication he swallowed.
   c. speeding absorption of the medication to move it quickly through his system.
   d. reassuring his mother that something is being done for her son.

3. When a parent like Mrs. Wilson is extremely upset, what is the best thing to do?
   a. Send the parent out of the room so she doesn't upset the child.
   b. Keep the parent in the room because the child will be upset if she leaves.
   c. Tell the parent to "calm down."
   d. Ask the parent to step aside and let you do your job.

EMERGENCY TRIP SHEET

TRIP #	
MEDIC #	
BEGIN MILES	
END MILES	
CODE __/__	PAGE __/__
UNITS ON SCENE	

NAME	SEX M F DOB __/__/__
ADDRESS	RACE
CITY STATE	ZIP
PHONE ( ) - PCP DR.	
RESPONDED FROM	CITY
TAKEN FROM	ZIP
DESTINATION	REASON
SSN - - MEDICARE #	MEDICAID #
INSURANCE CO INSURANCE #	GROUP #
RESPONSIBLE PARTY ADDRESS	
CITY STATE ZIP PHONE ( ) -	
EMPLOYER	

TIME	ON SCENE (1)	ON SCENE (2)	ON SCENE (3)	EN-ROUTE (1)	EN-ROUTE (2)	AT DESTINATION
BP						
PULSE						
RESP						
SpO2						
ETCO2						
EKG						

MEDICAL HISTORY

MEDICATIONS

ALLERGIES

C/C

EVENTS LEADING TO C/C

ASSESSMENT

TREATMENT

EMS SIGNATURE

BILLING USE ONLY

DAY				
DATE				
RECEIVED				
DISPATCHED				
EN-ROUTE				
ON SCENE				
TO HOSPITAL				
AT HOSPITAL				
IN-SERVICE				

CREW	CERT	STATE #

IV THERAPY
SUCCESSFUL Y N # OF ATTEMPTS _____
ANGIO SIZE _____ ga.
SITE _____
TOTAL FLUID INFUSED _____ cc
BLOOD DRAW Y N INITIALS

INTUBATION INFORMATION
SUCCESSFUL Y N # OF ATTEMPTS _____
TUBE SIZE _____ mm
TIME _____ INITIALS _____

CONDITION CODES				

TREATMENTS

TIME	TREATMENT	DOSE	ROUTE	INIT

GCS E__ V__ M__ TOTAL =

GCS E__ V__ M__ TOTAL =

HOSPITAL CONTACTED

CPR BEGUN BY B P TIME BEGUN

AED USED Y N BY:

RESUSCITATION TERMINATED - TIME

(   ) OSHA REGULATIONS FOLLOWED

Read the following scenario and think about how you would document this call if you were the EMT who responded to the scene. Then answer the multiple-choice questions and fill in the sample prehospital care report, basing your documentation on information from the scenario.

It is 11:30 P.M. on a cold winter night. You have just jumped into bed and are thinking about applying for the next paramedic program when the alarm sounds: "Unit 1 respond to 350 North Crystal Lake Drive for patient who is 'hearing voices.' Cross street Longfellow Boulevard. Time out 2330 hours." You are working with Bob Clayton, who has been an EMT for 15 years. You have learned a lot from him and respect his emergency medical skills. Bob meets you at the vehicle, and you advise dispatch that you are responding.

You arrive at a run-down home located in a working-class neighborhood. The porch light is on, and a female, who appears to be in her 20s, waves you down. You stop, park the rescue vehicle, and with Standard Precautions in place, approach the house. As you do so, the lady greets you with, "I'm sure glad you're here! It's my boyfriend. He took some LSD about 45 minutes ago, and he is just out of it. He hears voices and is acting weird." You introduce yourself and Bob, and ask, "Has your boyfriend been violent at all?" She asserts, "No, he is not the violent type at all. He is just acting strange." You ask her for her name and the patient's name. She tells you, "My name is April May and his name is Edward Bare."

You enter the home and are escorted to a bedroom located in the front of the house. When you go into the room, you see the patient sitting in a small chair next to the bed. He looks to be about 25 years of age. His eyes are open, and he is staring down at his lap. His hands are trembling. He does not acknowledge your presence. You say, "Good evening, Mr. Bare. We're EMTs, and we're here to help you. I'd like to talk with you." You maintain a distance of about 8 feet from the patient, who remains silent with his head lowered, continuing to stare at his lap. He is breathing adequately with no abnormal respiratory sounds noted. His skin color looks normal, and no signs of trauma are observed.

You continue by saying, "I'd like to try to help you understand what is happening to you." He looks up at you. You note that his pupils are dilated. He utters something that you can't understand. You say, "Ed, I'm sorry, what did you say? I didn't understand you. Could you repeat what you said?" Ed replies, "What the X*%$ are you doing here? I didn't want

you here or ask you to come! What? What's that you said? You think I'm a punk! Get out! Just get out!"

You and Bob calmly step outside and quickly request law enforcement backup. The two of you wait outside for the police to arrive, explaining to April that you need to wait for law enforcement assistance. They arrive on scene in about three minutes. Now you reenter the scene with law enforcement at your side. You calmly approach Ed and say, "Ed, April is worried about you. She says that you took some LSD and that you've been hearing things. What's happening to you is caused by the LSD, and it won't last forever. It's temporary. You must try to focus on the fact that this is temporary."

Ed breaks in, saying, "Did you call me a punk?" You reply, "No, Ed. I didn't say that. You're hearing things that are caused by the LSD you took. It won't last forever, Ed. You must focus on that. It won't last forever." Ed quietly says, "It won't last? Hearing the voices, I mean." You reply calmly and just as quietly, "No, Ed. Focus on that. It won't last forever. Ed, I want you to also understand that as the drug wears off, you may be confused at times and still hear voices. OK?" Ed says, "I'm hearing voices now, but I'm going to focus and it's not going to last!" You say, "Thanks, Ed!"

You continue, "Ed, we are going to take your blood pressure and pulse now and get you ready to go to the hospital. Bob is going to touch you. Is that OK?" Ed replies, "Yes, that's all right." Bob notes a red rash on Ed's arm and gathers the vital signs. His respirations are 18 per minute and normal; pulse is 100 per minute, strong, regular, and bounding; his skin color is normal, warm, and dry; his pupils are equal, dilated, and respond slowly to light; his blood pressure is 140/80; and the SpO_2 is 97%.

You speak with April to obtain additional information. You say, "April, I need to confirm some information with you. You said that Ed took some LSD about 45 minutes ago and that about 10 minutes ago he began acting strangely. Is that right?" She says, "That's right." You ask, "Did he have any other complaints?" "No," she states. You ask, "Does Ed have any allergies or take any medications?" "No," she says. You continue by asking, "Has Ed seen a doctor, or been sick in the past?" She replies, "No, Ed has always been very healthy." You ask April when Ed last ate. She says, "It was about an hour ago. He had a sandwich and a beer." You say, "Thanks, April, you've been a great help. We're going to take Ed to the hospital now." You place Ed on the cot and prepare him for transport.

1. The signs or symptoms of potential LSD use that Ed exhibited include
   a. red rash, dilated pupils, and blood pressure of 140/80.
   b. motor disturbance, dilated pupils, and hallucinations.
   c. SpO_2 of 97%, red rash, and dilated pupils.
   d. SpO_2 of 97%, motor disturbance, and dilated pupils.

2. The technique you used to communicate with and manage Ed is called the
   a. LSD management technique.
   b. violent patient technique.
   c. talk-down technique.
   d. drug abuse technique.

3. The technique used to communicate with and manage Ed would not be used if he had taken
   a. PCP.
   b. PCB.
   c. marijuana.
   d. alcohol.

4. The technique for communicating with and managing a patient on hallucinogens includes the steps in the following list. Based on the information provided in the scenario, did you accomplish each step with Ed? If you did, mark the step with a Y for yes. If you didn't, mark the step with an N for no.

   _____ a. Make the patient feel welcome.

   _____ b. Identify yourself clearly.

   _____ c. Reassure the patient that his condition is caused by the drug and will not last forever.

   _____ d. Reiterate simple and concrete statements.

   _____ e. Forewarn the patient about what will happen as the drug wears off.

   _____ f. Once the patient has been calmed, transport.

5. Was it appropriate for law enforcement backup to be requested in this incident?
   a. Yes, law enforcement should have been requested as described.
   b. Yes, but the EMTs should not have left the patient's side.
   c. No, the patient can be managed without law enforcement backup.
   d. No, law enforcement was not needed, so long as a way to exit the scene safely was anticipated.

EMERGENCY TRIP SHEET

TRIP #	
MEDIC #	
BEGIN MILES	
END MILES	
CODE___/___ PAGE___/___	
UNITS ON SCENE	

BILLING USE ONLY

DAY				
DATE				
RECEIVED				
DISPATCHED				
EN-ROUTE				
ON SCENE				
TO HOSPITAL				
AT HOSPITAL				
IN-SERVICE				

NAME	SEX M F DOB ___/___/___
ADDRESS	RACE
CITY STATE	ZIP
PHONE ( ) - PCP DR.	
RESPONDED FROM	CITY
TAKEN FROM	ZIP
DESTINATION	REASON
SSN - - MEDICARE #	MEDICAID #
INSURANCE CO INSURANCE #	GROUP #
RESPONSIBLE PARTY ADDRESS	
CITY STATE ZIP PHONE ( ) -	
EMPLOYER	

CREW	CERT	STATE #

TIME	ON SCENE (1)	ON SCENE (2)	ON SCENE (3)	EN-ROUTE (1)	EN-ROUTE (2)	AT DESTINATION
BP						
PULSE						
RESP						
SpO_2						
$ETCO_2$						
EKG						

IV THERAPY
SUCCESSFUL Y N # OF ATTEMPTS _____
ANGIO SIZE _____ ga.
SITE _____
TOTAL FLUID INFUSED _____ cc
BLOOD DRAW Y N INITIALS _____

INTUBATION INFORMATION
SUCCESSFUL Y N # OF ATTEMPTS _____
TUBE SIZE _____ mm
TIME _____ INITIALS _____

MEDICAL HISTORY

MEDICATIONS

ALLERGIES

C/C

EVENTS LEADING TO C/C

ASSESSMENT

TREATMENT

CONDITION CODES				

TREATMENTS

TIME	TREATMENT	DOSE	ROUTE	INIT

GCS E___V___M___TOTAL =
GCS E___V___M___TOTAL =

HOSPITAL CONTACTED

CPR BEGUN BY B P TIME BEGUN	
AED USED Y N BY:	
RESUSCITATION TERMINATED - TIME	

EMS SIGNATURE

(   ) OSHA REGULATIONS FOLLOWED

Abdominal, Hematologic, Gynecologic, Genitourinary, and Renal Emergencies

STANDARD

Medicine (Content Areas: Abdominal and Gastrointestinal Disorders; Gynecology; Genitourinary/Renal)

COMPETENCY

Applies fundamental knowledge to provide basic emergency care and transportation based on assessment findings for an acutely ill patient.

OBJECTIVES

After reading this chapter, you should be able to:

23-1. Define key terms introduced in this chapter.

23-2. Describe the anatomy and physiology of the structures of the abdominal cavity, including:
   a. Boundaries of the abdominal cavity
   b. Visceral and parietal peritoneum
   c. Intraperitoneal and retroperitoneal organs
   d. Relationship between the topographic anatomy of the four abdominal quadrants and nine abdominal regions to the location of the organs corresponding to them

23-3. Compare and contrast the general characteristics of hollow and solid organs and vascular structures found in the abdominal cavity.

23-4. List the general mechanisms and types of abdominal pain.

23-5. Describe the pathophysiology and the signs and symptoms associated with common causes of acute abdomen, including:
   a. Peritonitis
   b. Appendicitis
   c. Pancreatitis
   d. Cholecystitis
   e. Gastrointestinal bleeding
   f. Esophageal varices
   g. Gastroenteritis
   h. Ulcers
   i. Intestinal obstruction
   j. Hernia
   k. Abdominal aortic aneurysm

23-6. Describe the pathophysiology and the signs and symptoms associated with hematologic emergencies, including:

    a. Anemia

    b. Sickle cell anemia/sickle cell crisis

    c. Hemophilia

23-7. Explain the assessment-based approach to acute abdomen, including assessment and appropriate medical care.

23-8. Describe the basic anatomy and physiology of the female reproductive system.

23-9. Describe the pathophysiology and the signs and symptoms associated with common gynecologic conditions, including:

    a. Sexual assault

    b. Nontraumatic vaginal bleeding

    c. Menstrual pain

    d. Ovarian cyst

    e. Endometritis

    f. Endometriosis

    g. Pelvic inflammatory disease

    h. Sexually transmitted diseases

23-10. Explain the assessment-based approach to acute gynecologic emergencies, including assessment and appropriate medical care.

23-11. Describe genitourinary/renal structures and functions.

23-12. Describe the pathophysiology and the signs and symptoms associated with common genitourinary/renal conditions, including:

    a. Urinary tract infection

    b. Kidney stones

    c. Kidney failure

23-13. Describe the purpose of dialysis, how dialysis works, and dialysis emergency management.

23-14. Describe the purposes and types of urinary catheters and urinary catheter management.

23-15. Explain the assessment-based approach to genitourinary/renal emergencies, including assessment and appropriate medical care.

▌ KEY IDEAS

Acute abdominal pain may indicate a serious condition. This chapter reviews assessment and emergency care for the patient suffering from acute abdominal pain.

- Acute abdominal pain, also called *acute abdomen* or *acute abdominal distress,* is a common condition characterized by an acute onset of moderate to severe abdominal pain that may result from a variety of causes.

- All patients with an acute abdomen should be considered to have a life-threatening condition until proven otherwise.

- Internal bleeding, peritonitis, and diarrhea are conditions that often involve considerable fluid loss, leading to shock (hypoperfusion). A top priority during the assessment of a patient with an acute abdomen is to look for signs of shock.

- Rapid transport should be considered for the acute abdomen patient who meets any of the following criteria: poor general impression, unresponsive, responsive but not following commands, shock (hypoperfusion), or severe pain.

- Perform the examination of the abdomen carefully and gently. If the patient is a priority for rapid transport, the secondary assessment should be conducted en route to the hospital.

- Emergency medical care for the patient with an acute abdomen includes maintaining a patent airway, placing the patient in a position of comfort, administering oxygen, when needed, not giving anything by mouth, calming and reassuring the patient, being alert for shock, and initiating a quick and efficient transport.

TERMS AND CONCEPTS

1. Write the number of the correct term next to each definition.

1. Abdominal aorta
2. Acute abdomen
3. Guarded position
4. Involuntary guarding
5. Parietal pain
6. Peritoneum
7. Peritonitis
8. Referred pain
9. Rigidity
10. Umbilicus
11. Visceral pain
12. Voluntary guarding
13. Hematemesis
14. Hematochezia
15. Appendicitis
16. Cholecystitis
17. Dialysis
18. Gastroenteritis
19. Genitourinary system
20. Gynecology
21. Hematuria
22. Hernia
23. Melena
24. Pancreatitis
25. Renal calculi

_____ a. The navel

_____ b. Abdominal wall muscle contraction that the patient cannot control, caused by inflammation of the peritoneum

_____ c. The lining of the abdominal cavity

_____ d. Pain that is felt in a body part removed from its point of origin

_____ e. Moderate to severe abdominal pain with an acute onset

_____ f. A position generally adopted by patients with acute abdominal pain: knees drawn up and hands clenched over the abdomen

_____ g. A major division of the heart's primary artery that runs through the abdomen

_____ h. Abdominal wall muscle contraction that is controlled by the patient

_____ i. A localized, intense, sharp, constant pain associated with irritation of the peritoneal lining

_____ j. Inflammation or irritation of the peritoneum

_____ k. Constant involuntary abdominal muscle contraction that occurs as a result of peritonitis

_____ l. Poorly localized, intermittent, crampy abdominal pain associated with ischemia or distention of an organ

_____ m. Vomiting blood

_____ n. Bright red blood in the stool, normally signifying a rapid onset of gastrointestinal (GI) bleeding

_____ o. Inflammation of the gallbladder

_____ p. Inflammation of the stomach and small intestines

_____ q. Artificial process used to remove water and waste substances from the blood

_____ r. Male organ system that includes both the reproductive and urinary structures

_____ s. Blood in the urine

_____ t. Protrusion or thrusting forward of a portion of the intestine through an opening or weakness in the abdominal wall

_____ u. Branch of medicine that studies the health of female patients and their reproductive system

_____ v. Inflammation of the appendix

_____ w. Dark, tarry stools containing decomposing blood, normally from the upper GI system

_____ x. Inflammation of the pancreas

_____ y. Kidney stones

2. Match the correct organs of the abdomen with their function.

1. Bladder
2. Duodenum
3. Gallbladder
4. Kidneys
5. Large intestine
6. Liver
7. Pancreas
8. Small intestine
9. Spleen
10. Stomach

_____ a. A saclike, stretchable pouch located below the diaphragm, which receives food from the esophagus (a tubelike structure from the throat).

_____ b. The first part of the small intestine that connects to the stomach.

_____ c. A tubelike structure beginning at the distal end of the stomach and ending at the beginning of the large intestine. Its digestive function is to absorb nutrients from intestinal contents.

_____ d. A tubelike structure beginning at the distal end of the small intestine and ending at the anus. It reabsorbs fluid from intestinal contents, enabling the excretion of solid waste from the body.

_____ e. A large, solid organ located in the right upper quadrant (RUQ) just beneath the diaphragm, with a slight portion extending to the left upper quadrant (LUQ). It filters the nutrients from blood as it returns from the intestines, stores glucose (sugar) and certain vitamins, plays a part in blood clotting, filters dead red blood cells, and aids in the production of bile.

_____ f. A pear-shaped sac that lies on the underneath right side of the liver. This organ holds bile, which aids in the digestion of fats.

_____ g. An elongated, oval, solid organ located in the LUQ behind and to the side of the stomach. It aids in the production of blood cells, as well as in the filtering and storage of blood.

_____ h. A gland composed of many lobes and ducts located in both the RUQ and LUQ, just behind the stomach. It aids in digestion and regulates carbohydrate metabolism.

_____ i. Paired organs located behind the abdominal wall lining (retroperitoneal), one on each side of the spine. These organs excrete urine and regulate water, electrolytes, and acid-base balance.

_____ j. A saclike structure that acts as a reservoir for the urine received from the kidneys.

CONTENT REVIEW

1. The abdomen is the area below the diaphragm to the top of the pelvis. It is helpful to reference the abdomen by dividing it into quarters, or quadrants. The central reference point is the umbilicus. Correctly identify the following terms on the figure shown.

Diaphragm
Left lower quadrant (LLQ)
Left upper quadrant (LUQ)
Right lower quadrant (RLQ)
Right upper quadrant (RUQ)
Umbilicus

A _____
B _____
C _____
D _____
E _____
F _____

2. Dividing the abdominal cavity into regions is useful because the anatomical landmarks help identify the underlying organs' location. Correctly identify the following regions on the figure shown.

_____ Hypogastric region
_____ Umbilical region
_____ Epigastric region
_____ Right iliac region
_____ Right lumbar region
_____ Right hypochondriac region
_____ Left hypochondriac region
_____ Left lumbar region
_____ Left iliac region

3. Abdominal pain that is sharp, knifelike, or pinpoint and associated with irritation and inflammation of the peritoneal lining affects which nerve fiber?
   a. Phrenic nerve
   b. Optic nerve fiber
   c. Visceral nerve fiber
   d. Parietal (somatic) nerve fiber

4. A patient experiencing a rapid onset of abdominal pain can also be reported as suffering from which of the following?
   a. Acute abdomen
   b. Visceral pain
   c. Gastritis
   d. Parietal pain

5. All patients with abdominal pain should be considered
   a. to have a bowel obstruction until proven otherwise.
   b. to have a life-threatening condition until proven otherwise.
   c. to be stable until proven otherwise.
   d. to have a digestive system disorder until proven otherwise.

6. A person with an acute abdomen generally appears very ill. The patient will usually
   a. adopt a position on the side with legs straight.
   b. adopt a position lying on the stomach with legs flat.
   c. adopt a position lying flat on the back with legs flat.
   d. adopt a position with knees drawn up.

7. The patient with acute abdomen should be categorized as a priority for transport if he meets certain criteria. Which of the following should indicate a priority transport for the acute abdominal patient?
   a. Poor general appearance; responsive but not following commands; hypoperfusion
   b. Awake and alert to time and place; blood pressure above 120 systolic; headache
   c. Grimacing facial expression; blood glucose of 60; pulse oximeter reading of 96%
   d. Dazed look; patient presents in a Fowler position; hypertensive; diarrhea for two days

8. Which statement is true regarding the scene size-up for the acute abdomen patient?
   a. Patients experiencing abdominal pain are not likely to faint, and if they do, they usually faint after eating or drinking.
   b. You should not be concerned with looking for mechanisms of injury to rule out trauma as the cause of abdominal pain.
   c. Bloody vomitus is usually present in the majority of acute abdomen patients.
   d. Certain types of bleeding have a distinct smell that sometimes can be identified as you arrive at the patient's side.

9. When preparing to palpate the abdomen of the patient complaining of abdominal pain, you should
   a. have the patient point to the site of the pain, and palpate this quadrant last.
   b. have the patient point to the site of the pain, and palpate this quadrant first.
   c. have the patient point to the site of the pain, and do not palpate this quadrant.
   d. palpate all four quadrants, always with the upper quadrants first, then the lower quadrants.

10. Which of the following signs or symptoms is most likely associated with an acute abdomen?
    a. Localized right leg pain (referred pain)
    b. Soft abdomen that produces no pain on palpation
    c. Bloody vomitus or blood in the stool
    d. Normal vital signs and blood glucose level

11. Which of the following is appropriate management for the patient with an acute abdomen?
    a. Palpate the most painful quadrant first, moving clockwise thereafter.
    b. Position the patient in a supine position with legs flat.
    c. Perform a reassessment every 15 minutes for the unstable patient.
    d. Avoid giving anything to the patient by mouth.

12. Which of the following is a condition that can cause an acute abdomen?
    a. Cholecystitis
    b. Transient ischemic attack
    c. Bell syndrome
    d. Pneumothorax

13. While assessing your patient who complains of abdominal pain, you perform a modified Markle ("heel jar") test by knocking the heels together while the patient is supine. The patient responds with a facial grimace and moans, "That hurts my stomach." This positive test indicates
    a. peritonitis.
    b. abdominal aortic aneurysm.
    c. ruptured diaphragm.
    d. hemothorax.

14. While assessing your patient who complains of abdominal pain, you observe that the pulse pressure is narrowing, the heart rate has increased, and the skin has become pale, cool, and diaphoretic. You suspect
    a. acute inflammation of the appendix.
    b. inflammation of the peritoneal lining.
    c. constipation from a blocked large intestine.
    d. internal bleeding within the abdomen.

15. A bulging, engorgement, or weakening of the blood vessels in the lining of the lower part of the esophagus is known as
    a. hemothorax.
    b. esophageal varices.
    c. peritonitis.
    d. hematochezia.

16. The condition that presents with inflammation of the stomach and small intestines commonly associated with the presence of abdominopelvic pain is known as
    a. esophageal varices.
    b. hematemesis.
    c. hematochezia.
    d. gastroenteritis.

17. You are assessing your elderly male patient who complains of constant abdominal pain that radiates to the lower back. He describes it as a "tearing" pain. You note the skin of the lower extremities is mottled. You suspect this patient is suffering from
    a. abdominal aortic aneurysm.
    b. peritonitis.
    c. esophageal varices.
    d. hemothorax.

18. You are treating your patient who you suspect may have been sexually assaulted. Which of the following is considered inappropriate treatment or handling of this type of assault?
    a. Refrain from moving anything at the crime scene unless it impedes emergency medical care.
    b. Encourage the patient to shower to help prevent the possible spread of infection and to help deal with the psychological effects of the assault.
    c. If the patient has changed clothes, gather them and place them into a separate bag and transport them with the patient.
    d. When removing clothing to treat your patient, do not cut through any holes or tears in the clothing.

19. You are treating your patient who is bleeding heavily from her vagina. Which of the following is the appropriate and best way to control this type of bleeding?
    a. Carefully pack the vagina with a sterile gauze pad.
    b. Apply direct pressure with the gloved hand and a pad.
    c. Insert a sterile, nonporous pad into the vagina.
    d. Use a pad externally to absorb the blood flow.

20. You have been called to a doctor's office to transport a genitourinary patient that the doctor suspects of having an infection. The doctor states that the patient has had hematuria for the past two days. You know that hematuria is
    a. blood in the stool.
    b. blood in the urine.
    c. cloudy urine (not clear).
    d. discolored vaginal discharge.

21. Crystals of substances like calcium, uric acid, and struvite, that are formed from metabolic abnormalities and most frequently occur in men between the ages of 20 and 50, are known as
    a. renal calculi.
    b. urinary tract infection.
    c. hematuria.
    d. liver stones.

22. In which hematologic emergencies will patients likely develop kidney damage and have a higher rate of infections of the kidney, lung, bone, and central nervous system?
    a. Sickle cell
    b. Chronic anemia
    c. Hemophilia
    d. Gastrointestinal bleed

23. You are treating a 24-year-old who called you because of a nosebleed. While gathering the history, you learn that she has a history of hemophilia. You know
    a. this is a low-priority emergency and will likely resolve on its own.
    b. this condition affects the respiratory system and is not related to the nosebleed.
    c. this disorder most often afflicts African Americans and black Africans.
    d. this is a blood disorder that affects clotting and is a true emergency.

CASE STUDY

You and your partner, Jill, are busy washing the unit when the alarm sounds. You respond to a call for a patient complaining of abdominal pain. The scene appears safe as you arrive at a well-kept, one-story home. A man meets you at the curb and escorts you to the front door. As you follow him, you ask, "Why did you call the ambulance today?" He replies, "My wife's stomach hurts really bad!" As you enter the house, you see the patient. She appears to be about 25 years old. She is lying on her side on the floor with her knees drawn up to her chest. She is holding her lower abdominal area. She doesn't look at you as you enter. Your general impression is that she looks ill. Her skin color is pale. She responds to your questions slowly but appropriately. She tells you, "My stomach started hurting about an hour ago. I think I'm going to throw up!" Her respirations are rapid and shallow. Her radial pulse is weak and rapid, and her skin is cool and moist. Here SpO_2 is 92% and there is no sign of trauma, and no obvious bleeding is observed.

1. This patient
   a. is not showing serious signs. The patient does not require transport or additional treatment.
   b. is showing serious signs. However, the patient should be allowed to be transported by her husband to the hospital for additional evaluation.
   c. is not showing serious signs. However, the patient should be placed on oxygen and transported in a sitting-up position.
   d. is showing early signs of shock. The patient should be placed on oxygen, positioned with knees drawn up, and provided quick transport with suction unit ready.

2. When beginning the exam of the patient's abdomen, you should
   a. have the patient drink a glass of water to rehydrate.
   b. ask her to straighten her legs.
   c. ask her to point with one finger to the area that is most painful.
   d. reassure the patient that palpation of her abdomen will not hurt.

3. En route to the hospital, the patient vomits several times. The patient's emesis (vomitus)
   a. should be saved for possible testing at the hospital.
   b. should be saved, but only if it looks bloody or dark in color.
   c. should be disposed of immediately in an infectious waste container.
   d. should not be considered a serious sign of acute abdomen.

4. A reassessment of this patient should be performed every
   a. minute.
   b. 3 minutes.
   c. 5 minutes.
   d. 15 minutes.

CHAPTER 23 SCENARIO: DOCUMENTATION EXERCISE

Read the following scenario and think about how you would document this call if you were the EMT who responded to the scene. Then answer the multiple-choice questions and fill in the sample prehospital care report, basing your documentation on information from the scenario.

It is 10:00 P.M. on a Monday. You and your partner, Morris, are just returning to the station when dispatch calls: "Unit 3, respond to 4210 12th Place, cross street Aviation Avenue, for a 70-year-old male patient with abdominal pain." You advise dispatch that you are responding to the call. In about six minutes, you arrive on the scene. It is a residential area of mobile home parks. You knock on the door of a tidy mobile home and wait for an answer. A woman who appears to be in her mid-60s answers the door. With Standard Precautions taken, you and your partner enter. You introduce yourself and your partner, and you ask, "What's the problem today?" As you are walking toward a back bedroom, she tells you that her husband, Mr. Richter, has been complaining of severe abdominal pain.

You enter the room and observe Mr. Richter sitting up in bed, holding a small trash can between his legs. He leans over the trash can and retches but does not vomit. He briefly looks up at you as you enter the room. His skin looks pale, and you notice sweat on his forehead. He grabs his back and holds his flank area. He is breathing adequately, with no audible abnormal respiratory sounds. Moe quickly begins to take the vital signs as you begin a secondary assessment.

You begin your assessment by introducing yourself and Moe, and saying, "We are EMTs, and we're here to help you. What is the problem today?" Mr. Richter replies, "My stomach hurts!" You continue by asking, "When did the pain start? What were you doing when it started? Did it start all of a sudden?" Mr. Richter replies, "I was taking the trash out about two hours ago, and it started, all of a sudden. It really hurts!" You quickly say, "We'll do everything we can, but we need to ask you some more questions." Morris finishes taking Mr. Richter's pulse and tells you it is 124 per minute, regular, and weak. His skin is cool, clammy, and pale. Morris places the pulse oximeter, and you note his SpO_2 is 93%. You apply oxygen at 2 lpm by a nasal cannula.

You determine that ALS backup is required, and you advise dispatch of the need. Morris continues with the vital signs while you continue with the secondary assessment. You ask Mr. Richter, "Does anything make the pain better or worse?" He says, "No, it just hurts. I can't make it go away! Nothing seems to help it!" You ask, "Can you describe the discomfort you are having? Is it sharp or dull, pressing or squeezing? What does it feel like?" He says, "It feels like a ripping pain in my back and stomach. I don't know how else to describe it." Morris says that the patient's respirations are 20 per minute, full and regular, and breath sounds are clear and equal bilaterally. You continue with, "Does the pain

you are having move, or radiate, to any other part of your body?" He replies, "It starts in my lower gut and moves to my back. It hurts really bad." You ask Mr. Richter if the oxygen is helping him. "Well, no, it doesn't seem to be helping at all," he replies.

Mrs. Richter is visibly shaken by the events taking place. You look her in the eyes, place your hand on her shoulder, and say, "Mrs. Richter, we're doing everything we can right now, but I really need your help. Could you get together any medicines that Mr. Richter is currently taking and bring them to me?" She says, "I'll get them for you. All he takes is something for his high blood pressure."

Morris tells you the blood pressure is 140/70, and the pupils are equal and reactive. Mr. Richter's neck veins are flat. His abdomen is soft. You carefully palpate the abdomen and palpate a pulsating mass in the center of his lower abdomen. You quickly check for the equality of his femoral pulses. His right femoral pulse is stronger than his left. You don't see any swelling in his lower extremities or back region. You continue the secondary assessment. "Mr. Richter, have you ever had any pain like this before?" You wait for a response. "No, I don't think I have," he says. "On a scale of 1–10, with 10 being the worst pain you have ever had, how would you rate your current pain?" you ask. He replies, "It's at least a 9 or a 10. It really hurts." You ask, "Mr. Richter, when did this start? I know you told me it was about two hours ago. It's 10:10 P.M. now, so it started about 8:00 P.M., right?" He responds by saying, "Yes, that's right; it started about 8:00 P.M. tonight."

Mrs. Richter returns to the room with his medication, a hypertension medication for his blood pressure. You ask Mr. Richter if he is allergic to any medications, and he shakes his head no. "When did you last eat or drink anything?" you inquire. He says, "About 7:30 P.M. I ate a small bowl of soup. That was it." You hear the doorbell ring and hear the ALS crew entering the home. Paramedic Dave Johnson comes into the room. You introduce him to Mr. Richter and provide a patient report to Dave. You help move Mr. Richter to the ALS ambulance.

1. The most likely explanation for Mr. Richter's abdominal pain is
   a. intestinal obstruction.
   b. appendicitis.
   c. cholecystitis.
   d. abdominal aortic aneurysm.

2. Which statement best describes the inequality of Mr. Richter's femoral pulses?
   a. Acute appendicitis can result in obstruction of the aortic arch that limits blood flow.
   b. Cholecystitis results in inflammation and swelling of the aortic sheath, limiting flow.

    c. Intestinal obstruction results in swelling that constricts the lower aorta.

    d. An aortic aneurysm can result in obstruction of blood flow to the femoral arteries.

3. Mr. Richter's abdomen was palpated carefully. Why was careful palpation important for Mr. Richter?

    a. Deep palpation can cause rupture of an acute appendix.

    b. Deep palpation can cause rupture of the gallbladder.

    c. Deep palpation can cause rupture of the lower colon.

    d. Deep palpation can cause rupture of the aorta.

4. The condition that Mr. Richter is experiencing

    a. occurs in 20 percent of men over 50 years of age.

    b. occurs frequently in women over 60 years of age.

    c. occurs commonly in both sexes and all age groups.

    d. occurs in 50 percent of men at any age.

EMERGENCY TRIP SHEET

TRIP #	
MEDIC #	
BEGIN MILES	
END MILES	
CODE___/___ PAGE___/___	
UNITS ON SCENE	

DAY					
DATE					
RECEIVED					
DISPATCHED					
EN-ROUTE					
ON SCENE					
TO HOSPITAL					
AT HOSPITAL					
IN-SERVICE					

	CREW	CERT	STATE #

NAME   SEX M F DOB ___/___/___

ADDRESS   RACE

CITY   STATE   ZIP

PHONE ( )   -   PCP DR.

RESPONDED FROM   CITY

TAKEN FROM   ZIP

DESTINATION   REASON

SSN   -   -   MEDICARE #   MEDICAID #

INSURANCE CO   INSURANCE #   GROUP #

RESPONSIBLE PARTY   ADDRESS

CITY   STATE   ZIP   PHONE ( )   -

EMPLOYER

TIME	ON SCENE (1)	ON SCENE (2)	ON SCENE (3)	EN-ROUTE (1)	EN-ROUTE (2)	AT DESTINATION
BP						
PULSE						
RESP						
SpO$_2$						
ETCO$_2$						
EKG						

IV THERAPY
SUCCESSFUL Y N # OF ATTEMPTS _____
ANGIO SIZE _____ ga.
SITE _____
TOTAL FLUID INFUSED _____ cc
BLOOD DRAW Y N INITIALS

INTUBATION INFORMATION
SUCCESSFUL Y N # OF ATTEMPTS _____
TUBE SIZE _____ mm
TIME _____ INITIALS _____

MEDICAL HISTORY

CONDITION CODES

MEDICATIONS

ALLERGIES

C/C

EVENTS LEADING TO C/C

ASSESSMENT

TREATMENT

	TIME	TREATMENT	DOSE	ROUTE	INIT
TREATMENTS					

GCS E___V___M___TOTAL =

GCS E___V___M___TOTAL =

HOSPITAL CONTACTED

CPR BEGUN BY   B   P   TIME BEGUN

AED USED   Y   N   BY:

RESUSCITATION TERMINATED - TIME

EMS SIGNATURE

( ) OSHA REGULATIONS FOLLOWED

Environmental Emergencies

❚ STANDARD

Trauma (Content Area: Environmental Emergencies)

❚ COMPETENCY

Applies fundamental knowledge to provide basic emergency care and transportation based on assessment findings for an acutely injured patient.

❚ OBJECTIVES

After reading this chapter, you should be able to:

24-1. Define key terms introduced in this chapter.
24-2. Explain the importance of being able to recognize and provide emergency medical care for patients with environmental emergencies.
24-3. Describe the process by which the body maintains normal temperature.
24-4. Explain the mechanisms by which the body loses heat.
24-5. Explain the mechanisms by which the body gains heat.
24-6. Describe the pathophysiology of generalized hypothermia.
24-7. Recognize factors that contribute to a patient's risk for hypothermia, (including immersion hypothermia, urban hypothermia, and myxedema coma or hypothyroidism).
24-8. Describe the pathophysiology of local cold injury, including the stages of local cold injury.
24-9. Discuss the assessment-based approach to cold-related emergencies.
24-10. Describe the emergency medical care for generalized hypothermia.
24-11. Describe the emergency medical care for immersion hypothermia.
24-12. Describe the emergency medical care for local cold injury.
24-13. Describe the pathophysiology of heat-related emergencies.
24-14. Recognize factors that contribute to a patient's risk for hyperthermia.
24-15. Discuss the assessment-based approach to heat-related emergencies.
24-16. Describe the emergency medical care for a heat emergency patient with moist, pale, normal-to-cool skin.
24-17. Describe the emergency medical care for a heat emergency patient with hot skin that is moist or dry.
24-18. Describe the emergency medical care for heat cramps.
24-19. Describe the characteristics of common venomous snakes and factors that affect the severity of a snakebite.

24-20. Recognize the signs, symptoms, and patient history associated with bites or stings of the following:
  a. Black widow spiders
  b. Brown recluse spiders
  c. Scorpions
  d. Fire ants
  e. Ticks

24-21. Discuss the assessment-based approach to bites and stings.

24-22. Describe the signs and symptoms and the emergency medical care for anaphylactic shock resulting from a bite or sting.

24-23. Describe the signs and symptoms and the emergency medical care for a bite or sting.

24-24. Recognize the signs, symptoms, and patient history associated with the bite or sting of a marine animal and the emergency medical care for marine life poisoning.

24-25. Explain the pathophysiology of lightning strike injuries.

24-26. Given a scenario with a patient who has been struck by lightning, predict findings and complications associated with the mechanism of injury.

24-27. Describe the emergency medical care for a patient who has been struck by lightning.

24-28. Describe the signs, symptoms, and patient history associated with acute mountain sicknesses and emergency medical care for acute mountain sickness.

24-29. Describe the signs, symptoms, and patient history associated with high altitude pulmonary edema and emergency medical care for high altitude pulmonary edema.

24-30. Describe the signs, symptoms, and patient history associated with high altitude cerebral edema and emergency medical care for high altitude cerebral edema.

▎KEY IDEAS

Conditions brought on by interactions between people and the environment are reviewed in this chapter. The signs, symptoms, and expected emergency management of extremes of hot and cold, of bites and stings, and of altitude sickness are addressed.

■ Hypothermia occurs when the body loses more heat than it gains or produces. Heat loss occurs through five mechanisms: radiation, convection, conduction, evaporation, and respiration.

■ Exposure to cold can cause two kinds of emergencies. The first is generalized cold emergency (generalized hypothermia), which is an overall reduction in body temperature affecting the entire body. The second is local cold injury (commonly called *frostbite*) that results in damage to body tissues in a specific part or parts of the body.

■ Signs and symptoms of generalized hypothermia include decreasing mental status, decreasing motor and sensory function, and changing vital signs.

■ Emergency medical care for generalized hypothermia includes preventing further heat loss, rewarming the patient as quickly and safely as possible, and staying alert for complications. It is important to remove the patient from the cold environment, handle the patient gently, administer warm humidified oxygen to maintain an $SpO_2 > 94\%$, and be prepared to resuscitate the patient if he goes into cardiac arrest.

■ Local cold injury results from the freezing of body tissue. Local cold injury falls into two categories: early (superficial) or late (deep) injury.

■ Signs and symptoms of early (superficial) cold injury include blanching of the skin and loss of feeling. The skin and tissue beneath it remain soft. There may be a tingling sensation during rewarming.

■ Signs and symptoms of late (deep) cold injury include white, waxy skin; swelling; and blisters. The skin and tissues beneath the skin feel firm to frozen. If thawed, the skin may appear flushed or mottled.

■ Emergency medical care for local cold injury includes immediately removing the patient from the cold environment, avoiding thawing if there is danger of refreezing, administering warm humidified oxygen to maintain an SpO_2 of > 94%, removing jewelry or wet or restrictive clothing if not frozen to the skin, covering the skin with dressings or dry clothing, avoiding rubbing, and not permitting the patient to walk on an injured extremity.

■ Urban hypothermia occurs in individuals who have a predisposition, disability, illness, or medication usage that renders them more susceptible to hypothermia. It is subdivided into two general etiologies: internal and external causes. External hypothermia results from lack of protection from a cold environment, while internal hypothermia results chiefly from elderly patients' attempts to reduce their winter heating bills.

■ Hyperthermia occurs when the amount of heat that the body produces or gains exceeds the amount that it loses.

■ Signs and symptoms of a heat emergency may include elevated core temperature, muscle cramps, weakness, dizziness, heartbeat becoming progressively weak and rapid, deep breathing that becomes progressively shallow and weak, headache, seizures, loss of appetite, nausea or vomiting, altered mental status, and possible unresponsiveness. The skin may be moist and pale with a normal-to-cool temperature, or the skin may be hot and either dry or moist.

■ Emergency medical care for the patient with a heat emergency includes moving the patient to a cool place, administering oxygen to maintain an SpO_2 of 94%, removing as much clothing as possible, and cooling the patient. The patient should be placed supine. Consider elevating the feet. If the patient is fully responsive and not nauseated, the patient may drink cool water. (If the patient has an altered mental status or is nauseated or vomiting, do *not* give fluids.)

■ Hot skin (which may be either dry or moist, depending on how the sweat mechanisms are operating) represents a dire medical emergency. The patient requires rapid cooling and immediate transport.

■ Emergency care for bites and stings includes removing the stinger by scraping, washing the area, removing jewelry or other constricting objects, lowering the injection site slightly below the heart, and applying cold packs (except for marine stings and snakebites). It is important to be alert for and prepared to treat anaphylaxis. Keep the patient calm and transport.

TERMS AND CONCEPTS

1. Write the number of the correct term next to each definition.

1. Active rewarming
2. Conduction
3. Convection
4. Evaporation
5. Thermoreceptor
6. Hyperthermia
7. Hypothermia
8. Local cold injury
9. Myxedema coma
10. Passive rewarming
11. Radiation
12. Urban hypothermia
13. Water chill
14. Wind chill

_____ a. Technique of aggressively applying heat to a patient to increase the body temperature

_____ b. A sensory receptor that is stimulated by temperature

_____ c. Transfer of body heat through direct physical contact with nearby objects

_____ d. Abnormally low core body temperature

_____ e. Helping the body to increase temperature itself by simply placing the patient in a warm environment and covering with blankets

_____ f. Conversion of a liquid or solid into a gas

_____ g. The increase in rate of cooling in the presence of water or wet clothing

_____ h. Loss of body heat to the atmosphere when air passes over the body

_____ i. Transfer of heat from the surface of one object to the surface of another without physical contact between the objects

_____ j. The combined effect of wind speed and environmental temperature

_____ k. Abnormally high core body temperature

_____ l. Damage to body tissues in a specific part of the body resulting from exposure to cold

_____ m. A complication that occurs late in the progression of hypothyroidism

_____ n. Occurs in individuals who have a predisposition, disability, illness, or medication usage that renders them more susceptible to hypothermia; is subdivided into two general etiologies—external and internal

CONTENT REVIEW

1. There are five basic mechanisms by which the body loses heat. Which mechanism results in a loss of body heat to the atmosphere when air passes over it?
   a. Respiration
   b. Conduction
   c. Consolidation
   d. Convection

2. Exposure to cold can cause which of the following two kinds of emergencies?
   a. Generalized cold emergency and generalized hypothermia
   b. Generalized hypothermia and local cold injury
   c. Generalized hypovolemia and local cold injury
   d. Generalized hypovolemia and generalized hypothermia

3. Which factors may place a patient at greatest risk for developing generalized hypothermia?
   a. Drugs and alcohol
   b. Middle age and short exposure time
   c. Female gender and reduced activity level
   d. Asian descent and poor clothing

4. The stages of hypothermia are listed as follows. Next to each stage, place a number from 1 to 4 (earliest to latest) to indicate which stage it represents.

   _____ a. Pulse rate decreases by 50 percent

   _____ b. Shivering

   _____ c. Progressive decline in level of responsiveness

   _____ d. Pulse rate decreases by 80 percent

5. Emergency care for generalized hypothermia should include
   a. careful and gentle handling of the patient.
   b. asking the patient to walk about briskly to raise his body temperature.
   c. administering oxygen by a nonrebreather mask at 6 lpm.
   d. checking the patient's temperature with the EMT's hand on the patient's forehead.

6. Which statement best describes an appropriate technique for active rewarming?
   a. Heat should be added to the patient as quickly as possible.
   b. Increase the body temperature by no more than 1°F per hour.
   c. Immerse the patient in a hot tub of water or place in a hot shower.
   d. Apply heat first to the extremities, then the torso.

7. Immersion hypothermia should be considered in all cases of accidental immersion. Body temperature can drop to the water temperature in as little as
   a. 10 minutes.
   b. 15 minutes.
   c. 20 minutes.
   d. 25 minutes.

8. When managing the patient with immersion hypothermia, be sure to
   a. lift the patient from the water in a vertical position.
   b. ask the patient to swim to you as quickly as possible.
   c. ask the patient to remove all wet clothing quickly.
   d. provide treatment similar to that for generalized hypothermia.

9. The stages of local cold injury are
   a. frostbite and hypothermia.
   b. early (superficial) and late (deep).
   c. frostnip and frostbite.
   d. generalized and local.

10. Appropriate management of local cold injuries includes
    a. rubbing or massaging the affected skin.
    b. removing clothing that is frozen to the skin.
    c. initiation of thawing, even if refreezing is possible.
    d. the careful removal of clothing and jewelry.

11. Guidelines for rapid rewarming of local cold injuries include
    a. maintaining the water temperature between 120°F and 130°F.
    b. dressing the area with a nonsterile moist dressing and petroleum jelly.
    c. rewarming all injuries regardless of transport times or temperatures.
    d. keeping the tissue in warm water until it is soft and the color returns.

12. The term that best describes a grouping of heat-related emergencies is
    a. hypothermia.
    b. hyperthermia.
    c. hyperpyrexia.
    d. hyperenviron.

13. Which of the following is a factor that can increase an individual's reaction to a heat-related injury?
    a. Heart disease
    b. Gastrointestinal disorders
    c. Cigarette smoking
    d. Psychological disorders

14. A patient represents a dire medical emergency if he has been exposed to heat and has which of the following signs or symptoms?
    a. Cool, pale, moist skin
    b. Dizziness
    c. Muscle cramps
    d. Hot skin, either moist or dry

15. When cooling a heat emergency patient with hot skin that is moist or dry,
    a. cooling takes priority over all other emergency care procedures.
    b. one cooling method will generally be effective to cool the patient.
    c. be prepared to manage seizures and to prevent aspiration.
    d. place cold packs on the patient's hands and feet.

16. A heat emergency patient with moist, pale, normal-to-cool skin who is responsive and vomiting should be given
    a. cool water to drink.
    b. nothing by mouth.
    c. a half glass of water every 15 minutes.
    d. warm water to drink.

17. A heat emergency patient with moist, pale, normal-to-cool skin needs transport if the patient
    a. is sweating.
    b. has a temperature of 99°F.
    c. has a headache.
    d. has a history of medical problems.

18. The first step in the emergency medical care of any patient with a heat emergency is to
    a. administer oxygen at 15 lpm via a nonrebreather mask.
    b. place the patient supine and elevate the feet.
    c. move the patient to a cool place.
    d. remove as much clothing as possible.

19. Which of the following are grave indications that the heat emergency patient is deteriorating?
    a. The blood pressure falls, and the patient feels exhausted.
    b. The capillary refill time decreases, and respirations are labored.
    c. The pulse rate changes rapidly, and the mental status declines.
    d. The patient begins to shiver, and the skin becomes pale.

20. Which statement is most correct related to bites and stings?
    a. Snakebites are common and annually result in a large number of fatalities.
    b. Exercise caution during the scene size-up to protect yourself.
    c. Complications associated with airway and breathing never occur.
    d. Most insect bites result in major anaphylactic reactions.

21. Urban hypothermia
    a. is limited to individuals who live outdoors and are unable to escape the cold environment.
    b. is limited to the elderly who attempt to reduce their home heating bills.
    c. is limited to northern climates during the winter months.
    d. occurs in individuals with a predisposition to hypothermia.

22. Lightning strike injuries
    a. result in about 50 deaths per year.
    b. occur most frequently on Wednesdays.
    c. occur mostly in work-related or recreational situations.
    d. most often involve multiple patients.

23. Lightning strike patients
    a. are considered medical and trauma patients.
    b. do not routinely require spinal immobilization.
    c. are frequently talking on the telephone when struck.
    d. infrequently suffer damage to air-containing body cavities.

24. Dislocations and fractures associated with lightning strikes result from the
    a. thunder "blast wave" and the speed of the lightning strike.
    b. thunder "blast wave" and strong muscular contractions.
    c. burning effect of the lightning strike and strong muscular contractions.
    d. burning effect and the speed of the lightning strike.

25. What two types of poisonous snakes contribute to most snakebites in the United States?
    a. King cobras and coral snakes
    b. Coral snakes and pit vipers
    c. Pit vipers and king cobras
    d. King snakes and pit vipers

26. The signs and symptoms of a pit viper bite are
    a. usually delayed for up to eight hours.
    b. usually gauged by how much poison was injected.
    c. usually delayed for up to one hour.
    d. unrelated to the patient's size or weight.

27. Identify each of the following characteristics as belonging to either a poisonous (P) or a nonpoisonous (N) snake.

    _____ a. Triangular head that is larger than the neck

    _____ b. Pit between eye and mouth

    _____ c. Round head

    _____ d. Round pupils

    _____ e. Small teeth

    _____ f. Elliptical pupils

28. The black widow spider has a
    a. shiny black body, thin legs, and a crimson red hourglass on its abdomen.
    b. dull black body, thin legs, and a crimson red circle on its abdomen.
    c. shiny black body, short legs, and a white circle on its abdomen.
    d. dull black body, thin legs, and a red triangle on its back.

29. General signs and symptoms of a black widow spider bite include
    a. severe muscle spasms in the shoulders, back, chest, and abdomen.
    b. drooping eyelids with loss of eye movement and blinking.
    c. diminished saliva production and an inability to swallow.
    d. lower back pain and uncontrollable bowel movements.

30. This bite is usually painless for the first few hours. Several hours later, the site becomes bluish, surrounded by a red halo or "bull's-eye" pattern. The bite generally does not heal and may require surgical repair. These are characteristics of the bite of a
    a. southern fire ant.
    b. Rocky Mountain tick.
    c. brown recluse spider.
    d. scorpion.

31. The venom of aquatic organisms may be destroyed by the application of
    a. heat.
    b. rubbing alcohol.
    c. ice.
    d. tannic acid in the form of a tea bag.

32. Myxedema coma
    a. may make a person less susceptible to becoming hypothermic.
    b. occurs early in the progression of hyperthyroidism.
    c. occurs commonly in about 50 percent of all hyperthyroidism patients.
    d. is precipitated by exposure to cold, a recent illness, or infection and trauma.

▌CASE STUDY 1

You are standing by to provide medical coverage during a 10-kilometer running event on a hot summer day. You have responded to a call for a runner who is disoriented. The scene appears safe as you arrive at the finish line. As an event official leads you to the patient, you ask, "Why did you call the ambulance?" She replies, "This guy just finished the race, and he isn't acting right!"

As you approach the patient, you note that he looks to be about 25 years old. He is lying next to the finish line in full sunshine. He is wearing a polyester running suit. He is lying on his back, talking incoherently. He doesn't notice you as you kneel down beside him. Your general impression is that he looks ill. His skin color is red. He responds to your questions with inappropriate statements. His respirations are rapid and shallow, his radial pulse is weak and rapid, and his skin is hot to the touch and moist. There is no sign of trauma, and no bleeding is observed. You rapidly move the patient to the back of the ambulance, where the air conditioner is already turned on.

1. The next *best* action to take for this patient is to
    a. contact medical direction for treatment options.
    b. remove as much clothing as possible.
    c. fan the patient aggressively.
    d. give the patient cool water to drink.

You have removed the patient from the hot environment, performed the action taken in question 1, and begun to administer oxygen to maintain a SpO$_2$ of > 94%.

2. The next *best* action to take for this patient is to
   a. radio a report on the patient's condition to the receiving facility.
   b. place the patient in a position of comfort.
   c. pour tepid water over the patient's body.
   d. obtain a history.

You have begun rapid transport to the hospital.

3. The use of cold water should be avoided in this patient because it may
   a. stimulate the release of norepinephrine and increase the core temperature.
   b. stimulate central thermoreceptors and cause a reflex peripheral vasodilation.
   c. cause the acute onset of seizure activity.
   d. produce vasoconstriction and shivering.

I CASE STUDY 2

You are dispatched to the scene of a possible snakebite. The scene appears safe as you arrive at a hunting lodge in the woods. A man dressed in hunting clothing meets you at the gate and escorts you to the patient. As you follow him, you ask the hunter, "Why did you call the ambulance?" He replies, "Tony just finished for the day and was walking back to the lodge. He was walking across Crooked Creek and a cottonmouth got him! I blasted it and brought it and Tony back to the lodge. Then I called you."

As you approach the patient, you note that he appears to be about 35 years old. He is sitting in a chair, holding his leg. He looks at you as you enter the room. Your general impression is that he looks well, although he appears to be in pain. His skin color is normal. He responds to your questions appropriately. His respirations are normal, his radial pulse is strong and regular, and his skin is warm and dry. You examine the bite and observe two distinct puncture wounds on the lower leg. The wound is red and moderately swollen. There are no other signs of trauma, and no bleeding is observed. The snake (which is obviously dead) is lying next to the patient. Tony's friend puts it into a box so you can take it along to the hospital. You are extremely careful in handling the box, even though you are sure the snake is dead.

1. Appropriate treatment for this patient should include
   a. application of a commercial cold pack to the area.
   b. washing the area with a mild agent or strong soap solution.
   c. encouraging the patient to move about to reduce stress and anxiety.
   d. application of a commercial hot pack to the area.

2. What additional treatments should be provided for this patient?
   a. Lower the injection site slightly below the level of the heart.
   b. Cut and then suction the venom from the bite site.
   c. Administer epinephrine and then cut and suction the bite.
   d. Elevate the site slightly above the level of the heart.

3. This patient should be observed closely for signs of
   a. respiratory distress.
   b. hives.
   c. hypotension.
   d. anaphylaxis.

CASE STUDY 3

You are dispatched to a call for a woman down. It is the middle of winter, and the temperature is in the mid-20s. The scene appears safe as you arrive at a single-story residence. A well-dressed man who introduces himself as a neighbor meets you at the ambulance and escorts you to the patient. As you follow him, you ask, "Why did you call the ambulance?" He replies, "Mary is in her 80s and lives by herself. I stop by to check on her when I can. I found her on the floor of her garage, and I can't wake her up!"

As you enter the garage, you note that it is quite cold inside. The patient is lying on her side next to her car. She is dressed in a nightgown and a light bathrobe and slippers. She doesn't respond as you kneel down next to her. You apply a painful stimulus, but she does not respond. Your general impression is that she looks ill. Her skin color is gray. Her respirations are slow and shallow. Her radial pulse is slow and barely palpable. There is no sign of trauma, and no bleeding is observed. You move the patient to the back of the ambulance, where the heater is already on.

1. Assess the pulse in this patient for
   a. 10–20 seconds.
   b. 20–30 seconds.
   c. 30–45 seconds.
   d. 1–2 minutes.

2. You are more than 15 minutes from the receiving medical facility. The patient's body core temperature is 93.2° F. This patient requires which of the following?
   a. Active rewarming
   b. Passive rewarming
   c. Immersion in a tub of hot water or in a hot shower
   d. Active rewarming only if more than 30 minutes from the hospital

3. When moving this patient to the ambulance, you should
   a. move her as quickly as you can, using any possible method.
   b. try to keep her head elevated during movement, if possible.
   c. hyperventilate her during movement.
   d. handle her extremely gently.

CASE STUDY 4

You are dispatched to a call for a child with a local cold injury. It is mid-December and quite cold. The scene appears safe as you arrive at a small convenience store. Several children are standing next to the door as you arrive. You step out and ask, "Why did you call the ambulance?" One of the children replies, "I think my toes are frostbit! I called my mom and she's going to meet us here." The boy is 12 or 13 years old. He is dressed in a heavy coat and boots that look wet. He is alert and oriented to your questions. Your general impression is that he looks well. His skin color is normal. His respirations are normal. His radial pulse is strong and regular. There is no sign of trauma, and no bleeding is observed. You move the patient to the back of the ambulance, where the heater is already on. You remove his shoes and socks. He tells you his right big toe is numb. You examine his toe, and it looks somewhat white.

1. You would expect which of the following signs or symptoms to be present if the patient has suffered an early, or superficial, local cold injury?
   a. Good feeling and sensation in the toe
   b. Firm-to-frozen feeling when the skin is palpated
   c. When you palpate the skin, the normal color does not return
   d. Swelling and blisters

2. Which of the following is an appropriate treatment for this patient?
  a. Remove wet or restrictive clothing.
  b. Gently massage the area to increase blood flow.
  c. Administer oxygen at 6 lpm.
  d. Avoid splinting the area; this would reduce blood flow.

The toe has thawed in the warm ambulance. The tissue is soft. The color and sensation have returned to the toe.

3. It is now *most* important to
  a. elevate the affected extremity.
  b. prevent the possibility of refreezing.
  c. massage the affected area.
  d. dress the area with a moist, sterile dressing.

CHAPTER 24 SCENARIO: DOCUMENTATION EXERCISE

Read the following scenario and think about how you would document this call if you were the EMT who responded to the scene. Then answer the multiple-choice questions and fill in the sample prehospital care report, basing your documentation on information from the scenario.

It is 3:30 P.M. in midsummer. It is a very hot day, with the air temperature at 95°F and a humidity of 75 percent. You and your partner, Katy, just stopped to pick up a drink and are heading back to the station. The alert sounds: "Unit 6, respond to 500 Highlands Road for an altered mental status patient; cross street, Gachet Boulevard. Time out is 1530 hours." Katy tells dispatch that you are responding. You arrive in about two minutes at a small home that appears unkempt; the grass needs to be mowed, and the house is in need of basic repairs. Katy advises dispatch of arrival on scene. With Standard Precautions in place, you walk to the front of the home and knock. A girl of about 15 years of age answers the door and asks you to come in. You introduce yourself and Katy to her and find out that her name is Misty. She is a friend of the elderly woman who lives in the home. The elderly woman's name is Mrs. Holland. Misty tells you that she checked on Mrs. Holland this afternoon, and she was acting funny. Misty then called rescue for assistance.

It is quite hot in the house. The windows in the front of the house are open, but very little air is moving in the house. You walk to a back bedroom and see Mrs. Holland sitting in a chair next to her bed. She appears to be about 75 years of age. She is dressed in a long-sleeved shirt, a sweater, and long pants. She looks at you as you enter the room. Her skin looks flushed. She is breathing adequately, with no audible, abnormal respiratory sounds heard. Your initial impression is that she looks ill. Katy quickly begins to take the vital signs as you begin a history and physical exam.

You begin your assessment by introducing yourself and Katy, and saying, "We are EMTs, and we're here to help you. What's the problem today?" You place a nasal cannula on Mrs. Holland and set the oxygen flow rate at 3 lpm. She looks at you sleepily and replies, "Nothing. I'm just fine. Did you get my TV fixed?" You say, "Misty is concerned about you. She says that you seem confused about something." Mrs. Holland replies, "Well, Misty is a nice girl. I'm just glad you're here to get my TV fixed. Will it take you long? Misty, my head really hurts. Will you get me some aspirin?" You say, "Mrs. Holland, we are EMTs, and we are here to provide medical care for you. Misty is concerned about your health." You reach down to take her pulse and note that her skin is hot to the touch, and her pulse is rapid and bounding. Mrs. Holland retches as if to vomit. You hand her a small basin that is next to the bed. It is very warm in the room. You are sweating from the heat. You ask Misty if there is an air conditioner, and she says no, the house has no air conditioning. The bedroom windows are closed and you ask her to open the windows to try to get some air movement in the room.

You recognize that the situation is life threatening and request ALS backup. You ask Misty about Mrs. Holland's medical history and if she takes any medications. She tells you that she doesn't know if she takes any medications but that she has a history of a thyroid disorder. You tell Katy to get the cot. As Katy heads out to the rescue vehicle, she hands you a report form with the vitals recorded. The respirations are 24 per minute and rapid, the pulse is

120 strong and bounding, the skin is flushed and hot and dry to the touch, the pupils are equal and reactive to light, the blood pressure is 164/92, and the SpO_2 is 95%. You help Mrs. Holland take off her heavy sweater, and you ask Misty to fan her. Katy, out at the ambulance, wets a sheet with tepid water, places it on the cot, and turns the air conditioning on high. She removes the cot from the ambulance, closes the rear doors, and returns to the room with the cot. Katy and Misty remove all of Mrs. Holland's clothing and place two towels to cover her genitals and breasts. You move her to the cot and place cold packs in her armpits, on either side of her neck, and behind her knees. You encourage Misty to continue to fan Mrs. Holland aggressively.

The ALS crew arrives just as you are exiting the front door. Paramedic Darleen Brooks introduces herself to Mrs. Holland and looks to you for a report. You provide a quick report and help place Mrs. Holland in the ALS vehicle. You clean up your vehicle and advise dispatch that you are available for another call.

1. Mrs. Holland is mostly likely suffering from _____, which has a mortality rate ranging from _____.
   a. heat cramps/5 to 50 percent
   b. heat exhaustion/30 to 60 percent
   c. heat stroke/20 to 80 percent
   d. high fever/15 to 60 percent

2. The cooling of Mrs. Holland
   a. was appropriately performed.
   b. should have been performed by pouring ice water over Mrs. Holland's body.
   c. should have been performed by surrounding Mrs. Holland's torso with ice packs.
   d. should have included placing Mrs. Holland's hands and feet in ice water.

3. What information that you obtained would make you *most* likely to believe that Mrs. Holland was a priority patient who required rapid transport and ALS management?
   a. Environmental factors
   b. Mrs. Holland's confusion
   c. Mrs. Holland's headache
   d. Mrs. Holland's hot and dry skin

4. You and Katy did not provide any cool water for Mrs. Holland to drink. Was this appropriate?
   a. Yes, Mrs. Holland was nauseated and had an altered level of consciousness.
   b. Yes, Mrs. Holland had a headache and is over 65 years of age.
   c. No, Mrs. Holland should have been given a half glass of water every 15 minutes.
   d. No, Mrs. Holland should have been given one full glass of water.

5. An air temperature of 95°F and a relative humidity of 75 percent would represent a
   a. moderate danger on the heat-and-humidity risk scale.
   b. severe danger on the heat-and-humidity risk scale.
   c. caution status on the heat-and-humidity risk scale.
   d. safe area on the heat-and-humidity risk scale.

TRIP #			EMERGENCY	BILLING USE ONLY					
MEDIC #			TRIP SHEET						
● N MILES				DAY					
● D MILES				DATE					
CODE __/__	PAGE __/__			RECEIVED					
UNITS ON SCENE				DISPATCHED					

NAME		SEX M F DOB __/__/__	EN-ROUTE		
ADDRESS		RACE	ON SCENE		
CITY	STATE	ZIP	TO HOSPITAL		
PHONE ( ) -	PCP DR.		AT HOSPITAL		
RESPONDED FROM		CITY	IN-SERVICE		
TAKEN FROM		ZIP	CREW	CERT	STATE #
DESTINATION		REASON			
SSN - -	MEDICARE #	MEDICAID #			
INSURANCE CO	INSURANCE #	GROUP #			
RESPONSIBLE PARTY	ADDRESS				
CITY	STATE ZIP PHONE ( ) -		IV THERAPY		
EMPLOYER			SUCCESSFUL Y N # OF ATTEMPTS _____ ANGIO SIZE _____ga.		

TIME	ON SCENE (1)	ON SCENE (2)	ON SCENE (3)	EN-ROUTE (1)	EN-ROUTE (2)	AT DESTINATION	SITE _____
BP							TOTAL FLUID INFUSED _____ cc
PULSE							BLOOD DRAW Y N INITIALS
RESP							
SpO$_2$							INTUBATION INFORMATION
ETCO$_2$							SUCCESSFUL Y N # OF ATTEMPTS _____
EKG							TUBE SIZE _____ mm
							TIME _____ INITIALS _____

● EDICAL HISTORY	CONDITION CODES
	TREATMENTS
MEDICATIONS	TIME	TREATMENT	DOSE	ROUTE	INIT
ALLERGIES	
C/C	
EVENTS LEADING TO C/C	
ASSESSMENT	
TREATMENT	
	GCS E__ V__ M__ TOTAL =
	GCS E__ V__ M__ TOTAL =
	HOSPITAL CONTACTED
	CPR BEGUN BY B P TIME BEGUN
EMS SIGNATURE	AED USED Y N BY:
	RESUSCITATION TERMINATED - TIME
	( ) OSHA REGULATIONS FOLLOWED

Submersion Incidents: Drowning and Diving Emergencies

▌ STANDARD

Trauma (Content Area: Environmental Emergencies)

▌ COMPETENCY

Applies fundamental knowledge to provide basic emergency care and transportation based on assessment findings for an acutely injured patient.

▌ OBJECTIVES

After reading this chapter, you should be able to:

25-1. Define key terms introduced in this chapter.
25-2. Discuss ways to reduce the risk of submersion incidents.
25-3. Describe factors that can lead to submersion incidents in infants, children, adolescents, and adults.
25-4. Explain factors that affect the likelihood of survival from submersion incidents.
25-5. Describe the pathophysiology of drowning.
25-6. Discuss the association between shallow water diving and spinal injuries.
25-7. Explain actions you should take to protect your own safety when responding to a water emergency.
25-8. Explain the necessity of taking spinal precautions to any swimmer or diver who may have suffered trauma.
25-9. Given a scenario in which a patient has suffered a submersion incident, explain how to provide resuscitative care.
25-10. Explain the assessment-based approach to drowning and other water-related injuries, including emergency medical care for the drowning victim.
25-11. Explain the formation and relief of gastric distention in patients involved in submersion incidents.
25-12. Describe laws of physics as they relate to scuba or deepwater diving, including:
    a. Boyle law
    b. Dalton law
    c. Henry law
    d. Charles law
25-13. Explain the pathophysiology of decompression sickness.
25-14. Recognize the signs, symptoms, and patient history associated with:
    a. Type I decompression sickness
    b. Type II decompression sickness
    c. Arterial gas embolism

25-15. Explain the pathophysiology of barotrauma injuries.

25-16. Describe the emergency medical care of patients suffering from air embolism, decompression sickness, and barotrauma.

❙ KEY IDEAS

Drowning related to swimming is often assumed to be the major cause of death from water-related emergencies. Drownings related to swimming actually account for only a small number of water-related deaths. The rest are caused by diving and deepwater exploration, boating, water-skiing, and water-related deaths from motor vehicle crashes. This chapter reviews the statistics, signs, symptoms, and management of drowning and diving emergencies.

- Many drownings could be prevented if personal flotation devices (PFDs) were utilized in and around water, adult supervision was provided around swimming pools, and pools were fenced and locked.

- Always suspect a spinal injury in any swimmer who is found unresponsive in or out of the water, has signs of injury or alcohol intoxication, or has been diving or using a water slide.

- Never enter the water to rescue a patient unless you meet all the following criteria: you are a good swimmer; you are specially trained in water rescue techniques; you are wearing a personal flotation device; and you are accompanied by other rescuers.

- Use the reach, throw, row, and go strategy to reach a responsive, close-to-shore swimmer who requires rescue.

- All drowning patients require transport even if you think they are stable.

- Attempt resuscitation on any pulseless, nonbreathing patient who has been submerged in cold water for an extended time period.

- For the water-related-emergency patient, look for signs and symptoms of any of the following: airway obstruction, absent or inadequate breathing, pulselessness, spinal or head injury, soft tissue injuries, musculoskeletal injuries, external or internal bleeding, shock, hypothermia, or alcohol or drug abuse.

- The emergency care for drowning patients includes the following: If spinal injury is suspected, immobilize the patient. If no spinal injury is suspected, position the patient on the left side and suction the airway as needed. If the patient is in respiratory arrest or not breathing adequately, rapidly establish an airway. Begin positive pressure ventilation with supplemental oxygen (if pulseless and apneic, proceed with the automated external defibrillator (AED) protocol), watch for gastric distention, and transport quickly.

❙ TERMS AND CONCEPTS

1. Write the number of the correct term next to each definition.

   1. Drowning
   2. Gastric distention
   3. Mammalian diving reflex
   4. Surfactant
   5. Dysbarism

   _____ a. A substance responsible for maintaining surface tension in the alveoli

   _____ b. The body's natural response to submersion in cold water in which breathing is inhibited, the heart rate decreases, and blood vessels constrict in order to maintain cerebral and cardiac blood flow

   _____ c. Submersion causing primary respiratory impairment, whether the person survives or dies after the event

_____ d. The filling of the stomach with water and/or air, causing an enlarged abdomen, which makes ventilation difficult

_____ e. A medical condition that results from pressure changes that may occur when a person descends in water or ascends in altitude

▌ CONTENT REVIEW

1. Deaths from drowning
   a. occur only in deep water.
   b. are often associated with the use of alcohol.
   c. are not affected by the wearing of personal flotation devices.
   d. are not affected by adult supervision at swimming pools.

2. The two major age groups that are most at risk of death from drowning are
   a. children less than 2 years of age and young adults age 18–24.
   b. children less than 5 years of age and teenagers.
   c. children less than 8 years of age and adolescents age 15–18.
   d. children less than 10 years of age and adults age 65 and over.

3. Between 10 and 15 percent of drowning patients aspirate no water into their lungs during submersion. This is referred to as a
   a. hemostatic drowning.
   b. pernicious drowning.
   c. dry drowning.
   d. surfactant drowning.

4. Drowning patients may be placed into one of the following categories. Into which category should you place a patient with an altered mental status and a persistent cough?
   a. Asymptomatic
   b. Symptomatic
   c. Class I
   d. Near drowning

5. Abdominal thrusts should be used in the drowning patient
   a. routinely during resuscitation efforts.
   b. never, because it may lead to vomiting and aspiration.
   c. only if a foreign-body airway obstruction is suspected.
   d. only in salt-water immersion incidents.

6. If the responsive drowning patient is close to shore, the strategy you should use is
   a. reach, go, row, and tow.
   b. call, throw, tow, and go.
   c. reach, throw, row, and go.
   d. go, throw, reach, and row.

7. A patient is found unresponsive, floating in shallow water. Your _primary_ suspicion should be that
   a. the patient has a spinal injury.
   b. the patient is a poor swimmer.
   c. the patient was struck by a boat.
   d. the patient had a seizure.

8. You are evaluating a young patient who, you learn, has been submerged in cold water (68°F) for 30 minutes. You should
   a. not attempt resuscitation on this patient.
   b. not attempt resuscitation until ALS arrives on scene.
   c. attempt resuscitation of the patient with full efforts.
   d. provide a brief resuscitative effort for the benefit of the family.

9. Differences between saltwater and freshwater drowning
   a. pertain to whether or not surfactant is washed out.
   b. explain why there are more drownings in salt water than in fresh water.
   c. result in different degrees of respiratory distress suffered by the patient.
   d. do not play a major role in resuscitation of submersion patients.

10. When a person dives into water colder than 68°F, which controversial reflex may prevent death, even after prolonged submersion?
    a. Human diving reflex
    b. Beck diving reflex
    c. Mammalian diving reflex
    d. Momentary submersion reflex

11. Scuba diving emergencies
    a. never involve drowning.
    b. occur only in areas near the ocean.
    c. are increasing in incidence.
    d. can be managed only by a paramedic.

12. Which law of physics states that, at a constant temperature, the volume of a gas is inversely related to the pressure?
    a. Boyle law
    b. Dalton law
    c. Henry law
    d. Charles law

13. Decompression sickness (DCS)
    a. occurs as a result of bubbles formed from the expansion of nitrogen.
    b. has two primary effects: acting as emboli and reducing oxyhemoglobin loading.
    c. will be temporarily relieved by getting to a high altitude, as in an airplane.
    d. is more likely to occur while diving in warm water rather than cold water.

14. The joint in which pain associated with DCS is most commonly experienced is the
    a. hip.
    b. knee.
    c. shoulder.
    d. elbow.

15. DCS can be divided into three categories. Complete the following chart by indicating with a check mark if the sign or symptom is most likely associated with type I DCS, type II DCS, or arterial gas embolism (AGE). Since each may be associated with more than one category, you may use one, two, or three check marks for each sign or symptom.

Sign or Symptom	Type I DCS	Type II DCS	AGE
Pain in joints or tendons			
Low back pain			
Skin rash, itching			
Altered mental status			
Substernal burning sensation on inhalation			
Dyspnea			
Headache, visual disturbance			
Bloody sputum			
Nausea and vomiting			

16. The "squeeze" or barotrauma
    a. results from too rapid a descent.
    b. occurs during either ascent or descent.
    c. commonly occurs in divers with hypertension.
    d. results in a staggering gait or lack of coordination.

CASE STUDY 1

You are dispatched to a call for a drowning. You arrive at a small home located just outside of town. The scene appears safe as you arrive. A woman is frantically motioning to you. She screams at you as you exit the ambulance, "Please! Please! Hurry! My daughter! I just found her floating in the pool!" You follow the distraught mother to a backyard pool. As you approach the patient, you note that she looks to be about 4 years old. She is lying supine on the pool deck. CPR is being performed by a neighbor. The patient is located next to the shallow end of the pool. Your general impression is that she looks ill. Her skin color is cyanotic. She is unresponsive to pain. She has no respirations and no palpable carotid pulse. There is a small laceration on the front of her forehead, with minor bleeding.

1. Which of the following is the appropriate *initial* treatment for this patient?
    a. Determine the "downtime" before beginning resuscitation.
    b. Determine the "downtime" and the temperature of the water before beginning resuscitation.
    c. Begin resuscitation efforts after performing a detailed assessment.
    d. Begin resuscitation efforts immediately.

2. *Immediate* treatment for this patient should include which of the following?
    a. Checking for gastric distention
    b. Treating the patient for a possible spinal injury
    c. Controlling the bleeding from the laceration
    d. Administering oxygen by a nonrebreather mask

3. You have been providing positive pressure ventilation to the patient for a few minutes. You notice that the patient's abdomen is distended, and you cannot ventilate the patient effectively. You should
    a. reduce the volume and pressure delivered during your ventilations.
    b. continue with the ventilations and advise the ALS crew of the condition when they arrive.
    c. increase the volume and pressure delivered during your ventilations.
    d. turn the patient on her left side and apply pressure over the epigastric region; have suction available.

CASE STUDY 2

You are dispatched to the city pool for a drowning. Upon arrival, you observe a small crowd of people standing around a young boy who is sitting up in a chair. The scene appears safe as you walk to the patient. A lifeguard approaches and tells you, "I found this kid on the bottom of the pool. He couldn't have been under very long. I pulled him out and gave him one breath. He coughed, and then he woke up. I called his mom to come and get him. She should be here in a few minutes." As you approach the patient, you note that he appears to be about 11 years old. He looks up at you as you approach. He is coughing persistently. Your general impression is that he looks well. His skin color is normal. He answers your questions appropriately. His respirations are normal. His radial pulse is strong and regular. There is no sign of trauma, and no bleeding is observed. No other findings are made during the history and physical exam.

1. Should this patient be allowed to return home with his mother?
   a. Yes. The patient is stable. Allow him to return home.
   b. Yes, but only after you have described to his mother potential complications that can occur and what to watch for.
   c. No. Observe the patient at the scene for at least 30 minutes before making a decision.
   d. No. Fatal complications from a submersion can occur as long as 72 hours after the incident. He must be transported for evaluation by a physician.

2. Your care and treatment for this patient should include which of the following?
   a. No care is required. The patient will be allowed to return home.
   b. Administer oxygen to maintain an SpO_2 of 94% or greater, monitor carefully, and transport on his left side.
   c. Monitor carefully and transport sitting up.
   d. Administer oxygen to maintain an SpO_2 of 94% or greater, reevaluate his condition, and reach a decision following further observation.

3. This patient would be placed into which category?
   a. Asymptomatic
   b. Symptomatic
   c. Cardiac arrest
   d. Obviously dead

CHAPTER 25 SCENARIO: DOCUMENTATION EXERCISE

Read the following scenario and think about how you would document this call if you were the EMT who responded to the scene. Then answer the multiple-choice questions and fill in the sample prehospital care report, basing your documentation on information from the scenario.

It's 6:30 P.M. on a Thursday. You and your partner Tyler are just sitting down to supper when the alarm sounds: "Unit 5, respond to a vehicle accident at 3211 North Lucerne Park Road; cross street, Old Crossover Road. Time out 1830 hours." You take a bite of biscuit, grab your jacket, and quickly move to the vehicle. Tyler advises dispatch that you are responding. Dispatch tells you that a vehicle has plunged down a steep embankment; the local fire department, ALS backup, and law enforcement are responding.

You arrive on scene in six minutes. A police officer directs you to the side of the road. A group of people is crowded around a person lying on his side. With Standard Precautions in place, you and Tyler approach the crowd, introduce yourselves, and ask, "What happened?" The police officer replies, "The best I can make out at this time is that this guy was driving a car that went down that embankment. He was going too fast for the curve, and his car just lost it." A bystander quickly chimes in, "I saw the car flip at least three times, and I found it lying upside down in about five feet of water. These two guys [he points to two young men who are wet and have blankets draped around their shoulders] pulled him out of the car, started CPR, and carried him to the top of the hill."

Tyler is performing a primary assessment. He notes that the patient appears to be about 17 years of age. He is unresponsive to voice or pain; has a small laceration on his forehead; is breathing adequately, with no abnormal respiratory sounds audible; has a strong, regular radial pulse; and his skin is cold and wet. Oxygen via a nasal cannula at 3 lpm is placed. Tyler asks a trained Emergency Medical Responder to stabilize the cervical spine. You quickly inspect the neck for trauma and then place the cervical spine immobilization collar. Tyler checks the airway for secretions or foreign material and finds that the airway is clear. You quickly cut the clothing off the young man, inspect his back, position the spine board behind him, and carefully roll him onto the board. You place a heavy blanket on the patient.

Tyler starts taking the vital signs while you begin a rapid assessment. Your rapid assessment reveals a 3-inch laceration on his forehead, a large bruise on his left lateral chest, an intact pelvis, and a fracture of his left ankle. You check for a distal pulse and sensation in his ankle before and after you splint it.

Suddenly, the patient begins coughing and opens his eyes. You introduce yourself and Tyler, and say, "You've been in an accident. We've immobilized you just in case you may have other injuries. Please try to remain still. Could you tell me where you hurt?" The patient looks at you but does not respond. His coughing continues for about 30 seconds before it begins to diminish. Tyler has completed the vitals and reports that the patient's respirations are 20 per minute; the breath sounds are equal and clear; the

pulse is 90 per minute, strong, and regular; the skin is pale and cold; the pupils are equal and reactive and respond briskly to light; the blood pressure is 124/74; and the SpO_2 is 95%.

The police officer now tells you that the patient's name is Billy Wilson. He was on the way home from basketball practice and didn't make the curve. The officer also tells you that the two young men who pulled Billy from the car reported that he was in the water for at least 10 or 15 minutes before they were able to get him out of the car. The young man who pulled him free is standing behind the police officer and says, "We were coming back from the movies when we saw someone standing beside the road screaming and waving. We turned around and came back to help. He said a car went down the embankment. We found the spot where the car went off the road, and we went down to find the car. I can't believe how cold the water was. It came up to my chest. The car was turned over. I pulled the door open and kept grabbing until I felt something; I could feel it was a person, but he was jammed inside. I took my buddy's knife and cut the seat belt. We were pulling and pulling, and finally he came out. We pulled him to the bank, and we started CPR. After a few minutes, he coughed and started breathing. So then we pulled him up the bank to the road. He was in the water for at least 10 or 15 minutes."

You look up and see the ALS unit arriving on scene. It is a new paramedic whom you don't recognize. You quickly provide a report and assist with placing the patient in the ALS ambulance.

1. Treatment and management of Billy should be focused on
    a. hypothermia and traumatic injuries.
    b. drowning and traumatic injuries.
    c. drowning, hypothermia, and traumatic injuries.
    d. traumatic injuries only.

2. Billy's breath sounds on auscultation were clear and equal. How is this possible given his submersion?
    a. Spasm and tight closing of the larynx
    b. Relaxation of the laryngeal structures following hypoxia
    c. Upper bronchial tree spasm and contraction
    d. Alveolar spasm and massive production of surfactant

3. What effect did the very cold water temperature possibly have on Billy's condition?
    a. May have triggered aspiration of water via the mammalian diving reflex
    b. May have caused development of severe peripheral acidosis
    c. May have helped prevent brain damage while the brain cells were deprived of oxygen
    d. May have caused an increase in the heart rate and dilation of blood vessels

4. Management of Billy's condition should include
   a. removal from the cold environment.
   b. performance of a thermal rub.
   c. immediate immersion in hot water.
   d. placement of the AED.

5. Deaths due to complications of drowning occur. What is the likelihood that a patient such as Billy will die as a result of these complications?
   a. 5 percent
   b. 10 percent
   c. 15 percent
   d. 20 percent

EMERGENCY TRIP SHEET

TRIP #	
MEDIC #	
BEGIN MILES	
END MILES	
CODE___/___ PAGE___/___	
UNITS ON SCENE	

NAME	SEX M F DOB ___/___/___
ADDRESS	RACE
CITY	STATE	ZIP
PHONE ( ) -	PCP DR.
RESPONDED FROM	CITY
TAKEN FROM	ZIP
DESTINATION	REASON
SSN - -	MEDICARE #	MEDICAID #
INSURANCE CO	INSURANCE #	GROUP #
RESPONSIBLE PARTY	ADDRESS
CITY	STATE	ZIP	PHONE ( ) -
EMPLOYER	

BILLING USE ONLY

DAY			
DATE			
RECEIVED			
DISPATCHED			
EN-ROUTE			
ON SCENE			
TO HOSPITAL			
AT HOSPITAL			
IN-SERVICE			

CREW	CERT	STATE #

TIME	ON SCENE (1)	ON SCENE (2)	ON SCENE (3)	EN-ROUTE (1)	EN-ROUTE (2)	AT DESTINATION
BP						
PULSE						
RESP						
SpO$_2$						
ETCO$_2$						
EKG						

IV THERAPY
SUCCESSFUL Y N # OF ATTEMPTS _____
ANGIO SIZE _____ga.
SITE _____
TOTAL FLUID INFUSED _____ cc
BLOOD DRAW Y N INITIALS

INTUBATION INFORMATION
SUCCESSFUL Y N # OF ATTEMPTS _____
TUBE SIZE _____ mm
TIME _____ INITIALS _____

MEDICAL HISTORY

MEDICATIONS

ALLERGIES

C/C

EVENTS LEADING TO C/C

ASSESSMENT

TREATMENT

CONDITION CODES				

TREATMENTS

TIME	TREATMENT	DOSE	ROUTE	INIT

GCS E___ V___ M___ TOTAL =
GCS E___ V___ M___ TOTAL =
HOSPITAL CONTACTED

CPR BEGUN BY B P TIME BEGUN	
AED USED Y N BY:	
RESUSCITATION TERMINATED - TIME	

EMS SIGNATURE

( ) OSHA REGULATIONS FOLLOWED

Behavioral Emergencies

CHAPTER

26

STANDARD

Medicine (Content Area: Psychiatric)

COMPETENCY

Applies fundamental knowledge to provide basic emergency care and transportation based on assessment findings for an acutely ill patient.

OBJECTIVES

After reading this chapter, you should be able to:

26-1. Define key terms introduced in this chapter.

26-2. Explain the importance of recognizing and responding to patients suffering from behavioral emergencies.

26-3. Describe indications of danger associated with response to behavioral emergencies.

26-4. Discuss the underlying physical and psychological causes of behavioral emergencies.

26-5. Describe the focus of assessment and history taking for patients who have behavioral emergencies.

26-6. Recognize behavioral characteristics of the following conditions:
   a. Anxiety
   b. Phobias
   c. Depression
   d. Bipolar disorder
   e. Paranoia
   f. Psychosis
   g. Schizophrenia
   h. Agitated delirium

26-7. Describe risk factors associated with suicide and violence toward others.

26-8. Discuss basic principles related to the assessment and management of patients with behavioral emergencies.

26-9. Recognize indications of attempted suicide during scene size-up and patient assessment.

26-10. Prioritize patient care needs in terms of managing physical and behavioral problems.

26-11. Recognize indications for physical restraint of a patient and follow principles of safe physical restraint of patients.

26-12. Evaluate the need for law enforcement and medical direction involvement in a behavioral emergency situation.

26-13. Document all information pertinent to calls involving behavioral emergencies and patient restraint.

KEY IDEAS

This chapter focuses on the assessment and management of behavioral emergencies. Behavioral emergencies may be manifested in a variety of ways and require special considerations from the EMT. Key concepts include the following:

- A *behavioral emergency* is one in which the patient exhibits behavior that is not socially acceptable or tolerable to the patient, the family, or the community.

- The precipitating factor in a behavioral emergency may be extremes of emotion, a physical condition, or a psychological condition.

- The priority of the EMT at the scene of a behavioral emergency is to manage the patient's injuries or illness. What seems to be a behavioral emergency may arise from a traumatic or medical condition.

- Acts of violence against oneself or others are often associated with behavioral emergencies. Always remain vigilant on the scene and be aware of behavior changes in the patient.

- Every suicidal act or gesture should be taken seriously, and the patient should be transported for evaluation by a physician.

- When managing behavioral emergencies, the EMT should remember that interpersonal communications may have more impact on the outcome of the situation than emergency medical skills. These skills include using active listening skills, being supportive and empathetic, limiting interruptions in the interview, respecting the patient's space, and limiting physical touch until a rapport is established.

- Behavioral emergencies require special assessment and medical/legal considerations on the part of the EMT.

TERMS AND CONCEPTS

1. Write the number of the correct term next to each definition.

    1. Behavior
    2. Behavioral emergency
    3. Bipolar disorder
    4. Humane restraints
    5. Paranoia
    6. Phobia
    7. Reasonable force
    8. Schizophrenia
    9. Suicide
    10. Agitated delirium

    _____ a. The minimum amount of force required to prevent the patient from harming himself or others

    _____ b. The way a person acts

    _____ c. A willful act designed to end one's own life

    _____ d. Padded leather or cloth straps used to keep the patient from hurting himself or others

    _____ e. A situation in which a person exhibits "abnormal" behavior

    _____ f. Causes a patient to swing to opposite sides of the mood spectrum

    _____ g. A chronic mental illness in which a patient experiences distortions of speech and thought, bizarre delusions and hallucinations, social withdrawal, catatonic behavior, and lack of emotional expressiveness, and does not return to a premorbid level of functioning.

_____ h. Irrational fears of specific things, places, or situations

_____ i. A highly exaggerated or unwarranted mistrust or suspiciousness

_____ j. Mental state and physiological response characterized by unusual strength, pain tolerance, agitation, hostility, and hyperactive behavior.

CONTENT REVIEW

1. For each of the following signs or symptoms, indicate if it is potentially a clue of a physical (rather than a psychological) problem. Indicate yes (Y) if it is a potential clue of a physical problem. Indicate no (N) if it is not a potential clue of a physical problem.

   _____ a. The patient has auditory hallucinations.

   _____ b. The pupils are dilated.

   _____ c. The patient has intact memory and responsiveness.

   _____ d. The patient is incontinent.

   _____ e. The onset of symptoms was gradual.

   _____ f. The patient has excessive salivation.

   _____ g. The patient has an unusual breath odor.

2. _____ often presents with an overwhelming fear that is accompanied by rapid breathing, palpitations, dizziness, and carpal-pedal spasms.
   a. A panic attack
   b. Paranoia
   c. Bipolar disorder
   d. Schizophrenia

3. Deep feelings of sadness and worthlessness that are accompanied by fatigue, loss of appetite, and a sense of hopelessness may be due to which psychiatric disorder?
   a. Paranoia
   b. Schizophrenia
   c. Depression
   d. Anxiety

4. Which of the following best describes the chronic mental illness in which patients suffer debilitating distortions of speech and thought, bizarre delusions, hallucinations, social withdrawal, catatonic behavior, and lack of emotional expressiveness?
   a. Paranoia
   b. Schizophrenia
   c. Bipolar disorder
   d. Depression

5. For each of the following patients, indicate yes (Y) if the patient is in a high-risk category for suicide and no (N) if the patient is not in a high-risk category for suicide.

   _____ a. A 45-year-old man with a history of depression and other mental disorders

   _____ b. A 26-year-old who is recently married

   _____ c. A 20-year-old who has previously attempted suicide

   _____ d. A 24-year-old female with a history of child abuse

_____ e. A 75-year-old patient who recently had a stroke and is unable to care for herself

_____ f. A 65-year-old female who recently took a new job

_____ g. A 55-year-old male who is recently widowed

_____ h. A 40-year-old female who recently lost a job she had held for 20 years

6. When dealing with behavioral emergencies, it is important to understand that
   a. only certain people are susceptible to emotional injury.
   b. people have a more limited ability to cope with a crisis than they may think.
   c. primarily women and children are affected by disaster or injury.
   d. an emotional injury is just as real as a physical injury.

7. Your best protection against legal problems or false accusations when dealing with emotionally disturbed patients is
   a. careful documentation.
   b. use of restraints.
   c. a credible witness.
   d. use of a calm, reassuring voice.

8. Which of the following best describes the guidelines that apply when restraining a combative patient?
   a. Use as much force as possible to subdue the patient quickly.
   b. Never attempt restraint until you have sufficient help and an appropriate plan.
   c. Once you have determined that restraint is necessary, move slowly to avoid agitating the patient.
   d. Police-style metal handcuffs are a good way to restrain a combative patient to the stretcher.

9. The *first* priority in dealing with a behavioral emergency is to
   a. determine if the behavior is caused by a medical condition.
   b. establish and maintain an airway and oxygenation.
   c. protect yourself and others at the scene from harm.
   d. restrain the patient to protect him from harming himself.

10. Mark an X beside each of the following treatments that would be appropriate for a behavioral emergency. Leave the other blanks unmarked.

    _____ a. Avoid speaking directly to the patient.

    _____ b. Stay as close as you can to the patient.

    _____ c. Avoid making eye contact with the patient.

    _____ d. Avoid making any quick movements.

    _____ e. Do not play along with visual or auditory hallucinations.

    _____ f. Let the patient decide whether to involve family or friends.

    _____ g. Avoid spending long amounts of time on the scene.

    _____ h. Never leave the patient alone.

    _____ i. Force the patient to make decisions.

11. You respond to a call for a "man who is acting crazy." You arrive on scene and observe a 45-year-old male patient aggressively fighting with five police officers. You maintain a safe distance. While waiting for police to summon you, a bystander tells you that the patient has been drinking heavily and taking methamphetamine for the past day or two. The patient seems to exhibit super strength and is very agitated. The patient is most likely suffering from
    a. schizophrenia.
    b. bipolar disorder.
    c. agitated delirium.
    d. psychosis.

12. Agoraphobia is
    a. a fear of water.
    b. anxiety about or a fear of animals.
    c. anxiety about being in places or situations from which escape would be difficult.
    d. a fear of being alone.

13. Dystonia is
    a. a movement disorder.
    b. difficulty with speaking.
    c. difficulty with seeing clearly.
    d. a disorder associated with loud and accelerated speech.

CASE STUDY

You have been called to a dormitory at a local college. Your patient is a 20-year-old male who is cowering in the corner of the lobby. Bystanders report that his name is Jim and that just before your arrival, he was shouting, "Go away, leave me alone," and gesturing at someone or something that isn't there.

1. Your *first* action should be to do which of the following?
    a. Speak with authority and ask the patient to stand.
    b. Approach the patient to gain his trust.
    c. Stand directly in front of the patient to make eye contact.
    d. Scan the scene for potential hazards.

After you ask if you can come closer, Jim allows you to come within three feet of his location. You notice that he seems frightened. His hands are trembling slightly, and his breathing is rapid. You note that his skin is pink and dry, and you observe no obvious injuries. He tells you that he's hearing voices that are telling him to do "bad things."

2. Which technique would best help gain the trust of this patient?
    a. Maintain eye contact and speak calmly.
    b. Play along with visual or auditory disturbances.
    c. Leave the patient alone so he can rationalize his thoughts.
    d. Tell the patient what he wants to hear, even if it is not truthful.

3. What actions should your partner take?
    a. Keep you in his line of sight, move quickly to talk to bystanders, avoid eye contact with the patient, try to obtain additional information, and try to disperse bystanders.
    b. Keep you in his line of sight, speak in a loud and rapid voice, avoid eye contact with the patient, try to obtain additional information, and try to disperse bystanders.

c. Keep you in his line of sight, be alert that Jim may become violent, try to obtain additional information, and try to disperse bystanders.

d. Be alert that Jim may become violent, leave the room, and try to find witnesses who can provide additional information.

After 15 minutes of quiet conversation, you find that Jim has no past medical history but has had trouble concentrating and sleeping over the past several weeks. He denies that he has been injured recently. You ask Jim if he'll let you take him to the hospital to see the doctor. Jim agrees to accompany you. You help Jim to his feet and lead him out of the lobby and to your ambulance.

4. What should you do while en route to the hospital?

_____

_____

_____

_____

▌ CHAPTER 26 SCENARIO: DOCUMENTATION EXERCISE

Read the following scenario and think about how you would document this call if you were the EMT who responded to the scene. Then answer the multiple-choice questions and fill in the sample prehospital care report, basing your documentation on information from the scenario.

It is 10:30 P.M. on a Saturday. You and your partner, LaToya, are at the station watching TV. The alarm tone sounds: "Rescue 5, respond to 1626 Leighton Street, cross street Chatfield Street, for a possible suicide. Police are responding. Time out 2230 hours." You and LaToya quickly move to the rescue vehicle and advise dispatch that you are responding. Dispatch tells you that police are on the scene and that the patient is a 60-year-old female who is depressed. You arrive in about five minutes. LaToya tells dispatch, "Rescue Five on scene." Dispatch responds, "Rescue Five on scene at 2235 hours."

The home is a large block house in a pleasant, well-kept neighborhood. A police car, with parking lights on, is parked in front of the home. LaToya parks in the driveway. The door to the home is open, and you hear a TV blaring loudly. With Standard Precautions taken, you carefully enter and see a woman in her mid- to late 60s sitting in a chair. She is crying softly while leaning forward with her head in her hands. Your general impression is that she looks physically well. Two women are kneeling next to her and consoling her. A police officer is standing next to the front door holding a notepad.

You quickly introduce yourself to the police officer and ask what happened. He tells you, "This

lady's name is Mrs. Raunecker. She called the police department about 20 minutes ago and said that she was going to kill herself. I've been on scene for about 10 minutes. The two ladies are neighbors who came over when they saw my car. She seems to be pretty depressed." LaToya turns down the TV. You walk toward the patient and introduce yourself and LaToya to Mrs. Raunecker. You tell her, "We are EMTs, and we are here to help you." She lifts her head from her hands and quietly says, between sobs, "I just can't do it anymore. I can't take it. My husband died last year, I just found out that I'm going to be laid off at my job, and the police are here, so I guess I'm about to be arrested! I just can't keep going on."

You and LaToya are about six feet from Mrs. Raunecker. You kneel down, look her in the eyes, and say softly, "Mrs. Raunecker, we're concerned about your well-being. You called the police department and made a suicide threat. I can see that you're very depressed. We're here to help you. Would it be OK if LaToya took your vital signs?" Mrs. Raunecker nods her head yes. You move closer to Mrs. Raunecker, and LaToya begins to take her vital signs. One of the women consoling Mrs. Raunecker catches your eye and moves her head toward the kitchen. She heads to the kitchen, and you follow. She tells you that her name is Juanita Black and that she has lived next door to Mrs. Raunecker for many years. She tells you that Mrs. Raunecker has been depressed for the last three months. Juanita tried to get her to seek professional help, but she refused. Mrs. Black continues by saying that the patient has been drinking heavily since her husband died last year and that she made a similar suicide threat just last month. Mrs. Black says that she didn't take the threat seriously, and she told her to "go ahead and do it." She felt that this would shock her into reality.

You thank Mrs. Black for this information and head back to where the police officer is standing. You ask the officer to accompany you on a quick search of the home. You find nothing out of the ordinary except for two full pill bottles of a medication, prescribed for her husband, which was recently refilled. The containers were sitting on her nightstand. You return to the front of the house where Mrs. Raunecker is located. LaToya hands you a vitals report form. You quickly scan the sheet and review her vitals. She is alert and oriented to person, place, and time; respirations are normal at 14 per minute; pulse is 88, strong, and regular; skin color is normal, warm, and dry; pupils are equal and reactive; the blood pressure is 138/78; SpO_2 reads 96%.

LaToya tells you that she obtained a history and found out that the patient has no allergies, takes no medicines, and has no prior medical history. She last ate at about 6 P.M. Mrs. Raunecker says, "I don't think all this is necessary. I'm much better now. Thank you all for coming. I will be all right. I really don't need to go to the hospital." You reply, "Mrs. Raunecker, you called the police and made a threat to commit suicide, I found two bottles of pills next to your bed, and Mrs. Black told me that you made a similar suicide threat some months ago. All this must be taken very seriously. We are really concerned about your well-being. We can't leave you here under these circumstances. You must go to the hospital." She sobs and says, "Well, if you really think that I should, I guess I will." You place Mrs. Raunecker in the ambulance and transport her without incident.

1. When managing a patient who has made a suicide attempt, the EMT's primary concern is to
   a. manage the psychological aspects of the patient's condition.
   b. manage the well-being of the family and any bystanders.
   c. manage any injuries or medical conditions related to the suicide attempt.
   d. provide accurate documentation of the events.

2. Mrs. Raunecker appeared to improve and initially refused to be transported to the hospital. Was the action that you took to encourage her transport appropriate?
   a. Yes, Mrs. Raunecker was at great risk for following through on her threats.
   b. Yes, but Mrs. Raunecker should have been restrained for transport.
   c. No, Mrs. Raunecker is alert and oriented and should be allowed to refuse.
   d. No, Mrs. Raunecker should be placed under arrest and transported.

3. In questioning Mrs. Raunecker, what technique did you use?
   a. Avoided the use of "yes" or "no" questions
   b. Used the OPQRST method
   c. Made use of closed-ended questions
   d. Used a technique of rapid questioning

4. The interview with Mrs. Raunecker
   a. was appropriately conducted and performed professionally.
   b. should have been concluded by challenging her suicide gesture.
   c. should have taken place at the hospital rather than at her home.
   d. should have been conducted in a quiet surrounding, with limited people around.

5. The search of Mrs. Raunecker's home
   a. should not have been performed.
   b. should have been conducted only by law enforcement.
   c. was appropriate, given the circumstances.
   d. was inappropriate and required a search warrant.

EMERGENCY TRIP SHEET

TRIP #	
MEDIC #	
BEGIN MILES	
END MILES	
CODE___/___	PAGE___/___
UNITS ON SCENE	

NAME	SEX M F DOB __/__/__
ADDRESS	RACE
CITY	STATE ZIP
PHONE ( ) -	PCP DR.
RESPONDED FROM	CITY
TAKEN FROM	ZIP
DESTINATION	REASON
SSN - -	MEDICARE # MEDICAID #
INSURANCE CO	INSURANCE # GROUP #
RESPONSIBLE PARTY	ADDRESS
CITY	STATE ZIP PHONE ( ) -
EMPLOYER	

BILLING USE ONLY

DAY			
DATE			
RECEIVED			
DISPATCHED			
EN-ROUTE			
ON SCENE			
TO HOSPITAL			
AT HOSPITAL			
IN-SERVICE			

CREW	CERT	STATE #

TIME	ON SCENE (1)	ON SCENE (2)	ON SCENE (3)	EN-ROUTE (1)	EN-ROUTE (2)	AT DESTINATION
BP						
PULSE						
RESP						
SpO$_2$						
ETCO$_2$						
EKG						

IV THERAPY
SUCCESSFUL Y N # OF ATTEMPTS _____
ANGIO SIZE _____ga.
SITE _____
TOTAL FLUID INFUSED _____ cc
BLOOD DRAW Y N INITIALS

INTUBATION INFORMATION
SUCCESSFUL Y N # OF ATTEMPTS _____
TUBE SIZE _____ mm
TIME _____ INITIALS _____

MEDICAL HISTORY

MEDICATIONS

ALLERGIES

C/C

EVENTS LEADING TO C/C

ASSESSMENT

TREATMENT

CONDITION CODES

TREATMENTS				
TIME	TREATMENT	DOSE	ROUTE	INIT

GCS E___ V___ M___ TOTAL =
GCS E___ V___ M___ TOTAL =

HOSPITAL CONTACTED

CPR BEGUN BY B P TIME BEGUN

AED USED Y N BY:

RESUSCITATION TERMINATED - TIME

EMS SIGNATURE

( ) OSHA REGULATIONS FOLLOWED

Trauma Overview: The Trauma Patient and the Trauma System

▎ STANDARD

Trauma (Content Area: Trauma Overview)

▎ COMPETENCY

Applies fundamental knowledge to provide basic emergency care and transportation based on assessment findings for an acutely injured patient.

▎ OBJECTIVES

After reading this chapter, you should be able to:

27-1.   Define key terms introduced in this chapter.

27-2.   Explain why an understanding of kinetics is helpful to understanding injury and trauma.

27-3.   Describe the relationship of mass and velocity to kinetic energy, including the relative contribution of each to the amount of kinetic energy.

27-4.   Explain the effects of acceleration and deceleration on kinetic energy and the potential for injury.

27-5.   Describe the impacts that take place in a typical motor vehicle collision.

27-6.   List situations in motor vehicle collisions in which you should have a high index of suspicion for critical injuries.

27-7.   Explain the typical patterns of injury associated with each of the following types of motor vehicle impacts:
   a. Frontal
   b. Rear
   c. Lateral
   d. Rotational and rollover
   e. Vehicle–adult pedestrian
   f. Vehicle–child pedestrian

27-8.   Discuss the effects of the use of restraint systems in motor vehicle collisions.

27-9.   Explain the typical patterns of injury associated with motorcycle collisions.

27-10.   Describe factors that affect the pattern and severity of injury produced in falls.

27-11.   Compare and contrast injury patterns produced by low-, medium-, and high-velocity penetrating mechanisms of injury.

27-12.   Describe the mechanisms by which blast injuries produce injury.

27-13.   Describe the principles of care for multisystem trauma patients.

27-14. Explain the term "golden period" and identify indications for an on-scene time of 10 minutes (Platinum 10 minutes) or less when caring for trauma patients.

27-15. Differentiate the characteristics of Levels I, II, III, and IV trauma centers.

27-16. Identify patients who meet trauma triage criteria for transportation to a trauma center.

27-17. Discuss the "golden principles" and special considerations in trauma care.

KEY IDEAS

Maintaining a high index of suspicion for hidden injuries in the trauma patient is just as important as identifying obvious injuries. An understanding of the mechanism of injury (how the patient was injured) is the chief component of this crucial assessment skill.

- The amount of kinetic energy contained in a moving body depends on the body's mass (weight) and velocity (speed). Velocity is a much more significant factor than mass when evaluating the mechanism of injury.

- Motor vehicle collisions can be classified as frontal, rear-end, lateral, rotational, or rollover. Each type involves characteristic injuries.

- In a vehicle-pedestrian collision, the extent of injury depends on the speed of the vehicle, what part of the pedestrian's body was struck, how far he was thrown, the surface he lands on, and the body part that first impacts the ground. Also, children and adults will display different injury patterns.

- Motorcycle collisions are classified as head-on impact, angular impact, ejection, and "laying the bike down." Incidence of injury and death is greatly increased when the rider does not wear a helmet.

- Falls are the most common mechanism of injury. The severity of injury depends on the falling distance, landing surface, and the body part that impacts first. A fall of 20 feet or more onto an unyielding surface is considered severe for an adult. A fall greater than 10 feet or two to three times the height of the child is considered severe for a child.

- Penetrating injuries are classified as low velocity (knives), medium velocity (shotgun and handgun pellets or bullets), or high velocity (high-velocity rifles). Assess the patient for both entrance and exit wounds.

- Blast injuries are classified as primary phase (injuries due to the pressure wave), secondary phase (injuries due to flying debris), and tertiary phase (patient is thrown from the source of the blast) injuries. Keep a high index of suspicion for all three types of injuries when a patient has been involved in a blast.

- Start to evaluate the mechanism of injury during your scene size-up. This will assist you when making decisions regarding patient priorities and determining what injuries are possible, even when they are not apparent. During patient assessment, the mechanism of injury will help you determine if manual in-line stabilization of the patient's head and neck is necessary, how to proceed with the secondary assessment, and what problems may arise during transport. Be sure to give the hospital staff all relevant information about the patient's mechanism of injury.

TERMS AND CONCEPTS

1. Write the number of each term next to its definition.

   1. Cavitation
   2. Dissipation of energy
   3. Drag
   4. Kinetic energy
   5. Kinetics of trauma
   6. Mechanism of injury
   7. Profile
   8. Trajectory
   9. Fragmentation

_____ a. A cavity formed by a pressure wave resulting from the kinetic energy of a bullet traveling through body tissue; also called _pathway expansion_

_____ b. Refers to the size and shape of a bullet's point of impact; the greater the point of impact, the greater the injury

_____ c. The energy contained by an object in motion

_____ d. The factors and forces that cause traumatic injury

_____ e. The factors that slow a projectile

_____ f. The path of a projectile during its travel; it may be flat or curved

_____ g. The science of analyzing mechanisms of injury

_____ h. The way energy is transferred to the human body by the forces acting upon it

_____ i. Bullet that breaks up into small pieces or releases small pieces upon impact

CONTENT REVIEW

1. The amount of kinetic energy a moving body contains depends on which of the following two factors?
   a. Mass and weight
   b. Drag and mass
   c. Rate of acceleration and velocity
   d. Mass and velocity

2. Which of the following factors is most significant when evaluating the mechanism of injury?
   a. Mass
   b. Rate of acceleration
   c. Velocity
   d. Rate of deceleration

3. The rate at which a body in motion increases its speed is known as which of the following?
   a. Mass
   b. Deceleration
   c. Velocity
   d. Acceleration

4. The typical vehicular collision involves which of the following?
   a. One impact (vehicle)
   b. Two impacts (vehicle and body)
   c. Three impacts (vehicle, body, and organs)
   d. Four impacts (vehicle, body, organs, and vessels)

5. Which of the following is the most common mechanism of injury, accounting for over half of all trauma incidents?
   a. Vehicular collisions
   b. Falls
   c. Penetrating gunshots
   d. Explosions

6. Which of the following is the most lethal mechanism of injury, responsible for over one-third of all trauma deaths?
   a. Vehicular collisions
   b. Falls
   c. Penetrating gunshots
   d. Explosions

7. Which grouping is most likely to suffer injury from air bag deployment?
   a. Middle-aged adults
   b. Tall adults
   c. Short adults
   d. 14- to 18-year-olds

8. In a motor vehicle collision, the "up and over" and "down and under" pathways are examples of injury patterns associated with a _____ impact.
   a. frontal
   b. medial
   c. lateral
   d. rotational

9. When a passenger's head strikes the car windshield, the glass may crack in a typical _____ pattern.
   a. "cracked ice"
   b. "broken egg"
   c. "spiderweb"
   d. "halo"

10. The automobile driver's neck whips back, and the body is propelled forward, even while the head seems to remain at rest. This scenario best describes which of the following?
    a. A rotational impact
    b. A rear-end impact
    c. A lateral impact
    d. A frontal impact

11. In this type of motor vehicle collision, the body is struck from the side. This best describes which of the following?
    a. A rotational impact
    b. A rear-end impact
    c. A lateral impact
    d. A frontal impact

12. Which statement best describes injuries due to rotational or rollover impact?
    a. Multiple-system injury and possible ejection are likely if the patient was unrestrained.
    b. The head and neck are whipped back.
    c. Head injuries are common when passenger heads collide with one another.
    d. The "up and over" or "down and under" path is common.

13. A child who is about to be struck by an auto generally
    a. turns away from the oncoming auto.
    b. turns to the side of the oncoming auto.
    c. turns to face the oncoming auto.
    d. does not turn at all.

14. A common pattern of injuries to a child struck by an auto is injuries to the
    a. upper and lower extremities.
    b. femur, chest, abdomen, and head.
    c. phalanges, radius, and ulna.
    d. pelvis, chest, skull, and face.

15. Which of the following is correct regarding motor vehicle restraints?
    a. In a collision, a seat belt worn too low can cause lower-leg fractures.
    b. Properly applied lap belts and shoulder straps prevent lateral head movement.
    c. Air bags work well in multiple collision events.
    d. A deployed air bag should be lifted from the steering wheel.

16. Which of the following injuries is most likely the result of "laying the bike down," an evasive action meant to prevent ejection or separation of a motorcycle rider from his bike?
    a. Femur fracture
    b. Closed head injury
    c. Dislocated shoulder
    d. Leg burns

17. A fall of _____ feet onto an unyielding surface is considered severe for an adult. A fall of more than _____ feet can cause severe injuries to a child.
    a. 5/10
    b. 10/5
    c. 20/10
    d. 10/15

18. Experts say that a patient in a feet-first fall who falls _____ or more will likely have a spinal injury.
    a. two times his height
    b. three times his height
    c. four times his height
    d. five times his height

19. In a gunshot incident, the EMT should suspect both thoracic and abdominal injury if the entrance wound is
    a. between the nipple line and the waist.
    b. between the navel and the waist.
    c. between the trachea and the clavicle.
    d. between the nipple line and the sternum.

20. Primary phase, secondary phase, and tertiary phase injuries are related to
    a. motor vehicle collisions.
    b. blasts and explosions.
    c. low- and medium-velocity weapons.
    d. headfirst falls.

21. While assessing the scene of an accident, which of the following should increase your suspicion of serious traumatic injuries?
    a. Intrusion greater than 6 inches of the exterior of the car at the site opposite to the patient
    b. Intrusion greater than 8 inches of the interior of the car where the patient is riding
    c. Intrusion greater than 12 inches of the interior compartment where the patient is riding
    d. Intrusion greater than 10 inches of the exterior of the car at the site opposite to the patient

22. You are assessing a multisystem trauma patient. Which term best reflects the time period that is variable depending on the trauma patient's injury?
    a. "Golden period"
    b. "Golden hour"
    c. "Critical hour"
    d. "Critical period"

23. You have arrived on the scene of a multisystem trauma patient. Your EMS system uses the "platinum 10 minutes" as a goal for treatment. You know that this means that
    a. patient assessment and emergency care of life threats should be accomplished within 10 minutes of arriving on the scene.
    b. patient assessment, emergency care for life threats, and patient preparation for transport should all be accomplished within 10 minutes of arriving on the scene.
    c. treatment for life threats and splinting of suspected fractures should be accomplished within 10 minutes after leaving the scene.
    d. treatment for all life-threatening injuries should be accomplished within 10 minutes of assessing the patient's condition.

24. You have responded to a trauma patient who has suffered a fall. Which of the following is an indication for an on-scene time of 10 minutes or less and rapid transport to the trauma hospital?
    a. Glasgow Coma Scale (GCS) score of 15 or more
    b. Respiratory rate of 22 breaths each minute
    c. A single fracture to the lower leg
    d. Sensory deficit to the lower leg

25. Match the correct level of trauma center with the description of each level.
    _____ Level I
    _____ Level II
    _____ Level III
    _____ Level IV
    a. An Area Trauma Center can manage most trauma with surgical capabilities 24 hours a day, seven days a week. They are capable of stabilizing more specialized trauma patients and then transferring them to a level I center.
    b. A Community Trauma Center has some surgical capability and specially trained emergency department personnel to manage trauma. This type of center focuses on stabilizing the seriously injured trauma patient and then transferring to a higher-level center.
    c. A Regional Trauma Center can manage all types of trauma 24 hours a day, seven days a week.
    d. A Trauma Facility is typically a small community hospital in a remote area capable of stabilizing seriously injured trauma patients and then transferring them to a higher-level trauma center.

26. According to the golden principles of prehospital trauma care, the use of pneumatic antishock garments (PASGs) is considered in which of the following situations?
    a. Decompensated shock (systolic blood pressure, 90 mmHg) with suspected pelvic fracture
    b. Lower limb fractures with a heart rate greater than 100 beats per minute
    c. Head-injured patients with a suspected traumatic brain injury (TBI) with unresponsiveness
    d. Traumatic injury to a pregnant female with a heart rate of less than 60 beats each minute

27. You are treating a trauma patient who has sustained a large open wound to the upper arm. The wound is bleeding profusely. You know that in order to prevent or reverse shock, you must stop this bleeding quickly. You immediately apply direct pressure. If this is not effective, your next action should be to
    a. elevate the arm.
    b. apply a warm compress.
    c. compress the pressure point.
    d. apply a tourniquet.

28. As you approach your trauma patient and start to perform your primary assessment, you find arterial bleeding of the upper arm. You should
    a. continue to assess the airway.
    b. assess the breathing for adequacy.
    c. determine the quality of the pulse.
    d. apply immediate direct pressure to the bleeding.

29. You have determined that your multisystem trauma patient needs to be transported to a trauma center. The patient has sustained multiple fractures to both legs and one arm. The trauma helicopter is approximately five minutes from landing. What should you do next?
    a. Utilize the backboard to stabilize the fractures and prepare the patient for transport.
    b. Splint the lower legs by utilizing long board splints because stabilization is required before transport.
    c. Wait until the helicopter crew has made patient contact to determine if splinting is necessary.
    d. Splint the fractures because this must be done before transport in the multisystem trauma patient.

▌ CASE STUDY 1

You are at the scene of a one-car, high-speed motor vehicle collision. The driver is dead, ejected from the vehicle sometime during several rollovers. A woman about 20 years old approaches you and identifies herself as a passenger in the vehicle. She tells you she walked to a gas station to call for help, then returned. Your general impression is that she looks well, although she has a small laceration over her left eye. She is holding her left upper abdominal and chest region. Her skin color appears to be normal. She responds to your questions appropriately, although somewhat slowly.

1. Which of the following describes the most appropriate treatment for the patient?
    a. The patient should be carefully assessed and monitored for any injuries.
    b. The patient should be advised of potential serious signs and symptoms to watch for and released.
    c. The patient should be assessed, immobilized, monitored carefully, and transported.
    d. The patient should be transported by a family member for evaluation at a local hospital.

2. Which of the following regarding the patient's mental status is correct?
    a. It should concern you, but only if her mental status deteriorates further.
    b. It should concern you, since an altered mental status is one of the earliest signs of brain injury.
    c. It should not concern you, since it appears to be normal or only slightly altered.
    d. It should not concern you, since the mechanism of injury has been identified.

CASE STUDY 2

You have been dispatched to a residential area to assist a worker who fell from a tree. The 35-year-old patient is lying on his right side in a soft, grassy area. His eyes are open. You ask him, "What happened?" He tells you that he was trimming the tree when the branch he was standing on gave way.

1. Which of the following questions is most important in determining the patient's potential injuries?
   a. How long have you been lying here?
   b. Where do you hurt the most?
   c. What is your doctor's name?
   d. How did you land?

2. The patient tells you that he landed feet first with his knees locked, and then he broke his forward fall with his hands. What potential injuries should you suspect?
   a. Spine injury in the lumbar, midthoracic, and cervical regions, and also head trauma
   b. Injuries to the femur, hips, pelvis, spine, midthoracic and cervical regions, and wrists
   c. Spinal injury in the cervical and lumbar region, plus chest and shoulder injury
   d. Injuries to the hands and knees

CASE STUDY 3

A teenage gunshot victim is lying on her back next to the front door of her house. Her eyes are open. You ask, "What happened?" She replies, "I was just standing here, and these guys drove by and shot me." There is noticeable bleeding to her left lower chest, and she is holding the area with her right hand. Her skin is pale, cool, and moist. Respirations are normal, and radial pulse is weak, rapid, and regular.

1. Given this description of the patient's injury, which of the following statements is correct?
   a. Lung tissue is intolerant of cavitation caused by projectiles.
   b. Pneumothorax is an uncommon result of injury to the chest and/or lung.
   c. You should evaluate the patient for both thoracic and abdominal injury.
   d. The presence of associated rib fractures is unlikely.

2. You dress the wound to the patient's lower chest. What have you forgotten to do?
   a. Look for and treat any additional (entrance or exit) wounds.
   b. Probe the wound to see if the bullet has lodged in the body.
   c. Pour an antiseptic solution into the wound prior to bandaging.
   d. Provide oxygen therapy via a nasal cannula at 6 lpm.

Bleeding and Soft Tissue Trauma

▍ STANDARD

Trauma (Content Areas: Bleeding; Soft Tissue Trauma)

▍ COMPETENCY

Applies fundamental knowledge to provide basic emergency care and transportation based on assessment findings for an acutely injured patient.

▍ OBJECTIVES

After reading this chapter, you should be able to:

28-1. Define key terms introduced in this chapter.

28-2. Explain the importance of recognizing and providing emergency medical care to patients with soft tissue injuries to control bleeding, prevent or treat shock, and to prevent contamination of wounds.

28-3. Recognize the severity and type of external bleeding.

28-4. Describe methods of controlling external bleeding.

28-5. Describe the assessment-based approach to external bleeding, including emergency medical care.

28-6. Explain why bleeding from the nose, ears, or mouth is of special concern and describe the appropriate care for bleeding from the nose, ears, or mouth.

28-7. Recognize indications of the severity of internal bleeding and describe the assessment-based approach to internal bleeding, including medical care to maintain perfusion and treat for shock.

28-8. Explain factors that may increase bleeding.

28-9. Define hemorrhagic shock and describe the assessment-based approach to hemorrhagic shock, including emergency medical care.

28-10. List types of closed soft tissue injuries and describe the assessment-based approach to closed soft tissue injuries, including emergency medical care.

28-11. List types of open soft tissue injuries and describe the assessment-based approach to open soft tissue injuries, including emergency medical care.

28-12. Explain special considerations and appropriate care for chest injuries, abdominal injuries, impaled objects, amputations, and large neck injuries.

28-13. Describe various types of dressings and bandages, including the purpose and methods of applying pressure dressings, and discuss general principles of dressing and bandaging.

KEY IDEAS

This chapter focuses on the emergency management of bleeding and soft tissue trauma. As an EMT, you must be able to recognize the signs and symptoms of internal and external bleeding and be able to treat soft tissue injuries. Failure to quickly recognize and treat bleeding of either type has the potential to lead to rapid patient deterioration, shock, and death. A soft tissue injury is an injury to skin, muscles, nerves, blood vessels, or organs.

- It is imperative that the EMT always take appropriate Standard Precautions and practice good hand washing when caring for any patient.

- Differentiation of the type of bleeding (arterial, venous, or capillary) is based on the color of the blood and the nature of blood flow. Each type can be life threatening.

- Only airway and breathing have a higher priority than the control of severe bleeding.

- External bleeding is controlled by the use of direct pressure and/or a tourniquet.

- Always suspect internal bleeding in patients exhibiting signs or symptoms of unexplained hypovolemic shock.

- The goal of emergency medical care for internal bleeding is to recognize its presence quickly, maintain the body's perfusion, and provide rapid transport to an appropriate medical facility.

- Shock, also known as *hypoperfusion* or *hypoperfusion syndrome,* is the direct result of inadequate perfusion of tissue from the loss of blood volume.

- Soft tissue injuries are categorized as closed, open, single, or multiple.

- In general, emergency care of closed injuries includes taking Standard Precautions, ensuring an open airway and adequate breathing, treating for shock, and splinting suspected fractures.

- In general, emergency care of open injuries includes taking Standard Precautions, ensuring an open airway, adequate breathing and oxygenation, exposing the wound, controlling bleeding, preventing further contamination, dressing and bandaging the wound, keeping the patient calm, and treating for hypovolemic shock.

- Special considerations for the emergency care of soft tissue injuries include using occlusive dressings on open chest wounds, abdominal eviscerations, and large, open neck injuries; securing objects impaled in the body (except the cheek); and caring for amputated parts.

- Dressings cover open wounds, and bandages hold dressings in place. A pressure (or bulky) dressing can be used to control bleeding. General principles of dressing and bandaging include using materials that are sterile (or at least clean); bandaging only when bleeding has stopped; adequately covering the entire wound with a dressing and the entire dressing with a bandage; removing all jewelry from injured parts; bandaging not too loosely or tightly (checking distal pulses, motor function, and sensory function before and after bandage application); on an extremity, bandaging a larger area than the wound to avoid creating a pressure point; and applying a tourniquet if bleeding is not controlled with direct pressure.

MEDICAL TERMINOLOGY

Term	Prefix	Word Root Combining Form	Suffix	Definition
abrasion (uh-BRAY-zhun)	ab- (away from)	ras (to scrape)	-ion (process)	An open injury to the epidermis caused by a scraping away, rubbing, or shearing away of the tissue
epistaxis (ep-uh-STAKS-is)	epi- (upon, over, above)		-staxis (dripping, trickling)	Bleeding from the nose; a nosebleed

Term	Prefix	Word Root Combining Form	Suffix	Definition
hemophilia (hee-moh-FEEL-yuh)		hem/o (blood)	-philia (attraction)	Disease that prevents activation of the normal clotting mechanism
avulsion (uh-VUL-shun)	a- (no, not, without, lack of)	vuls (to pull)	-ion (process)	An open injury characterized by a loose flap of skin and soft tissue that has been torn loose or pulled off
dermis (DER-miss)		derm (skin)	-is (pertaining to)	The second layer of skin; the layer of skin below the epidermis
embolism (EM-boh-lizm)		embol (to cast, to throw)	-ism (condition of)	Obstruction of a blood vessel by a foreign substance
epidermis (ep-uh-DER-miss)	epi- (upon, over, above)	derm (skin)	-is (pertaining to)	The outermost or top layer of skin; the layer above the dermis
hematoma (hee-muh-TOH-muh)		hemat (blood)	-oma (tumor)	A closed injury to the soft tissues characterized by swelling and discoloration caused by a mass of blood below the epidermis
pneumothorax (nu-moh-THOR-aks)		pneum/o (lung, air) thorax (chest)		Collection of air or gas in the pleural cavity
subcutaneous (sub-kyu-TAY-nee-us)	sub- (below, under, beneath)	cutane (skin)	-ous (pertaining to)	The third layer of skin; the layer below the dermis

1. The medical term *abrasion* refers to an open injury to the epidermis caused by scraping. You know that the prefix *ab-* means
   a. skin.
   b. toward.
   c. away from.
   d. scrape.

2. The medical term *avulsion* contains the word root *vuls,* which means
   a. to pull.
   b. to cut.
   c. flap.
   d. skin.

3. You use the medical term *dermis* in your prehospital care report. The word root *derm* means
   a. skin.
   b. blood.
   c. above.
   d. toward.

4. The medical term *hematoma* contains the word root *hemat*, which means
   a. cut.
   b. bump.
   c. tumor.
   d. blood.

5. The medical term *subcutaneous* contains the word root *cutane*, which means
   a. lung.
   b. skin.
   c. below.
   d. finger.

6. The medical term *epistaxis*, referring to a nosebleed, contains the suffix *-staxis*. You know this means
   a. flowing, rushing.
   b. dripping, trickling.
   c. uncontrolled.
   d. surge, flood.

7. The medical term *hemophilia* contains the word root *hem/o,* which refers to
   a. blood.
   b. heart.
   c. clotting.
   d. vessel.

TERMS AND CONCEPTS

1. Write the number of the correct term next to each definition.
   1. Abrasion
   2. Air embolism
   3. Avulsion
   4. Contusion
   5. Crush injury
   6. Evisceration
   7. Hematoma
   8. Laceration
   9. Occlusive dressing
   10. Penetration/puncture

   _____ a. An open injury usually caused by forceful impact with a sharp object and characterized by a wound whose edges may be linear or stellate in appearance

   _____ b. A protrusion of organs from a wound

   _____ c. A closed or an open injury to soft tissues and underlying organs that is the result of a crushing force applied to the body

   _____ d. An open injury to the outermost layer of the skin caused by a scraping, rubbing, or shearing away of the tissue

   _____ e. An open injury caused by a sharp, pointed object being forced into the soft tissues

   _____ f. An air bubble that obstructs a blood vessel

_____ g. A closed injury to the cells and blood vessels contained within the dermis that is characterized by discoloration, swelling, and pain; a bruise

_____ h. A closed injury to the soft tissues characterized by swelling and discoloration caused by a mass of blood beneath the epidermis

_____ i. A dressing that can form an airtight seal over a wound

_____ j. An open injury characterized by a loose flap of skin and soft tissue that has been torn loose or pulled completely off

❙ CONTENT REVIEW

1. Write the number of the correct term beside its description.
   1. Arterial bleeding
   2. Venous bleeding
   3. Capillary bleeding

   _____ a. Dark red blood that flows steadily from a wound

   _____ b. Dark red blood that slowly oozes from a wound

   _____ c. Bright red blood that spurts from a wound

2. Your patient is not breathing and has life-threatening bleeding from a large, open wound. What is the treatment priority?
   a. Airway, breathing, and then bleeding control
   b. Breathing, airway, and then bleeding control
   c. Bleeding, airway, and then breathing control
   d. Patient is critical; no priority of sequence

3. Your patient has a large wound to his right lower leg, which is bleeding profusely. There is no deformity of the extremity. Which of the following best describes the *first* steps in emergency management of this injury?
   a. Use a tourniquet.
   b. Use a swathe.
   c. Use direct pressure.
   d. Use the femoral pressure point.

4. You are treating a patient who has a large laceration. You note that the vessels have been cut across, or perpendicular to, the vessel. A vessel that has been cut in this manner has a tendency to
   a. retract and clot off.
   b. spasm and dilate.
   c. open and hemorrhage.
   d. contract, then expand.

5. A tourniquet is used to control bleeding
   a. when there is spurting arterial bleeding.
   b. when there is an amputated extremity.
   c. when nerves, muscles, and blood vessels are damaged.
   d. when direct pressure fails to control the bleeding.

6. You are treating a patient who has sustained a large wound and has an altered mental status. You apply direct pressure to the wound and assess the patient. The patient's breathing is adequate, so you should
   a. apply oxygen via a nasal cannula at 6 lpm.
   b. administer oxygen via a simple face mask at 8 lpm.
   c. provide oxygen via a nonrebreather mask at 15 lpm.
   d. deliver positive pressure ventilations by bag-valve mask (BVM).

7. List at least three causes of internal bleeding.
   1. _____
   2. _____
   3. _____

8. Which of the following is considered inappropriate emergency medical care for the patient whom you suspect of having an internal bleed?
   a. Administer high-concentration oxygen.
   b. Splint potential fractures.
   c. Never estimate the severity of internal bleeding based on signs and symptoms.
   d. Provide immediate transport.

9. Hemostatic agents used to control bleeding
   a. are designed only as a dressing that promotes clotting.
   b. have shown poor results when applied to wounds with major arterial and venous bleeding.
   c. are used without a pressure dressing to control arterial and venous bleeding.
   d. are usually reserved for prolonged transport times.

10. The layers of the skin from the outermost to the innermost are the
    a. dermis, epidermis, and subcutaneous layer.
    b. subcutaneous, epidermis, and dermis layer.
    c. subcutaneous, dermis, and epidermis layer.
    d. epidermis, dermis, and subcutaneous layer.

11. Which of the following descriptions are considered functions of the skin?
    1. Aids in the elimination of water and various salts
    2. Serves as a sensory receptor organ
    3. Produces white blood cells
    4. Protects the body from the environment
    a. 1, 2, 3
    b. 1, 2, 4
    c. 1, 3, 4
    d. 2, 3, 4

12. Which of the following injuries is considered an open injury?
    a. Contusion
    b. Amputation
    c. Hematoma
    d. Crush injury

13. Which of the following dressings may contain fibrinogen and thrombin, chitosan, or other substances on the surface, which promote clotting when applied to wounds?
    a. Occlusive dressing
    b. Hemostatic dressing
    c. Hemorrhagic dressing
    d. Tamponade dressing

14. Which of the following is the correct order for treatment of closed soft tissue injuries?
    a. Airway, breathing and oxygenation, Standard Precautions, shock, injured extremities
    b. Standard Precautions, shock, airway, breathing and oxygenation, injured extremities
    c. Standard Precautions, airway, breathing and oxygenation, shock, injured extremities
    d. Injured extremities, Standard Precautions, airway, breathing and oxygenation, shock

15. You are treating a patient who has sustained a chest wound. Which of the following dressings is used to prevent air from entering the chest cavity?
    a. Nonelastic, self-adhering
    b. Multitrauma
    c. Bulky
    d. Occlusive

16. While treating a patient who has sustained an open chest wound, how should you tape the dressing?
    a. On the top and bottom only
    b. On three sides only
    c. On all four sides
    d. Down the middle only

17. An incomplete amputation typically bleeds more than a complete amputation.
    a. The statement is true unless circumferential abrasions of the appendage are present.
    b. The statement is false unless a clean cut through the vessels and tissues has occurred.
    c. The statement is true.
    d. The statement is false.

18. Which of the following is the correct order of steps for emergency care of a patient with an impaled object?
    1. Use a bulky dressing to help stabilize the object.
    2. Manually secure the object.
    3. Control bleeding.
    4. Expose the wound area.
    a. 2, 4, 3, 1
    b. 4, 3, 2, 1
    c. 3, 1, 2, 4
    d. 4, 2, 3, 1

19. Which of the following is considered an inappropriate treatment for an amputated part and may cause further tissue damage?
    a. Place the part directly on an ice pack or ice.
    b. Wrap the part in dry, sterile dressing.
    c. Wrap or bag the part in plastic.
    d. Keep the part cool.

20. Bleeding control and prevention of an air embolism are the major goals of emergency care of a large, open neck wound. What type of dressing would help to prevent an air embolism?
    a. Occlusive
    b. Trauma
    c. Porous
    d. Bulky

21. List the steps for applying a pressure dressing.

    a. _____

    b. _____

    c. _____

    d. _____

22. For circumferential bandages, which of the following should you check before and after bandaging?
    a. Distal pulses, skin color, and temperature
    b. Capillary refill, skin color, and temperature
    c. Distal pulses, motor function, and sensory function
    d. ABCs, motor function, and sensory function

23. Which of the following are the proper dressings for an abdominal evisceration?
    a. Sterile, moist gauze, then an occlusive dressing
    b. Self-adhering roller bandage, then an occlusive dressing
    c. Any sterile absorbent material, then an occlusive dressing
    d. Bulky dressing, then an occlusive dressing

24. You have ruled out potential spinal injury in a patient with abdominal evisceration. Your partner asks you to flex the patient's hips and knees during transport. Why?
    a. It helps stabilize the abdominal organs.
    b. It will prevent the development of an embolism.
    c. It reduces the tension on the abdominal muscles.
    d. It helps to increase oxygen to the vital organs.

25. You are called to a patient who has been bitten by a large dog. You know that the most dangerous bites are those in which the injury occurs
    a. over nerve tissue.
    b. over fat tissue.
    c. over vascular areas.
    d. over bones or joints.

26. You are treating a 5-year-old patient who has placed his hand into the mouth of a small jar and now is unable to remove it. Which of the following would be considered inappropriate treatment for this situation?
    a. Apply lubricant and try to remove the hand.
    b. Raise the hand and the jar above the patient's head.
    c. Transport the patient with the hand in the jar to the hospital.
    d. Wrap a towel around the jar and gently break it to remove the hand.

CASE STUDY 1

You are dispatched to a local bar for a stabbing. The patient is a female, about 25 years old. She is sitting at a table, her hand to her neck, with dark red blood flowing steadily through her fingers. Your general impression of her is good; however, her skin is pale, warm, and slightly moist. As your partner begins to control the bleeding, you find that respirations are adequate, with good tidal volume. The radial pulse is strong and regular. There are no other obvious signs of trauma or bleeding present.

1. The bleeding from the patient's neck wound is likely which of the following?
   a. Capillary bleeding
   b. Arterial bleeding
   c. Venous bleeding
   d. Combination of arterial/capillary bleeding

2. Which of the following lists the correct procedures in the correct order for emergency care for this wound?
   a. Gloved hand over the wound, then an occlusive dressing, and finally a pressure dressing
   b. Occlusive dressing over the wound, then a pressure dressing, and finally your gloved hand
   c. Pressure dressing over the wound, then an occlusive dressing, and finally your gloved hand
   d. Gloved hand over the wound, then a pressure dressing, and finally an occlusive dressing

CASE STUDY 2

You are at the scene of a shooting. The 20-year-old patient is supine and responsive. A law enforcement officer has told you that three shots were fired, the weapon was a .357-caliber handgun, and the patient was shot from 30 to 40 yards away. There is obvious bleeding coming from the patient's right upper chest region, and a sucking sound is heard with each breath. As your partner proceeds to control bleeding, you find that the patient is cyanotic, respirations are shallow and rapid, the radial pulse is weak and regular, and the skin is cool and slightly moist.

1. In addition to this patient's obvious injury, you should suspect which of the following?
   a. Ring avulsion
   b. Spinal injury
   c. Lower airway obstruction
   d. Cardiac tamponade

2. In addition to treatment for this patient's obvious injury, treatment also includes
   a. splinting of upper extremities.
   b. care of large, open neck injuries.
   c. methodically assessing for closed wounds.
   d. assessing for other entry and exit wounds.

Read the following scenario and think about how you would document this call if you were the EMT who responded to the scene. Then answer the multiple-choice questions and fill in the sample prehospital care report, basing your documentation on information from the scenario.

It's 6:00 P.M. You and your partner, Lt. Rodriguez, are preparing a healthful dinner at your station. The workday has been steady with typical medical calls. As you prepare the salad, the station alerting system sounds. "Squad 7, Engine 7, EMS Battalion Chief, respond to an industrial accident at 1215 82nd Avenue for a possible amputated arm." You acknowledge the call and ask dispatch to notify the trauma center and to place the helicopter on standby. En route to the scene, Lt. Rodriguez double-checks the address in the map book. After a short emergency response, you arrive on scene at a large manufacturing plant. As you both scan for obvious hazards, you apply gloves, mask, and eye protection. You pull the stretcher from the ambulance, place all the equipment you may need on it, and walk briskly toward the building.

You approach the entryway and are met by an anxious manager of the facility, who says, "You must hurry. His whole arm has been cut off by the equipment." Lt. Rodriguez asks the manager if the patient is entrapped and if the equipment has been shut down. He answers, "He's not trapped, and all of the equipment has been shut down and secured with lockout locks so the equipment cannot be restarted inadvertently."

As you and Lt. Rodriguez approach, you see the middle-aged male patient lying supine on the floor with a coworker holding a towel over the end of a right arm severed at about the midshaft area of the humerus. The patient also has a deep laceration to the right side of the neck, which is bleeding profusely with a steady flow of dark red blood. The patient's eyes meet yours with a terrified look.

You ask the patient his name as you apply a large sterile trauma dressing to the amputated site. He responds, "Bill." You introduce yourself and Lt. Rodriguez and reassure him that you are going to take good care of him. Lt. Rodriguez places his gloved hand directly over the wound on the patient's neck. Bill is quite restless. You explain that, since he has a serious injury, he will be transported to the trauma center in a nearby town by helicopter. You ask Bill what his age is and if he has any medical history or takes any medications. He replies, "I'm

48, and I haven't been to a doctor in 10 years." You ask him if he is allergic to anything, and he states, "Not that I know of."

Lt. Rodriguez asks dispatch to launch the helicopter and issue a trauma alert to the trauma center so they can prepare for the arrival of a serious patient. Lt. Rodriguez performs a quick initial assessment. There are no stridorous or crowing sounds with inhalation or exhalation. Bill's breathing is normal at about 20 breaths per minute. His chest is rising and falling, with adequate air flowing in and out of the mouth without the use of accessory muscles. You apply high-concentration oxygen with a nonrebreather mask at 15 lpm.

You ask the manager what happened, and he says that Mary, a coworker, witnessed the incident. The manager calls Mary over. She is visibly upset. You explain that it is very important that she quickly explain what happened. She says, "Bill was working on the conveyor belt when his hand got pulled into the mechanisms. He got pulled hard against the conveyor belt when his arm was cut off, and that's how his neck got slashed." You ask her if he was knocked out, and she states, "No, he has remained awake the whole time."

The firefighters arrive on the scene and ask what they can do to help. You instruct the firefighter lieutenant to see if they can locate the severed arm. You instruct another firefighter to maintain in-line stabilization of the spine while you apply a dressing to the neck.

You feel for a radial pulse and find a weak pulse at 110 beats per minute. The skin is cool and diaphoretic, the capillary blanch is delayed at 4 seconds and the SpO_2 is 92%. Lt. Rodriguez begins a rapid trauma assessment. The head reveals no deformities; the pupils are equal and react briskly to light. The nose, mouth, and ears are all clear of blood or fluid. The neck is soft with a large, deep laceration to the right side; there is no noted subcutaneous emphysema. The trachea is midline, and there is no deformity or pain to the posterior neck. He palpates the chest and notes equal chest rise and fall with no signs of trauma or use of accessory muscles. He inspects the axillary area, and no trauma is noted. Inspection of the abdomen reveals no obvious injuries, distention, or pain with palpation. Lt. Rodriguez quickly inspects the pelvis for deformity, contusions, abrasions, or penetrating injuries, and none are found. He rapidly assesses the extremities and finds no injuries to the other arm or legs. The amputated arm is a clean cut, with little bleeding. Bill indicates that he can feel him touching each of the unaffected extremities, and he has good movement. Lt. Rodriguez remarks, "I have good but weak distal pulses." He examines the posterior body and finds no trauma or sacral edema. The patient does not complain of any pain when the spine is palpated.

You and Lt. Rodriguez maintain in-line stabilization and place the patient on a backboard, using a c-collar, and then secure him with straps. The fire lieutenant approaches you and says, "We found it. We found the missing arm." With a squeamish look on his face, he hands the detached arm to you, wrapped in a towel. You ask Lt. Rodriguez and the firefighters to load the patient into the ambulance while you prepare the severed arm for transport.

With the severed arm in the ambulance, you instruct the firefighter to drive carefully in an emergency response mode to a local baseball field, where your battalion chief has instructed the helicopter to land. En route to the landing zone, you obtain baseline vital signs: pulse 124 beats per minute, weak but regular; blood pressure 102/86; respirations 20 each minute with good tidal volume; skin pale, cool, and diaphoretic, no cyanosis noted; pupils equal and slightly sluggish; pulse oximeter reading at 96% on high-concentration oxygen. You arrive at the landing zone area and are met by the flight crew, Missy and Dave. You give a quick report to Missy and help to transfer the patient to the waiting helicopter. Missy thanks you and says, "We'll have Bill at the trauma center in approximately 15 minutes." With a thumbs-up gesture, she slides the door closed on the helicopter and lifts off en route to the trauma center.

1. The neck wound is bleeding profusely with a dark red blood that flows steadily. You suspect that the patient has sustained what type of injury?
   a. Laceration to the carotid artery
   b. Laceration to the pulmonary artery
   c. Laceration to the jugular vein
   d. Laceration to the pulmonary vein

2. Why did Lt. Rodriguez place his gloved hand directly over the wound on the patient's neck?
   a. There was a danger of air being sucked into the neck vein.
   b. This prevents clots from forming and occluding the airway.
   c. He was assessing the blood flow through the severed vessel.
   d. The gloved hand will prevent the area from becoming infected.

3. You recognize the laceration to the patient's neck to be very serious. Which of the following dressings is appropriate for this type of injury?
   a. An all-purpose sterile cotton bandage held in place with circumferential rolled meshed gauze
   b. A universal or multitrauma dressing that is sterile and usually bulky, taped on two sides
   c. A commercially wrapped sterile gauze pad that is the same size as the wound and is self-adhering
   d. An occlusive dressing that extends beyond the edge of the laceration, taped on all four sides

4. If the bleeding soaks through the original pressure dressing that was applied to the severed right arm, indicating continued severe bleeding, what should you do?
   a. Without removing the original bandage, apply additional bandages on top of the previous ones and then rewrap the wound.
   b. Remove the bandages and apply direct fingertip pressure. Once the bleeding is controlled, apply a dressing and bandage to cover the wound again.
   c. Remove all of the original bandages, apply a wide tourniquet proximal to the severed site, and tighten until the bleeding has stopped.
   d. Without removing the original bandages, apply a circumferential constricting band and tighten until the bleeding has slowed.

5. Prior to loading the patient and his severed arm onto the helicopter, you prepared the arm for transport. You know that the proper handling of the amputated arm can have a significant impact on the success of surgical reattachment. Which of the following is the appropriate treatment for an amputated body part?

a. Wrap the amputated part in a pressure dressing and place on ice.
b. Place the amputated part into a plastic bag and fill the bag with ice.
c. Wrap in sterile gauze, place in a plastic bag, and keep the amputated part cool.
d. Place the amputated part directly on ice or a chemical ice pack, then wrap with gauze.

TRIP #						EMERGENCY				BILLING USE ONLY				

EMERGENCY TRIP SHEET

TRIP #	
MEDIC #	
BEGIN MILES	
END MILES	
CODE___/___ PAGE___/___	
UNITS ON SCENE	

BILLING USE ONLY
DAY
DATE

RECEIVED				
DISPATCHED				
EN-ROUTE				
ON SCENE				
TO HOSPITAL				
AT HOSPITAL				
IN-SERVICE				

NAME	SEX M F DOB ___/___/___
ADDRESS	RACE
CITY	STATE	ZIP
PHONE ( ) -	PCP DR.
RESPONDED FROM	CITY
TAKEN FROM	ZIP
DESTINATION	REASON
SSN - -	MEDICARE #	MEDICAID #
INSURANCE CO	INSURANCE #	GROUP #
RESPONSIBLE PARTY	ADDRESS
CITY	STATE	ZIP	PHONE ( ) -
EMPLOYER	

	CREW	CERT	STATE #

TIME	ON SCENE (1)	ON SCENE (2)	ON SCENE (3)	EN-ROUTE (1)	EN-ROUTE (2)	AT DESTINATION
BP						
PULSE						
RESP						
SpO_2						
$ETCO_2$						
EKG						

IV THERAPY
SUCCESSFUL Y N # OF ATTEMPTS _____
ANGIO SIZE _____ga.
SITE _____
TOTAL FLUID INFUSED _____ cc
BLOOD DRAW Y N INITIALS

INTUBATION INFORMATION
SUCCESSFUL Y N # OF ATTEMPTS _____
TUBE SIZE _____ mm
TIME _____ INITIALS _____

MEDICAL HISTORY	

CONDITION CODES				

TREATMENTS

MEDICATIONS	

TIME	TREATMENT	DOSE	ROUTE	INIT

ALLERGIES
C/C

EVENTS LEADING TO C/C

ASSESSMENT

TREATMENT

GCS E___ V___ M___ TOTAL =

GCS E___ V___ M___ TOTAL =

HOSPITAL CONTACTED

EMS SIGNATURE	CPR BEGUN BY B P TIME BEGUN
	AED USED Y N BY:
	RESUSCITATION TERMINATED - TIME

( ) OSHA REGULATIONS FOLLOWED

Burns

STANDARD

Trauma (Content Area: Soft Tissue Trauma)

COMPETENCY

Applies fundamental knowledge to provide basic emergency care and transportation based on assessment findings for an acutely injured patient.

OBJECTIVES

After reading this chapter, you should be able to:

29-1. Define key terms introduced in this chapter.

29-2. Explain the concept that burns are not just "skin deep."

29-3. Describe the effects of burns on the following body systems:
   a. Circulatory
   b. Respiratory
   c. Renal
   d. Nervous and musculoskeletal
   e. Gastrointestinal

29-4. Explain the classification of burns by depth and by body surface area involved, for both adult and pediatric patients.

29-5. Discuss considerations of burn depth, location, body surface area involved, the patient's age, and any preexisting medical conditions in determining the severity of burn injuries.

29-6. Discuss each of the following types of burns:
   a. Thermal
   b. Inhalation
   c. Chemical
   d. Electrical
   e. Radiation

29-7. Discuss each of the following mechanisms of burn injuries:
   a. Flame
   b. Contact
   c. Scald
   d. Steam
   e. Gas
   f. Electrical
   g. Flash

29-8. Describe the assessment-based approach to burns.

29-9. Describe special considerations in the scene size-up when responding to calls involving burned patients.

29-10. Explain the concept of stopping the burning process.

29-11. Identify indications of inhalation injury.

29-12. Discuss special considerations for dressing burns, including burns to specific anatomical areas.

29-13. Describe special considerations in responding to, assessing, and managing chemical and electrical burns.

KEY IDEAS

Burn injuries can do more than burn the skin. They can impair the body's fluid and chemical balance, its temperature regulation, and its musculoskeletal, circulatory, and respiratory functions. In order to care for burns properly, you need to have a basic understanding of the various kinds of burns; how burn injuries are classified; and how they affect adult, child, and infant patients.

- Burns are classified according to the depth of the injury. A superficial burn affects the epidermis. A partial-thickness burn affects the epidermis and portions of the dermis. A full-thickness burn involves all layers of the skin and can extend into the muscle, bone, or organs below.

- Burns are also classified by severity of injury—critical, moderate, or minor. The most important factors in determining burn severity are percentage and location of body surface area involved, the patient's age, and preexisting medical conditions.

- Assessment and emergency care of burn patients includes removing the patient from the source of the burn and stopping the burning process, being especially alert for compromise of the airway, estimating the severity of the burns, and determining whether the patient is a priority for transport.

- When called to care for chemical burns, be prepared to protect yourself from exposure to hazardous materials. Remember to flush chemicals from the patient, when appropriate, for at least 20 minutes. Brush off dry chemicals before flushing.

- Special considerations for care of electrical burns include making sure that power sources have been shut down before rescue and emergency care, monitoring the patient for respiratory and cardiac arrest, and assessing for both entrance and exit wounds.

TERMS AND CONCEPTS

1. Write the number of each term next to its definition.

   1. Circumferential burn
   2. Eschar
   3. Full-thickness burn
   4. Partial-thickness burn
   5. Rule of nines
   6. Superficial burn

   _____ a. Standardized format used to identify quickly the amount or percentage of skin or body surface area that has been burned

   _____ b. Burn that involves all the layers of the skin and can extend beyond the subcutaneous layer into the muscle, bone, or organs below

   _____ c. The hard, tough, leathery, dead soft tissue formed as a result of a full-thickness burn

   _____ d. A burn that encircles a body area

_____ e. A burn that involves only the epidermis

_____ f. A burn that involves the epidermis and portions of the dermis

CONTENT REVIEW

1. List six functions of the skin.

   _____

   _____

   _____

   _____

   _____

   _____

2. In discussing burn assessment, the letters BSA stand for
   a. body surface area.
   b. burn severity assessment.
   c. blistered surface area.
   d. burn surface analysis.

3. Which of the following classifications of burns is usually caused by a flash flame, a hot liquid, or the sun?
   a. Superficial burn (first-degree)
   b. Eschar burn
   c. Full-thickness burn (third-degree)
   d. Circumferential burn

4. You are treating a patient who has sustained a burn. Which of the following would indicate that the patient has most likely sustained a deep partial-thickness burn?
   a. Thin-walled blisters are present.
   b. Skin is red and blanched white.
   c. Skin is soft and tender to touch.
   d. Capillary refill to the burn site is normal.

5. Which one of the following kinds of burns damages the blood vessels, causing plasma and tissue fluid to collect between layers of the skin?
   a. Superficial burn (first-degree)
   b. Partial-thickness burn (second-degree)
   c. Eschar burn
   d. Circumferential burn

6. Burns to the face are considered
   a. minor.
   b. moderate.
   c. critical.
   d. fatal.

7. You are treating a patient who has sustained an electrical injury with a deep burn that extends into the muscle, blood vessels, and nerves. This type of burn can be categorized as which of the following?
   a. Neuromuscular burn
   b. Partial-thickness, second-degree burn
   c. Circumferential burn
   d. Fourth-degree burn

8. In a child, partial-thickness burns of 10–20 percent BSA are considered
   a. minor.
   b. moderate.
   c. critical.
   d. fatal.

9. Which of the following age groups are less tolerant of burn injuries?
   a. Children under age 3 and adults over age 33
   b. Children under age 4 and adults over age 44
   c. Children under age 5 and adults over age 55
   d. Children under age 6 and adults over age 66

10. Briefly list the steps of emergency medical care of burn injuries.

   _____

   _____

   _____

   _____

   _____

   _____

11. When treating a burn patient, it is inappropriate to apply the rule of nines to which type of burn?
   a. Superficial burns
   b. Superficial partial-thickness burns
   c. Deep partial-thickness burns
   d. Full-thickness burns

12. Separate burned fingers or toes with dry, sterile dressings to prevent
   a. scarring of burned areas.
   b. adherence of burned areas.
   c. further contamination of burned areas.
   d. potential blistering of burned areas.

13. Your patient has sustained a burn to his right eye. Which of the following is an appropriate treatment for this patient?
   a. Apply firm pressure to the right eye.
   b. Treat the burn by applying burn ointment.
   c. Apply a dry, sterile dressing to both eyes.
   d. Cover the burned eye with a moist, sterile dressing.

14. Which of the following statements pertaining to the care of a patient who has sustained a chemical burn is considered inappropriate?
    a. Chemical burns may involve hazardous materials, so protect yourself first.
    b. Dry chemicals should be immediately flushed off the patient.
    c. Some chemicals may produce combustion when in contact with water.
    d. Chemical burns require immediate care.

15. You are treating a patient who has sustained a superficial partial-thickness burn from touching a hot exhaust pipe on a vehicle. What type of mechanism caused this burn?
    a. Flame burn
    b. Gas burn
    c. Flash burn
    d. Contact burn

16. Which of the following is correct about the assessment and care of an electrical burn patient?
    a. Always assume that the power source has been shut down.
    b. Rescue all patients in contact with an electrical source.
    c. All tissues between the entrance and exit wounds may be injured.
    d. Injuries caused by an electrical burn always have a rapid onset.

17. You arrive on the scene minutes after your patient sustained critical burns. You find your patient in a state of hypoperfusion. You should suspect
    a. direct blood loss from an associated external hemorrhage or internal hemorrhage.
    b. a large fluid shift outside of the vessels and into the spaces surrounding the cells.
    c. protein has traveled from the muscle tissue into the vascular system.
    d. indirect loss of fluid into the vascular space through osmosis.

18. You are treating a patient who has been severely burned. You know that the burns will
    a. cause fluid to leak into the cells.
    b. increase capillary permeability.
    c. increase blood flow to the kidneys.
    d. protect against fluid loss.

19. Which one of the following conditions is incorrect and unlikely to be seen in the burn patient?
    a. Leakage of fluid from body cells will cause severe edema (swelling).
    b. Circumferential burns can interfere with respiration by preventing chest expansion.
    c. Scarring from burns can cause long-term muscle wasting and joint dysfunction.
    d. Gastrointestinal dysfunction is caused by increased blood flow to the gastrointestinal system.

CASE STUDY

You are called to the scene of a burned child. You note that the patient's pajamas are still smoldering. The patient is crying loudly.

1. After soaking the pajamas with water, you try to remove them. However, the plastic booties have adhered to the patient's feet. You should
    a. gently try to remove the plastic from the skin.
    b. gently cut around the area with bandage scissors.
    c. transport to the hospital with the clothes left on.
    d. call medical direction for help with this situation.

2. Your partner notices singed nasal hairs in the patient; the SpO$_2$ is 92% on room air. After requesting ALS backup, you should provide
   a. oxygen via a nasal cannula at 6 lpm.
   b. oxygen via a simple mask at 8 lpm.
   c. oxygen via a nonrebreather mask at 15 lpm.
   d. positive pressure ventilations with oxygen.

The mother tells you that she heard the 4-year-old child's screams and found him on fire in the garage. She suspects that lighter fluid may have been involved. You determine that the burns are all partial-thickness burns that cover the entire right leg and foot. You begin to transport the patient to the hospital, which is also a burn center.

3. What is the estimated body surface area affected by the burn, and what is the severity classification?
   a. 1 percent and moderate
   b. 9 percent and critical
   c. 14 percent and critical
   d. 18 percent and moderate

4. You continue the emergency care en route to the hospital. Which of the following is most appropriate?
   a. Cover the burned area with a sterile, dry dressing, and keep the patient cool.
   b. Cover the burned area with a sterile, dry dressing, and keep the patient warm.
   c. Cover the burned area with a sterile, moist dressing, and keep the patient cool.
   d. Cover the burned area with a sterile, moist dressing, and keep the patient warm.

CHAPTER 29 SCENARIO: DOCUMENTATION EXERCISE

Read the following scenario, and think about how you would document this call if you were the EMT who responded to the scene. Then answer the multiple-choice questions and fill in the sample prehospital care report, basing your documentation on information from the scenario.

It's near dinnertime on your shift duty day. You and your partner, Becky, are picking up groceries from the store for tonight's dinner. Suddenly your portable radio squawks: "Unit 4, respond to a possible burned child at 1500 Ninth Street South West." You and Becky quickly place the groceries at the front counter, telling the cashier that you have a call and will return later. You both walk briskly toward the ambulance and, after confirming the address location on the onboard computer, you mark en route.

After a short emergency response, you arrive at a modest home. You quickly scan the area, looking for hazards, as you both put on your gloves and eye protection. You are pulling the stretcher and equipment from the rear of the ambulance when a frantic mother, carrying her daughter, meets you at the back of the ambulance. Her daughter is wearing shorts and a T-shirt with socks and tennis shoes. Quickly you lower the stretcher and help the mother to lay the injured child supine on the stretcher. The visibly upset mother tells you, "I was frying chicken in a pan of hot oil when the whole pan caught fire. I tried to carry the flaming pan outside the house when my daughter came in to see what was the matter. I bumped into her, and the hot oil spilled all down the front of her. Please help her."

The patient gazes into your eyes with a frightened look and says, "I hurt real bad." You quickly introduce Becky and yourself to the patient and ask her how old she is and what her name is. She replies with a trembling voice, "My name is Ashley, and I'm 9 years old." You quickly place Ashley into the ambulance with the mother sitting by her side. Becky explains that you will be doing a lot of things quickly to help her, and if she has any questions, she should just ask.

Becky explains to Ashley that she will need to cut off all of her clothes and place cool water on her burns. She also describes how she will place special bandages on her burns. Becky carefully cuts the clothing off, and you find that the burned area has thick-walled blisters, some of which have ruptured. The burned area is red with blanched white patches. You gently press on an area of the burn and find that the capillary refill is delayed, but the patient can feel pressure at the site. You begin to cool the burns with sterile saline while Becky performs a primary assessment.

The burns encompass the patient's anterior trunk, bilateral anterior legs, and genitalia area. You advise the mother that you will be transporting her daughter to a local hospital that specializes in the treatment of burn patients. There are no stridorous or crowing sounds with inhalation or exhalation. Ashley's breathing is slightly shallow and rapid at approximately 24 breaths per minute. The chest is rising and falling, with adequate air flowing in and out of the mouth, without the use of accessory muscles. The pulse oximeter reads an SpO_2 of 93%. Becky applies oxygen. You feel for a radial pulse and find a strong, rapid pulse at 120 beats per minute. The unaffected skin is warm and dry, with a capillary refill of less than two seconds.

You begin a rapid physical exam. Ashley's head reveals no injuries or deformities; the pupils are equal and react briskly to light. The nose, mouth, and ears are all clear of blood, fluid, or burns. The neck is soft and free of any burns, and there is no noted subcutaneous emphysema. The trachea is midline, and there is no deformity or pain to the posterior neck. The chest and abdomen reveal the burns found in the primary assessment. You remember to inspect the axillary area, and no trauma or burns are noted. The same type of burn extends down from the chest and abdomen and covers the pelvis and genital area. You assess the extremities and find no injuries to the arms, but the anterior portions of both legs are burned. The patient's feet were protected from the hot oil by her socks and shoes, and no burns are found on her feet. You remark, "I have good distal pulses in all extremities." You promptly examine the posterior body and find no burns, trauma, or sacral edema. The patient does not complain of any pain when her spine is palpated.

You say to Becky, "Let's get going. I'll finish the rest en route." Becky moves to the driver's seat and marks en route to the burn center with dispatch. On the way to the burn center, you apply dressings to the burns. Ashley says that she feels cold, so you cover her and adjust the interior temperature of the ambulance to keep her warm and comfortable. You now have time to gather additional information, including a history that will be helpful to the burn center team. Ashley's mother tells you that Ashley has no known allergies, takes no medications, and has no past medical history. You notify the burn center by radio that you are en route with an approximately 10-minute arrival time, and you brief the burn team on your patient's condition.

After a short emergency response, you arrive at the burn center. Ashley once again looks into your eyes for reassurance. You tell her that she is at a special hospital, and they will take good care of her. She cracks a small smile, acknowledging that she understands. You and Becky whisk her through the emergency department doors with her mother still by her side.

1. This burn was caused by hot oil that was spilled onto the patient. What type of burn resulted from this incident?
   a. Flash burn
   b. Steam burn
   c. Gas burn
   d. Scald

2. When you assessed the burn area, you found thick-walled blisters, some of which had ruptured. The burned area was red with blanched white patches. When you gently pressed on the area of the burn, you found that the capillary refill was delayed and the patient could feel pressure at the site. From this description, you would suspect that the patient is suffering from which classification of burn?
   a. Superficial partial-thickness burn (second-degree)
   b. Deep partial-thickness burn (second-degree)
   c. Full-thickness burn (third-degree)
   d. Full-thickness burn (fourth-degree)

3. This patient's burns cover her anterior trunk, bilateral anterior legs, and genitalia area. By the rule of nines, what percentage of the total BSA best represents this patient's burns?
   a. 19 percent
   b. 28 percent
   c. 37 percent
   d. 55 percent

4. Which statement best describes this patient's condition?
   a. The patient's burns are critical because they comprise over 20 percent partial-thickness burns.
   b. The patient's burns are critical because they comprise over 10 percent full-thickness burns.
   c. The patient's burns are moderate because they comprise 10–20 percent partial-thickness burns.
   d. The patient's burns are moderate because they comprise 15–25 percent full-thickness burns.

5. For treating this patient's burns, which of the following dressings would be considered appropriate?
   a. Wet, sterile, particle-free dressing
   b. Dry, sterile, particle-free dressing
   c. Dry, sterile dressing with burn cream
   d. Moist cotton-batting-type dressing

EMERGENCY TRIP SHEET

TRIP #	
MEDIC #	
BEGIN MILES	
END MILES	
CODE___/___ PAGE___/___	
UNITS ON SCENE	

BILLING USE ONLY				
DAY				
DATE				
RECEIVED				
DISPATCHED				
EN-ROUTE				
ON SCENE				
TO HOSPITAL				
AT HOSPITAL				
IN-SERVICE				

NAME _____ SEX M F DOB ___/___/___
ADDRESS _____ RACE
CITY _____ STATE ___ ZIP
PHONE ( ) ___ - ___ PCP DR.
RESPONDED FROM _____ CITY
TAKEN FROM _____ ZIP
DESTINATION _____ REASON
SSN ___ - ___ - ___ MEDICARE # ___ MEDICAID #
INSURANCE CO ___ INSURANCE # ___ GROUP #
RESPONSIBLE PARTY ___ ADDRESS
CITY ___ STATE ___ ZIP ___ PHONE ( ) ___ - ___
EMPLOYER

	CREW	CERT	STATE #

TIME	ON SCENE (1)	ON SCENE (2)	ON SCENE (3)	EN-ROUTE (1)	EN-ROUTE (2)	AT DESTINATION
BP						
PULSE						
RESP						
SpO$_2$						
ETCO$_2$						
EKG						

IV THERAPY
SUCCESSFUL Y N # OF ATTEMPTS _____
ANGIO SIZE _____ ga.
SITE _____
TOTAL FLUID INFUSED _____ cc
BLOOD DRAW Y N INITIALS _____

INTUBATION INFORMATION
SUCCESSFUL Y N # OF ATTEMPTS _____
TUBE SIZE _____ mm
TIME _____ INITIALS _____

MEDICAL HISTORY

CONDITION CODES

MEDICATIONS

TREATMENTS

TIME	TREATMENT	DOSE	ROUTE	INIT

ALLERGIES
C/C

EVENTS LEADING TO C/C

ASSESSMENT

TREATMENT

GCS E___ V___ M___ TOTAL =
GCS E___ V___ M___ TOTAL =

HOSPITAL CONTACTED

CPR BEGUN BY B P TIME BEGUN _____
AED USED Y N BY:
RESUSCITATION TERMINATED - TIME _____

EMS SIGNATURE

( ) OSHA REGULATIONS FOLLOWED

Musculoskeletal Trauma and Nontraumatic Fractures

▌ STANDARD

Trauma (Content Area: Orthopedic Trauma; Content Area: Nontraumatic Musculoskeletal Disorders)

▌ COMPETENCY

Applies fundamental knowledge to provide basic emergency care and transportation based on assessment findings for an acutely injured or ill patient.

▌ OBJECTIVES

After reading this chapter, you should be able to:

30-1. Define key terms introduced in this chapter.

30-2. Describe the structures and functions of the musculoskeletal system, including:
  a. Bones
  b. Skeletal muscle
  c. Tendons
  d. Ligaments
  e. Cartilage
  f. Joints

30-3. Describe each of the following types of injuries and their associated signs and symptoms:
  a. Fractures
  b. Strains
  c. Sprains
  d. Dislocations

30-4. Give examples of direct, indirect, and twisting forces that can produce musculoskeletal injuries.

30-5. Explain why fractures of the femur and pelvis are considered to be critical fractures.

30-6. Describe the assessment-based approach to bone and joint injuries.

30-7. Establish the priority for assessing and treating musculoskeletal injuries with respect to a patient's overall condition.

30-8. Discuss the significance of assessing a musculoskeletal injury for each of the following findings:
  a. Pain
  b. Pallor
  c. Paralysis

    d. Paresthesia

    e. Pressure

    f. Pulses

30-9. Explain the rationale for splinting musculoskeletal injuries.

30-10. Compare and contrast the characteristics and uses of various types of splints, including:

    a. Rigid splints

    b. Pressure (air or pneumatic) splints

    c. Traction splints

    d. Formable splints

    e. Vacuum splints

    f. Sling and swathe

    g. Spine board

    h. Improvised splints

30-11. Discuss hazards of improper splinting.

30-12. Discuss special considerations in splinting long bone injuries, splinting joint injuries, and traction splinting.

30-13. Discuss special considerations in splinting pelvic fractures.

30-14. Describe the basic pathophysiology of compartment syndrome.

30-15. Describe the pathophysiology of nontraumatic fractures.

30-16. Describe the management of nontraumatic fractures.

KEY IDEAS

Musculoskeletal injuries are frequently encountered in the field. Most of these injuries are simple and not life threatening. Appropriate management can prevent further painful injury and even prevent permanent disability or death. This chapter provides a review of the musculoskeletal system and discusses musculoskeletal injuries and their appropriate management.

- The functions of the musculoskeletal system are to give the body shape, to protect the internal organs, and to provide for movement.

- The six basic components of the skeletal system are the skull, spinal column, thorax, pelvis, lower extremities, and upper extremities.

- The forces that may cause bone and joint injuries are direct, indirect, and twisting forces.

- Bone and joint injuries can be either open or closed.

- Any painful, swollen, or deformed extremity should be immobilized.

- Splinting prevents movement of bone fragments, bone ends, or dislocated joints, thereby reducing the chance for further injury, and it reduces pain and minimizes complications.

- The general rules of splinting include the following: Check pulse, motor function, and sensation (PMS) before and after splinting; immobilize the joints above and below a long bone injury, or immobilize the bones above and below a joint injury; remove clothing and jewelry; cover all wounds before splinting; never replace bone ends; splint before moving the patient; and when in doubt, splint the injury and pad the splints.

- If there is severe deformity or the distal extremity is cyanotic or pulseless, then make one attempt to realign the limb. If pain, resistance, or crepitus increases, stop and transport immediately.

- If a patient shows signs of shock, align the patient in the normal anatomical position, treat for shock, and transport immediately without taking the time to apply a splint.

- The general types of splints are rigid, traction, pressure, improvised, and sling and swathe.

TERMS AND CONCEPTS

1. Write the number of each term next to its definition.

   1. Crepitus
   2. Direct force
   3. Indirect force
   4. Paresthesia
   5. Splint
   6. Twisting force
   7. Osteoporosis

   _____ a. A force that rotates a bone while one end is held stationary

   _____ b. The sound or feel of broken fragments of bone grinding against each other

   _____ c. A force that causes injury some distance away from the point of impact

   _____ d. A force that causes injury at the point of impact

   _____ e. Any device used to immobilize a body part

   _____ f. A prickling or tingling feeling that indicates some loss of sensation

   _____ g. Degenerative bone disorder associated with an accelerated loss of minerals, primarily calcium, from the bone

CONTENT REVIEW

1. Three of the following are functions of the musculoskeletal system, and one is the function of the circulatory system. Which is a function of the circulatory system?
   a. Gives the body shape
   b. Produces platelets
   c. Protects the internal organs
   d. Provides for movement

2. List the six basic components of the skeletal system.

   _____

   _____

   _____

   _____

   _____

   _____

3. Which of the following are forces that cause bone and joint injury?
   a. Direct, partial, and indeterminate
   b. Direct, indirect, and frontal
   c. Direct, indirect, and twisting
   d. Direct, primary, and secondary

4. Which of the following is considered to be a serious condition when distal to an injured extremity?
   a. Swelling and tenderness
   b. Coolness and paleness
   c. Pain and flushing
   d. Pulselessness and cyanosis

5. If a fracture is suspected, which of the following is considered to be a critical injury that must be managed in a manner that not only immobilizes the bone, but also reduces the associated bleeding?
   a. Radius or ulna
   b. Tibia or fibula
   c. Scapula or clavicle
   d. Femur or pelvis

6. A patient has an injured extremity. The patient is unresponsive, with a suspected spinal injury and other life-threatening injuries unrelated to the extremity injury. You and your partner have established manual in-line stabilization of the head and spine, ensured an open airway and adequate breathing, controlled major bleeding, and completed a rapid physical exam. There is no one at the scene who can provide a history, and you will assess vital signs en route. In addition, you perform the steps in the following list. Number the list in the proper order from 1 to 4 to show the order of priority for performing these steps.

   _____ Splint the injured extremity.

   _____ Perform further management of the life-threatening injuries and reassess every five minutes.

   _____ Immobilize the patient to a spine board.

   _____ Initiate transport.

7. The skin over the fracture site has been broken, and the bone may or may not protrude through the skin. Which type of injury does this statement best describe?
   a. A spiral injury
   b. An open injury
   c. A closed injury
   d. A simple injury

8. List at least five signs and symptoms of bone or joint injury.

   _____

   _____

   _____

   _____

   _____

9. Which of the following, if fractured, can easily cause the loss of 1 to 2 liters of blood around the bone?
   a. Humerus
   b. Mandible
   c. Femur
   d. Radius

10. If an injured extremity is painful, swollen, and deformed, which of the following should you do?
    a. Apply warm packs to the site.
    b. Restrict blood flow.
    c. Splint the extremity.
    d. Position the extremity below the heart.

11. The patient's distal pulses, motor function, and sensation should be checked
    a. before splinting.
    b. after splinting.
    c. before and after splinting.
    d. just before arrival at the hospital.

12. A general rule for the immobilization of an injury to a long bone is to immobilize
    a. the joints above and below the injury site.
    b. the joint above the injury site only.
    c. the joint below the injury site only.
    d. only the bone, not the adjacent joint.

13. In a patient who may have sustained a fracture to the pelvis, the pneumatic antishock garment (PASG) performs two functions. One function is to stabilize the fracture; the other is to
    a. decrease the compartment into which the pelvis can bleed.
    b. apply direct pressure to the anterior olecranon.
    c. pull the femur away from the pelvic girdle.
    d. apply downward and lateral pressure to the pelvis.

14. If there is severe deformity in an extremity, the distal pulses are absent, or the extremity is cyanotic, you should
    a. make no attempt to align the extremity.
    b. make one attempt to align the extremity.
    c. persist until the extremity is aligned.
    d. apply the splint before attempting to align.

15. Which of the following is considered an inappropriate action when splinting an injured extremity?
    a. Maintain manual traction until after the splint has been applied.
    b. Push protruding bones back into the skin.
    c. Cover all open wounds before splinting.
    d. Cut clothing away and remove jewelry from the site.

16. When forced to use an improvised splint, ensure that the splint is
    a. heavy, but flexible and soft.
    b. short, extending just the length of the bone.
    c. narrower than the thickest part of the injured limb.
    d. well padded on the inner surface.

17. A sling and swathe is commonly used to provide stability to a painful and tender
    a. leg injury.
    b. shoulder injury.
    c. cervical spine injury.
    d. pelvic injury.

18. When splinting an extremity, the hand or foot must be immobilized in the position of function. The position of function for the hand can be attained by
    a. extending the hand over the end of the splint.
    b. securing the hand to the splint in a palm-up position.
    c. bandaging the hand in a clenched-fist position.
    d. putting a roll of bandage in the patient's hand.

19. In which of the following situations should you use a traction splint?
    a. The injury is within 1 or 2 inches of the knee.
    b. The knee has been injured.
    c. The thigh is painful, swollen, or deformed.
    d. The hip or pelvis has been injured.

20. Which statement describes how the traction splint achieves stabilization?
    a. It applies circumferential pressure to the femur.
    b. It stabilizes the bone ends by producing negative torque.
    c. It pulls on the thigh and realigns the broken femur.
    d. It pushes the bones together and "resets" the fracture.

21. Your patient injured her right ankle and foot when she stepped off a curb while crossing the street. Which of the following assessment techniques will give you the same results as if the entire foot were tested?
    a. Checking PMS
    b. Having the patient push and pull back the great (big) toe
    c. Palpating for a brachial pulse
    d. Pushing upward on the bottom (plantar) of the patient's foot

22. Which of the following splints can be used to help stabilize a suspected fractured pelvis?
    a. Bipolar traction splint
    b. Sling and swathe
    c. Short padded-board splint
    d. PASG

23. The condition that occurs when the pressure in the space around the capillaries exceeds the pressure needed to perfuse the tissues and then causes the blood flow to be cut off, leading to cellular hypoxia, is known as
    a. compartment syndrome.
    b. extremity necrosis syndrome.
    c. system dysfunction syndrome.
    d. capillary pressure syndrome.

24. A fracture that is caused by a disease that degrades and dramatically weakens the bone and makes it prone to fracture is known as
    a. systemic fracture.
    b. causation fracture.
    c. simplex fracture.
    d. pathologic fracture.

25. While gathering your patient's medical history, you note that there is a history of osteoporosis. From the following, which is correct pertaining to osteoporosis?
    a. There is a thickening of the bone wall from the addition of calcium.
    b. The condition is caused by plaque buildup in the arteries and veins of the elderly.
    c. It is a degenerative disorder associated with an accelerated loss of minerals.
    d. This condition occurs most often in elderly men and precedes menopause.

26. Overstretching or tearing of muscle fibers that causes pain that typically increases with muscle use is known as
    a. strain.
    b. sprain.
    c. dislocation.
    d. fracture.

27. You are assessing a 21-year-old patient with a suspected isolated leg fracture. When assessing an extremity for the possibility of a fracture or dislocation, there are six "Ps" to remember to assess. List and briefly describe the six Ps.

    1. _____
    2. _____
    3. _____
    4. _____
    5. _____
    6. _____

28. Nontraumatic fractures will likely present with which of the following?
    a. Abrasions
    b. Lacerations
    c. Hematomas
    d. History of cancer

▌CASE STUDY 1

You are dispatched to a high school to assist a 17-year-old soccer player who is injured. The patient is sitting on a bench on the sideline of the field, holding his left shoulder and leaning forward. You sit down next to him and ask, "What happened?" He replies, "I was moving down to score and tripped. I put my arm out to catch myself, and I felt something snap in my shoulder." Your general impression is a noncritical injured patient. He responds to your questions appropriately and is alert and oriented. His respirations are normal; radial pulse is strong and regular; and skin is a good color, warm, and dry. You examine his shoulder and observe deformity over his left clavicle. The area is tender to touch and obviously swollen. He denies any other complaints or injuries.

1. The immediate action to take for this patient should be to
   a. immobilize the shoulder with an air splint, splinting the entire arm.
   b. evaluate the PMS
   c. splint the shoulder with a sling and swathe.
   d. immobilize the shoulder with a rigid splint on the entire arm.

2. What is the best way to evaluate this patient's sensory function?
   a. Ask if he can feel you pinch him on the back.
   b. Ask him to wiggle his fingers without looking.
   c. Ask him to tell you which finger you are touching without looking.
   d. Ask him if he can feel you prick him with a sharp object.

3. This patient's injury is most likely due to what type of force?
   a. Direct
   b. Indirect
   c. Twisting
   d. Secondary

CASE STUDY 2

You are at the scene of a motorcycle collision with a car. About 20 yards from the vehicles, a male biker is sitting and holding his right leg. He looks to be about 30 years old. You ask, "What happened?" He replies, "That car stopped in front of me. I hit the rear, flew off the bike, and landed on my leg." You maintain in-line stabilization of the head and c-spine. Respirations are normal; radial pulse is strong and regular; skin color is normal, warm, and dry. You cut away his pant leg so you can evaluate his injury. The thigh region is deformed, swollen, and tender to touch. He denies any other complaints or injuries. You ask your partner to initiate manual traction to the right leg.

1. Manual traction on the patient's leg
   a. should be continued until you arrive at the hospital.
   b. should be continued until you are ready to position the splint.
   c. should be continued until the splint is applied.
   d. should not have been initiated.

2. When checking the pulse distal to the injury site on this patient, use which of the following?
   a. Pedal or posterior tibial pulse
   b. Radial or brachial pulse
   c. Popliteal or femoral pulse
   d. Carotid or femoral pulse

CASE STUDY 3

You are dispatched to a call for an elderly patient who is lying on the kitchen floor. She is 70 years old and in severe pain. She tells you that when she fell, she heard a "loud pop." There is bruising to the right hip region, and the patient complains of severe pain there upon palpation. She also tells you that her leg feels numb and is tingling. She denies any additional complaints or injuries. You apply a padded rigid splint that extends from below the foot to above the hip.

1. The patient's complaint of numbness and tingling in her right leg
   a. may indicate some loss of sensation.
   b. may indicate an additional injury to the lower leg.
   c. may require the application of a full leg air splint.
   d. is to be expected after this type of injury.

2. The patient's foot should be immobilized in a position of function. Which statement best describes the position of function for the foot?
   a. Toes curled toward the sole of the foot
   b. Foot bent at a normal angle to the leg
   c. Foot pushed downward to align with the shin
   d. Foot bent upward toward the shin

3. To evaluate this patient's motor function, ask her to do which of the following?
   a. Lift the leg and rotate it outward.
   b. Rotate the leg outward and tense the foot.
   c. Tighten the kneecap and move the foot up and down.
   d. Tighten the buttocks and lift the leg.

CHAPTER 30 SCENARIO: DOCUMENTATION EXERCISE

Read the following scenario and think about how you would document this call if you were the EMT who responded to the scene. Then answer the multiple-choice questions and fill in the sample prehospital care report, basing your documentation on information from the scenario.

You and your newly promoted partner, Lt. Rackard, are working as the EMT crew at a local horse show. A show official runs up to your ambulance and tells you that a horse in a barn kicked a person. Lt. Rackard notifies dispatch of the possible injury as you drive the ambulance to the barn. While putting on your eyewear and gloves, you both scan the general area looking for obvious hazards, but none are observed. As you are removing the stretcher from the rear of the ambulance, the show official runs up to you, saying in a stern voice, "You must hurry. She is in a lot of pain." You reassure her and walk briskly toward the barn door. As you enter the large open door, you once again scan the area for hazards. The official leads you toward an open stall door. You ask if the horse has been removed and secured in another area, and she replies, "The horse has been removed to a corral outside."

As you enter the stall area, you find a young adult female lying supine on the floor. She is holding her right leg above the knee and is screaming in agony. She appears slightly pale and extremely anxious. You approach her and quickly introduce yourself and Lt. Rackard. You reassure her and explain that you are there to help her. Lt. Rackard asks her name and what happened, and she says, "My name is Jennifer, and I was cleaning the stall when the horse spooked and kicked me in the thigh. It really hurts!" You mention to your partner that a kick from a horse can be violent, with potential for other injuries. Lt. Rackard positions herself to maintain in-line stabilization of the patient's head, neck, and spine. You observe that the patient is breathing approximately 22 times each minute. Her chest is rising and falling, with adequate air flowing in and out of the mouth, and without the use of accessory muscles. You feel for a radial pulse and find a strong, rapid pulse at 100 beats per minute. Her skin is warm and dry. You notice a small blood spot on the patient's jeans. The spot is on the right thigh midway between the knee and hip.

Because of the potential for other injuries, you begin a rapid physical exam. You quickly expose the patient by cutting the clothes, being careful to protect her modesty. The head reveals no injuries or deformities, and the pupils are equal and react briskly to light. The nose, mouth, and ears are all clear of blood or fluid. The neck is soft, with no trauma or subcutaneous emphysema noted. The trachea is midline, and there is no deformity or pain to the posterior neck. You palpate the chest and note equal chest rise and fall. There is no sign of trauma or use of accessory muscles. You inspect the axillary area, noting that it is without injury. Inspection of the abdomen reveals no obvious injuries, distention, or pain with palpation. You quickly inspect the pelvis for deformity, contusions, abrasions, or penetrating injuries, and none are found.

You assess the lower extremities and find that the left leg is not injured, but the right has a large contusion and open wound that is oozing blood. The injury is to the anterior midposition of the thigh. You do not observe any bone ends protruding from the open wound. When you palpate the affected leg, you feel broken bone fragments grinding against each other, which sends an uncomfortable shiver up your spine. The right leg appears to be having muscle spasms, and it appears to be larger than the unaffected left leg. The upper extremities are uninjured. You ask Jennifer if she can feel you touching her extremities, and she replies, "Yes." You then ask her to wiggle her toes and fingers, and she does. Next, you check all four distal pulses and find them to be strong and regular.

This appears to be an isolated injury to the right leg. However, you and Lt. Rackard agree to maintain in-line stabilization of the spine as a precaution. You apply a cervical collar and solicit assistance from two bystanders to help you with moving the patient onto the backboard. While placing the patient on the backboard, you support the affected leg and examine the posterior body, finding no injuries or sacral edema. The patient does not complain of any pain when the spine is palpated. She is quickly secured to the backboard.

Lt. Rackard repositions herself and tells the patient that she will help to relieve the pain to her right leg by applying manual traction. She replies in a stern, loud voice, "Don't touch my leg. It hurts too bad!" She reassures her that it is necessary and the pain should decrease when traction is pulled, she states, "OK, I understand." Lt. Rackard reassesses the PMS of the injured leg and then stabilizes the injured leg by applying manual traction. Jennifer grimaces and says, "Ouch! Oh! That does feel much better!" You prepare and apply the bipolar traction splint. After the leg has been placed in the splint, you attach the "S" hook and start to apply mechanical traction. After the splint has been applied, the patient states that she still feels the pain but it is more tolerable now. After you apply a dressing to the open wound site, you place cold packs on and around the injury.

You and Lt. Rackard lift the backboard, place the patient on the stretcher, and make your way toward the ambulance. You advise the patient that it will take about 25 minutes to reach the hospital and you will try to give her a smooth ride. The show official asks Jennifer if there is anyone she should notify to inform them that she has been taken to the hospital,

and Jennifer gives her the contact information. You both load the patient into the back of the ambulance, and Lt. Rackard positions herself in the driver's seat.

While en route to the hospital, you gather additional information, including a history. Jennifer tells you that she is allergic to penicillin and takes albuterol through a metered-dose inhaler for her asthma. You obtain vital signs, which are blood pressure 118/60, pulse rate 94 and regular, and respirations 18 each minute with good tidal volume. The pulse oximeter reveals an SpO_2 of 98% on oxygen. You notify the hospital by radio that you are en route with an approximately 20-minute arrival time and quickly brief them on the patient's condition.

1. When you palpated the affected leg, you felt the broken fragments of bone grinding against each other. What is the medical term for this finding?
   a. Atelectasis
   b. Kyphosis
   c. Eupnea
   d. Crepitus

2. When Lt. Rackard applied manual traction, the pain to the affected leg decreased. In addition to reducing pain, application of manual traction
   a. reduces the diameter of the thigh, which increases pressure on the bleeding bones, slowing bleeding.
   b. pulls the arteries, which decreases the size of the vessel, reducing the associated bleeding.
   c. applies direct pressure to the fractured ends of the femur, cutting off the flow of blood.
   d. slows bleeding by circumferential direct, as well as indirect, pressure from the snug ischial strap.

3. If this patient were to become unresponsive, how would you know when full traction was achieved when applying mechanical traction with the bipolar traction splint?
   a. The injured leg will be 3 to 5 centimeters longer than the uninjured leg.
   b. The injured leg should be the same length as the uninjured leg.
   c. The size of the injured thigh will increase slightly over that of the uninjured thigh.
   d. The unresponsive patient will grimace when full traction has been achieved.

4. Which of the following actions would be considered inappropriate for this patient?
   a. Application of ice packs to the injury site
   b. Pulling traction to a suspected open fracture
   c. Pulling manual traction while the splint is readied
   d. Elevating the injured extremity to reduce swelling

5. It was proper to evaluate the PMS distal to the injury before and after the splint was applied. How often should you reevaluate the PMS after the splint is applied?
   a. Every 2 minutes
   b. Every 5 minutes
   c. Every 10 minutes
   d. Every 15 minutes

EMERGENCY TRIP SHEET		BILLING USE ONLY				

TRIP #

MEDIC #

BEGIN MILES

END MILES

CODE___/___   PAGE___/___

UNITS ON SCENE

BILLING USE ONLY			
DAY			
DATE			
RECEIVED			
DISPATCHED			

NAME ___ SEX M F DOB ___/___/___

ADDRESS ___ RACE

CITY ___ STATE ___ ZIP

PHONE ( )   - ___ PCP DR.

RESPONDED FROM ___ CITY

TAKEN FROM ___ ZIP

DESTINATION ___ REASON

SSN   -   - ___ MEDICARE # ___ MEDICAID #

INSURANCE CO ___ INSURANCE # ___ GROUP #

RESPONSIBLE PARTY ___ ADDRESS

CITY ___ STATE ___ ZIP ___ PHONE ( )   -

EMPLOYER

EN-ROUTE	
ON SCENE	
TO HOSPITAL	
AT HOSPITAL	
IN-SERVICE	

CREW	CERT	STATE #

TIME	ON SCENE (1)	ON SCENE (2)	ON SCENE (3)	EN-ROUTE (1)	EN-ROUTE (2)	AT DESTINATION
BP						
PULSE						
RESP						
SpO$_2$						
ETCO$_2$						
EKG						

IV THERAPY
SUCCESSFUL Y N # OF ATTEMPTS _____
ANGIO SIZE _____ga.
SITE _____
TOTAL FLUID INFUSED _____ cc
BLOOD DRAW Y N INITIALS

INTUBATION INFORMATION
SUCCESSFUL Y N # OF ATTEMPTS _____
TUBE SIZE _____ mm
TIME _____ INITIALS _____

MEDICAL HISTORY

MEDICATIONS

ALLERGIES

C/C

EVENTS LEADING TO C/C

ASSESSMENT

TREATMENT

CONDITION CODES				

TREATMENTS

TIME	TREATMENT	DOSE	ROUTE	INIT

GCS E___ V___ M___ TOTAL =

GCS E___ V___ M___ TOTAL =

HOSPITAL CONTACTED

CPR BEGUN BY   B   P   TIME BEGUN

AED USED Y N BY:

RESUSCITATION TERMINATED - TIME

EMS SIGNATURE

( ) OSHA REGULATIONS FOLLOWED

Head Trauma

▌ STANDARD

Trauma (Content Area: Head, Facial, Neck, and Spine Trauma)

▌ COMPETENCY

Applies fundamental knowledge to provide basic emergency care and transportation based on assessment findings for an acutely injured patient.

▌ OBJECTIVES

After reading this chapter, you should be able to:

31-1. Define key terms introduced in the chapter.

31-2. Explain the importance of recognizing and providing emergency medical care to patients with injuries to the head.

31-3. Identify the anatomy of the skull.

31-4. Identify the meningeal layers and the spaces into which intracranial bleeding can occur in relationship to the meninges, skull, and brain.

31-5. Associate each of the major anatomical portions of the brain with its functions.

31-6. Explain the pathophysiology and key signs and symptoms of injuries to the scalp, skull, and brain, including:
  a. Scalp lacerations
  b. Skull fractures
  c. Cerebral concussion and diffuse axonal injury
  d. Cerebral contusion
  e. Coup/contrecoup injury
  f. Cerebral and intracranial hematomas
  g. Cerebral laceration

31-7. Identify and, where possible, manage factors that can worsen traumatic brain injuries, including:
  a. Hypoxia
  b. Hypercarbia
  c. Hypoglycemia
  d. Hyperglycemia
  e. Hyperthermia
  f. Hypotension

31-8. Describe the goals of emergency treatment of patients with traumatic brain injuries.

31-9. Describe the pathophysiology and key signs of increased intracranial pressure and brain herniation.

31-10. Describe the neurological assessment of patients with suspected traumatic brain injury.

31-11. Discuss the focus of history taking and assessment for patients with injuries to the head.

31-12. Assess and provide emergency treatment to patients with injuries to the head.

31-13. Explain the importance of reassessment of the patient with an injury to the head.

31-14. Document information relevant to the assessment and management of patients with injuries to the head.

KEY IDEAS

Injury to the skull, which contains the brain, can have severe consequences for the patient. Since head injuries may occur weeks before signs and symptoms appear, it is important to recognize both potential and actual injury at the scene.

- The brain and spinal cord make up the central nervous system, which controls the body's systems.

- The skull, which protects the brain, is made up of the cranial skull, the facial bones, and the basilar skull. Cerebrospinal fluid and the meninges help protect the brain inside the skull.

- The brain is made up of three parts: the cerebrum (conscious and sensory functions, emotions, and the personality), the cerebellum (muscle movement and coordination), and the brain stem (most autonomic and vital functions).

- Head injuries may involve the scalp, skull, and/or the brain and are classified as open or closed. Both open and closed injuries of the head may involve extensive damage to the brain. Injury to the brain that results from shearing, tearing, and stretching of nerve fibers is called diffuse axonal injury (DAI).

- Brain injury may be direct (from penetrating trauma), indirect (from a blow to the skull), or secondary (for example, from lack of oxygen, buildup of carbon dioxide, or a change in blood pressure).

- Unresponsiveness or an altered mental status, especially in trauma patients, should always suggest the possibility of head injury. Nontraumatic injury may be caused by clots or hemorrhaging and also may result in an altered mental status.

- Emergency medical care of head injury includes in-line stabilization of the spine; maintaining a patent airway, adequate breathing, and oxygenation; close monitoring of airway, breathing, oxygenation and mental status for changes or deterioration; and immediate transport.

TERMS AND CONCEPTS

1. Write the number of each term next to its definition.

   1. Anterograde amnesia
   2. Battle sign
   3. Cerebellum
   4. Cerebrospinal fluid
   5. Concussion
   6. Coup/contrecoup injury
   7. Cushing reflex
   8. Extension or decerebrate posturing
   9. Flexion or decorticate posturing
   10. Meninges
   11. Raccoon sign
   12. Subarachnoid hemorrhage

_____ a. The patient extends arms and legs and sometimes arches the back, which may be a sign of serious brain injury.

_____ b. The patient is unable to remember circumstances after the incident.

_____ c. Three layers of tissue that enclose the brain.

_____ d. Discoloration of the mastoid, suggesting basilar skull fracture.

_____ e. Discoloration of tissue around the eyes.

_____ f. Sometimes called the "little brain"; it controls equilibrium and coordinates muscle activity.

_____ g. Clear fluid that protects the brain.

_____ h. Hypertension, bradycardia, and altered respiratory pattern.

_____ i. The patient flexes the arms across the chest and extends the legs, which may be a sign of serious brain injury.

_____ j. Damage at the point of a blow to the head and/or damage on the side opposite the blow as the brain is propelled against the opposite side of the skull.

_____ k. Temporary loss of brain function.

_____ l. Bleeding that occurs between the arachnoid membrane and the surface of the brain.

▌CONTENT REVIEW

1. Injury to the brain that results from shearing, tearing, and stretching of nerve fibers is called
   a. DAI.
   b. cerebral contusion.
   c. cerebral hematoma.
   d. cerebral laceration.

2. The single most important sign in cases of suspected head injury is
   a. decreasing blood pressure.
   b. altered respiratory pattern.
   c. decreasing mental status.
   d. increasing pulse rate.

3. This is a tool that uses numerical values to monitor a patient's level of consciousness carefully. It is called the
   a. Common Coma Scale.
   b. AVPU Scale.
   c. Glasgow Coma Scale.
   d. Bond Responsiveness Scale.

4. Which technique should be used to maintain the airway of a patient with a possible head injury who has a decreased level of responsiveness?
   a. Head-tilt, chin-lift maneuver
   b. Jaw-thrust maneuver
   c. Crossed-finger technique
   d. Two-rescuer ventilation

5. The mental status response that is likely to indicate the most serious head injury is
   a. alertness.
   b. responsiveness to verbal stimulus.
   c. responsiveness to painful stimulus.
   d. unresponsiveness.

6. Any patient whose mental status worsens at any stage of the assessment or treatment process needs
   a. treatment for anaphylactic shock.
   b. palpation of the head and neck.
   c. immediate transport and monitoring.
   d. history and rapid assessment.

7. A flexion response or decorticate posturing
   a. indicates a lower-level brain stem injury.
   b. results in extension of the arms and arching of the back.
   c. is also called a *purposeful response.*
   d. results in flexing of arms across the chest and extension of the legs.

8. When managing a patient with a suspected head injury
   a. a lowered SpO_2 is always an indication of a head injury.
   b. oxygenation and ventilation are not of critical importance.
   c. it is critical to determine a baseline mental status.
   d. who had a brief period of unconsciousness, evaluation is not necessary.

9. Mark an X beside each of the following options that is a potential sign of increasing intracranial pressure.

   _____ a. Systolic blood pressure is high or rising.

   _____ b. Systolic blood pressure is low or dropping.

   _____ c. Pulse is slow or decreasing.

   _____ d. Pulse is fast or increasing.

   _____ e. Respiratory pattern is altered.

   _____ f. Respiratory pattern remains unchanged.

10. Emergency care of a patient with a severe brain injury and herniation should include
    a. ventilation at 12/minute.
    b. application of a snug pressure dressing to any open skull injury.
    c. scant or little attention to airway and breathing status.
    d. anticipation of potential seizure activity.

11. Complete the following chart by indicating with a check mark if each listed sign or symptom is associated with each type of brain injury (concussion, contusion, subdural hematoma, or epidural hematoma). You may use one or up to four check marks for each sign or symptom.

Sign or Symptom	Concussion	Contusion	Subdural Hematoma	Epidural Hematoma
Momentary confusion				
Abnormal respiratory pattern				
Retrograde and anterograde amnesia				

Sign or Symptom	Concussion	Contusion	Subdural Hematoma	Epidural Hematoma
Loss of responsiveness, followed by a return of responsiveness and then rapid deterioration				
Weakness or paralysis on one side of the body				
Dilation of one pupil				
Fixed and dilated pupil				
Posturing (withdrawal or flexion)				
Repeated questioning about what happened				
Increasing systolic blood pressure				
Decreasing pulse rate				
Seizures				
Cushing reflex				
Vomiting				
Headache				

12. A mild form of DAI, which generally presents with an altered mental status that progressively improves, is called a(n)
   a. concussion.
   b. contusion.
   c. epidural hematoma.
   d. subdural hematoma.

13. A contusion of the brain is usually caused by two types of injuries. They are
   a. blunt lateral injury and anterior/posterior injury.
   b. coup/contrecoup injury and acceleration/deceleration injury.
   c. medial/central injury and acceleration/deceleration injury.
   d. explosive/implosive injury and radical/conservative injury.

14. This brain injury is typically the result of low-pressure venous bleeding that occurs above the tissue of the brain between the dura mater and the arachnoid layer. It is called a(n)
   a. concussion.
   b. contusion.
   c. epidural hematoma.
   d. subdural hematoma.

15. A subdural hematoma
   a. is the least common type of head injury.
   b. occurs in 10 percent of all severe head injuries.
   c. is more common in patients older than 40 years of age.
   d. is more likely in patients with abnormally long blood-clotting times.

16. The two types of subdural hematomas are
   a. hemolytic and venous.
   b. acute and occult.
   c. acute and chronic.
   d. hemolytic and arterial.

CASE STUDY 1

You have been called to the scene of a four-wheeler all-terrain vehicle (ATV) accident. The patient is a 16-year-old male who hit a small hole and was thrown from the vehicle. A bystander who witnessed the accident states that the driver was thrown about 30 feet and that he landed on his back and struck his head on the ground. As you approach the patient, his eyes are closed and he appears to be in critical condition. His skin color is normal, and his respirations appear to be rapid, deep, and full, without any audible abnormal respiratory sounds. His pulse is slow, regular, and weak. His blood pressure is 130/80; the pulse is 60/minute, weak, and regular; his respirations are 24/minute, deep, and full; his pupils are unequal and slow to respond to light; and the SpO_2 is 96%. The vital signs are repeated in five minutes and are as follows: respirations are 24/minute and irregular; pulse is 50/minute, weak, and regular; skin color is normal, warm, and dry; SpO_2 is 96%, pupils remain unequal and slow to respond to light; and blood pressure is 140/86.

1. This patient is exhibiting signs of _____ reflex, which is a sign of brain herniation.
   a. Bank
   b. Historic
   c. Cushing
   d. Corral

2. The reflex described in the preceding answer consists of a "triad" of signs. These three signs are
   a. decrease in systolic blood pressure, increasing pulse, and rapid respirations.
   b. increasing systolic blood pressure, slowing pulse, and alteration in respirations.
   c. increasing systolic blood pressure, increasing pulse, and alteration in respirations.
   d. decrease in systolic blood pressure, slowing pulse, and rapid respirations.

3. This patient may be managed by ventilations delivered at a rate of _____.
   a. 10 per minute
   b. 12 per minute
   c. 20 per minute
   d. 28 per minute

CASE STUDY 2

You have been called to the scene of a fall. The caller, the patient's neighbor, says that he found Mrs. McDonald, a 70-year-old female, lying at the bottom of her basement stairs. He has not moved her. She is unresponsive with good skin color, her skin is warm and dry, and the pulse is slow and regular. You observe a large deformity at the back of Mrs. McDonald's head. Her pupils are dilated and slow to respond to light. She has bruising around both eyes and over the mastoid process. You find no blood or fluid in the nose, but a clear fluid is draining from her left ear. She is unresponsive to painful stimuli. There is no other evidence of injury. Baseline vitals are blood pressure 178/72, pulse 68, respirations regular and full at 18/minute, and SpO_2 93%.

1. The bruising around Mrs. McDonald's eyes is a late sign of a skull fracture and is called
   a. the Battle sign.
   b. a raccoon sign.
   c. orbital bruising.
   d. the Barry sign.

2. The bruising over the mastoid area is also a late sign of a skull fracture and is called
   a. the Battle sign.
   b. a raccoon sign.
   c. mastoid bruising.
   d. the Barry sign.

3. Mark an X next to each treatment in the following list that should be provided for Mrs. McDonald.

_____ a. Maintain manual in-line spinal stabilization.

_____ b. Apply a cervical spine immobilization collar (CSIC).

_____ c. Perform a head-tilt, chin-lift maneuver to open the airway.

_____ d. Place an oropharyngeal airway.

_____ e. Administer oxygen to maintain the SpO$_2$ at 94% or greater.

_____ f. Consider controlled hyperventilation at 20 per minute.

_____ g. Immobilize to a spine board.

_____ h. Pack gauze into her left ear.

_____ i. Continue to evaluate her mental status.

_____ j. Apply pressure to the head deformity.

CHAPTER 31 SCENARIO: DOCUMENTATION EXERCISE

Read the following scenario and think about how you would document this call if you were the EMT who responded to the scene. Then answer the multiple-choice questions and fill in the sample prehospital care report, basing your documentation on information from the scenario.

It is 5:00 P.M. on a Thursday. You are backing into the station after completing a call for an elderly woman with respiratory distress when the alarm sounds: "Unit 3, respond to 1186 U.S. Highway 92 East for a car that struck a bicycle. Time out 1700 hours." Your partner, Susan, advises dispatch that you are responding. You arrive on the scene in about six minutes. As you prepare to park, you observe a man who appears to be in his mid-30s lying supine on the side of the roadway. You exit the rescue vehicle with Standard Precautions taken and walk toward the patient. A mangled bicycle is lying in the roadway underneath a pickup truck. The truck is about 75 feet from where the patient is lying. As you and Susan walk by the truck, you notice that the front of the hood has significant damage. You quickly confirm that ALS backup has been dispatched.

As you approach the patient, you observe three bystanders kneeling next to him. One is holding a towel on the man's forehead while the other two motion for you and Susan to hurry. Your initial impression is that the patient is in critical condition. A woman kneeling next to him identifies herself as an Emergency Medical Responder and says, "I saw the accident happen!" The patient's eyes are closed as you approach, and he has gurgling respirations that seem shallow and slow. You tell your partner, "Susan, we need to roll him on his side and suction the mouth!" "OK," she replies. You ask Susan to maintain the cervical spine and enlist the help of the bystanders to roll the patient on his side quickly. You suction a small amount of vomitus from his nose and mouth. You quickly size and place an oropharyngeal airway, and no gag reflex is observed.

You position the spine board behind the patient, cut off his clothing, and roll him onto the board. You ask the Emergency Medical Responder on the scene to once again assume manual cervical spine control so that Susan can strap the patient to the board. You quickly assess the patient's breathing and note that the respirations are shallow and rapid. His skin color is cyanotic. You attach the bag-valve-mask (BVM) device to oxygen and begin to ventilate the patient at 20 respirations per minute. The Emergency Medical Responder is helping to maintain the head in neutral alignment. You ask her what she saw. She tells you, "I was driving along behind the pickup truck that struck him. The truck veered right off the road and struck him. It threw him about 60 or 70 feet. He landed on the top of his head. He wasn't wearing a helmet. I stopped to help, and he was unconscious when I got to him."

Susan performs a rapid physical assessment and finds a depressed area of his skull on the right parietal region, blood in his right ear, a fracture of his left ankle, and a large bruise on his upper right abdomen. The abdomen appears to be slightly distended. His right pupil is fixed and dilated, and the left is slow to respond to light. His skin is cool and clammy, he has a weak and rapid radial pulse, the breath sounds are clear and equal bilaterally, and his SpO$_2$ is 95%. Susan checks for a pain response. The patient responds by moving his arms across his chest, and his hands rotate inward, his back arches, and his feet extend. You are relieved to look up and see paramedic Ed Nixon and his partner, Connie Buck, approaching. You give a report to Ed and quickly help place the patient in the ALS ambulance. You return to the station, clean up your ambulance, and prepare for another call.

1. Rolling the patient quickly on his side to suction his airway
   a. should have been delayed until after the oropharyngeal airway was placed.
   b. should not have been performed until after ALS took over management.
   c. was an appropriate and important action to take.
   d. should have been delayed until he was immobilized on the long spine board.

2. This patient is most likely suffering from
   a. a high-level brain stem injury.
   b. injury to the lateral cerebrum.
   c. a low-level brain stem injury.
   d. injury to the cerebral cortex.

3. The patient may be ventilated at _____ ventilations/minute.
   a. 12
   b. 14
   c. 18
   d. 20

4. This patient is likely suffering from
   a. hypoperfusion from bleeding into a body cavity.
   b. hypoperfusion from bleeding into the head.
   c. shock from the fractured left ankle.
   d. spinal shock from the head injury.

5. The patient's fractured ankle
   a. should have been immobilized prior to placement on the long spine board.
   b. should have been immobilized with a splint prior to transport by ALS.
   c. should not have been immobilized because it would delay transport.
   d. should have been stabilized with sandbags and tape.

TRIP #		EMERGENCY	BILLING USE ONLY			

EMERGENCY TRIP SHEET

			BILLING USE ONLY
TRIP #			
MEDIC #			DAY
BEGIN MILES			DATE
END MILES			RECEIVED
CODE___/___	PAGE___/___		DISPATCHED
UNITS ON SCENE			

NAME			SEX M F DOB ___/___/___	EN-ROUTE
ADDRESS			RACE	ON SCENE
CITY	STATE		ZIP	TO HOSPITAL
PHONE ( ) -		PCP DR.		AT HOSPITAL
RESPONDED FROM			CITY	IN-SERVICE

TAKEN FROM	ZIP	CREW	CERT	STATE #
DESTINATION	REASON			
SSN - -	MEDICARE #	MEDICAID #		
INSURANCE CO	INSURANCE #	GROUP #		
RESPONSIBLE PARTY	ADDRESS			
CITY	STATE ZIP PHONE ( ) -			
EMPLOYER				

IV THERAPY
SUCCESSFUL Y N # OF ATTEMPTS _____
ANGIO SIZE _____ga.
SITE _____
TOTAL FLUID INFUSED _____ cc
BLOOD DRAW Y N INITIALS

TIME	ON SCENE (1)	ON SCENE (2)	ON SCENE (3)	EN-ROUTE (1)	EN-ROUTE (2)	AT DESTINATION
BP						
PULSE						
RESP						
SpO$_2$						
ETCO$_2$						
EKG						

INTUBATION INFORMATION
SUCCESSFUL Y N # OF ATTEMPTS _____
TUBE SIZE _____ mm
TIME _____ INITIALS _____

MEDICAL HISTORY	CONDITION CODES				
	TREATMENTS				

MEDICATIONS		TIME	TREATMENT	DOSE	ROUTE	IN
ALLERGIES						
C/C						

EVENTS LEADING TO C/C

ASSESSMENT

TREATMENT

	GCS E___V___M___TOTAL =
	GCS E___V___M___TOTAL =
	HOSPITAL CONTACTED

	CPR BEGUN BY B P TIME BEGUN
EMS SIGNATURE	AED USED Y N BY:
	RESUSCITATION TERMINATED - TIME

( ) OSHA REGULATIONS FOLLOWED

Spinal Column and Spinal Cord Trauma

| STANDARD

Trauma (Content Area: Head, Facial, Neck, and Spine Trauma)

| COMPETENCY

Applies fundamental knowledge to provide basic emergency care and transportation based on assessment findings for an acutely injured patient.

| OBJECTIVES

After reading this chapter, you should be able to:

32-1. Define key terms introduced in this chapter.

32-2. Describe the structure and function of the spinal column, spinal cord, and tracts within the spinal column.

32-3. Recognize common mechanisms of spinal injury and describe the incidence of neurological deficits in patients with spinal column trauma.

32-4. Give examples of forces that would produce each of the following mechanisms of spinal injury:
   a. Compression
   b. Flexion
   c. Extension
   d. Rotation
   e. Lateral bending
   f. Distraction
   g. Penetration

32-5. Differentiate spinal column injury and spinal cord injury.

32-6. Describe the concept of complete spinal cord injury and differentiate between the concepts of spinal shock and neurogenic hypotension.

32-7. Describe the concept of incomplete spinal cord injury and syndromes that may result from incomplete spinal cord injury.

32-8. Use scene size-up, patient assessment, and patient history to develop an index of suspicion for spinal injuries.

32-9. Given a series of scenarios, demonstrate the assessment-based management of patients suspected of having an injury to the spine.

32-10. Demonstrate the assessment of pulse, motor function, and sensory function in the extremities of a patient who is suspected of having an injury to the spine.

32-11. Recognize signs and symptoms of injury to the spinal column and spinal cord.

32-12. Explain how complications of spinal injury may result in inadequate breathing, paralysis, and inadequate circulation.

32-13. Describe appropriate emergency medical care for the patient with suspected spinal injury.

32-14. Describe correct immobilization techniques for the following:
   a. Supine or prone patient
   b. Standing patient
   c. Seated patient

32-15. Describe the indications for rapid extrication and the correct procedures for rapid extrication.

32-16. Explain special handling and immobilization considerations when spinal injury is suspected for the following:
   a. Helmet removal
   b. Football injuries, including removal of face mask and immobilization
   c. Infants and children, including extrication from a car seat

KEY IDEAS

As an EMT, you may encounter patients with potential spinal injuries in a wide variety of settings. Each encounter must be grounded in the recognition that improper movement and handling of such patients could easily lead to permanent disability or even death. This chapter focuses on the assessment and management of spinal injuries.

- The spinal column, which serves to protect the spinal cord, is the principal support system of the body. It is made up of 33 vertebrae; each pair of vertebrae is separated by a disc.

- Common mechanisms of spinal injury include compression, flexion, extension, rotation, lateral bending, distraction, and penetration, which may occur as a result of collisions, falls, diving accidents, and so on.

- A spinal (vertebral) column injury is an injury to the portion of the spine composed of bone. A spinal cord injury involves damage to the nervous tissue contained within the spinal cord. A spinal column injury will generally result in a complaint of pain or tenderness somewhere along the length of the spine and is a potential indicator of spinal column fracture. A patient with a spinal cord injury may have a complete or incomplete spinal cord injury.

- A complete spinal cord injury is a result of complete transection of the spinal cord. The injury does not allow motor or sensory impulses to pass down the cord; therefore, there is a total loss of motor and sensory function below the level of injury. Incomplete spinal cord injury occurs when the spinal cord is injured, but not completely. The three most common types of incomplete spinal cord injury are the central cord syndrome, anterior cord syndrome, and Brown-Séquard syndrome.

- Suspicion of injury to the spine or spinal cord is based primarily on the assessment findings and sets the standard for subsequent emergency care for the patient. All assessment and care must be conducted with extreme caution to avoid excessive movement and manipulation of the body. In-line spinal stabilization must be maintained throughout the entire patient contact.

- Once established, manual stabilization must not be released until the patient is securely strapped to a backboard with head and neck immobilized.

- The goal of emergency management of suspected spinal cord injury is to ensure that life-threatening conditions are cared for, that the possibility of further injury is reduced through careful handling, and that the patient is properly immobilized and expeditiously transported.

- The tools associated with spinal immobilization include cervical spine immobilization collars, full-body spinal immobilization devices, and short spinal immobilization devices.

TERMS AND CONCEPTS

1. Write the number of each term next to its definition.

1. Autonomic nervous system
2. Central nervous system
3. Peripheral nervous system
4. Voluntary nervous system

_____ a. The portion of the nervous system that influences deliberate muscle movement

_____ b. The structures of the nervous system located outside the brain and spinal cord

_____ c. The portion of the nervous system that influences involuntary muscles and glands

_____ d. The portion of the nervous system consisting of the brain and the spinal cord

2. Label the diagram with the following spinal column divisions:

Cervical spine
Coccyx
Lumbar spine
Sacral spine
Thoracic spine

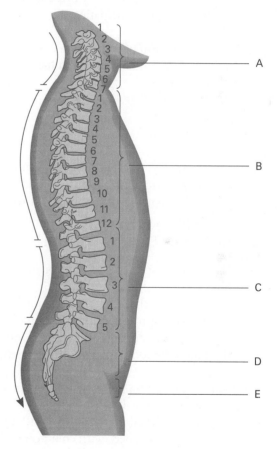

CONTENT REVIEW

1. Mark an X beside each mechanism of injury or type of emergency scene that should make you especially alert to the possibility of spinal injury.

_____ a. Electrical injury

_____ b. Blunt trauma

_____ c. Fall

_____ d. Heart attack

_____ e. Motorcycle crash

_____ f. Gunshot wound to the head, neck, chest, abdomen, back, or pelvis

_____ g. Acute asthmatic attack

_____ h. Hanging

_____ i. Diving accident

_____ j. Unresponsive trauma patient

2. Which of the following would apply to a patient who is found lying unresponsive in an alley beside an apartment building?
   a. Assume that the patient has a psychological problem.
   b. Maintain a high index of suspicion for spinal injury.
   c. Manage the patient by placing the patient directly on the stretcher and transporting rapidly.
   d. Quickly place the patient in a lateral recumbent position.

3. This mechanism of spinal injury occurs when the vertebrae and spinal cord are stretched or pulled apart and is common in hangings. It is called
   a. flexion.
   b. lateral bending.
   c. extension.
   d. distraction.

4. Which statement is correct regarding the signs and symptoms associated with spinal injury?
   a. Diaphragmatic breathing is indicative of a thoracic spine injury.
   b. The patient should move about to try to locate the area of spinal pain.
   c. Priapism, if present, is a classic sign of cervical spine injury.
   d. Obvious deformity of the spine upon palpation is a common finding.

5. When assessing for pulses, motor function, and sensory function in the patient with a spine injury, you should
   a. bilaterally check the brachial and popliteal pulses for strength and equality.
   b. assess motor function by having the patient lift his shoulders and feet slightly.
   c. check the sensory function by lightly touching both knees and elbows.
   d. pinch the foot and hand to determine a sensory response if the patient is unresponsive.

6. When positioning the patient for manual spinal stabilization, the nose should be aligned with the navel, and the head should be
   a. slightly flexed forward in a "sniffing" position.
   b. slightly extended, with chin pointing up.
   c. neither flexed nor extended.
   d. both flexed and extended.

7. Which of the following regarding cervical spine immobilization collars (CSICs) is correct?
   a. Soft collars permit needed lateral movement.
   b. The collar provides complete immobilization of the spine.
   c. The size of the collar is important, but not critical.
   d. The collar should be applied by two rescuers.

8. For each type of patient listed in the following table, indicate with an X or a check mark the appropriate device or technique required to immobilize the patient properly.

Patient Type	Standing Immobilization Technique	Rapid Extrication	Apply Vest-Type Immobilization Device	Immobilize to Backboard
Standing patient				
Seated patient with critical injuries				
Seated patient with no critical injuries				
Supine or prone patient				

9. Mark an X beside each treatment that would be an appropriate management technique for a patient with a spine injury.

_____ a. The EMT must attempt to diagnose the condition and locate the exact site of spinal injury.

_____ b. If in doubt as to whether a spinal injury is present, always immobilize the patient.

_____ c. Manual in-line spinal stabilization should be established as soon as patient contact is made.

_____ d. If the patient complains of severe neck or spine pain or the head does not easily move, the patient's head should be immobilized in the position found.

_____ e. Use the head-tilt, chin-lift airway maneuver to maintain the airway.

_____ f. Following immobilization, reassess, record, and document the pulses, motor function, and sensory function in all extremities.

10. When performing the log roll technique of spinal immobilization,
a. you must always use four rescuers.
b. avoid placing padding on the board to prevent slipping.
c. the CSIC should be placed before movement.
d. immobilize the patient's head to the board before the torso is immobilized.

11. The steps in the following list describe the procedure for immobilizing a supine or prone patient. Number the steps in the proper order from 1 to 7.

_____ Place pads in the spaces between the patient and the board.

_____ Establish and maintain in-line manual stabilization.

_____ Apply a CSIC.

_____ Immobilize the patient's torso to the board with straps.

_____ Log-roll the patient onto the long spine board.

_____ Secure the patient's legs to the board.

_____ Immobilize the patient's head to the board.

12. Identify the best description of immobilization of a standing patient.
    a. Walk him to the cot and have him lie on the backboard placed there.
    b. Immobilize him from a standing position while maintaining alignment.
    c. Have him sit on the backboard and then carefully help him lie down.
    d. Patients who are able to stand or walk do not require immobilization.

13. A short spinal immobilization device
    a. is chiefly used to immobilize a critical sitting patient with a spinal injury.
    b. does not require the use of a long spine board.
    c. does not generally require the use of a CSIC.
    d. requires that the torso be secured prior to the head.

14. Rapid extrication is indicated if
    a. the patient's condition is stable.
    b. the patient is on a scene that is safe.
    c. the patient blocks access to a critical patient.
    d. the patient complains of severe pain.

15. Safe and effective rapid extrication requires which of the following?
    a. Constant cervical spine stabilization
    b. Application of a short spine board or vest-type immobilization device
    c. Application of only a cervical spine immobilization collar with no manual stabilization
    d. At least one rescuer

16. Removal of a helmet
    a. should, generally, not be attempted if the helmet fits well.
    b. is always required, even if the patient is breathing adequately.
    c. can be adequately performed by one rescuer working carefully.
    d. should be performed only on motorcycle helmets, not football helmets.

17. Which of the following describes what is generally the *best* care for a football player with potential spinal injury?
    a. Leave the helmet and shoulder pads in place.
    b. Remove the helmet, but leave the shoulder pads in place.
    c. Cut away and remove all clothing and equipment.
    d. Remove both the helmet and the shoulder pads.

18. Spinal shock usually results from injury of the _____ region of the spine.
    a. cervical
    b. thoracic
    c. lumbar
    d. sacral

19. Which of the following findings is commonly associated with neurogenic shock?
    a. Moist, cool, clammy skin
    b. Pulse rate of 60–80/minute
    c. Irregular respirations of 12–20/minute
    d. Pale skin color

20. Neurogenic shock results in
   a. a "relative" hypovolemia.
   b. massive vasoconstriction.
   c. excessive fluid loss.
   d. a temporary fluid overload.

21. A patient who has been involved in a motor vehicle crash complains of neck pain, weakness, and loss of pain sensation in the upper extremities, while the lower extremities have good function. The patient most likely has
   a. anterior cord syndrome.
   b. central cord syndrome.
   c. anterio-lateral syndrome.
   d. Brown-Séquard syndrome.

22. Identify with an X the following physical findings as being associated with complete spinal cord injury, anterior cord syndrome, central cord syndrome, or Brown-Séquard syndrome.

Findings	Complete Spinal Cord Injury	Anterior Cord Syndrome	Central Cord Syndrome	Brown-Séquard Syndrome
Upper extremity loss of motor and sensory function				
Lower extremity loss of motor and sensory function				
Loss of bowel and bladder control				
Upper extremity weakness or paralysis and loss of pain sensation, with motor and sensory functions normal in the lower extremities				
Loss of ability to feel pain and crude touch/ loss of motor function; will retain the ability to feel light touch below the injury site				
Loss of motor function and light touch sensation but retain sensation to pain on one side of the body, while experiencing a loss of pain on the opposite side but retaining motor function and light touch sensation				

❘ CASE STUDY

You have been dispatched for a young woman injured in a softball game. You arrive at a local college softball complex and observe a 20-year-old female softball player lying supine on the ground next to home plate. The coach tells you that she was the catcher and was accidentally struck in the head with a bat. She was unconscious for about a minute. She regained consciousness and is now alert and oriented. She complains of neck and head pain.

1. When immobilizing this patient,
   a. only prevention of lateral movement is required.
   b. pad voids under the head and torso.
   c. use a vest-type device in addition to the long spine board.
   d. carefully pad behind the CSIC.

2. Manual in-line stabilization can be released
   a. following application of the CSIC.
   b. just prior to movement onto the long spine board.
   c. following placement of the patient on the long spine board, but just prior to immobilization of the head to the board.
   d. following immobilization of the head to the long spine board.

3. A minimum of _____ straps should be used to ensure proper immobilization.
   a. two
   b. three
   c. four
   d. five

CHAPTER 32 SCENARIO: DOCUMENTATION EXERCISE

Read the following scenario and think about how you would document this call if you were the EMT who responded to the scene. Then answer the multiple-choice questions and fill in the sample prehospital care report, basing your documentation on information from the scenario.

It is 2:45 A.M. on a Saturday night—or actually Sunday morning. You have been asleep since 1:00 A.M., when you returned from a call for a hit pedestrian. The alarm sounds and wakes you from a deep sleep: "Unit 4, respond to 6th Street NW and Avenue D NW for a two-car collision. Time out 0245 hours." You jump out of bed and arrive at the rescue vehicle at the same time as your partner, Carly. You advise dispatch that you are responding, and dispatch advises that Engine One and law enforcement are also responding. You arrive on scene in about three minutes.

Two cars are involved: a silver Cadillac and a white Toyota Camry. The Cadillac struck the Camry in the passenger-side door. The Cadillac does not appear to be damaged. The impact broke the glass in the Camry's door and pushed the door about a couple of inches into the passenger compartment. The air bags deployed in both vehicles. The firefighters on scene advise you that the driver of the Cadillac fled the scene, and the driver of the Camry is the only patient. Jack, a burly firefighter, waves you over to the Camry, where the driver of the vehicle is sitting behind the steering wheel with his seat belt on. Jack walks around to the rear driver-side door and positions himself behind the driver. He establishes manual in-line stabilization of the driver's cervical spine, explaining to the driver who he is and why he is holding his head. You and Carly circle the car quickly to check for additional hazards and mechanisms of injury. No other damage is noted to the car other than the damage on the passenger side.

The driver appears to be about 25 years old. His eyes are open. He has a small laceration on his forehead. His skin color is normal, and he appears to be in stable condition. You introduce yourself and Carly to the driver, and say, "We are EMTs, and we're here to help you. Where do you hurt?" You reach down and feel his radial pulse, which is rapid and strong. His skin is warm and dry. He is breathing adequately, and there are no audible, abnormal respiratory sounds. The patient is keeping his head and neck very still as he says, "My neck. It really hurts! It started just after the crash. That idiot! He ran the red light! I was just driving along, and he slams into me. Then he jumps out of his car and takes off. What a jerk! . . . My neck really hurts!" You say, "Do you hurt anyplace else?" "No," he says.

"What is your name?" you ask. "Wardell Johnson," he replies. You say, "Wardell, I need you to keep your head and neck still and don't move at all. I know Jack told you that's why he's holding your head, to help you keep still. Carly and I are going to take some vital signs and ask you some additional questions. Then we are going to place you in a special immobilization device that will help to keep your head and neck from moving. We are concerned that you may have damaged your spine, and—again—it is important to keep your head and neck still. Do you understand this? Do you have any questions?" He moves his eyes to look at you and says, "Yes, I understand. I'll keep my head as still as I can. I really appreciate you guys helping me!" You say, "We're glad to help you, Wardell."

Carly climbs in the passenger side of the car and performs a rapid physical exam. She tells you that she finds nothing and quickly checks the neck again before placing a cervical spine immobilization collar on Wardell. She starts to take vital signs while you begin a history. You ask, "Wardell, you don't hurt anyplace else? Is that correct?" "That is right," Wardell says. You ask, "Are you allergic to any medications?" "Not a thing!" Wardell replies. You next ask, "Are you taking any medications, or have you ever been injured or sick before?" Wardell quickly responds, "Nope!" You continue by saying, "OK, so when was the last time you ate or drank something?" He says, "Well, I guess it was about 1:00 A.M. or so. I stopped at The Clock restaurant and grabbed something to eat after I got off work. I had a burger, a soda, and some fries." Carly reports Wardell's vital signs. He is alert and oriented to person, place, and time; his respirations are normal at 14 per minute; his skin is warm, dry, and of normal color; his pupils are equal and reactive and respond briskly to light; his blood pressure is 124/68; and his SpO$_2$ is 96%.

You ask Carly to get the cot, the short spinal immobilization device, and the long spine board while you continue with your assessment. You say to Wardell, "Don't try to, but can you move your hands and feet?" "Yes, I can," he says. "Do you have any numbness or tingling sensations in your arms or legs?" you ask. "Well, I do have some weakness in both arms but not my legs," Wardell states in a tentative voice. "Did you move about after the accident?" you continue. "No, I knew that I was hurt. I didn't move a bit," Wardell replies.

"All right, Wardell, I'm going to ask you to perform some tasks for me. It involves checking for pulses, the ability to move your fingers and toes, and sensation in both your arms and legs. I'm going to start with your hands." You assess for pulses in each extremity, for sensation (pain and light touch) in each extremity, and for motor movement. Wardell's pulses are present and equal, and he has weakness and loss of a pain response in his upper extremities and good sensation to pain and light touch in his lower extremities. He is able to perform all tests for motor function appropriately. Carly returns with the equipment, and you prepare to immobilize Wardell. You carefully immobilize him with the short spine immobilization device and move him to the cot for transport to the hospital.

1. The injury sustained by Wardell is most likely the result of
   a. compression.
   b. flexion.
   c. extension.
   d. lateral bending.

2. Improper management and stabilization of Wardell's injury could produce complications. Three major complications of spinal injury are
   a. inadequate breathing effort, hemiplegia, and inadequate circulation.
   b. cerebral hypoxia, hemiplegia, and inadequate circulation.
   c. inadequate breathing effort, paralysis, and inadequate circulation.
   d. cerebral hypoxia, paralysis, and circulatory overload.

3. The presence of weakness in Wardell's arms is
   a. not an important physical finding.
   b. a significant finding of a spinal injury.
   c. not generally important unless accompanied by paralysis.
   d. most likely the result of a stress reaction.

4. Following immobilization of Wardell in the short spinal immobilization device, you and Carly should
   a. rapidly transport Wardell to the hospital.
   b. reevaluate the pulse, motor function, and sensory function.
   c. place Wardell on the long spine board.
   d. tie Wardell's hands together.

5. When securing Wardell to the long spine board, straps (at a minimum) should be positioned at the
   a. hips and above the knees.
   b. hips, above the knees, and below the knees.
   c. arms, hips, and below the knees.
   d. chest, hips, and above the knees.

EMERGENCY TRIP SHEET

TRIP #	
MEDIC #	
BEGIN MILES	
END MILES	
CODE___/___ PAGE___/___	
UNITS ON SCENE	

BILLING USE ONLY

DAY				
DATE				
RECEIVED				
DISPATCHED				
EN-ROUTE				
ON SCENE				
TO HOSPITAL				
AT HOSPITAL				
IN-SERVICE				

NAME   SEX M F DOB ___/___/___

ADDRESS   RACE

CITY   STATE   ZIP

PHONE ( )   -   PCP DR.

RESPONDED FROM   CITY

TAKEN FROM   ZIP

CREW	CERT	STATE #

DESTINATION   REASON

SSN   -   -   MEDICARE #   MEDICAID #

INSURANCE CO   INSURANCE #   GROUP #

RESPONSIBLE PARTY   ADDRESS

CITY   STATE   ZIP   PHONE ( )   -

IV THERAPY
SUCCESSFUL Y N # OF ATTEMPTS _____
ANGIO SIZE _____ga.
SITE _____
TOTAL FLUID INFUSED _____ cc
BLOOD DRAW Y N INITIALS

EMPLOYER

INTUBATION INFORMATION
SUCCESSFUL Y N # OF ATTEMPTS _____
TUBE SIZE _____ mm
TIME _____ INITIALS _____

TIME	ON SCENE (1)	ON SCENE (2)	ON SCENE (3)	EN-ROUTE (1)	EN-ROUTE (2)	AT DESTINATION
BP						
PULSE						
RESP						
SpO$_2$						
ETCO$_2$						
EKG						

MEDICAL HISTORY

CONDITION CODES				

TREATMENTS

TIME	TREATMENT	DOSE	ROUTE	INIT

MEDICATIONS

ALLERGIES

C/C

EVENTS LEADING TO C/C

ASSESSMENT

TREATMENT

GCS E___ V___ M___ TOTAL =

GCS E___ V___ M___ TOTAL =

HOSPITAL CONTACTED

CPR BEGUN BY   B   P   TIME BEGUN

AED USED   Y   N   BY:

RESUSCITATION TERMINATED - TIME

EMS SIGNATURE

( ) OSHA REGULATIONS FOLLOWED

Eye, Face, and Neck Trauma

▌ STANDARD

Trauma (Content Area: Head, Facial, Neck, and Spine Trauma)

▌ COMPETENCY

Applies fundamental knowledge to provide basic emergency care and transportation based on assessment findings for an acutely injured patient.

▌ OBJECTIVES

After reading this chapter, you should be able to:

33-1. Define key terms introduced in this chapter.

33-2. Describe the anatomy and function of the eye, face, and structures of the neck.

33-3. Discuss special considerations in the assessment and management of patients with injuries to the eye, face, and neck, including:
   a. Airway compromise
   b. Profuse bleeding
   c. Potential that injuries may be self-inflicted or due to violence
   d. Patient fears associated with these injuries

33-4. Discuss the assessment-based management of patients with injuries to the eye, face, and neck.

33-5. Demonstrate the assessment and management of specific injuries of the eye, including:
   a. Foreign body in the eye
   b. Injury of the orbit
   c. Injury to the eyelid
   d. Injuries to the globe of the eye
   e. Chemical burns to the eye
   f. Impaled objects in the eye
   g. Extruded eyeball

33-6. Explain the indications and procedure for removing contact lenses from an injured eye.

33-7. Demonstrate the assessment and management of specific injuries of the face, including:
   a. Facial fracture
   b. Avulsed tooth
   c. Impaled object in the cheek
   d. Injury to the nose
   e. Injury to the ear

33-8. Demonstrate the assessment and management of specific injuries of the neck, including:
   a. Penetrating injury to the neck
   b. Blunt injury to the neck

▌ KEY IDEAS

Injuries to the eyes, face, or neck have a high probability of causing airway compromise, severe bleeding, and shock. Injuries to the face and neck also are associated with spinal injury. When the potential for these life-threatening conditions exists, establish manual stabilization of the head and neck, open the airway with the jaw-thrust maneuver, and suction as needed. Consider ALS backup for advanced airway care. If necessary, administer supplemental oxygen to maintain an SpO₂ of 94% or greater.

■ Basic rules for emergency care of eye injuries include the following: Consult medical direction before irrigating foreign objects from the eye and before removing contact lenses, do not remove blood or blood clots from the eye, do not apply salve or medicine, do not try to force the eyelid open unless chemicals must be flushed out, flush a chemically burned eye for at least 20 minutes, stabilize an object that is impaled in the eye, cover both the injured eye and the uninjured eye to prevent unnecessary movement, give the patient nothing by mouth, and always transport for evaluation by a physician.

■ Injuries to the face include injury to the midface, jaw, nose, and ear, and objects impaled in the cheek. For severe injuries to the face, suspect and treat for cervical spine injury and immediately manage airway, breathing, and circulation problems. Consider advanced life support to provide advanced airway care. An object impaled in the cheek should be stabilized with bulky dressings. If the object has penetrated the cheek all the way and it may obstruct the airway, remove the object.

■ With any blunt or penetrating trauma to the neck, maintain a high index of suspicion for cervical spine injury. Due to the possibility of swelling, crushed airway structures, debris, and clotted blood, maintaining an airway also is extremely important.

▌ TERMS AND CONCEPTS

1. Write the number of each term next to its definition.
   1. Aqueous humor
   2. Conjunctiva
   3. Cornea
   4. Iris
   5. Pupil
   6. Lens
   7. Retina
   8. Sclera
   9. Vitreous humor

   _____ a. Portion of the eye that covers the pupil and the iris

   _____ b. Fluid that fills the anterior chamber of the eye

   _____ c. Clear jelly that fills the large chamber of the eye

   _____ d. Back of the eye

   _____ e. Outer coating of the eye; the white of the eye

   _____ f. Colored portion of the eye that surrounds the pupil

   _____ g. Thin covering of the inner eyelids and exposed portion of the sclera of the eye

   _____ h. The dark center of the eye

   _____ i. The portion of the eye that focuses light on the retina

2. Label the diagram of the eye with the appropriate terms from the following list.

aqueous humor

conjunctiva

cornea

iris

lens

pupil

retina

sclera

vitreous humor

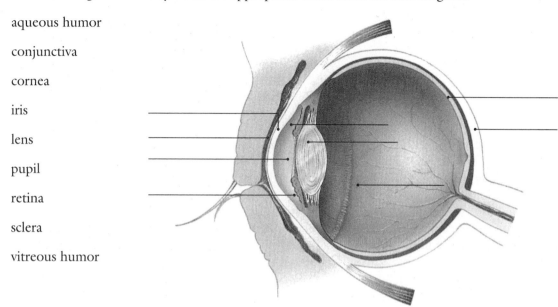

▌ CONTENT REVIEW

1. When conducting the secondary assessment and physical exam on a patient with an eye injury,
   a. evaluate the pupils for size by applying direct pressure to the globe.
   b. check for appropriate eye movement up and down only.
   c. check the lids for bruising, swelling, and laceration by direct visualization.
   d. check the globe for redness and abnormal coloring by pulling the eyelid open.

2. During the primary assessment of a patient with facial trauma, establish manual stabilization of the head and neck
   a. after assessing the facial trauma.
   b. on first contact with the patient.
   c. following application of oxygen.
   d. while examining the eyes with a penlight.

3. Suspect significant damage to the eye if
   a. vision improves only after blinking.
   b. the field of vision increases.
   c. there is an injury to the forehead or cheek.
   d. there is unusual sensitivity to light.

4. Which of the following is considered appropriate when treating an injured eye?
   a. Remove blood clots from the sclera with a sterile dressing.
   b. Force the eyelids open, if necessary, to examine the pupils.
   c. Have the patient walk or lean forward to reduce pressure on the eye.
   d. Transport the patient for evaluation covering both eyes.

5. Only attempt to remove foreign particles that are lodged in which of the following?
   a. Conjunctiva
   b. Cornea
   c. Globe
   d. Retina

6. You are treating a patient with a lacerated eyelid. Your treatment and management of this patient should include
   a. covering the eye with a dry, sterile dressing.
   b. application of direct pressure to control bleeding.
   c. frequently checking for visual acuity in the uninjured eye.
   d. preserving any avulsed skin and transporting with the patient.

7. Your patient, who presents with double vision (diplopia), a marked decrease in vision, and loss of sensation above the eyebrow, over the cheek, or in the upper lip, is most likely suffering from a(n)
   a. chemical eye burn.
   b. orbital fracture.
   c. laceration to the eyelid.
   d. laceration of the globe.

8. When should you begin treatment of a suspected chemical burn of the eye?
   a. During the primary assessment
   b. After a rapid trauma assessment
   c. After the secondary assessment and physical exam
   d. During the reassessment

9. You are treating a patient with a chemical burn to the eyes. The eyes should be flushed from the inside corner to the outside edge for at least
   a. 5 minutes.
   b. 10 minutes.
   c. 15 minutes.
   d. 20 minutes.

10. In which of the following positions would you place the patient with an impaled or extruded eye injury?
    a. Fowler position
    b. Lateral recumbent position
    c. Supine position
    d. Prone position

11. Contact lenses
    a. are never worn by people who wear glasses.
    b. are always worn in both eyes.
    c. can be clearly seen by using a penlight.
    d. should not be removed in chemical burns to the eye.

12. You are treating a patient who has sustained an eye injury and is wearing soft contacts. Which of the following is the correct way to remove a soft contact lens?
    a. Pinch the lens between your thumb and index finger.
    b. Press the lower eyelid under the bottom edge of the lens.
    c. Apply a moistened suction cup.
    d. Slide a fingernail under the edge of the lens and lift.

13. Your patient presents with a painful, deformed, and swollen jaw and has dentures that are still intact and in place. How should this be managed?
    a. Leave the dentures in place.
    b. Remove dentures if the patient requests it.
    c. Contact medical direction for instructions.
    d. Dentures should always be removed.

14. Your patient is suffering from facial trauma with exposed nerves and tendons. You should do which of the following?
    a. Apply a moist, sterile dressing to the injury.
    b. Apply a dry, sterile dressing to the injury.
    c. Do not cover; it may damage the nerves.
    d. Cover exposed tissues with an occlusive dressing.

15. Your patient has presented you with an avulsed tooth resulting from facial trauma. You should
    a. scrub it with water and place it in a saline solution.
    b. rinse it with saline and place it in a saline solution.
    c. scrub it with saline and place it in dry gauze.
    d. rinse it with water and place it in an alcohol solution.

16. Your patient has an impaled nail that has penetrated the cheek all the way through and is loose. What should you do?
    a. Stabilize it, and be prepared to remove it from the airway.
    b. Stabilize it with bulky dressings, and transport.
    c. Pull it out in the same direction from which it entered.
    d. Push it out in the direction opposite to the way it entered.

17. To prevent a patient from swallowing a dressing that is packed between the teeth and cheek, you should do which of the following?
    a. Place a gloved index finger into the mouth to hold the dressing.
    b. Have the patient hold onto one end of the dressing.
    c. Tape some of the dressing material to the outside of the mouth.
    d. Never place a dressing into the mouth because it may block the airway.

18. You suspect your patient has a nasal fracture. Which of the following is the most appropriate for treating this type of injury?
    a. Gently pull to align the nose, and transport.
    b. Apply cold compresses, and transport.
    c. Apply a pressure dressing, and transport.
    d. Pack the nostrils, and transport.

19. You are assessing your patient and notice a clear fluid draining from the ear. You should do which of the following?
    a. Pack the ear with dressings.
    b. Apply pressure dressings.
    c. Apply direct pressure.
    d. Place a loose dressing across the opening.

20. Your patient has a severed blood vessel in the neck. You should
    a. apply pressure to both sides of the neck at the same time.
    b. use a loosely placed, moist, sterile dressing.
    c. use a figure-eight wrap to secure the dressing.
    d. position the patient on his left side, head up.

21. You are assessing your patient who has an eye injury and notice blood in the anterior chamber of the eye. You know this condition as
    a. bipolar.
    b. hyphema.
    c. hemophilia.
    d. myopia.

22. You are preparing to treat a critically injured patient with a midfacial injury. Your initial management priorities should be to
    a. establish spinal stabilization with a cervical collar, control bleeding, ensure a patent airway, and assist breathing.
    b. ensure a patent airway, establish stabilization of the cervical spine, support breathing, and obtain baseline vital signs.
    c. establish manual spinal stabilization, ensure a patent airway, support breathing, and control life-threatening bleeding.
    d. manage life-threatening bleeding, manage the cervical spine, ensure a patent airway, and support breathing.

▌ CASE STUDY

You and your partner are at the scene of an overturned car. Your patient is a 22-year-old male. He is responsive and supine, with battery acid burns to the eyes and a deep laceration to the left side of the neck that is bleeding heavily. Your partner will maintain manual stabilization of the head and neck.

1. Should you consider advanced life support backup for this patient? Explain your answer.

2. Which of the following best describes the sequence that should be followed?
    a. Assess the patient, provide emergency care, and then transport.
    b. Assess the patient, provide emergency care, and wait for the paramedics.
    c. Provide emergency care for life-threatening injuries first, assess the patient, treat other injuries, and then transport.
    d. Transport immediately, provide emergency care, and meet the paramedics en route.

3. Which of the following describes the best treatment for this patient's injuries?
    a. Immediately begin flushing the eyes with saline. Simultaneously, place a gloved hand over the neck wound to control bleeding and administer high-concentration oxygen.
    b. Immediately begin flushing the eyes with saline. Probe the neck wound to locate and apply pressure to the carotid artery, then administer high-concentration oxygen.
    c. Immediately stop the profuse bleeding from the neck wound. Then begin flushing the eyes with saline. Administer high-concentration oxygen as soon as you can.
    d. Once bleeding is under control and you have administered oxygen, check with medical direction to find out if you can flush the patient's eyes with saline.

CHAPTER 33 SCENARIO: DOCUMENTATION EXERCISE

Read the following scenario and think about how you would document this call if you were the EMT who responded to the scene. Then answer the multiple-choice questions and fill in the sample prehospital care report, basing your documentation on information from the scenario.

It's about 10:30 P.M. on a warm summer evening. You and your partner, Prudence, are completing a continuing education program homework assignment. The alarm sounds and startles you: "Unit 7, respond to the Wild Buck Club at 8204 Bush Boulevard, cross street Lincoln Avenue, for a fight. Law enforcement is responding. Time out 2230 hours." You meet your partner at the vehicle, quickly remove the shoreline (the electrical connection from the station to the ambulance that provides electrical power to charge batteries and to run heaters, computers, lights, and so on), and advise dispatch that you are responding. Dispatch tells you law enforcement advises that the scene is secure and one patient has been stabbed. You arrive in front of a nightclub that is located in a formerly abandoned retail shopping center. The parking lot is full of patrons. A large crowd is milling about near two police cars parked in front of the club. You tell dispatch of your arrival on scene. Dispatch responds, "Affirmative. Unit 7 on scene at 2237 hours."

With Standard Precautions taken, you exit the vehicle and walk toward the crowd. A police officer waves you over to his location. The crowd moves so that you can get to the patient. You observe what appears to be a 20-year-old male patient lying in a supine position. A bystander is holding a towel on the left side of the patient's neck. There is a large pool of blood next to the patient. The patient's left eye is swollen shut. The right eye is open, and the patient acknowledges your presence by moving his right hand. His skin color is good, and he appears to be breathing adequately, with no obvious respiratory sounds heard. You and Prudence kneel down next to the patient. You reach down and feel his radial pulse, which is rapid and weak. You introduce yourself and Prudence, and say, "We are EMTs, and we're here to help you. Can you tell me what happened?"

You note a strong odor of alcohol as the patient says, "I was trying to talk to this girl that I just met, and this guy runs up to me and hits me in the face with his fist, and then he stabs me in my neck! I'm really worried about my eye. I was seeing double before my eye got so swollen." You ask his name. He tells you it is Richard Mraz. Prudence inspects the neck wound and finds bleeding from a laceration on Richard's left neck about an inch lateral to the trachea at the level of the larynx. Prudence quickly covers the wound with a dressing and applies direct pressure to control the bleeding. You tell dispatch that you need an ALS unit. Dispatch lets you know that they are responding and are about five minutes away from the scene. Prudence asks a bystander, who identified himself as an EMR, to assume direct pressure on the neck wound while another EMR stabilizes the neck. Prudence then takes the vital signs while you prepare to immobilize the patient to the long spine board.

You begin a rapid trauma assessment. Your assessment reveals that the left eye is swollen shut and that the patient complains of numbness just above the left eye. The bleeding from the wound on the patient's neck is controlled, the trachea is midline, breath sounds are clear and equal bilaterally, and a small laceration is found on his right hand. You place a CSIC on the patient, cut his clothing away, and roll him onto the long spine board. You obtain a history from Richard and determine that he is complaining of pain in the eye and neck and denies any other pain or complaint. He has no allergies and doesn't take any medications. He has no prior medical history. He last ate about 7:00 P.M. and had a large meal. Prudence reports the vital signs: Respirations are 20 per minute, full, and normal; the pulse is 98 per minute, weak, and regular; the skin color is pale, warm, and moist; the right pupil responds normally to light; the blood pressure is 100/80; and the SpO$_2$ is 97%.

You place Richard on the stretcher just as the ALS unit arrives. You provide a brief patient report to the paramedic and assist in placing the patient in the ALS unit.

1. When assessing Richard's pupils, Prudence should
   a. perform a normal pupil check.
   b. carefully check both eyes for visual acuity.
   c. cover both eyes and not check the pupils.
   d. check the pupil in the right eye and then cover both eyes.

2. Which of the following best describes how to secure a figure-eight bandage over the neck wound?
   a. Over the dressing, around the neck, under the armpit on the side of the injury, back around the neck, and anchored at the shoulder
   b. Over the dressing, across one shoulder, across the back, under the opposite armpit, and anchored at the shoulder
   c. Over the dressing, around the neck, and anchored at the neck
   d. Over the dressing, around the neck, under the armpit on the side of the injury, and anchored at the shoulder

3. Richard complained about numbness over his left eye and double vision (diplopia). These complaints are most likely the result of
   a. the injury to the neck.
   b. an injury to the orbit of the eye.
   c. trauma to the globe of the eye.
   d. hypoperfusion.

4. Prudence should apply what kind of dressing to Richard's neck injury?
   a. Gauze
   b. Self-adhering
   c. Porous
   d. Occlusive

5. Richard's neck injury
   a. is not serious since Richard is alert and oriented.
   b. is not serious unless Richard has difficulty in speaking or a loss of voice.
   c. is not serious since the trachea remains at midline.
   c. must be carefully observed for swelling and airway compromise.

TRIP #							BILLING USE ONLY			

EMERGENCY TRIP SHEET

TRIP #				BILLING USE ONLY			
MEDIC #							
BEGIN MILES				DAY			
MILES				DATE			
CODE___/___	PAGE___/___			RECEIVED			
UNITS ON SCENE				DISPATCHED			
NAME		SEX M F DOB ___/___/___		EN-ROUTE			
ADDRESS		RACE		ON SCENE			
CITY	STATE	ZIP		TO HOSPITAL			
PHONE ( ) -	PCP DR.			AT HOSPITAL			
RESPONDED FROM		CITY		IN-SERVICE			
TAKEN FROM		ZIP		CREW	CERT	STATE #	
DESTINATION		REASON					
SSN - -	MEDICARE #	MEDICAID #					
INSURANCE CO	INSURANCE #	GROUP #					
RESPONSIBLE PARTY	ADDRESS						
CITY	STATE ZIP PHONE ( ) -			IV THERAPY			
EMPLOYER				SUCCESSFUL Y N # OF ATTEMPTS ____			

TIME	ON SCENE (1)	ON SCENE (2)	ON SCENE (3)	EN-ROUTE (1)	EN-ROUTE (2)	AT DESTINATION
BP						
PULSE						
RESP						
SpO$_2$						
ETCO$_2$						
EKG						

ANGIO SIZE _____ga.
SITE _____
TOTAL FLUID INFUSED _____ cc
BLOOD DRAW Y N INITIALS

INTUBATION INFORMATION
SUCCESSFUL Y N # OF ATTEMPTS ____
TUBE SIZE _____ mm
TIME _____ INITIALS _____

MEDICAL HISTORY

CONDITION CODES

MEDICATIONS

TREATMENTS

TIME	TREATMENT	DOSE	ROUTE	INIT

ALLERGIES

C/C

EVENTS LEADING TO C/C

ASSESSMENT

TREATMENT

GCS E___V___M___TOTAL =

GCS E___V___M___TOTAL =

HOSPITAL CONTACTED

CPR BEGUN BY B P TIME BEGUN

EMS SIGNATURE

AED USED Y N BY:

RESUSCITATION TERMINATED - TIME

( ) OSHA REGULATIONS FOLLOWED

Chest Trauma

STANDARD

Trauma (Content Area: Chest Trauma)

COMPETENCY

Applies fundamental knowledge to provide basic emergency care and transportation based on assessment findings for an acutely injured patient.

OBJECTIVES

After reading this chapter, you should be able to:

34-1. Define key terms introduced in this chapter.
34-2. List the major structures of the thoracic cavity.
34-3. Define and list specific types of open chest injury.
34-4. Define and list specific types of closed chest injury.
34-5. Explain the pathophysiology of each of the following injuries:
    a. Flail segment
    b. Pulmonary contusion
    c. Open pneumothorax, tension pneumothorax, hemothorax
    d. Traumatic asphyxia
    e. Cardiac contusion
    f. Pericardial tamponade
    g. Rib injury
    h. Commotio cordis
34-6. Discuss an assessment-based approach to manage patients with chest trauma.
34-7. Discuss the following aspects of chest trauma care:
    a. General emergency care for chest trauma
    b. Specific emergency care for an open chest wound
    c. Specific emergency care for a flail segment

KEY IDEAS

Injuries to the chest can be easily overlooked in the physical assessment because clothing hides potential physical findings unless the areas are exposed for examination. Injury to vital organs in the chest can quickly cause lethal disturbances in respiration, oxygen exchange, and circulation. The EMT must rely on the mechanism of injury, a high index of suspicion, and careful physical examination in order to anticipate and manage these potential life threats.

- A closed chest injury is the result of blunt trauma to the chest, and an open chest wound is the result of a penetrating injury, both of which can cause extensive damage to ribs and the underlying internal organs.

- Remember these points when assessing the patient with a chest injury: Establish and maintain in-line spinal stabilization and administer oxygen; quickly expose the chest and examine it; note any sign of respiratory distress; immediately seal any open wound with a gloved hand; and if there is paradoxical movement, continuous positive airway pressure (CPAP) or positive pressure ventilation with supplemental oxygen is the ideal treatment. A patient with an open chest wound sealed with an occlusive dressing requires careful monitoring of respiratory status. Patients with chest injuries are a high priority; immediate transport with assessment and care continuing en route is required. Early recognition and prompt transport is key.

- Emergency care of an open chest injury includes the points already described and, additionally, observing for signs of a developing tension pneumothorax: difficulty breathing with increasing respiratory distress, tachypnea, severely decreased or absent breath sounds on the injured side, tachycardia, decreasing blood pressure with a narrowing pulse pressure, jugular vein distention, tracheal deviation, unequal movement of the chest wall, and increasing resistance to positive pressure ventilation.

- Significant findings for a chest injury include a mechanism of injury involving either blunt or penetrating trauma, signs of trauma, early signs and symptoms of shock, cyanosis, dyspnea, absent or decreased breath sounds on auscultation, tachypnea or bradypnea, hemoptysis, pulsus paradoxus, jugular vein distention, systolic blood pressure that drops by more than 10 mmHg during inhalation, and tracheal deviation.

- Specific chest injuries include flail segment, pulmonary contusion, pneumothorax, open pneumothorax, tension pneumothorax, hemothorax, traumatic asphyxia, cardiac tamponade, and rib injury.

MEDICAL TERMINOLOGY

Term	Prefix	Word Root Combining Form	Suffix	Definition
atelectasis (at-uh-LEK-tuh-sis)		atel (imperfect)	-ectasis (dilation, distention)	Condition in which the lungs have collapsed or are airless
eupnea (yoop-NEE-uh)	eu- (good, normal)	-pnea (breathing)		Good or normal breathing
hemopneumothorax (HEE-moh-NEW-moh-THOR-aks)		hem/o (blood); pneum/o (lung, air); thorax (chest)		Accumulation of blood and air in the thoracic cavity, causing collapse of a portion of the lung
hemoptysis (hee-MOP-tuh-sis)		hem/o (blood)	-ptysis (to spit, spitting)	Spitting up of blood

Term	Prefix	Word Root Combining Form	Suffix	Definition
hemorrhage (HEM-uh-rij)		hem/o (blood)	-rrhage (to burst forth, bursting forth)	Excessive bleeding
hemothorax (hee-moh-THOR-aks)		hem/o (blood); thorax (chest)		Accumulation of blood in the thoracic cavity, causing collapse of a portion of the lung
orthopnea (or-THOP-nee-uh)		orth/o (straight)	-pnea (breathing)	Inability to breathe unless in an upright position
pneumothorax (new-moh-THOR-aks)		pneum/o (lung, air); thorax (chest)		Accumulation of air in the thoracic cavity, causing collapse of a portion of the lung
pulmonectomy (pull-mohn-EK-tuh-mee)		pulmon (lung)	-ectomy (surgical excision)	Surgical removal of the lung or part of the lung (synonym: pneumonectomy)
tracheostomy (tray-kee-OSS-tuh-mee)		trache/o (trachea)	-stomy (new opening)	New opening created into the trachea

1. The home health nurse tells you that your patient had an episode of hemoptysis. You know that the word root *hemo* means "blood" and the suffix *-ptysis* refers to
   a. vomiting.
   b. spitting.
   c. artery.
   d. lung.

2. In your patient care report, you describe your patient's breathing as *eupnea*. What does the prefix *eu-* mean?
   a. Clear, unremarkable
   b. Loud, noisy
   c. Difficult, labored
   d. Good, normal

3. Your patient is suffering from a hemothorax. The word root *thorax* refers to
   a. chest.
   b. blood.
   c. air, lung.
   d. abdomen.

4. While transferring your patient to the hospital staff, you hear the nurse state that the patient suffers from orthopnea. You know that the parts of this word—the word root *ortho* and the suffix *-pnea*—mean
   a. blood, lung.
   b. damaged, lung.
   c. difficult, breathing.
   d. straight, breathing.

5. While reviewing your patient's medical records at a local care facility, you note that the patient has a tracheostomy. You know the word root *trache/o* means trachea and the suffix *-stomy* means
   a. inflammation of.
   b. new opening.
   c. surgical removal.
   d. constriction, closing.

TERMS AND CONCEPTS

1. Write the number of each term beside its definition.
   1. Flail segment
   2. Paradoxical movement
   3. Pneumothorax
   4. Sucking chest wound
   5. Tension pneumothorax
   6. Pericardial tamponade

   _____ a. A segment of the chest wall that moves inward during inhalation and outward during exhalation

   _____ b. An open injury to the chest that permits air to enter the thoracic cavity during inhalation

   _____ c. Two or more consecutive ribs that are fractured in two or more places

   _____ d. Air in the chest cavity, outside the lungs

   _____ e. A condition in which the buildup of air and pressure in the thoracic cavity on the injured side is so severe that it begins to shift the lung on that side to the uninjured side, resulting in compression of the heart, vessels, and the uninjured lung

   _____ f. A condition in which the fibrous sac around the heart fills with blood and decreases the ability of the ventricles to fill and eject blood effectively

CONTENT REVIEW

1. A hollow area located in the middle of the thoracic cavity between the right and left lungs is called the
   a. central chest cavity.
   b. medial chest region.
   c. mediastinum.
   d. pneumocentric.

2. The pleura consist of the visceral pleura and parietal pleura. Which statement describes the parietal pleura?
   a. The parietal pleura is the outermost layer of the pleura.
   b. The parietal pleura is in contact with the lungs.
   c. The parietal pleura lines the abdominal cavity.
   d. The parietal pleura is where gas is exchanged in the lungs.

3. Jugular veins that engorge during inhalation may be a sign of a
   a. developing flail segment.
   b. pericardial tamponade.
   c. simple pneumothorax.
   d. hemothorax.

4. You are treating a patient who has been stabbed in the chest. There is a puncture wound that penetrates the parietal and visceral pleura, with air being sucked into the pleural space. As the pleural space expands, you would suspect which of the following to occur?
   a. The expanding pressure will cause a hemothorax.
   b. The space will expand, resulting in a hematoma.
   c. A pneumothorax will develop, leading to a collapsed lung.
   d. The internal and external pressures will equalize, causing a flail chest.

5. While treating your patient, you find that a section of the anterior chest wall moves in a direction opposite to the rest of the chest wall. You identify this as a
   a. paradoxical segment.
   b. lateral chest syndrome.
   c. pleural cavity segment.
   d. flail segment.

6. The mechanism of injury suggests an open chest injury. You should quickly expose and examine the patient's chest during which phase of the patient assessment?
   a. Primary assessment
   b. Physical examination
   c. Secondary assessment
   d. Reassessment

7. Some patients with chest wall injury will breathe with extremely shallow, rapid breaths. What is the probable reason?
   a. The patient is hyperventilating.
   b. It is an attempt to reduce pain.
   c. It is an attempt to relieve hypoxia.
   d. The patient is hyperglycemic.

8. Upon palpation of your patient's neck, you feel a crackling sensation. You also observe an inflated appearance to the same region. What is the condition described, and what is the potential cause?
   a. Pneumocutaneous pooling; blood pooling in the subcutaneous tissue of the neck
   b. Pneumocutaneous syndrome; air flowing upward and being trapped under the skin
   c. Subcutaneous phenomenon; blood pooling in the subcutaneous tissue of the neck
   d. Subcutaneous emphysema; air flowing upward and being trapped under the skin

9. Which of the following is the correct way to identify tracheal deviation?
   a. Palpate the trachea immediately above the cricoid cartilage.
   b. Palpate the trachea immediately above the suprasternal notch.
   c. Inspect the trachea visually above the cricoid cartilage.
   d. Inspect the trachea visually just inferior to (below) the suprasternal notch.

10. Your patient is exhibiting signs and symptoms of a flail segment with paradoxical movement of the chest. What is the ideal way to treat this condition?
    a. Place a nonporous dressing over the site.
    b. Place the patient on the uninjured side.
    c. Provide CPAP.
    d. Place a gloved hand over the injured site.

11. Which of the following best describes auscultated lung sounds produced during a tension pneumothorax?
    a. Absent breath sounds on the uninjured side; decreased breath sounds on the injured side
    b. Absent breath sounds at the lower lobes; decreased breath sounds at the upper lobes
    c. Absent breath sounds on the injured side; decreased breath sounds on the uninjured side
    d. Absent breath sounds at the upper lobes; decreased breath sounds at the lower lobes

12. Which of the following describes physical findings that suggest an ominous sign of a severe chest injury requiring immediate transport?
    a. A decreasing heart rate, decreasing blood pressure, and increasing respiratory distress
    b. An increasing heart rate, decreasing blood pressure, and increasing respiratory distress
    c. An increasing heart rate, increasing blood pressure, and increasing respiratory distress
    d. A decreasing heart rate, increasing blood pressure, and increasing respiratory distress

13. The serious condition often caused by blunt trauma, which causes bleeding to occur in and around the alveoli and into the interstitial space that separates the capillaries and alveoli, is known as
    a. pulmonary contusion.
    b. pneumatic hematoma.
    c. pneumohemorrhage.
    d. pulmonic tension.

14. Which traumatic chest injury may result in a narrowing pulse pressure?
    a. Cardiac contusion
    b. Traumatic asphyxia
    c. Hemothorax
    d. Pericardial tamponade

15. Your patient presents with severe chest pain upon movement and breathing. There is tenderness and crepitus on palpation of the right lateral chest, and you suspect simple rib fractures. Which of the following is considered an appropriate technique for managing this injury?
    a. Apply a sling and swathe to the arm located on the opposite side of the chest injury.
    b. The patient holds a book firmly over the site, applying heavy pressure.
    c. The patient guards the injury by placing his arm tightly over the injury site.
    d. Apply a swathe or tape circumferentially, snugly, and completely around the chest.

16. You arrive on the scene where a 12-year-old boy was struck in the chest by a baseball during a game. The patient was successfully resuscitated from cardiac arrest by use of an on-site AED. You suspect the young man was suffering from which of the following?
    a. Cardiac tamponade
    b. Commotio cordis
    c. Tension pneumothorax
    d. Paradoxical syndrome

| CASE STUDY

You and your partner are on the scene of a fall. An injured tree trimmer is lying on the ground among fallen branches. You immediately take in-line spinal stabilization. You introduce yourself and your partner. The patient can speak only a word or two at a time and must breathe in between. Your partner quickly exposes the patient's body to find an open chest wound under the left breast. You immediately call for advanced life support backup.

1. Which of the following is the correct immediate treatment for the chest wound?
   a. Place an occlusive dressing on the wound during the primary assessment.
   b. Place an occlusive dressing on the wound during the secondary assessment.
   c. Seal the wound with a gloved hand during the primary assessment.
   d. Seal the wound with a gloved hand during the secondary assessment.

The patient is now unresponsive and requires ventilatory assistance. Your partner states that it is becoming increasingly harder to squeeze the bag-valve-mask (BVM) device to ventilate the patient. You note cyanosis of the fingertips and quickly palpate the trachea through the examination hole in the cervical spine immobilization collar (CSIC). The trachea appears to be deviated or shifted to the right side. Further examination reveals jugular vein distention. You quickly auscultate the lungs and find that breath sounds are absent on the left and decreased on the right.

2. The changes in respiratory status of this patient indicate which possible condition, and what steps should be taken to rectify the problem?
   a. Flail segment with paradoxical movement; support with pressure from your hand.
   b. Flail segment with paradoxical movement; continue to provide positive pressure ventilations.
   c. Tension pneumothorax; transport immediately.
   d. Tension pneumothorax; lift the corner of the occlusive dressing on the chest wound to allow air to escape and transport immediately.

CHAPTER 34 SCENARIO: DOCUMENTATION EXERCISE

Read the following scenario and think about how you would document this call if you were the EMT who responded to the scene. Then answer the multiple-choice questions and fill in the sample prehospital care report, basing your documentation on information from the scenario.

While receiving the report from the previous shift's crew, you and your partner, EMT Meads, are preparing to inventory the ambulance when the station alerting system sounds: "Unit 4, respond to 3344 Ocean Drive for a person who fell from a ladder. ALS backup is not, repeat not, available." Meads acknowledges the call as you both walk to the front of the ambulance. While en route to the call, you approach the railroad tracks and notice that the guard gates are down and a train is approaching. You advise dispatch that you will have a train delay. After the short train has passed, you advise dispatch that you are back en route to the call.

You soon arrive on the scene of a construction site and notify dispatch. As you and Meads quickly scan the area for obvious hazards, you see a bystander motioning you to the area where the patient is lying. After you pull up, you both take Standard Precautions and proceed to the rear of the ambulance. You place all of the equipment that you may need on the stretcher and quickly make your way toward the patient. You find the patient lying on his left side on the ground next to a tall ladder. A worker states, "Fred was up on the ladder about 12 feet when he and the ladder fell to the ground." Meads positions herself at the patient's head and maintains in-line stabilization of the spine as he asks the patient his name and age. The patient responds, "Fred. I'm 22." Meads introduces you and herself to Fred, then asks him where he hurts. Fred replies, "My left chest hurts a lot!"

Meads says, "He is breathing about 26 times a minute with shallow breathing. There is adequate air flowing in and out of the mouth." A quick check of the pulse reveals a strong, regular pulse at approximately 100 beats per minute. The skin is warm and dry, with a capillary refill of less than 2 seconds. You palpate the neck. It is soft, with no trauma or subcutaneous emphysema noted. The trachea is palpated and found to be midline, and there is no deformity or pain to the posterior neck. As you place the cervical collar on the patient, Meads explains how you will be placing him on the backboard. Because the patient is already lying on his left side, you quickly cut his shirt to expose the back. No deformities are noted or felt. You place the backboard next to the patient and carefully roll him onto the board with the assistance of two coworkers. The patient is quickly secured to the backboard, and you and Meads begin a rapid secondary assessment.

You quickly cut away the clothing to the patient's anterior body. Meads states that the head reveals no injuries or deformities; the pupils are equal and react briskly to light. The nose, mouth, and ears are all clear of blood or fluid. The neck was assessed prior to application of the cervical collar. Meads palpates the chest and notes an area of the left chest that moves inward when the patient inhales and outward when the patient exhales. The patient is breathing with small, fast breaths and says, "It hurts when I take a deep breath." Lung sounds are diminished but equal. You inspect the axillary area. It is without injury. You quickly inspect the pelvis for deformity, contusions, abrasions, or penetrating injuries, and none is found. You assess the upper and lower extremities, and there is no deformity or pain on palpation. You proceed to check pulse, motor function, and sensory function, asking Fred if he can feel you touching his extremities. He replies, "Yes." You then ask him to wiggle his fingers and toes, and he does. Next, you check all four distal pulses and find them to be strong and regular.

Meads immediately begins to provide positive pressure ventilation with the BVM with supplemental oxygen. Next, you obtain vital signs while Meads continues to ventilate the patient. The blood pressure is 128/68; the pulse is 104 and regular. Respirations are supported at about 20 breaths each minute. The pulse oximeter reveals an SpO_2 at 98% with the BVM. Reassessment of the PMS reveals no changes. You ask Fred if he has any medical history, is on any medication, or is allergic to anything, and he responds, "No." You ask him what happened that caused him to fall; he explains that he lost his footing on the ladder, and it just went out from under him. You ask when his last oral intake was, and he states, "I had breakfast cereal about two hours ago."

Meads states that she feels increased resistance to positive pressure ventilation. Fred's breathing becomes more labored with severe tachypnea. You check but do not note any tracheal tugging or deviation. You quickly auscultate his chest and find diminished lung sounds on the left side. You notice slight cyanosis around his lips. A quick check of the pulse oximeter reveals an SpO_2 of 84%. After a short emergency response, you arrive at the trauma center.

1. When Meads palpated the chest, she noted an area of the left chest that moved inward when the patient inhaled and outward when the patient exhaled. What type of injury did Meads discover?
   a. Pneumothorax
   b. Flail segment
   c. Pericardial tamponade
   d. Hemothorax

2. Which action would be considered appropriate treatment for this patient?
   a. Splint the unstable chest segment in an outward position with the gloved hand.
   b. Place a circumferential splint made from the tightly applied swathe to the chest.
   c. Continue to provide positive pressure ventilations with the BVM while transporting.
   d. Position the patient on the injured side to help splint the flail segment.

3. EMT Meads stated that she felt increased resistance while providing positive pressure ventilation. You should suspect which of the following?
   a. The patient has developed pericardial tamponade.
   b. The diaphragm has ruptured.
   c. A tension pneumothorax has likely developed.
   d. The patient has developed a hemothorax.

4. Which of the following best describes a flail segment?
   a. Two or more consecutive ribs have been fractured in two or more places.
   b. A single rib has been fractured in two or more places.
   c. Three or more successive ribs have been fractured in one place, producing crepitus.
   d. Two or more ribs on the affected side have at least one fracture each.

EMERGENCY TRIP SHEET

TRIP #	
MEDIC #	
BEGIN MILES	
END MILES	
CODE____/____ PAGE____/____	
UNITS ON SCENE	

DAY			
DATE			
RECEIVED			
DISPATCHED			
EN-ROUTE			
ON SCENE			
TO HOSPITAL			
AT HOSPITAL			
IN-SERVICE			

NAME	SEX M F DOB ____/____/____
ADDRESS	RACE
CITY STATE	ZIP
PHONE ( ) - PCP DR.	
RESPONDED FROM	CITY
TAKEN FROM	ZIP
DESTINATION	REASON
SSN - - MEDICARE #	MEDICAID #
INSURANCE CO INSURANCE #	GROUP #
RESPONSIBLE PARTY ADDRESS	
CITY STATE ZIP PHONE ( ) -	
EMPLOYER	

CREW	CERT	STATE #

TIME	ON SCENE (1)	ON SCENE (2)	ON SCENE (3)	EN-ROUTE (1)	EN-ROUTE (2)	AT DESTINATION
BP						
PULSE						
RESP						
SpO$_2$						
ETCO$_2$						
EKG						

IV THERAPY
SUCCESSFUL Y N # OF ATTEMPTS _____
ANGIO SIZE _____ga.
SITE _____
TOTAL FLUID INFUSED _____ cc
BLOOD DRAW Y N INITIALS

INTUBATION INFORMATION
SUCCESSFUL Y N # OF ATTEMPTS _____
TUBE SIZE _____ mm
TIME _____ INITIALS _____

MEDICAL HISTORY

MEDICATIONS

ALLERGIES

C/C

EVENTS LEADING TO C/C

ASSESSMENT

TREATMENT

CONDITION CODES					

TREATMENTS

TIME	TREATMENT	DOSE	ROUTE	INIT

GCS E___ V___ M___ TOTAL =

GCS E___ V___ M___ TOTAL =

HOSPITAL CONTACTED

CPR BEGUN BY   B   P   TIME BEGUN

EMS SIGNATURE

AED USED   Y   N   BY:

RESUSCITATION TERMINATED - TIME

(   ) OSHA REGULATIONS FOLLOWED

Abdominal and Genitourinary Trauma

STANDARD

Trauma (Content Area: Abdominal and Genitourinary Trauma)

COMPETENCY

Applies fundamental knowledge to provide basic emergency care and transportation based on assessment findings for an acutely injured patient.

OBJECTIVES

After reading this chapter, you should be able to:

35-1. Define key terms introduced in this chapter.
35-2. Describe the anatomy of the abdominal cavity and its contents.
35-3. Differentiate hollow and solid organs and vascular structures in the abdomen.
35-4. Give examples of both blunt and penetrating mechanisms of abdominal trauma and discuss the potential for severe internal bleeding.
35-5. Discuss an assessment-based approach to management of the patient with open and closed abdominal injury, including evisceration and impaled objects.
35-6. Recognize signs and symptoms associated with injuries to the abdomen.
35-7. Explain the general emergency medical care for abdominal trauma.
35-8. Explain the emergency medical care for abdominal evisceration.
35-9. Explain the special considerations in management of trauma to the male and female genitalia.

KEY IDEAS

Like chest injuries (discussed in the previous chapter), abdominal injuries can be easily overlooked in the physical assessment because clothing hides potential physical findings unless the areas are exposed for examination. Injury to vital organs in the abdomen can quickly cause lethal disturbances in respiration, oxygen exchange, and circulation. The EMT must rely on the mechanism of injury, a high index of suspicion, and careful physical examination in order to anticipate and manage these potential life threats.

- Abdominal injuries are broadly classed as open or closed injuries. Open wounds to the abdomen include evisceration, in which organs protrude through the skin. Closed abdominal injuries can crush, tear, or rupture a large number of organs, causing severe internal bleeding.

- Assessment of abdominal injury includes recognizing that such injury can cause excruciating pain, so much so that other injuries or problems may not be noticed by the patient. A mechanism of injury that involves either blunt or penetrating trauma, signs of trauma, early signs and symptoms of shock, shallow and rapid respirations, and abdominal pain and rigidity is showing significant signs of serious abdominal injury.

- Emergency care of both open and closed abdominal injuries includes aggressive management and monitoring of the airway, breathing, oxygenation, and circulation. Early recognition and prompt transport is key. In abdominal evisceration, apply a moist dressing over protruding organs, cover with an occlusive dressing, and add a second dressing over that. Secure the dressings in place with tape, cravats, or a bandage.

- While injuries to the genitalia are rarely life threatening, they are typically extremely painful and embarrassing. They may have a number of causes, including sexual assault. Treat such injuries as you would any soft tissue injury.

| MEDICAL TERMINOLOGY

Term	Prefix	Word Root Combining Form	Suffix	Definition
visceral (VISS-er-ul)		viscer (body organs)	-al (pertaining to)	Pertaining to a body organ
retroperitoneal space (retro-peri-TON-e-al) space	retro- (backward, behind)	peritoneal (the membrane that lines the walls of the abdominal cavity)		Space located behind the peritoneum
evisceration ee-VIS-cer-a-shun	e-	viscer (body organs)	-al (pertaining to)	Body organs protrude through an open wound

1. The retroperitoneal space is located
   a. in front of the peritoneum.
   b. behind the peritoneum.
   c. lateral to the peritoneum.
   d. within the peritoneum.

2. *Viscer* refers to
   a. body organs.
   b. internal body chemical reactions.
   c. a skin condition.
   d. a disorder related to the lower bowel.

TERMS AND CONCEPTS

1. Write the number of each term beside its definition.

   1. Abdominal evisceration
   2. Peritonitis
   3. Peritoneal cavity
   4. Retroperitoneal cavity
   5. Kehr sign

   _____ a. The space located behind the peritoneal cavity

   _____ b. Abdominal organ protrusion through an open wound to the lower torso

   _____ c. Irritation and inflammation of the abdominal lining

   _____ d. The anterior abdominal cavity that houses the majority of the abdominal organs and is lined by the peritoneum

   _____ e. Severe shoulder pain referred from a hemorrhaging injury within the abdominal cavity and associated irritation of the diaphragm

CONTENT REVIEW

1. Identify each organ in the following list as either a hollow (H) or a solid (S) organ.
   _____ Stomach
   _____ Liver
   _____ Gallbladder
   _____ Kidneys
   _____ Fallopian tubes
   _____ Spleen
   _____ Ureters
   _____ Pancreas

2. Which organ is located in the retroperitoneal cavity?
   a. Liver
   b. Spleen
   c. Duodenum
   d. Superior vena cava

3. The major complication associated with the laceration, or tearing, of a solid organ is
   a. major bleeding.
   b. diaphragmatic rupture.
   c. the release of highly acidic gastric juices.
   d. intense pain.

4. A patient presents with signs of abdominal trauma and complains of shoulder pain. This is a referred pain and may be caused by blood irritating the diaphragm. This is called the
   a. Van Camp sign.
   b. Callie sign.
   c. Kehr sign.
   d. Davis sign.

5. Often abdominal injuries produce only subtle signs and symptoms. Therefore, you must base your treatment and transport decisions on which of the following?
   a. The patient's motor response
   b. The patient's sensory response
   c. The mechanism of injury
   d. Bystander information

6. When assessing a patient with abdominal pain, start palpating the abdomen
   a. without regard to the pain.
   b. at the upper right quadrant.
   c. closest to or directly over the pain.
   d. farthest from the pain.

7. If no injury to the lower extremities, hips, pelvis, or spine is suspected, place a patient with a closed abdominal injury in a
   a. lateral recumbent position with both legs flexed.
   b. Trendelenburg position with the legs flexed at the hips.
   c. supine position with the legs flexed at the knees.
   d. Fowler position with the legs straight.

8. Which of the following dressings is most appropriate to use with an abdominal evisceration?
   a. Sterile, dry paper dressing covered with plastic wrap or aluminum foil
   b. Sterile, absorbent cotton soaked in saline and covered with an occlusive dressing
   c. Sterile dressing soaked in saline and covered with plastic wrap as an occlusive dressing
   d. Sterile dressing soaked in saline and covered by a bulky dressing

9. You are treating a female who has a laceration to her external genitalia. Which of the following is the correct way to control the bleeding?
   a. Apply direct pressure, using a moistened sterile compress.
   b. Apply direct pressure, using your gloved hand.
   c. Pack the vagina with a sterile moist dressing.
   d. Place a moist dressing on the laceration and cover with plastic wrap.

10. Hollow organs typically
    a. contain substances that can be spewed out and cause severe damage or infection.
    b. cause little harm or damage if ruptured or lacerated.
    c. are very vascular and bleed heavily if ruptured or lacerated.
    d. are not typically ruptured, damaged, or injured.

11. The outermost layer of the abdominal cavity is lined by the
    a. visceral peritoneum.
    b. parietal peritoneum.
    c. sagittal peritoneum.
    d. lateral peritoneum.

12. The muscle that separates the abdominal and chest cavity is the
    a. rectus abdominal.
    b. lateral abdominal.
    c. diaphragm.
    d. abdominal dome muscle.

13. During exhalation, at what anatomical level is the structure described in question 12 located?

   a. At the level of the umbilicus
   b. Just inferior to the umbilicus level
   c. Just below the nipple line
   d. At the nipple line

CASE STUDY

You and your partner are on the scene of a bar fight. An intoxicated patron was attacked and was cut in the genitalia region. The injured man is sitting in a chair as you approach. You observe a significant amount of blood on the ground, in the chair, and on the man's clothing. You introduce yourself and your partner. The patient looks at you and appears to be in severe pain. Your partner helps the man to the stretcher, quickly exposes the area, and uses direct pressure to control moderate bleeding. The patient's penis has been amputated.

   1. Which of the following is the best method of transporting an amputated male genital body part?

   a. Wrap it in a dry, sterile dressing and put in a plastic bag with ice chips or cubes.
   b. Wrap it in a dry, sterile dressing, cover with an occlusive dressing, and place on ice.
   c. Wrap it in a saline-moistened, sterile dressing and cover with an occlusive dressing.
   d. Wrap it in a saline-moistened, sterile dressing, put this in a plastic bag, and place the bag on a cold pack.

   2. What is the best method to control bleeding with this patient?

   a. Use a cold compress.
   b. Use direct pressure.
   c. Use a pressure point.
   d. Use a tourniquet.

CHAPTER 35 SCENARIO: DOCUMENTATION EXERCISE

Read the following scenario and think about how you would document this call if you were the EMT who responded to the scene. Then answer the multiple-choice questions and fill in the sample prehospital care report, basing your documentation on information from the scenario.

While you are talking to your supervisor about a previous call at the station, the alerting system sounds: "Unit 6, respond to 1640 Lake Hollingsworth Drive for a person who fell from a roof. ALS backup is responding. Time out 1510 hours." Your partner, Sandy, acknowledges the call as you both walk to the front of the ambulance and jump in. Sandy confirms the location as you pull from the station.

You arrive in about four minutes and are at the scene of a large home that appears to be in the process of having the roof replaced. You notify dispatch that you are on scene. As you and Sandy scan the area for obvious hazards, you see a bystander waving you to the area where the patient is lying. You both take Standard Precautions, gather your gear

from the ambulance, and walk to the patient. You find the patient lying on his back on the ground next to a ladder leaning against the house. He has an obvious abdominal evisceration with a large segment of intestine protruding from his abdomen. Moderate bleeding is noted. He looks up at you as you approach. A worker tells you, "Bill was on the roof working with some sheet metal. He stepped off the side of the roof and I guess the metal cut him when he hit the ground." Sandy positions herself at the patient's head and maintains in-line stabilization of the spine as she asks the patient his name and age. The patient responds, "Bill and I'm 35." Sandy introduces you both to Bill and then asks him where he hurts. Bill replies, "I think it's pretty obvious. My belly hurts! My guts are hanging out!" Sandy asks if he hurts any place else. "Well my lower back hurts as well. I guess I hurt that when I fell, too. My stomach hurts a lot!"

Sandy says, "He is breathing about 20 times a minute with shallow breathing. There is adequate air flowing in and out of the mouth." You apply oxygen via a nasal cannula at 3 lpm. A quick check of the radial pulse reveals a strong, regular pulse at approximately 90 beats per minute. You notice the front of Bill's shirt has a bloodstain on the center of the abdominal area. The skin is warm and dry, with a capillary refill less than 2 seconds. You palpate the neck. It is soft, with no trauma or subcutaneous emphysema noted. The trachea is palpated and found to be midline, and there is no deformity or pain to the posterior neck. As you place the cervical collar on the patient, Sandy explains how you will be placing him on the backboard. You cut his shirt to expose the chest and abdomen. No deformities are noted or felt. You dress the abdominal injury and prepare him for transport. You request ALS backup.

A First Responder arrives on scene and takes over spinal immobilization for Sandy. You place the backboard next to the patient and prepare to move him on the long spine board. Sandy continues with a rapid secondary assessment.

Sandy states that the head reveals no injuries or deformities; the pupils are equal and react briskly to light. The nose, mouth, and ears are all clear of blood and fluid. The neck was assessed prior to application of the cervical collar.

Sandy palpates the chest, and Bill denies any pain on palpation. The patient is breathing normally. Bill breaks your routine when he tells you, "It's really strange, but my left shoulder hurts, right at the tip of my shoulder."

You make note of his complaint and then check lung sounds. They are equal bilaterally. You quickly inspect the pelvis for deformity, contusions, abrasions, or penetrating injuries, and none are found.

You assess the upper and lower extremities, and there is no deformity or pain on palpation. You proceed to check pulse, motor function, and sensory function, asking Bill if he can feel you touching his extremities. He replies, "Yes." You then ask him to wiggle his fingers and toes, and he is able to do so. You check all four distal pulses and find them to be strong and regular.

Next, you obtain vital signs. The blood pressure is 136/78; the pulse is 96 and regular. Respirations are 20 breaths each minute. The pulse oximeter reveals an SpO_2 at 97%. Reassessment of the PMS reveals no changes. You ask Bill if he has any prior medical history or is on any medication or is allergic to anything, and he responds, "No." You ask him what caused him to fall; he explains that he wasn't watching what he was doing and just stepped off the edge of the roof. You ask when he last ate or drank something. He says, "I had lunch about 4 hours ago and a bottle of water about 30 minutes ago."

Sandy prepares to log roll Bill onto the long spine board. Bill is immobilized to the long board. You recheck the abdominal wound. The ALS ambulance arrives, and paramedic Steve Bedsole approaches you and asks how he can help. You advise him that you will need his assistance moving the patient to the ambulance. The patient is moved to the ambulance, and the driver marks en route to the trauma center with dispatch.

While moving Bill to the ambulance, you explain what he should expect at the trauma center. You wish Bill well and close the doors to the ambulance. You clean up and prepare for the next call. You advise dispatch that you are returning to the station.

1. What type of dressing should you apply to the abdominal evisceration?
   a. Sterile dressing soaked with saline covered with an occlusive dressing
   b. Dry, sterile, absorbent cotton covered with a pressure dressing
   c. Saline-soaked sterile dressing covered with aluminum foil
   d. Occlusive dressing covered with a saline-soaked sterile dressing

2. Which action would be considered inappropriate treatment for this patient?
   a. Covering the abdominal dressing with an occlusive dressing
   b. Maintaining complete spinal immobilization
   c. Administering oxygen to maintain the SpO_2 at 94% or greater
   d. Flexing the legs up toward the chest to relieve pressure on the abdominal muscles

3. Bill's complaint of shoulder pain
   a. is not significant and likely just indicates trauma to the shoulder.
   b. may indicate abdominal trauma by pain referred from diaphragmatic irritation.
   c. may indicate chest trauma by pain referred from a rib fracture.
   d. may indicate head trauma by pain referred from a head injury.

EMERGENCY TRIP SHEET

TRIP #	
MEDIC #	
BEGIN MILES	
MILES	
CODE___/___ PAGE___/___	
UNITS ON SCENE	

BILLING USE ONLY			
DAY			
DATE			
RECEIVED			
DISPATCHED			
EN-ROUTE			
ON SCENE			
TO HOSPITAL			
AT HOSPITAL			
IN-SERVICE			

CREW	CERT	STATE #

NAME   SEX M F DOB ___/___/___

ADDRESS   RACE

CITY   STATE   ZIP

PHONE (   )   -   PCP DR.

RESPONDED FROM   CITY

TAKEN FROM   ZIP

DESTINATION   REASON

SSN   -   -   MEDICARE #   MEDICAID #

INSURANCE CO   INSURANCE #   GROUP #

RESPONSIBLE PARTY   ADDRESS

CITY   STATE   ZIP   PHONE (   )   -

EMPLOYER

IV THERAPY
SUCCESSFUL Y N # OF ATTEMPTS _____
ANGIO SIZE _____ga.
SITE _____
TOTAL FLUID INFUSED _____ cc
BLOOD DRAW Y N INITIALS

TIME	ON SCENE (1)	ON SCENE (2)	ON SCENE (3)	EN-ROUTE (1)	EN-ROUTE (2)	AT DESTINATION
BP						
PULSE						
RESP						
SpO$_2$						
ETCO$_2$						
EKG						

INTUBATION INFORMATION
SUCCESSFUL Y N # OF ATTEMPTS _____
TUBE SIZE _____ mm
TIME _____ INITIALS _____

MEDICAL HISTORY

CONDITION CODES

MEDICATIONS

TREATMENTS

TIME	TREATMENT	DOSE	ROUTE	INIT

ALLERGIES

C/C

EVENTS LEADING TO C/C

ASSESSMENT

TREATMENT

GCS E___ V___ M___ TOTAL =

GCS E___ V___ M___ TOTAL =

HOSPITAL CONTACTED

CPR BEGUN BY   B   P   TIME BEGUN

AED USED Y N BY:

RESUSCITATION TERMINATED - TIME

EMS SIGNATURE

(   ) OSHA REGULATIONS FOLLOWED

Multisystem Trauma and Trauma in Special Patient Populations

STANDARD

Trauma (Content Area: Multisystem Trauma; Special Considerations in Trauma)

COMPETENCY

Applies fundamental knowledge to provide basic emergency care and transportation based on assessment findings for an acutely injured patient.

OBJECTIVES

After reading this chapter, you should be able to:

36-1. Define key terms introduced in this chapter.

36-2. Discuss the increased morbidity and mortality associated with multisystem trauma.

36-3. Describe the importance of the golden principles of prehospital multisystem trauma assessment, care, and transport.

36-4. Summarize anatomical and physiological changes of pregnancy that create special considerations in assessing, managing, and transporting pregnant trauma patients.

36-5. Describe the relationship of maternal injuries to fetal distress and death.

36-6. Summarize anatomical and physiological changes in children that create special considerations in assessing, managing, and transporting pediatric trauma patients.

36-7. Summarize anatomical and physiological changes in the elderly that create special considerations in assessing, managing, and transporting geriatric trauma patients.

36-8. Discuss special considerations in assessing, managing, and transporting cognitively impaired trauma patients.

36-9. Discuss the assessment-based approach to multisystem trauma and trauma in special patient populations.

KEY IDEAS

In previous chapters, you have learned how to assess and manage an adult trauma patient properly. However, not every trauma patient is the same. Some trauma patients have multiple body systems that have been injured, which makes their assessment and care more challenging. Other patients may be a member of a special population, such as pregnant women, children, the elderly, and people with cognitive impairments, that can also require additional assessment and management skills. If the patient is a member of a special population, the EMT should be able to incorporate knowledge about that particular type of patient into the assessment and emergency care.

In this chapter, you will apply your knowledge of the patient with multiple body systems affected by trauma and the patient who is part of the special population affected by trauma. After completion of this chapter, you should be able to recognize life-threatening problems and properly treat the trauma patient, as well as ensure effective management and transport to a special receiving hospital. It is important to do the following:

- Ensure the safety of the rescue personnel and the patient.
- Understand that the EMT may determine the need for additional resources.
- Understand kinematics. Knowing the mechanism of injury can help the EMT anticipate injuries that the patient may have.
- Identify and manage life threats. Airway, ventilation, and oxygenation are key elements to the successful management of a multisystem trauma patient.
- Know the techniques for ventilating patients with and without suspected spinal injury.
- Know techniques to control external hemorrhage and treat for shock.
- Splint musculoskeletal injuries and maintain spinal immobilization on a long spine board.
- Understand the importance of performing a secondary assessment and obtaining a medical history.

❙ CONTENT REVIEW

1. You are assessing your patient, whom you suspect may have multisystem trauma injuries. You note that the steering wheel of the vehicle is bent and the windshield has an interior strike damage area. This type of observation is known as
   a. injury appraisal and damage assessment.
   b. trauma evaluation diagnosis test.
   c. understanding kinematics or the mechanism of injury.
   d. vehicle damage interpretation assessment.

2. As you approach your multisystem trauma patient and make patient contact, you immediately find arterial bleeding from the lower leg. You should
   a. immediately control the bleeding.
   b. assess the patient's mental status.
   c. assess the airway and ventilation effort.
   d. immediately assess the carotid pulse.

3. You are attending to a multisystem trauma patient involved in a fall. Which of the following must be performed simultaneously during the "rapid physical exam"?
   a. Insert an oral or nasogastric airway while applying the nonrebreather mask.
   b. Apply the appropriate flow of oxygen while assessing for disabilities.
   c. Control bleeding while assessing the pulse rate and rhythm.
   d. Manage the airway while maintaining cervical spinal stabilization.

4. Your multisystem trauma patient is breathing approximately six times a minute, with inadequate tidal volume. Your immediate action should be to
   a. apply oxygen via a nasal cannula.
   b. apply oxygen via a nonrebreather mask.
   c. ventilate with a bag-valve mask (BVM).
   d. ventilate with a Venturi mask.

5. You are treating a patient who has sustained a large leg wound that is bleeding profusely. You know that this condition can lead to cellular hypoxia and anaerobic metabolism. The loss of which of the following reduces the ability of the blood to carry and deliver oxygen to the cells?
   a. Hemoglobin
   b. Surfactant
   c. Serum
   d. Platelets

6. Your unstable multisystem trauma patient has sustained bilateral upper arm fractures. When should you stabilize and splint the arm fractures?
   a. While backboarding the patient
   b. Before assessing the pulse
   c. After the rapid physical exam
   d. While en route to the hospital

7. You are assessing a pregnant woman who you suspect has sustained traumatic injuries. There is a higher incidence of tension pneumothorax in the pregnant patient because
   a. the diaphragm is elevated.
   b. the lungs are weaker.
   c. the patient retains fluid.
   d. the intercostal muscles are weakened.

8. While treating a trauma patient who is in her second or third trimester of pregnancy, you know that placing her lying flat on her back can result in
   a. supine bradycardia.
   b. supine hypotension.
   c. supine fetal distress.
   d. supine tachypnea.

9. An expectant mother in her third trimester has fallen down a flight of steps. During your assessment, you find that she is having uterine contractions. You should
   a. gently massage the lower abdomen.
   b. pack the vagina to control bleeding.
   c. place the patient in the prone position.
   d. assess for crowning or bleeding.

10. You arrive on the scene of a late-term pregnant woman who was involved in a car crash. You find her pulseless. You should
    a. provide resuscitative efforts and transport to the medical facility for an attempt of resuscitation of the fetus.
    b. transport to the hospital without resuscitative efforts so the patient can be pronounced dead by the medical doctor.
    c. not move the patient from the scene and place a clean protective covering over the patient to preserve the scene.
    d. await the arrival of the ALS unit to determine if the patient is able to be resuscitated.

11. You have responded to a young child who will not stop crying. Which of the following leads you to suspect that the child may be a victim of abuse?
    a. The child's crying is continuous and relentless.
    b. The child has multiple injuries in various healing stages.
    c. You find a closed fracture of the upper arm.
    d. You note abrasions to both knees.

12. Which of the following statements pertaining to the anatomical and physiological differences between the adult and pediatric patient is true?
    a. The pediatric patient's body surface area is less than the adult patient's body surface area; thus, the child retains heat better.
    b. The pediatric patient's head weighs less; however, the neck muscles are more developed than in the adult patient.
    c. The location of the pediatric patient's internal organs, such as the spleen, makes the child less susceptible to injury.
    d. The pediatric patient's chest wall is more flexible and can allow for internal injuries with few external signs of injury.

13. Which side of the pediatric assessment triangle (PAT) developed by the American Academy of Pediatrics or the initial impression components found in the American Heart Association's Pediatric Advanced Life Support represents the "child's overall mental status"?
    a. Circulation or color
    b. Breathing
    c. Appearance or consciousness
    d. Cognitive ability

14. You are assessing a 9-month-old trauma patient involved in a fall. Your partner is assessing the pulse rate. Which pulse point is most appropriate for this patient?
    a. Brachial
    b. Carotid
    c. Femoral
    d. Radial

15. A 2-year-old pediatric patient has sustained multisystem trauma injuries from a motor vehicle crash. From the following, which is an unreliable way to assess the patient's perfusion status?
    a. Mental status
    b. Skin color
    c. Blood pressure
    d. Capillary refill

16. You are preparing to provide spinal immobilization for a 7-year-old trauma patient. Which of the following is an appropriate treatment for this patient?
    a. Place a pad beneath the patient from the shoulders to the hips.
    b. Apply a soft cervical collar to stabilize the neck and spine.
    c. Position the patient on a backboard, securing the head first.
    d. Apply manual traction to the cervical spine by pulling with steady pressure.

17. While assessing a pediatric trauma patient, you hear stridor. You know that this is
    a. an abnormal heart sound found in the trauma patient.
    b. caused by inadequate tissue perfusion.
    c. an indication of upper airway obstruction.
    d. a normal sound in the trauma patient.

18. You are treating an elderly trauma patient with a history of kyphosis. While placing the patient on the long backboard, you notice voids or space between the board and the patient's upper back. You should
    a. roll the patient to the left side and support the spine.
    b. remove the patient from the backboard and transport.
    c. gently assist the patient into a neutral position and secure.
    d. add padding to the voids to help stabilize the space.

19. While treating a cognitively impaired trauma patient, you note that he seems to be uncooperative. You should
    a. include the patient's caregiver in the emergency treatment to gain trust.
    b. position yourself slightly above the patient in an authoritative position.
    c. speak firmly while maintaining direct eye contact.
    d. gently use the power of touch to gain the patient's approval and trust.

▌CASE STUDY

You and your partner, Ivan, are preparing dinner at the station when the station alerting system sounds: "Unit 2 respond to an automobile accident with injuries at Beachland Boulevard and Ocean Drive." As you approach the scene and don your protective equipment, you scan the scene for hazards. You find a single car that has struck a utility pole. There is one patient lying supine on the ground next to the vehicle. The patient is obviously pregnant. The patient is unresponsive and breathing inadequately. She does not respond to verbal or painful stimulation.

1. You should perform which of the following immediately during the rapid physical examination?
    a. Splint any suspected fractures as they are discovered and assessed.
    b. Manage the airway while maintaining cervical spinal stabilization.
    c. Assess the patient's mental status by questioning what she can recall about the incident.
    d. Apply the cervical collar and position the patient on the backboard, utilizing cross straps.

Further examination indicates that the patient has sustained multiple fractures to the extremities. She also has a large wound to her right lower abdomen area that is bleeding profusely. Recognizing this is a critical patient, you call for additional resources, including a trauma helicopter to transport her to the appropriate hospital.

2. Your next immediate action should be to
    a. place the patient on the long backboard utilizing the log roll technique.
    b. carefully splint the suspected fractures, checking for pulses before and after splinting.
    c. continue to maintain the cervical spine immobilization until the helicopter arrives.
    d. direct your partner to control the bleeding by direct pressure with a bulky dressing.

3. As you place the late-term pregnancy patient on a long backboard, to help prevent supine hypotension, you should
    a. place the patient lying supine on the board with a large pillow placed under the flexed knees.
    b. tilt the backboard with the patient slightly toward the left side.
    c. position the backboard and patient with the head lower than the feet approximately 30 degrees.
    d. use pillows and rolled sheets to pad the voids to prevent pressure on the abdominal arteries.

4. As the helicopter is landing, the patient becomes pulseless and apneic. You should
    a. immediately begin resuscitative efforts, including CPR and ventilations.
    b. wait for the helicopter crew to approach the patient and decide the next action.
    c. stop all efforts to treat this patient. She is a trauma patient and will not survive.
    d. immediately call your supervisor or the hospital before further treatment is provided.

Obstetrics and Care of the Newborn

▌ STANDARD

Special Patient Populations (Content Area: Obstetrics; Neonatal Care)

▌ COMPETENCY

Applies fundamental knowledge of growth, development, and aging and assessment findings to provide basic emergency care and transportation for a patient with special needs.

▌ OBJECTIVES

After reading this chapter, you should be able to:

37-1. Define key terms introduced in this chapter.
37-2. Describe the anatomy of pregnancy, the menstrual cycle, and the prenatal period.
37-3. Describe physiological changes in pregnancy, including changes to the following systems:
    a. Reproductive
    b. Respiratory
    c. Cardiovascular
    d. Gastrointestinal
    e. Urinary
    f. Musculoskeletal
37-4. Describe the pathophysiology, assessment, and emergency care of patients with antepartum emergencies, including:
    a. Spontaneous abortion
    b. Placenta previa
    c. Abruptio placentae
    d. Ruptured uterus
    e. Ectopic pregnancy
    f. Preeclampsia/eclampsia
    g. Pregnancy-induced hypertension
    h. Supine hypotensive syndrome
37-5. Describe the assessment-based approach to antepartum emergencies.
37-6. Describe the stages of labor.
37-7. Describe the assessment-based approach to a patient in active labor with normal delivery.
37-8. Describe the steps of assisting with a normal prehospital obstetric delivery.

37-9. Discuss reassessment of the postpartum patient for blood loss.

37-10. Describe the assessment-based approach to a patient in active labor with abnormal delivery.

37-11. Take steps to manage abnormal prehospital obstetric deliveries, including:

  a. Prolapsed umbilical cord

  b. Breech and limb presentations

  c. Multiple births

  d. Meconium staining

  e. Premature birth

  f. Post-term pregnancy

  g. Precipitous delivery

  h. Shoulder dystocia

  i. Preterm labor

  j. Premature rupture of membranes

37-12. Take steps to manage postpartum complications, including:

  a. Postpartum hemorrhage

  b. Embolism

37-13. Demonstrate the steps of assessing and managing the newborn, including:

  a. Initial care, including drying, wrapping, suctioning, and positioning

  b. Apgar scoring and stimulation to breathe if necessary

  c. Apgar scoring

37-14. Recognize signs that indicate the need for neonatal resuscitation.

37-15. Apply the concepts of the neonatal resuscitation pyramid to the care of neonates in need of resuscitative measures.

▎KEY IDEAS

This chapter focuses on the assessment and management of obstetric emergencies and care of the newborn. The EMT does not frequently encounter obstetric emergencies, so these are often stressful calls. In this chapter, you learn how to recognize and provide emergency care for obstetric emergencies and provide initial care for the newborn. Key concepts include the following:

- The anatomical structures associated with pregnancy include the ovaries, fallopian tubes, uterus, placenta, amniotic sac, umbilical cord, cervix, and vagina.

- Antepartum emergencies include conditions causing hemorrhage (spontaneous abortion, placenta previa, abruptio placentae, ruptured uterus, ectopic pregnancy) or conditions causing seizures or blood pressure disturbances (preeclampsia/eclampsia, pregnancy-induced hypertension, and supine hypotensive syndrome).

- The three stages of labor are dilation, expulsion, and placental.

- Recognition of a predelivery emergency is based on information obtained from the history and physical exam that relates to the reported abnormality, such as pain, discomfort, or bleeding.

- The priorities for care do not change at the scene of an obstetric emergency. Use the same assessment and treatment techniques as you would use on any patient who is not pregnant.

- Imminent delivery is recognized by crowning, the frequency and duration of contractions, and the sensation of bowel movement (urge to push).

- The role of the EMT during childbirth is to assist in the delivery and to recognize and treat life-threatening problems for the mother or baby.

- *Gravida* refers to pregnancy, while *para* refers to a woman who has given birth. When a Roman numeral is added, it indicates the number for each. For example, a patient who is pregnant for the third time is reported as gravida III, and a woman who has given birth once is referred to as para I (or primipara).

- Abnormal deliveries include intrapartum (onset of labor to the delivery of the neonate) emergencies (prolapsed cord, breech birth, limb presentation, multiple births, meconium staining, premature birth, postterm pregnancy, precipitous delivery, shoulder dystocia, preterm labor, and premature rupture of membranes) and postpartum (period following delivery) complications (hemorrhage and embolism).

■ The Apgar score is reported 1 minute and 5 minutes after birth. A change in the Apgar score may indicate improvement (higher score), worsening (lower score), or no change. Assessed are the newborn's appearance (0-1-2), pulse (0-1-2), grimace (0-1-2), activity (0-1-2), and respiration (0-1-2). A newborn with a score of 7–10 should be active and requires routine care. A score of 4–6 indicates a moderately depressed newborn that requires stimulation and oxygenation. A score of 0–3 points indicates a severely depressed newborn that requires bag-valve-mask (BVM) ventilation and cardiopulmonary resuscitation (CPR).

■ The essential emergency care of the newborn includes the establishment and maintenance of an adequate airway, breathing, oxygenation, and circulation, and the prevention of heat loss.

▍ TERMS AND CONCEPTS

1. Write the number of the correct term next to each definition.
   1. Amniotic sac
   2. Braxton-Hicks contractions
   3. Fetus
   4. Perineum
   5. Placenta
   6. Primigravida
   7. Prolapsed cord
   8. Umbilical cord

   _____ a. An unborn infant

   _____ b. Placental extension that supplies nourishment to the fetus

   _____ c. Organ of pregnancy for the exchange of oxygen and waste products

   _____ d. When the umbilical cord is the presenting part

   _____ e. Transparent membrane forming the sac that holds fluid and the fetus

   _____ f. Area of skin between a female's vagina and anus

   _____ g. Woman who is pregnant for the first time

   _____ h. Painless, short duration, irregular contractions

▍ CONTENT REVIEW

1. Which of the following is the lowest portion of the birth canal?
   a. Cervix
   b. Uterus
   c. Vagina
   d. Perineum

2. Uterine contractions that expel the fetus and placenta are generally referred to as
   a. labor.
   b. the Braxton-Hicks phase.
   c. the dilation phase.
   d. the fetal expulsion phase.

3. The final stage of labor is generally described as the
   a. dilation stage.
   b. expulsion stage.
   c. placental stage.
   d. fundal stage.

4. A woman who is gravida III
   a. is pregnant for the fourth time.
   b. has delivered three times.
   c. is pregnant for the third time.
   d. has delivered for the fourth time.

5. Postmaturity syndrome
   a. occurs when the gestation of the fetus extends beyond 32 weeks.
   b. occurs when the gestation of the fetus extends beyond 36 weeks.
   c. causes improved placental blood flow and nutrient delivery to the fetus.
   d. causes a hardened fetal skull, leading to a more difficult delivery.

6. Your supine, third-trimester pregnant patient is noted to have a lowered systolic blood pressure. You suspect that this may be due to which of the following?
   a. Supine hypotensive syndrome
   b. Lateral emergent syndrome
   c. Prone hypertensive syndrome
   d. Supine hyperglycemic syndrome

7. Management specific to the situation noted in question 6 should include
   a. placing the patient in the Trendelenburg position.
   b. beginning chest compressions.
   c. positioning the patient on her side.
   d. applying the automated external defibrillator (AED).

8. Your 30-year-old female patient is four months pregnant. She complains of cramping, abdominal pain, and bright red vaginal bleeding. Your treatment should include
   a. packing the vagina with sanitary pads to control bleeding.
   b. elevation of the patient's head to prevent aspiration.
   c. the administration of oxygen at 6 lpm.
   d. providing general management for shock.

9. Your 20-year-old patient is eight months pregnant. Prior to your arrival, she had a seizure that lasted about two minutes. You find her to have an altered mental status, with a patent airway and adequate respirations and perfusion. Care of this patient should include
   a. administration of low-flow oxygen by a nonrebreather mask.
   b. withholding positive pressure ventilation.
   c. transporting the patient in a supine position.
   d. minimization of noise, light, and movement to prevent further seizures.

10. Which of the following is a sign of an imminent delivery?
    a. Contractions that occur every two minutes or closer and last 60–90 seconds
    b. Contractions that occur every two minutes and last 30–60 seconds
    c. Contractions that occur every four minutes and last 30–60 seconds
    d. Contractions that occur every four minutes and last 60–90 seconds

11. Number the following list in the proper order from 1 to 5 to show, after taking appropriate Standard Precautions and positioning the patient, the emergency care of a patient during active labor for a normal delivery.

_____ Suction the infant's airway if obvious obstruction to breathing exists. Support the body as the infant delivers; then again suction the infant's airway if obvious obstruction to breathing exists. Dry, wrap, warm, and position the infant.

_____ Observe for the delivery of the placenta. As it delivers, grasp it gently. Place it in a plastic bag for transport to the hospital.

_____ Support the bony part of the infant's skull and exert gentle pressure against the perineum as the head delivers. Determine the position of the umbilical cord.

_____ Keep the infant at or above the level of the vagina. Have your partner assume care of the infant. Wait 30 seconds prior to cutting the cord, clamp or tie, and then cut the umbilical cord.

_____ Place one or two sanitary pads at the vaginal opening. Record the time of delivery and then transport. Keep mother and infant warm en route.

12. Your patient has just delivered a healthy baby boy. Following the delivery of the placenta, her vaginal bleeding seems to increase. Which of the following best describes what you should do to provide emergency care for this patient?
    a. Massage the uterus, and position your patient on her side.
    b. Administer oxygen, and firmly massage the uterus.
    c. Massage the uterus, and pack the vagina to control bleeding.
    d. Administer oxygen, and pack the vagina with sanitary pads.

13. Which of the following is a sign of an abnormal delivery emergency?
    a. Fetal presentation of the head
    b. Colorless amniotic fluid
    c. Labor before the 46th week of pregnancy
    d. Recurrence of contractions after the infant is born

14. Management of a breech birth presentation includes
    a. positioning the mother in a supine head-down, pelvis-elevated position.
    b. administering low-flow oxygen by a nonrebreather mask.
    c. placing a hand in the vagina to delay delivery.
    d. delaying transport for safe delivery on the scene.

15. Which of the following best describes an abnormal delivery situation where there may be compression of the cord against the walls of the vagina and the bony pelvis by the pressure of the infant's head or buttocks?
    a. Crowning
    b. Limb presentation
    c. Breech
    d. Prolapsed cord

16. How should you manage the situation in question 15?
    a. Immediately push the cord back into the vagina.
    b. Insert a gloved hand into the vagina to relieve pressure on the cord.
    c. Cover the cord with a dry, sterile towel to prevent infection.
    d. Push on the mother's abdomen to expedite delivery.

17. Meconium staining of the amniotic fluid in a newborn that is depressed or nonvigorous with a heart rate less than 100 per minute or has inadequate respirations should be managed
    a. immediate transport to the hospital for evaluation by a physician.
    b. administration of oxygen to the mother to resolve fetal distress.
    c. quickly suctioning the mouth and nose and immediately begin positive pressure ventilation.
    d. stimulating the infant to cough to clear meconium from the airway.

18. In addition to the usual care for a newborn, care of the premature infant requires
    a. vigorous suctioning to maintain the airway.
    b. direct administration of supplemental oxygen by a face mask.
    c. immediate transport for resuscitation.
    d. vigilant attention to prevent heat loss or contamination.

19. The Apgar scoring assessment of the newborn
    a. ranges from 0 to 10.
    b. includes assessment of the newborn's affect.
    c. ranges from 3 to 10.
    d. is performed at 1 and 2 minutes following birth.

20. Which of the following is a sign of a severely depressed newborn?
    a. Respiratory rate of over 50 per minute
    b. Apgar score of 7–10 points
    c. Cyanotic body (core and extremities)
    d. Heart rate over 120 per minute or under 80 per minute

21. You have assisted with the delivery of a baby girl. She has labored respirations and a heart rate that is less than 90 beats per minute. Which of the following best describes your emergency care for this patient?
    a. Administer "blow-by" oxygen and monitor pulse for 60 seconds.
    b. Assist ventilations with a BVM and reassess in 30 seconds.
    c. Administer high-concentration oxygen with a nonrebreather mask.
    d. Assist ventilations with a BVM and begin chest compressions.

22. Meconium staining
    a. that is thick and dark in color is associated with increased fetal risk.
    b. rarely occurs in a term, male fetus.
    c. rarely occurs in a term, female fetus.
    d. requires rapid suctioning of the infant's nose and then the mouth.

23. The Apgar score is initially performed at _____ after birth and repeated at _____ after birth.
    a. 30 seconds, 3 minutes
    b. 60 seconds, 5 minutes
    c. 90 seconds, 6 minutes
    d. 30 seconds, 4 minutes

24. Irregular contractions that vary in intensity and duration are called
    a. Braxton-Hicks contractions.
    b. normal predelivery contractions.
    c. Braddock-McKoy contractions.
    d. postdelivery contractions.

25. Placenta previa results from
    a. uterine trauma and subsequent placental separation from the uterine wall.
    b. rupture of blood vessels under the placenta and subsequent separation.
    c. an abnormal implantation of the placenta.
    d. hypertension and separation of the placenta from the uterine wall.

26. A predisposing factor for the development of placenta previa is
    a. fewer than two deliveries.
    b. younger than 20 years of age.
    c. no history of vaginal bleeding.
    d. bleeding following intercourse.

27. The hallmark sign of placenta previa is
    a. second-trimester, painless vaginal bleeding.
    b. third-trimester, painless bright red vaginal bleeding.
    c. third-trimester, painless vaginal bleeding.
    d. third-trimester, painless dark red vaginal bleeding.

28. Abruptio placentae results from
    a. uterine trauma and subsequent placental separation from the uterine wall.
    b. the rupture of blood vessels under the placenta and subsequent separation.
    c. an abnormal implantation of the placenta.
    d. hypertension and separation of the placenta from the uterine wall.

29. Predisposing factors for an abruptio placentae are
    a. a history of fewer than two deliveries.
    b. an abnormally long umbilical cord.
    c. fever and use of psychotropic drugs.
    d. smoking and hypertension.

30. The hallmark sign of abruptio placentae is
    a. vaginal bleeding that is associated with constant abdominal pain.
    b. lower abdominal pain without vaginal bleeding.
    c. lower back pain and cramping.
    d. signs and symptoms of hypovolemic shock.

31. Preeclampsia
    a. is a common condition that affects one in five women.
    b. occurs most frequently in the first trimester of pregnancy.
    c. frequently affects pregnant women over the age of 40.
    d. chiefly affects women with a history of hypertension or diabetes.

32. The primary clinical signs of preeclampsia are
    a. vomiting and pulmonary edema.
    b. hypertension and swelling in the extremities.
    c. abdominal pain and severe headache.
    d. reactive airway disease and pulmonary edema.

33. The third-leading cause of maternal death, which is most common in women 25–34 years of age, is
    a. abruptio placentae.
    b. placenta previa.
    c. preeclampsia/eclampsia.
    d. ectopic pregnancy.

34. Factors that predispose an individual to develop an ectopic pregnancy include
    a. smoking.
    b. cardiac disease.
    c. pelvic inflammatory disease.
    d. inactivity.

35. A sign or symptom of an ectopic pregnancy emergency is
    a. an intense urge to urinate.
    b. sharp, knifelike lower abdominal pain localized to one side.
    c. a bluish discoloration around the umbilicus immediately following rupture.
    d. bilateral lower abdominal pain that is described as a tearing pain.

▍CASE STUDY

You have been dispatched to the scene of a single vehicle accidentally driven into a river. A jogger and another bystander dived into the river and were able to rescue the driver. Your patient is a woman in her 30s who is obviously pregnant. By the size of her abdomen, you suspect she is near term. Your initial assessment reveals an unresponsive female with rapid, shallow respirations. Her pulse is slow and irregular. Her skin is cool. There are no obvious signs of injury.

1. Initial management of this patient should first include
    a. assisting respirations by a BVM with oxygen.
    b. completing a physical exam.
    c. covering with a blanket to maintain body heat.
    d. immobilization on a long spine board.

2. The patient is immobilized on a long spine board. How should the potential for supine hypotensive syndrome be managed in this patient?
    a. Keep the spine board in a flat position.
    b. Position a blanket or pillow under the side of the spine board.
    c. Position a blanket or pillow under the head of the spine board.
    d. Position a blanket or pillow under the foot end of the board.

Two blocks from the hospital, your patient stops breathing and becomes pulseless.

3. What is the best action to take?
    a. Start vigorous CPR.
    b. Withhold CPR, the baby must be surgically delivered.
    c. Contact the hospital for instructions.
    d. Speed your response time to the hospital.

Your patient is successfully resuscitated at the hospital and undergoes surgical delivery of a baby girl.

CHAPTER 37 SCENARIO: DOCUMENTATION EXERCISE

Read the following scenario and think about how you would document this call if you were the EMT who responded to the scene. Then answer the multiple-choice questions and fill in the sample prehospital care report, basing your documentation on information from the scenario.

It is 3:30 A.M. You are sleeping soundly when the alarm sounds: "Unit 3, respond to 1451 U.S. Highway 98 South, cross street Highway 540A, for an unknown medical emergency." You climb out of bed, get dressed, and meet your partner, Jack, in the rescue vehicle. Dispatch tells you that your patient is in a car parked on the northbound lane of Highway 98 and is a female patient in labor. You advise dispatch that you are responding. You arrive on scene in about eight minutes. You pull up behind a car with its hood up, and you park. A young man is in the back seat of the car and motions you to hurry.

You walk toward the car with your Standard Precautions on. You look inside and observe a young woman lying in a supine position in the back seat of the car. She is lying with her legs spread apart and her head against the door. She is covered by a small blanket and is moaning loudly as you approach the car. You introduce yourself and Jack to the young man, and say, "We are EMTs. We're here to help. What's the problem tonight?" He anxiously says, "I was taking Mary to the hospital when my car broke down. She has been in labor for about two hours. She's going to have the baby! You've got to help us!" You reply, "We will do everything we can."

You quickly jump into the back seat to evaluate Mary. Mary, who appears to be about 30 years old, is alert and screaming, "It's coming! It's coming!" You administer oxygen via a nasal cannula and set the flow rate at 4 lpm. You quickly remove the blanket and cut off her underpants so you can examine the vaginal area. Crowning is present with each contraction.

Mary says, "I feel like I have to move my bowels. I really need to push." You tell her to try not to push until you can get things set up. You place a folded sheet under her hips and open up the sterile obstetrical kit that Jack brings you. You create a sterile area by placing a sterile sheet under her buttocks and place a sterile sheet on her lower abdomen. You then put the Obstetrical kit within easy reach.

She yells once again, "I've gotta push now!" You tell her to go ahead and push. You place your gloved, spread fingers on the infant's skull and exert gentle, steady pressure. The head is bulging from the vagina and is covered with a thin, semitransparent membrane. You quickly use a clamp from the OB kit to tear the membrane and push it away from the infant's head and face. The head delivers quickly and is in a "nose down" position. You use two fingers to check down the neck of the infant. The head is completely delivered and has rotated in such a manner as to now be facing the mother's right leg. You quickly examine the newborn's airway; no secretions appear to be present. The infant's torso is expelled. You support the head and torso with your hands and grasp the infant's feet as the delivery proceeds. You again check the newborn's airway; it seems clear. The infant begins to cry.

You tell Mary, "It's a girl!" You dry the infant with a sterile towel and place her on her back with her head in a sniffing position on the car seat even with the mother's vagina. You place two clamps on the umbilical cord and use a sterile scalpel to cut the cord between the clamps. You hand the baby to Jack to manage. Jack wraps the baby in a warm receiving blanket, shows her to the ecstatic father, and takes the baby to the ambulance to keep her warm and evaluate her. You continue to manage the mother. You clean her up while preparing for delivery of the placenta. You observe some bleeding from the vagina and control it with sanitary pads. You take the vital signs on the mother.

You ask Mary if she has been under prenatal care. She states, "Yes, Dr. Menendez has been taking care of me. Everything has been quite normal, up to now. He is at the hospital waiting for us." Mary is alert and oriented; her respirations are 14 per minute and of normal depth; the pulse is 100 per minute, strong, and regular; the skin is warm and dry; pupils are equal and reactive and respond briskly to light; the blood pressure is 130/80; and her SpO_2 is 96%. In about 10 minutes, the placenta appears at the vagina, and you take hold of it and gently support it as it is expelled. You place the placenta in a plastic bag. You inspect the perineum for tearing and place sanitary pads over the vaginal opening. You ask the mother to put her legs together, and you record the time of birth.

You find out that Mary has had four pregnancies and has delivered three live births, including this newborn. Jack has been managing the infant baby girl. He obtained the following findings from the 1-minute Apgar: *appearance*—blue hands and feet with pink skin at the body core; *pulse*—140 per minute; *grimace*—stimulation causes a cry; *activity*—newborn moves around; *respiration*—good respirations and strong cry. He maintains the infant's warmth and repeats the Apgar at 5 minutes.

The following findings are noted: *appearance*— the skin of the extremities as well as the trunk are pink; *pulse*—150 per minute; *grimace*—stimulation causes a cry; *activity*—newborn moves around; *respiration*—good respirations and strong cry.

You transport mother and daughter to the hospital while continuing to monitor both closely. The father rides along in the front of the ambulance, planning to call the car repair service from the hospital.

1. Immediately after cutting and clamping the umbilical cord, you should
   a. document the time on the run report.
   b. place a second umbilical clamp on the mother.
   c. place a second umbilical clamp on the infant.
   d. check to make sure that no bleeding is taking place.

2. What physical findings or symptoms let you know that delivery was imminent?
   a. Her age and general attitude
   b. Need to push and crowning
   c. Prior number of births
   d. Length of time in labor for prior births

3. What is the 1-minute Apgar score?
   a. 6
   b. 7
   c. 8
   d. 9

4. What is the 5-minute Apgar score?
   a. 7
   b. 8
   c. 9
   d. 10

5. The bleeding that occurs following the birth of Mary's baby girl is normal and expected. Bleeding, however, should typically not exceed _____.
   a. 200 mL (cc)
   b. 300 mL (cc)
   c. 400 mL (cc)
   d. 500 mL (cc)

EMERGENCY TRIP SHEET

TRIP #	
MEDIC #	
BEGIN MILES	
END MILES	
CODE ___/___	PAGE ___/___
UNITS ON SCENE	

BILLING USE ONLY	
DAY	
DATE	
RECEIVED	
DISPATCHED	

NAME	SEX M F DOB ___/___/___
ADDRESS	RACE
CITY STATE	ZIP
PHONE ( ) -	PCP DR.
RESPONDED FROM	CITY
TAKEN FROM	ZIP
DESTINATION	REASON
SSN - -	MEDICARE # MEDICAID #
INSURANCE CO	INSURANCE # GROUP #
RESPONSIBLE PARTY	ADDRESS
CITY STATE ZIP	PHONE ( ) -
EMPLOYER	

EN-ROUTE		
ON SCENE		
TO HOSPITAL		
AT HOSPITAL		
IN-SERVICE		
CREW	CERT	STATE #

TIME	ON SCENE (1)	ON SCENE (2)	ON SCENE (3)	EN-ROUTE (1)	EN-ROUTE (2)	AT DESTINATION
BP						
PULSE						
RESP						
SpO$_2$						
ETCO$_2$						
EKG						

IV THERAPY
SUCCESSFUL Y N # OF ATTEMPTS _____
ANGIO SIZE _____ga.
SITE _____
TOTAL FLUID INFUSED _____ cc
BLOOD DRAW Y N INITIALS

INTUBATION INFORMATION
SUCCESSFUL Y N # OF ATTEMPTS _____
TUBE SIZE _____ mm
TIME _____ INITIALS _____

MEDICAL HISTORY	CONDITION CODES
MEDICATIONS	TREATMENTS
ALLERGIES	
C/C	
EVENTS LEADING TO C/C	
ASSESSMENT	
TREATMENT	

TIME	TREATMENT	DOSE	ROUTE	INIT

GCS E___ V___ M___ TOTAL =
GCS E___ V___ M___ TOTAL =

HOSPITAL CONTACTED

CPR BEGUN BY   B   P   TIME BEGUN

EMS SIGNATURE

AED USED   Y   N   BY:

RESUSCITATION TERMINATED - TIME

(   ) OSHA REGULATIONS FOLLOWED

Pediatrics

STANDARD

Special Patient Populations (Content Area: Pediatrics)

COMPETENCY

Applies fundamental knowledge of growth, development, and aging and assessment findings to provide basic emergency care and transportation for a patient with special needs.

OBJECTIVES

After reading this chapter, you should be able to:

38-1. Define key terms introduced in this chapter.

38-2. Explain the special considerations in dealing with the caregiver of a sick or injured child.

38-3. Describe the major developmental characteristics and modifications of patient assessment and management techniques recommended for patients in each of the following age groups:
   a. Neonates
   b. Infants
   c. Toddlers
   d. Preschoolers
   e. School-age children
   f. Adolescents

38-4. Describe the major anatomical and physiological differences in children with regard to the following:
   a. Airway
   b. Head
   c. Chest and lungs
   d. Respiratory system
   e. Cardiovascular system
   f. Abdomen
   g. Extremities
   h. Metabolic rate
   i. Skin and body surface area

38-5. Discuss the normal vital signs for children in various age groups.

38-6. Use the Pediatric Assessment Triangle (PAT) to determine a pediatric patient's status.

38-7. Discuss special considerations for the following elements of the pediatric secondary assessment:
   a. Physical exam
   b. Vital sign assessment
   c. History taking
38-8. Recognize signs of respiratory distress, respiratory failure, and respiratory arrest in pediatric patients.
38-9. Discuss the guidelines for emergency care of the following:
   a. Respiratory emergencies
   b. Foreign body airway obstruction
38-10. Describe the presentation and emergency medical care for pediatric patients with the following conditions:
   a. Croup
   b. Epiglottitis
   c. Asthma
   d. Bronchiolitis
   e. Pneumonia
   f. Congenital heart disease
   g. Shock
   h. Cardiac arrest
38-11. Explain the assessment steps and emergency care protocol for a respiratory or cardiopulmonary emergency in the pediatric patient.
38-12. Describe the presentation and emergency medical care for pediatric patients with the following conditions:
   a. Seizures, including status epilepticus
   b. Altered mental status
   c. Drowning
   d. Fever
   e. Meningitis
   f. Gastrointestinal disorders
   g. Poisoning
   h. Apparent life-threatening emergencies (ALTE)
   i. Sudden infant death syndrome (SIDS)
38-13. Describe special considerations in the scene size-up, emergency medical care, and assisting family members in case of suspected SIDS and the importance of the presence of parents during pediatric resuscitation.
38-14. Integrate consideration of a pediatric patient's size and anatomy into the assessment of mechanisms of injury.
38-15. Demonstrate removal of a pediatric patient from a child car seat.
38-16. Demonstrate proper spinal immobilization of a pediatric patient.
38-17. Explain the importance of injury prevention programs to reduce pediatric injuries and deaths.
38-18. Discuss the purpose of the federal Emergency Medical Services for Children (EMSC) program and the concept of family-centered care.
38-19. Discuss factors that can increase EMS providers' stress on pediatric calls and ways of managing the stress that may be associated with a pediatric call.

▌ KEY IDEAS

This chapter focuses on the unique assessment and emergency medical management considerations that the EMT must take into account when providing care to ill or injured infants and children. Most EMS providers find such situations among the most stressful of any emergency call that they encounter. A good understanding of the basics about caring for infants and children will go a long way toward increasing your confidence and decreasing your stress.

- The ill or injured infant or child is not your only patient. The caregiver will also need your attention.
- The developmental classifications of the infant or child patient include neonate (birth–1 month), infant (1 month–1 year), toddler (1–3 years), preschooler (3–6 years), school-age child (6–12 years),

and adolescent (12–18 years). The developmental characteristics related to age will affect your assessment and treatment activities. Management of most infant and child emergencies is identical to the management of the adult patient; however, modifications may need to be made based on the anatomical, physiological, and psychological development of the infant or child.

- The Pediatric Assessment Triangle (PAT) is a visual assessment performed as you approach the pediatric patient. It consists of rapidly assessing appearance (tone, interactivity, consolability, look or gaze, and speech or cry), work of breathing (abnormal sounds or posture, retractions, nasal flaring, and head bobbing), and circulation to skin (pallor, mottling, cyanosis, and petechiae).

- The primary goal in treating any infant or child patient is to anticipate and recognize respiratory problems and to support any function that is compromised or lost.

- The skin color, temperature, and condition and capillary refill time provide valuable information about the perfusion status of infants and children.

- Fever is a common emergency for infants and children and may be due to infection or heat exposure.

- Sudden infant death syndrome (SIDS) is the leading cause of death among infants from 1 month to 1 year old. Blunt trauma is the most common injury in children.

- Child abuse may take a variety of forms, including physical, emotional, and sexual abuse and neglect.

- The EMT can alleviate some of the personal stress of caring for children through advance preparation and by seeking out help when necessary.

┃ TERMS AND CONCEPTS

1. Fill in the following chart. Include at least two characteristics for each stage.

Developmental Stage	Age Group	Characteristics
a. Neonate		
b. Infant		
c. Toddler		
d. Preschooler		
e. School-age child		
f. Adolescent		

┃ CONTENT REVIEW

1. Which of the following is a generally helpful method of dealing with caregivers at the scene of an emergency for an infant or a child?
   a. The use of technical terms will reassure caregivers that you are qualified to care for their child.
   b. Acknowledge caregivers' concerns and, when appropriate, allow them to assist you in caring for their child.
   c. Immediately remove the child from the scene so that caregivers cannot interfere with your care.
   d. Even if the child is seriously injured, reassure caregivers that "everything will be fine" to help keep them calm.

2. Which statement best describes the anatomical difference between a child and an adult airway?
   a. Newborns and infants are obligate mouth breathers.
   b. Infants have proportionally smaller tongues than adults when compared to the size of their mouths.
   c. The smallest level of the airway in the child is at the level of the vocal cords.
   d. The epiglottis is much higher in the child airway than in the adult airway.

3. The child's skin surface is large compared to body mass, thus making children more susceptible to which of the following?
   a. Hyperventilation
   b. Hyperglycemia
   c. Hypothermia
   d. Hypovolemia

4. Infants and children have faster _____ rates than adults; therefore, they use oxygen from the bloodstream faster than adults do.
   a. lymphatic
   b. metabolic
   c. abdominal musculature
   d. central nervous system

5. The primary goal in treating any infant or child patient is the anticipation and recognition of _____ problems and support of any compromised or lost function.
   a. central nervous system
   b. cardiovascular system
   c. respiratory system
   d. urinary system

6. Which is a sign of early respiratory distress?
   a. Warm skin temperature
   b. Nasal flaring
   c. Flushed skin color
   d. SpO$_2$ reading of 97%

7. Your infant patient is lethargic and has decreased muscle tone, grunting respirations at 80 per minute with obvious use of accessory muscles, and head bobbing. You suspect which of the following?
   a. Early respiratory distress
   b. Supraclavicular retractions
   c. Decompensated respiratory failure
   d. Cardiopulmonary arrest

8. Which of the following occurs when the compensatory mechanisms designed to maintain oxygenation of the blood have failed and the body is just moments away from complete cardiopulmonary arrest?
   a. Decompensated respiratory failure
   b. Early cardiopulmonary arrest
   c. Respiratory arrest
   d. Hypotension

9. Which of the following is most correct regarding the respiratory assessment of the infant or child?
   a. Normal respiration ranges from 30–50/minute in an infant.
   b. Normal respiration ranges from 15–30/minute in a child.
   c. Measure respiratory rate by counting for 15 seconds and multiplying by 4.
   d. Adults generally breathe faster than children and infants.

10. When assessing breath sounds in an infant or child, auscultate in the
    a. midclavicular line on the anterior chest.
    b. midscapular line on the posterior chest.
    c. midaxillary line on the lateral chest.
    d. midsternal line on the anterior chest.

11. If perfusion is adequate, pulses, skin color and temperature, capillary refill, mental status, and _____ will be normal.
    a. respiratory effort
    b. urinary output
    c. motor function
    d. intercostal motion

12. Number the following list in the proper order from 1 to 4 to show the steps for managing a foreign body airway obstruction in a responsive infant. The following assumes that the infant is responsive and unable to cough or make any sound.

    _____ Support the infant in a prone, head-down position on your forearm.

    _____ Repeat back slaps and chest thrusts until the obstruction is dislodged.

    _____ Deliver five sharp back slaps between the shoulder blades.

    _____ Transfer the patient to a supine position and deliver five chest thrusts using two fingertips.

13. Regarding seizures in infants and children, which of the following is correct?
    a. Seizures are generally not caused by conditions that cause seizures in adults.
    b. Children over age 12 have an especially high risk of seizures.
    c. Seizures are caused by fever in about 50 percent of cases.
    d. Seizures can result in loss of bladder and bowel control.

14. Status epilepticus is defined as a seizure that lasts for
    a. at least 20 minutes, with a recovery period.
    b. longer than 5 minutes, or that recurs without a recovery period.
    c. at least 2 minutes, with a recovery period and a recurrence.
    d. any period of time over 15 minutes, with or without a recovery period.

15. Management of the infant or child with a fever includes
    a. being concerned if the fever is over 104°F–105°F.
    b. administering antipyretics.
    c. cooling by sponging with ice or cold water.
    d. recognizing that all high temperatures produce seizures.

16. Regarding shock or hypoperfusion in children, which of the following is correct?
    a. It is common in children because their blood vessels are unable to constrict efficiently.
    b. It can occur in older children due to loss of body heat and an immature thermoregulatory system.
    c. When it leads to cardiac arrest in a child, it is generally due to cardiac compromise.
    d. The pediatric patient deteriorates faster and more severely than an adult.

17. Management of an infant or a child in shock includes
    a. keeping the patient warm and calm.
    b. performing a reassessment every 10 minutes.
    c. administering oxygen to maintain an SpO_2 of 90% or greater.
    d. providing positive pressure ventilation without supplemental oxygen.

18. SIDS
    a. is also known as "sleeping death."
    b. is the leading cause of death in infants age 12–18 months.
    c. occurrence cannot be predicted.
    d. is easy to diagnose in the field.

19. Management of SIDS should include
    a. avoiding resuscitation efforts until law enforcement is present.
    b. not providing false reassurances to the family.
    c. discouraging the caregivers from talking and telling their story.
    d. delaying transport until law enforcement is present.

20. You are assessing your pediatric patient for possible shock. How should you perform the capillary refill test on your patient?
    a. Compress the soft tissue of the kneecap.
    b. Compress the tissue under the fingernail.
    c. Compress the tissue under the toenail.
    d. Compress the tissue of the forehead.

21. Trauma in children
    a. is the leading cause of death from age 12–20 years.
    b. is caused primarily by bicycle-related accidents.
    c. results in death within the first hour in 10 percent of all cases.
    d. is most commonly caused by blunt trauma.

22. Which of the following mechanisms of injury would require transporting to a pediatric trauma center, if one is available?
    a. Motor vehicle crash in which another occupant is killed
    b. Pedestrian struck at 5 mph
    c. Restrained occupant of a vehicle traveling 10 mph
    d. Fall from 5 feet onto concrete

23. The National Highway Traffic Safety Administration 2012 recommendations for the safe transport of children in ground ambulances
    a. are divided into eight different situations involving children at the scene of an emergency.
    b. recommend transporting an infant or a child on the squad bench.
    c. provides standards enforced by federal regulation.
    d. do not allow the caregiver to hold the infant/child in his/her arms during transport.

24. Which statement is correct relating to infants and children?
    a. A common cause of hypoxia is the tongue obstructing the airway.
    b. Hypoperfusion is typically a sign of a closed head injury.
    c. Infants' and children's ribs are less pliable than adults' ribs.
    d. The capillary refill test is the only reliable assessment finding for shock.

25. Infant and child burn patients are at more risk of hypothermia and _____, in part because of their greater skin surface in relation to body mass.
    a. respiratory compromise
    b. fluid loss
    c. fever
    d. scarring

26. Which statement is most correct regarding child abuse?
    a. Physical abuse is the provision of inadequate attention.
    b. Neglect is when an improper action causes an injury.
    c. The abused child will seldom exhibit fear when questioned about the injury.
    d. In many cases, the child will be the victim of both abuse and neglect.

27. You suspect child abuse by a local caregiver. Which of the following best describes how you should proceed?
    a. Question neighbors about your suspicions, and flag your prehospital care report by writing "suspected child abuse" on it.
    b. Refuse to leave the scene until the police arrive to investigate the caregivers.
    c. Record your objective observations, follow local reporting protocols, and maintain total confidentiality.
    d. Record all details of your observation, confront the caregiver, and contact the local child protective service agency.

28. You are preparing to assess your pediatric patient by using the PAT. Which of the following best describes the PAT?
    a. It can be performed from across the room prior to patient contact.
    b. It is performed during the physical exam of the patient.
    c. It is composed of appearance, work of breathing, and blood pressure.
    d. It requires specific knowledge of the anatomy of the pediatric patient.

29. Pediatric patients compensate for a reduction in cardiac output by
    a. dilating blood vessels.
    b. increasing the strength of contractions.
    c. increasing the heart rate.
    d. increasing the respiratory rate.

30. The use of pulse oximetry in children
    a. is not recommended.
    b. should be cautiously used for anything other than noting trends.
    c. if above a reading of 92%, does not require the administration of oxygen.
    d. is only cautiously recommended.

31. Your pediatric patient presents with signs of shortness of breath but is still maintaining adequate respiratory depth and rate. This patient is considered to be in
    a. respiratory arrest.
    b. decompensated respiratory distress.
    c. early respiratory distress.
    d. impending apneic distress.

32. You are treating a pediatric patient for shortness of breath when you note that the tidal volume has become inadequate. You should
    a. apply oxygen with a nonrebreather mask.
    b. continue your treatment; this is not uncommon.
    c. decrease the oxygen; your patient is hyperventilating.
    d. immediately ventilate with a bag-valve mask (BVM) with oxygen.

33. While treating your child patient, you notice that the wheezing has resolved without the use of medication. This often indicates that
    a. the child has worsened and is no longer moving adequate air to create wheezes.
    b. the child's compensatory response has been initiated and the wheezes are relieved.
    c. the hypoxic drive has increased the respiratory effectiveness and has relieved the wheezes.
    d. the bronchioles are constricting, lessening the restrictions in the airway.

34. You arrive on the scene, and the parents of a small child rush to meet you and hand you a limp, unresponsive 2-year-old patient. The parent's state that he choked on a hot dog, then became unresponsive. After you open the airway using the head-tilt, chin-lift maneuver, you should next
    a. open the mouth and look for a foreign body in the oropharynx.
    b. perform a blind finger sweep of the mouth.
    c. perform two back slaps while in the supine position.
    d. position the patient in a Fowler's position and attempt to ventilate.

35. Croup
    a. typically results from a bacterial infection of the upper airway.
    b. has a rapid onset of symptoms accompanied by a high fever.
    c. produces stridor on inhalation with a harsh "seal bark."
    d. patients should be administered non-humidified oxygen.

36. Epiglottitis
    a. is a viral infection that causes swelling of the epiglottis.
    b. most commonly affects 2- to 7-year-olds.
    c. causes drooling, and the patient sits up and leans forward.
    d. if left untreated, has a 10 percent mortality rate.

37. Asthma
    a. occurs when the bronchioles dilate.
    b. causes a decrease in airway resistance.
    c. sufferers may assume a "tripod" position.
    d. attacks generally result in localized wheezes on auscultation.

38. A severe attack of asthma that cannot be managed with medication is known as
    a. acute asthma.
    b. chronic asthma.
    c. pernicious asthma.
    d. status asthmaticus.

39. A condition that affects children younger than 2 years of age and that is caused when the small bronchi in the lungs become inflamed by a viral infection is called
    a. asthma.
    b. croup.
    c. bronchiolitis.
    d. chronic lung disease.

40. Chest compressions in children may be necessary if the heart rate drops below _____ with signs of poor perfusion.
    a. 90/minute
    b. 80/minute
    c. 70/minute
    d. 60/minute

41. An infection of the brain and spinal cord by a virus or bacteria is called
    a. meningitis.
    b. bronchiolitis.
    c. croup.
    d. epiglottitis.

42. NHTSA recommends using the car seat that a child was in during a crash if
    a. the vehicle can be driven from the crash site.
    b. the airbags did not deploy.
    c. there is no visible damage to the safety seat.
    d. all of these, plus there were no injuries to occupants and the door nearest the safety seat is undamaged.

43. The AHA's Pediatric Advanced Life Support (PALS) initial impression uses what three assessment criteria?
    a. Revised Glasgow Coma Scale (GCS), airway, and color
    b. Consciousness, breathing, and color
    c. Oxygenation status, consciousness, and color
    d. Oxygenation saturation, breathing, and color

▌CASE STUDY

You are dispatched to a women's shelter for "baby not breathing." Upon arrival, the patient's mother reports that her five-month-old male infant has had a cold and has been fussy for the past two days. Today, the child had episodes of coughing that "made him vomit." About 10 minutes ago, he appeared to stop breathing briefly, and she called 911. The infant is lying quietly in his mother's arms. He is awake but lethargic, with decreased muscle tone. Eyes appear "glassy." Airway is patent, with very rapid, shallow, grunting respirations at 60 per minute. Skin is pale, very warm, and dry. The brachial pulse is strong and regular at 90 per minute. The anterior fontanelle appears to be sunken. Capillary refill is greater than 2 seconds. There are no obvious injuries or signs of trauma.

1. The infant is exhibiting signs of
    a. decompensated respiratory failure.
    b. gastric distention and distress.
    c. early respiratory distress.
    d. progressive dehydration syndrome.

2. What is the most appropriate immediate treatment for the infant?
    a. Provide oxygen at 15 lpm and administer oral fluids.
    b. Provide oxygen at 15 lpm and immediate transport.
    c. Provide oral fluids in small amounts and rapid transport.
    d. Provide immediate positive pressure ventilation with oxygen and transport.

During the history taking, the mother reports that the patient was born seven weeks premature but has been doing fine. The patient is taking no medications and has no known allergies. She says that she fed him about three hours ago, but he has vomited several times since then. He has not had a wet diaper since this morning. She starts to cry and says it's her fault that the baby is so sick, but she couldn't afford to take him to the doctor when he "caught his cold."

3. In addition to the problem identified in the case, the infant is most likely suffering from
   a. dehydration.
   b. fever.
   c. seizure.
   d. flu.

CHAPTER 38 SCENARIO: DOCUMENTATION EXERCISE

Read the following scenario and think about how you would document this call if you were the EMT who responded to the scene. Then answer the multiple-choice questions and fill in the sample prehospital care report, basing your documentation on information from the scenario.

It is 11:30 P.M. on a cold winter evening. You and your partner have just finished cleaning the jump kit following a call for a vehicle versus a pedestrian when the station alarm sounds: "Unit 2, respond to 879 Venice Way for a child that has fallen; cross street, Edgewood Drive. Time out 2330 hours." You quickly return the contents to the jump kit and head to the rescue vehicle. Your partner, John, acknowledges the call and advises dispatch that you are responding.

You arrive at an upper-class residential area and quickly locate the home. It is a large three-story house. A man is standing out in the front yard waving you down. You pull into a circular driveway, step out of the vehicle with your Standard Precautions in place, and are immediately met by the man. He quickly says, "Thank goodness you're here! It's my son. He fell and hit his head. He's not moving at all. You've got to hurry, please!" You introduce yourself and John, and say, "We are EMTs, and we're here to help you and your son. What is your name, sir?" He says, "It's Ed River." As you remove the jump kit, oxygen, the pediatric immobilization device, and other equipment, you ask, "Mr. River, how old is your son?" He replies as you are walking toward the front door, "He just turned 18 months old." You continue your questioning. "How did he fall, and from how high did he fall?" As the father opens the front door, he says, "The only thing we can figure out is that he fell from the second-story area. I think he must have climbed over the railing and fell to the first floor.

I found him on the hallway floor. He hasn't moved at all. You asked about how high he fell from. I think it must be at least 15 feet, because we have really high ceilings on the first floor."

You call dispatch to request ALS, and they advise that the ALS unit is about six minutes away. You enter the front door and see a small boy lying on his right side. You estimate his weight at about 30 pounds. The mother is softly crying and holding the child's hand. When your eyes meet, you can see that she is terrified. As you move toward the child, you look up and observe the upper living area from which it is assumed that the child fell. As Mr. River had said, it is at least 15 feet up. The child's respirations appear to be adequate with no abnormal respiratory sounds present. John sets down the jump kit and immobilization device and places a simple face mask on the child, adjusting the flow to 4 lpm. The child does not move. His eyes are closed and remain closed. He has a large laceration on the right frontal area of his head. The mother is holding pressure on the wound, and the bleeding appears to be controlled.

John quickly cuts the clothing from the boy and positions the pediatric immobilization device next to him. He holds manual stabilization of the cervical spine while you roll the child onto the immobilization device. The child is secured to the immobilization device with a cervical collar in place. You check for a pain response and observe an extension response to pain. Both arms and legs move. You size and place an oropharyngeal airway, and a gag reflex is not triggered.

You check the brachial pulse and find it strong and regular. The skin is warm, and the skin color is good. The capillary refill is less than 2 seconds. You perform a rapid secondary assessment while John takes the vital signs. You observe the laceration on the child's forehead. The child's pupils are unequal: the right pupil is fixed and dilated, and the left eye responds slowly to light. The eyes are deviated to the right. The ears and nose are clear of blood and fluid. On palpation of the skull, you feel a depressed area over the right parietal region. No obvious deformities of the neck are noted, and the trachea is in the midline. The breath sounds are clear and equal bilaterally. You note a probable closed fracture of the right forearm. No other physical findings are observed.

John completes the vital signs and tells you, "His breathing is 24 per minute and appears to be of normal depth. His pulse is 130 per minute and strong and regular. His pupils are unchanged from your assessment. The blood pressure is 96/48; his skin color is good; the radial and brachial pulses are strong. The capillary refill time is less than 2 seconds. The SpO$_2$ is 96%." You obtain a history from the father. He tells you that his son has no allergies, takes no medications, has no prior medical history, and last ate about 30 minutes ago.

You hear a knock at the door and see Paramedic Beck walk into the house. You give the paramedic a quick patient report and help place the patient into the ALS ambulance.

1. You requested ALS when the child's father told you that the child fell from a height of about 15 feet. You knew that any fall of at least _____ feet is a mechanism of injury that requires transport of the pediatric patient to a level 1 pediatric trauma center.
   a. 5
   b. 10
   c. 12
   d. 15

2. The average pulse in this 18-month-old patient is expected to be
   a. 140 per minute.
   b. 130 per minute.
   c. 120 per minute.
   d. 110 per minute.

3. When providing spinal immobilization for this patient,
   a. do not apply a spinal immobilization collar.
   b. check for pulses, motor function, and sensation before and after immobilization.
   c. place padding under the head to account for the large occiput.
   d. secure the head to the immobilization device before the torso.

4. The child in this case could be more accurately referred to as a(n)
   a. neonate.
   b. infant.
   c. toddler.
   d. preschooler.

5. The child in this case would be assigned a Pediatric GCS score of
   a. 3.
   b. 4.
   c. 5.
   d. 6.

<table>
<tr><td>TRIP #</td><td colspan="3" rowspan="6"><h1>EMERGENCY
TRIP SHEET</h1></td><td>BILLING USE ONLY</td></tr>
</table>

TRIP #		BILLING USE ONLY
MEDIC #		
BEGIN MILES		DAY
END MILES		DATE
CODE___/___ PAGE___/___		RECEIVED
UNITS ON SCENE		DISPATCHED

EMERGENCY TRIP SHEET

NAME	SEX M F DOB ___/___/___	EN-ROUTE
ADDRESS	RACE	ON SCENE
CITY	STATE ZIP	TO HOSPITAL
PHONE ( ) - PCP DR.		AT HOSPITAL
RESPONDED FROM	CITY	IN-SERVICE
TAKEN FROM	ZIP	CREW / CERT / STATE #
DESTINATION	REASON	
SSN - - MEDICARE #	MEDICAID #	
INSURANCE CO INSURANCE #	GROUP #	
RESPONSIBLE PARTY ADDRESS		
CITY STATE ZIP PHONE ( ) -		
EMPLOYER		

TIME	ON SCENE (1)	ON SCENE (2)	ON SCENE (3)	EN-ROUTE (1)	EN-ROUTE (2)	AT DESTINATION
BP						
PULSE						
RESP						
SpO$_2$						
ETCO$_2$						
EKG						

IV THERAPY
SUCCESSFUL Y N # OF ATTEMPTS _____
ANGIO SIZE _____ga.
SITE _____
TOTAL FLUID INFUSED _____ cc
BLOOD DRAW Y N INITIALS

INTUBATION INFORMATION
SUCCESSFUL Y N # OF ATTEMPTS _____
TUBE SIZE _____ mm
TIME _____ INITIALS _____

MEDICAL HISTORY

MEDICATIONS

ALLERGIES

C/C

EVENTS LEADING TO C/C

ASSESSMENT

TREATMENT

CONDITION CODES				

TREATMENTS

TIME	TREATMENT	DOSE	ROUTE	INIT

GCS E___ V___ M___ TOTAL =
GCS E___ V___ M___ TOTAL =

HOSPITAL CONTACTED

CPR BEGUN BY   B   P   TIME BEGUN

EMS SIGNATURE

AED USED   Y   N   BY:

RESUSCITATION TERMINATED - TIME

(   ) OSHA REGULATIONS FOLLOWED

Geriatrics

STANDARD

Special Patient Populations (Content Area: Geriatrics)

COMPETENCY

Applies fundamental knowledge of growth, development, aging, and assessment findings to provide basic emergency care and transportation for a patient with special needs.

OBJECTIVES

After reading this chapter, you should be able to:

39-1. Define key terms introduced in this chapter.
39-2. Summarize age-related anatomical and physiological changes for each of the following systems:
   a. Cardiovascular
   b. Respiratory
   c. Neurological
   d. Gastrointestinal
   e. Endocrine
   f. Musculoskeletal
   g. Renal
39-3. Discuss characteristic findings and emergency care steps for common medical emergencies in the elderly population, including:
   a. Myocardial infarction
   b. Congestive heart failure
   c. Pulmonary edema
   d. Pulmonary embolism
   e. Pneumonia
   f. Stroke
   g. Chronic obstructive pulmonary disease
   h. Stroke and transient ischemic attack
   i. Seizure
   j. Syncope
   k. Hyperosmolar hyperglycemic nonketotic syndrome (HHNS)
   l. Drug toxicity

m. Dementia and delirium

n. Alzheimer's disease

o. Trauma or shock

p. Gastrointestinal bleeding

q. Environmental emergencies

r. Abuse

39-4. Describe modifications that may be necessary to effectively assess and treat geriatric patients.

KEY IDEAS

This chapter focuses on the assessment of the geriatric patient, which is a person over the age of 65. Since this is the fastest-growing segment of the population in the United States, and because the majority of EMS calls involve geriatric patients, it is important to understand the characteristics of this age group and how to tailor your assessment to their special needs. Key concepts include the following:

- The elderly are at greater risk for nearly all types of injuries and illness.

- Due to physiological changes caused by aging, the geriatric patient will present with different signs and symptoms than you would expect to find if your patient were younger.

- Geriatric patients often have one or more coexisting long-term conditions or health problems that can mask or change the presentation of their current problem.

TERMS AND CONCEPTS

1. Write the number of the correct term next to each definition.

   1. Arteriosclerosis
   2. Cardiac hypertrophy
   3. Chronic
   4. Dementia
   5. Kyphosis
   6. Osteoporosis
   7. Silent heart attack
   8. Syncope
   9. Stenosis
   10. Neuropathy

   _____ a. Heart attack that causes little or no chest pain

   _____ b. Chronic condition resulting in the malfunctioning of normal cerebral processes

   _____ c. Long term, progressing gradually

   _____ d. Abnormal curvature of the spine

   _____ e. Disease process that causes the loss of elasticity in the vascular walls

   _____ f. Disease characterized by an abnormal loss of bone minerals

   _____ g. A brief period of unconsciousness due to lack of blood flow to the brain

   _____ h. Thickening of the cardiac walls without an increase in the size of the chamber

   _____ i. Any disease of the nerves

   _____ j. Abnormal narrowing of a body canal, vessel, or passageway

CONTENT REVIEW

1. Which of the following statements related to aging is accurate?
   a. Changes in body physiology associated with aging typically begin at about age 50.
   b. The trend is that people are not living as long with chronic disease.
   c. The aging body has fewer reserves with which to combat diseases and traumatic injuries.
   d. Illness is an inevitable part of aging.

2. Cardiovascular system changes associated with aging include
   a. increased arterial elasticity that speeds reaction to stimulation.
   b. a conduction system that carefully maintains heart rate and rhythm.
   c. increased cardiac output due to cardiac hypertrophy.
   d. increased systolic blood pressure due to increased vascular resistance.

3. Aging causes a generalized deterioration of the respiratory system. This is characterized by decreased flexibility of the rib cage, alveolar degeneration, decreased elasticity of the lung tissue, and
   a. increased resistance to infection.
   b. blunted sensitivity to hypoxia.
   c. increased gas exchange through diffusion.
   d. enhanced cough and gag reflex.

4. Which of the following is the most significant musculoskeletal change associated with aging?
   a. Arthritis
   b. Kyphosis
   c. Fibrosis
   d. Osteoporosis

5. Slowing of reflexes commonly seen in the elderly is due to
   a. degeneration of nerve cells.
   b. increased muscle elasticity.
   c. increased impulse transmission.
   d. increased brain mass and weight.

6. Aging of the gastrointestinal system contributes to a variety of medical conditions, as well as
   a. enhanced drug absorption.
   b. increased peristalsis.
   c. malnutrition.
   d. obesity.

7. Which statement best describes changes related to the renal system in the elderly compared to other age groups?
   a. The kidneys become larger in size and weight.
   b. An increase in nephrons in the elderly allows for more blood to be filtered.
   c. It is more common for the elderly to suffer from drug toxicity if they take too much medication.
   d. Elderly patients' renal systems are more resistant to failure during acute illness or injury.

8. Which statement is most correct related to the scene size-up phase of an emergency call involving an elderly patient?
   a. Always wear a HEPA mask when treating a nursing home patient with a cough.
   b. Elderly patients' diminished sensitivity to temperature changes means cold- or heat-related emergencies are less common for these patients.
   c. When you enter a nursing home, focus only on the patient that you have been called to treat.
   d. Elderly patients are unlikely to suffer a medical and a traumatic problem at the same time.

9. Which of the following is a sign of dehydration in the elderly?
   a. The eyes appear to bulge in the orbits.
   b. The mucous membranes appear cyanotic.
   c. The lips appear swollen.
   d. The tongue appears furrowed.

10. Geriatric patients as a group
    a. deteriorate less quickly than other age groups.
    b. are more sensitive to pain than other age groups.
    c. suffer depression less than other age groups.
    d. abuse alcohol more than other age groups.

11. Which statement related to the assessment or management of the geriatric patient is correct?
    a. A sudden onset of altered mental status is common and is called *dementia*.
    b. A narrowed, more rigid esophagus means a reduced incidence of choking on food.
    c. You should never attempt to perform a jaw-thrust maneuver in an elderly patient.
    d. A resting respiratory rate of greater than 20 per minute may be normal.

12. You are treating a 75-year-old woman with an altered mental status and no history of trauma. She should be transported
    a. in a Fowler's position.
    b. lying on her side to protect her airway.
    c. immobilized on a long spine board after applying a cervical collar.
    d. wearing a cervical collar but placed in a position of comfort.

13. You are treating a 78-year-old who fell from a ladder onto his concrete patio and is complaining of back and neck pain. Because of his severe kyphosis, he should be transported
    a. in whatever position is most comfortable.
    b. fully immobilized on a long spine board, wearing a rigid cervical collar.
    c. on a long spine board, using blankets to fill the void from the curvature of the spine.
    d. lying on his left side to prevent aspiration of stomach contents.

14. Due to depressed pain perception, geriatric patients may have a "silent heart attack." Rather than experiencing chest discomfort, they may more commonly complain of
    a. lower abdominal pain.
    b. lower back pain.
    c. weakness and fatigue.
    d. tingling in the fingers.

15. Congestive heart failure commonly occurs in older patients because the heart no longer pumps effectively and blood begins to "back up" into the lungs or peripheral vessels. Results may include fatigue and difficulty breathing. Treatment includes administering oxygen and expediting transport
    a. immobilized to a long spine board.
    b. in a Fowler's position (sitting up).
    c. lying on the side to prevent aspiration.
    d. supine on the stretcher.

16. Your 80-year-old patient suffers from chronic obstructive pulmonary disease (COPD). She is alert and complains of increasing difficulty breathing over the past few days. She denies having any pain. Emergency care for your patient would include administering oxygen to maintain an SpO_2 reading of 94% or greater in the patient with adequate breathing and
    a. assisting her in taking nitroglycerin.
    b. assisting her ventilations with positive pressure.
    c. transporting her in a supine position.
    d. assisting her in using a metered-dose inhaler.

17. You are treating a 77-year-old patient who is complaining of a sudden onset of difficulty breathing and chest pain that is localized and does not radiate. His breathing is labored at 16 per minute. He has a history of heart problems and recently had surgery. Your first priority in emergency treatment is
    a. administering oxygen to maintain an SpO_2 reading of 94% or greater.
    b. administering positive pressure ventilation.
    c. having him sit up with pillows behind his back.
    d. placing him in a lateral recumbent position.

18. After you perform the emergency treatment in question 17, your patient's respiratory rate decreases to 8 per minute. Your most accurate conclusion would be that
    a. your treatment has caused his condition to improve, and no further treatment is required.
    b. your treatment has caused his condition to deteriorate, and you will contact medical direction for advice.
    c. his condition is deteriorating because he is unable to sustain the labor of breathing, and you need to provide positive pressure ventilation.
    d. his condition is improving because these spells come and go spontaneously.

19. An altered mental status in the geriatric patient is
    a. usually a difficult condition to manage.
    b. generally caused by senility.
    c. most often accompanied by a headache.
    d. most often due to hypotension.

20. For each item in the following list, write Y (yes) or N (no) to indicate if it is a common cause of altered mental status in the elderly.
    _____ a. Change in blood glucose level
    _____ b. HIV and HIV-related complexes
    _____ c. Hypothermia or hyperthermia
    _____ d. Respiratory disorders and hypoxia
    _____ e. Medical or traumatic head injury
    _____ f. Infection

21. Key treatment of a stroke includes
    a. maintaining oxygen saturation at an SpO$_2$ reading of 94% or greater.
    b. complete immobilization of the head and neck.
    c. rapid transport to the medical receiving facility with delayed assessment en route.
    d. administering fluids to maintain hydration and perfusion.

22. Which statement is correct related to drug toxicity in the elderly patient?
    a. Younger patients are more at risk for drug toxicity than older patients.
    b. Younger patients buy more prescription drugs than older patients.
    c. Treatment for drug toxicity is based on treating the drug's effects.
    d. You should leave over-the-counter and prescription drugs at the patient's home.

23. You are treating your elderly patient from a nursing facility. As you gather a history from the nurse, she states that the patient has a medical history of "cardiac hypertrophy." You know this to be
    a. a thickening of the cardiac walls without any increase in atrial or ventricular chamber size, which decreases stroke volume.
    b. a thinning (reduction) of the heart walls, increasing the atrial or ventricular chambers, thus increasing stroke volume.
    c. a deterioration in the conduction system of the heart, resulting in the inability of the heart to initiate and transmit a normal impulse.
    d. a systemic increase in the conduction system of the heart, resulting in the ability of the heart to adapt to increased load and demand on the heart.

24. A drop in the systolic blood pressure and an elevation of the heart rate when the elderly patient goes from a lying to a standing position is known as
    a. Trendelenburg hypotension.
    b. supine hypotension.
    c. hemostatic hypotension.
    d. orthostatic hypotension.

25. Which of the following factors contributes to the development of environmental emergencies among the elderly?
    a. Aging enhances the body's ability to control temperature.
    b. Limitations on mobility allow the elderly to maintain body warmth.
    c. Medications that the elderly take have little impact on the ability to control temperature.
    d. Situational factors, such as fixed income, lead to environmental emergencies.

26. Number the following list in the proper order from 1 to 5 to provide emergency care to an elderly patient who is suffering from hypothermia.

    _____ Remove wet clothing.

    _____ Remove the patient from the environment.

    _____ Protect the airway.

    _____ Wrap the patient in a dry blanket.

    _____ Maintain normal breathing and circulation.

27. In the elderly patient, which of the following receptors become less sensitive in detecting hypoxia or carbon dioxide levels in the blood?
    a. Baroreceptors
    b. Chemoreceptors
    c. Oxygen receptors
    d. Kodiak receptors

28. The characteristic curvature of the spine that is caused by narrowing of the vertebral disks in the elderly patient is known as
    a. lumbarosis.
    b. spineosis.
    c. curveosis.
    d. kyphosis.

CASE STUDY

It is early one Sunday afternoon, and the emergency services are relaxing by watching the Buccaneers play the Saints. The Buccaneers have just scored a touchdown when you are dispatched to an 88-year-old woman, Mrs. Walter, who has suffered a fall. As you enter the house, Mrs. Walter's daughter tells you that her mother had pneumonia three months ago but has been doing well since then. No hazards are present. You find your patient seated on the couch holding her right arm very carefully across her chest. She has a large bruise on the left frontal region of her forehead. When you introduce yourself and your partner, Mrs. Walter apologizes for bothering you on a Sunday afternoon. She goes on to say that she lost her balance and fell while coming down a flight of stairs. You find Mrs. Walter to be alert and oriented. Her airway is patent, and her breathing is regular at 16 per minute, with good air exchange. Core and peripheral pulses are strong and regular at 78 per minute and her SpO_2 is 96%. Her skin is slightly pale and moist but warm to the touch. Your partner auscultates her blood pressure at 168/98 in her left arm. Mrs. Walter complains that her right shoulder is very painful where she hit the wall as she fell. You note that there is an obvious deformity near her shoulder and that her right arm seems to droop at an unnatural angle, even though she is supporting it with her left hand.

1. Which statement best describes how you should next proceed with Mrs. Walter's care?
   a. Establish and maintain stabilization of the head and neck.
   b. Provide positive pressure ventilation.
   c. Apply a splint to the injured arm.
   d. Contact adult protective services.

2. Which of the vital sign findings is of concern related to Mrs. Walter's condition?
   a. Pulse
   b. Respirations
   c. Skin color and condition
   d. Blood pressure

Patients with Special Challenges

STANDARD

Special Patient Populations (Content Area: Patients with Special Challenges)

COMPETENCY

Applies fundamental knowledge of growth, development, aging, and assessment findings to provide basic emergency care and transportation for a patient with special needs.

OBJECTIVES

After reading this chapter, you should be able to:

40-1. Define key terms introduced in this chapter.

40-2. Explain the importance of understanding the care of patients with special challenges.

40-3. Give examples of special challenges and their causes.

40-4. Describe accommodations and modifications to patient assessment and management required for patients with sensory impairments.

40-5. Describe accommodations and modifications to patient assessment and management required for patients with cognitive and emotional impairments.

40-6. Describe accommodations and modifications to patient assessment and management required for paralyzed patients.

40-7. Describe accommodations and modifications to patient assessment and management required for obese patients.

40-8. Describe accommodations and modifications to patient assessment and management required for homeless or poor patients.

40-9. Describe accommodations and modifications to patient assessment and management required for abused patients.

40-10. Describe accommodations and modifications to patient assessment and management required for patients who are dependent on the following types of technology:
   a. Airway and respiratory devices
   b. Vascular devices
   c. Renal dialysis
   d. Gastrointestinal and genitourinary devices
   e. Intraventricular shunts

40-11. Describe accommodations and modifications to patient assessment and management required for patients who are terminally ill and describe the philosophy of hospice care.

KEY IDEAS

The EMT is called to manage patients with special needs when their preexisting condition worsens, when a medical device fails, or when the patient experiences some other emergency. Patients that were once primarily cared for in the hospital are increasingly cared for in the patient's home with the use of in-home medical devices. Since EMS is the first agency that is called to care for these special needs patients, the EMT must have a basic understanding of the equipment and special patient requirements.

- When dealing with patients who have sensory impairments of hearing, vision, or speech, use good communication techniques. Speak clearly, position yourself so your face is in clear view, communicate in writing if needed, use a family member to interpret, allow patients the time to respond to questioning, and never pretend that you understand something the patient said if you don't.

- Managing a patient with a mental or emotional impairment, developmental disability, or brain injury requires relying on the caregiver (family or professional health care provider) for information about how the patient's present condition has changed. This will help to determine if the current problem is a chronic or an acute presentation.

- Care for the paralyzed patient depends upon the degree of paralysis. Consult with family or caregivers about the best way to move these patients. When possible, transport assisting devices. Take special care not to dislodge catheters, lines, or tubes.

- Obese patients require special positioning to ensure adequate breathing. Notify the receiving facility about morbidly obese patients and enlist additional personnel during patient moves.

- Individuals who live at or near the poverty level are more likely to be subject to accidental trauma, physical abuse, or crimes and to develop chronic medical conditions. Don't be judgmental. Treat your patients because they need your help, and be familiar with local support services.

- The categories of home medical devices commonly found in homes include airway and respiratory, medical oxygen, pulse oximetry, tracheostomy tubes, continuous positive airway pressure (CPAP) and bilevel positive airway pressure (BiPAP), ventilators, vascular access devices (central intravenous catheters, central lines, and implanted ports), gastrointestinal and genitourinary devices, and intraventricular shunts.

MEDICAL TERMINOLOGY

Term	Prefix	Word Root or Combining Form	Suffix	Definition
hydrocephalus (high-droh-SEFF-ah-lus)	hydro- (water)	cephal (head)		Excessive accumulation of cerebrospinal fluid
intraventricular (in-trah-VEN-trik-u-lar)	Intra (within)	ventricul (ventricle)		Within the ventricle
paraplegia (pair-ah-PLEE-jee-ah)	para (beside)		-plegia (paralysis or stroke)	Paralysis from the waist down
retinopathy (RET-in-op-a-thee)	retin- (retina)		-pathy (disease)	Disease of the retina

1. Atn intraventricular shunt is used to drain excessive cerebrospinal fluid from the brain. The prefix *intra-* means
   a. dry.
   b. life.
   c. cell.
   d. within.

2. In the medical term *diabetic retinopathy*, the suffix *-pathy* refers to
   a. vision.
   b. disease.
   c. swelling.
   d. condition of.

3. In the terms *paraplegia* and *quadriplegia*, the suffix *-plegia* refers to
   a. swelling.
   b. small vessel.
   c. stroke, paralysis.
   d. strength.

TERMS AND CONCEPTS

1. Write the number of each term by its definition.
   1. Acute renal failure (ARF)
   2. Central intravenous catheters
   3. Cataract
   4. Chronic kidney disease (CKD)
   5. Diabetic retinopathy
   6. Intraventricular shunt
   7. Ostomy bag
   8. Surgically implanted medication delivery devices
   9. Tracheostomy

   _____ a. A rapid loss of renal function that results in poor urine production, electrolyte disturbance, and fluid balance disturbance

   _____ b. Damage to the small blood vessels of the eye due to the long-term effects of diabetes mellitus

   _____ c. A long, hollow, tubelike device that is surgically placed in a ventricle of the brain and extends to a blood vessel in the neck, heart, or abdomen in order to drain excess cerebrospinal fluid and keep the intracranial pressure within an acceptable level

   _____ d. A condition in which the lens of the eye becomes cloudy due to pathologic changes within the lens itself

   _____ e. A progressive loss of kidney function over a period of months to years

   _____ f. A pouch or bag that is attached outside the body to help remove feces from the body by directing it through the abdominal wall and into the bag or pouch

   _____ g. Devices that are placed while the patient is in the hospital and are designed to deliver medication into the central circulation of the body

   _____ h. A surgical opening in the trachea

   _____ i. Medication administration devices that are surgically placed beneath the skin, but outside the rib cage

CONTENT REVIEW

1. Which of the following statements best describes the concept of "compression of morbidity"?
   a. It is a general concept of disease prevention that is gaining prominence in the national public health sector.
   b. The term denotes a general trend of lower life spans occurring in certain elderly populations.
   c. The term refers to maximizing healthy years and simultaneously minimizing years of disease or disability at the end of life.
   d. The term refers to deaths that occur among population groups such as those with special needs or challenges.

2. Which of the following terms is paired with its correct definition?
   a. Glaucoma—condition in which the lens of the eye becomes cloudy
   b. Dysarthria—the inability to effectively communicate verbally
   c. Diabetic retinopathy—damage occurring to the vocal cords and larynx
   d. Cataracts—abnormal increase in intraocular pressure

3. Speech impairment chiefly occurs because of four reasons: articulation disorders, voice production disorders, language disorders, and
   a. fluency disorders.
   b. mentation processing disorders.
   c. neurovascular disorders.
   d. glossal function disorders.

4. Which statement is most correct when caring for a patient with a speech impairment?
   a. Ask open-ended questions that require extensive dialogue.
   b. Finish words or statements for the patient in order to limit frustration.
   c. Pretend to understand what the patient is saying, even though you do not understand.
   d. Allow the patient adequate time to respond to your questions.

5. In many patients with special challenges, it may be difficult to determine what is "normal" for the patient. Presenting signs and symptoms may be categorized as
   a. emergent or urgent.
   b. trauma or medical.
   c. chronic or acute.
   d. antegrade or retrograde.

6. Which of the following is not one of the problems commonly encountered by a patient who is paralyzed?
   a. Dementia
   b. Respiratory infections
   c. Urinary tract infections
   d. Bed sores

7. The branch of medicine that deals with the management of obese patients is called
   a. adipositics.
   b. lipidgnosis.
   c. steatpheresis.
   d. bariatrics.

8. It is estimated that about _____ percent of the adults in the United States are either obese or overweight.
   a. 40
   b. 50
   c. 60
   d. 70

9. Morbidly obese patients weigh 50 to 100 percent over their ideal body weight, or more than _____ pounds over their ideal weight.
   a. 200
   b. 175
   c. 150
   d. 100

10. Which statement is most correct in regard to homelessness and poverty in America?
    a. In January 1997, the U.S. Department of Housing and Urban Development reported that there were more than 100,000 people in the United States who meet the definition for homelessness.
    b. The health of a person living in the United States is strongly correlated with the state that the person or family lives in.
    c. A total of 5% of people below the poverty level are older than 65 years of age.
    d. Patients who live at or near the poverty level are more likely to be subject to accidental trauma, physical abuse, or crimes, and to develop chronic medical conditions.

11. Management of the homeless patient
    a. requires the EMT to become familiar with local homeless support services.
    b. should not begin before obtaining payment for services.
    c. should include counseling the patient to seek employment.
    d. requires treatment different from that given to other patients.

12. The most common medical equipment used for patients with special challenges can be categorized into five general groups. Four of the five groupings are listed next. Which common grouping is missing from this list?

    Airway and respiratory devices

    Vascular access devices

    Dialysis shunts

    Gastrourinary support devices

    a. Renal filtering device
    b. Occular equipment
    c. Intraventricular shunts
    d. Fecal containment devices

13. It is impossible to know about all types and makes of medical technology used in patients' homes. The EMT should always approach the special needs patient that is utilizing in-home medical devices by asking the following questions. For each question, insert the key word that is missing.
    1. Where would I get the best _____ from regarding this piece of equipment?
    2. What does this _____ do for the patient?
    3. Can I replicate its _____ should the device fail?
    4. Will this equipment have an effect on how I _____ the patient, or on the findings I may discover?
    5. Has this _____ ever occurred previously, and if so, what fixed it?
    6. Has anyone attempted already to _____ the problem?
    7. Are there specific considerations I need to make when deciding how to best prepare the patient for _____ and transport the patient?

14. The three sources of oxygen for the patient at home are
    a. cylinder, massification, and liquid.
    b. oxygenesis, concentrator, and liquid.
    c. cylinder, concentrator, and liquid.
    d. cylinder, concentrator, and carbogenic transference.

15. The most common cause for an EMS response to a patient dependent upon home oxygen is
    a. operator error.
    b. environmental conditions.
    c. equipment failure.
    d. impure gas.

16. An apnea monitor is
    a. commonly found in the homes of elderly patients.
    b. a device that monitors a patient's tidal volume and ventilates the patient when the tidal volume falls below preset values.
    c. commonly found in the homes of patients with renal, hepatic, or adrenal failure.
    d. designed to monitor the patient's breathing and emit a warning if breathing stops.

17. Which medical device is most likely to be found in the home of a patient with a medical need to keep the oxygen concentration within a specific range?
    a. Apnea monitor
    b. Pulse oximeter
    c. CPAP device
    d. BiPAP device

18. Emergencies involving a patient with a tracheostomy tube generally result from two problems. What are these two problems?
    a. The tube fails or ruptures, or the tube becomes dislodged.
    b. The tube splits horizontally from excessive airway pressures or becomes occluded.
    c. The tube becomes plugged with mucus, or the tube becomes dislodged or occluded.
    d. The tube softens, or the tube becomes occluded by foreign material.

19. The primary purpose of this device is to keep the small bronchiole airways open during exhalation. This improves oxygenation and ventilation and lowers the work of breathing. The device that accomplishes this is called
    a. CPAP.
    b. PAPD.
    c. OPBD.
    d. FiO_2.

20. Which statement is most correct in regard to home ventilators?
    a. They typically have two or three controls: ventilatory rate, tidal volume, and oxygen concentration.
    b. The high-pressure alarm is activated when lung compliance is increased.
    c. The low-pressure alarm is usually set to activate when the tidal volume falls below 10–40 mL, below the tidal volume.
    d. The low FiO_2 alarm will sound when lung compliance is increased.

21. This medication administration device is surgically placed beneath the skin but outside the rib cage. What is the device?
    a. Central venous line
    b. Implanted port
    c. Central intravenous catheter
    d. Vascular access device

22. The two primary types of dialysis are
    a. hemodialysis and ureglobin.
    b. urepathic and peritoneal.
    c. glycodialysis and ureglobin.
    d. hemodialysis and peritoneal.

23. Which statement is most correct in regard to the dialysis patient?
    a. Ureglobin dialysis complications generally involve a displaced catheter, inflammation at the site, or infection of the site.
    b. The EMT should remove the patient from the dialysis machine rapidly without supervision of the dialysis staff when needed during an emergent situation.
    c. The EMT should never attempt to obtain a blood pressure in any extremity with an AV shunt, fistula, or graft.
    d. Glycodialysis patients can bleed excessively and commonly have an AV shunt implanted.

24. Patients that are receiving their nourishment by a feeding tube are said to be receiving
    a. enteral feeding.
    b. external feeding.
    c. enterotubular feeding.
    d. gastro feeding.

25. Orogastric tubes are
    a. slightly smaller than nasogastric tubes.
    b. inserted through the nose.
    c. inserted through the mouth.
    d. slightly shorter than nasogastric tubes.

CASE STUDY 1

You have been dispatched to a dialysis center for a patient who is feeling ill during a dialysis treatment. You arrive on scene and observe a white female about 45 years of age who is lying on a bed, waiting for your arrival. The dialysis center nurse advises you that your patient feels nauseated and lightheaded following her dialysis treatment. The nurse also tells you that the patient has an AV shunt on her left arm.

1. Given this information, you know that
   a. the patient has been undergoing dialysis for some time.
   b. the patient has been undergoing dialysis for a short time.
   c. the patient is most likely suffering from volume overload or volume deficit.
   d. given a few minutes of rest, the patient will most likely not require transport.

2. When taking the patient's diagnostic and vital signs, avoid
   a. taking the patient's blood pressure.
   b. taking the patient's blood pressure in her left arm.
   c. pulse oximeter use in her left arm.
   d. taking the pulse in her left arm.

3. This patient is undergoing
   a. hemodialysis.
   b. peritoneal dialysis.
   c. blood-fluid dialysis.
   d. micturitcentesis dialysis.

CASE STUDY 2

You are transporting a male, special needs patient with an indwelling urinary catheter.

1. Which statement is most correct when transporting a patient with an indwelling urinary catheter?
   a. Transport the collection bag on the stretcher between the patient's legs.
   b. Don't empty the collection bag prior to transport.
   c. Transport the collection bag on the patient's stomach.
   d. Empty the collection bag before moving and document any irregularities in urine color or smell.

2. Indwelling urinary catheters are prone to causing infection
   a. due to patient dislodgment or patient movement.
   b. because the catheter allows a portal of entry for bacteria.
   c. only in elderly patients confined to extended care facilities.
   d. only in immunosuppressed or immunocompromised patients.

3. The patient is disoriented and suddenly pulls on the catheter, dislodging it. You should
   a. quickly replace the catheter.
   b. replace the catheter using sterile technique.
   c. document the incident and report it to the receiving facility staff.
   d. transport the patient without reporting or documenting the incident.

CHAPTER 40 SCENARIO: DOCUMENTATION EXERCISE

Read the following scenario and think about how you would document this call if you were the EMT who responded to the scene. Then answer the multiple-choice questions and fill in the sample prehospital care report, basing your documentation on information from the scenario.

It is 5:30 P.M. on a clear, warm, sunny day. You and your partner, Rebecca, just completed a call and are heading back to the station. The alert sounds: "Unit 5, respond to 826 Chatfield Street for a quadriplegic with ventilator problems; cross street, Cleveland Heights Boulevard. Time out is 1730 hours." Rebecca tells dispatch that you are responding. You arrive in about four minutes at a large, well-kept home in an upper-class neighborhood. A wheelchair ramp snakes up to the front door. Rebecca advises dispatch of arrival on scene. With Standard Precautions in place, you both walk to the front of the home and ring the doorbell.

A well-dressed lady of about 55 years of age answers the door and asks you to come in. You hear an alarm sounding in the back portion of the house: a repetitive sound of three beeps, a pause, and then three more beeps. As you walk toward the beeps, you introduce yourself and Rebecca to the woman and find out that her name is Mrs. Wheaton. She is the patient's mother. The patient's name is Lynn. Lynn is a 26-year-old quadriplegic who is dependent upon a home ventilator device.

Mrs. Wheaton tells you that the high-pressure alarm on Lynn's ventilator triggered about 10 minutes ago, and she is unable to reset the alarm. A nurse normally cares for Lynn, but he had to leave for a few minutes. She states that she has a backup ventilator, if this is needed. She continues by telling you that she is just not sure what is going on. You enter the patient's room and observe Lynn. He is in a hospital bed, in a semi-Fowler's position. The alarm continues to sound, with three beeps, a pause, and then three more beeps. A large blue tube is connected to his tracheostomy tube, which is also connected to the portable ventilator. Lynn looks up at you as you enter the room, and you introduce yourself and Rebecca to him. Rebecca begins a primary survey.

The ventilator's faceplate identifies the device as a Puritan Bennett, Achevia PSO2. You look on the front panel. A red light is flashing the following symbol: **P**–y. Mrs. Wheaton tells you that according to the nurse's notes, this is a high-pressure alarm that sounds when Lynn's tracheostomy tube requires suctioning or when the patient circuit (the blue tube) becomes kinked.

Rebecca is completing the primary assessment. The patient appears to be in moderate distress. He opens his eyes and responds appropriately to commands. His skin color is pale. Rebecca removes the blue tube (patient circuit) from the tracheostomy tube, connects the bag-valve ventilator to the standard connection on the tracheostomy tube, and begins bag-valve ventilation at a rate of 12 ventilations per minute. As she squeezes the bag-valve device, she notes difficulty squeezing the bag and a fluid sound coming from the tracheostomy tube. No kinks are evident in the patient circuit. You tell Rebecca to prepare to suction the patient's tracheostomy tube. You prepare the suction device. Rebecca removes the inner cannula by rotating the tube to the left until a click is felt. She removes the tube while you prepare to suction the outer cannula. You suction the outer cannula while Mrs. Wheaton tells you she will clean the inner cannula that you just removed. The inner cannula appears to be partially filled with clear mucus.

Rebecca replaces the bag-valve device on the proximal connector and continues to ventilate the patient. She reports that it is now much easier to ventilate the patient. Mrs. Wheaton reconnects Lynn's patient circuit to the tracheostomy tube and resets the alarm. The alarm is silenced. You begin to reassess Lynn while Rebecca takes Lynn's vital signs. You talk to Lynn and explain what you are doing. His eyes follow your actions. You perform a secondary assessment and find a red area on Lynn's left heel and observe that the urine in Lynn's urinary catheter bag is cloudy. No other positive assessment findings are noted.

Rebecca reports that the respirations are 14 per minute; the pulse is 96, strong, and regular; the skin is slightly pale, warm to the touch, and dry; the pupils are equal and reactive to light; the blood pressure is 130/80; and the SpO_2 is 98%.

Mrs. Wheaton is relieved that the problem is resolved quickly and thanks you for your help. Lynn's nurse enters the room, and you explain to him what happened. He makes a quick check of the ventilator settings, checks Lynn's tracheostomy tube, and compliments you both on doing a great job. You ask the nurse if Lynn requires transport to the hospital. The nurse advises you that he is fine now. You complete a patient refusal-of-treatment-and-transportation form and ask Mrs. Wheaton to sign the form. She does so and thanks you both once again for your assistance.

You clean up your equipment and advise dispatch that you are available for another call.

1. What is the best way to determine the proper depth of insertion for the suction catheter?
   a. Measure the width of the patient's hand.
   b. Measure the length of the patient's tracheostomy obturator.
   c. The suction catheter does not need to be sized; just insert it deeply and firmly.
   d. Measure the distance from the tip of the patient's nose to the suprasternal notch.

2. The cloudy nature of Lynn's urine in the urinary catheter bag is
   a. appropriate given Lynn's condition.
   b. inappropriate and may be a sign of a urinary tract infection.
   c. a sign of neglect and should be reported at once.
   d. a sign of diabetes and is not a significant finding.

3. The sore on Lynn's heel is
   a. not significant to report and note.
   b. a sign of a urinary tract infection.
   c. a bed sore and should be reported.
   d. a sign of excessive physical therapy.

4. The proximal end of the tracheostomy tube
   a. requires a special, U-shaped adapter to connect to the bag-valve ventilation device.
   b. fits a bag-valve ventilation device.
   c. is color coded to identify it as a potential infection hazard.
   d. requires a special air filter to limit inhalation of foreign materials.

5. Suctioning Lynn's tracheostomy tube
   a. should be limited to no more than 45–60 seconds.
   b. should be limited to no more than 30–45 seconds.
   c. should be limited to no more than 10–15 seconds.
   d. may be conducted without regard to a specific time limit.

EMERGENCY TRIP SHEET

TRIP #	
MEDIC #	
BEGIN MILES	
⬤ MILES	
CODE ___/___ PAGE ___/___	
UNITS ON SCENE	

BILLING USE ONLY

DAY			
DATE			
RECEIVED			
DISPATCHED			

NAME	SEX M F DOB ___/___/___
ADDRESS	RACE
CITY STATE	ZIP
PHONE ( ) -	PCP DR.
RESPONDED FROM	CITY
TAKEN FROM	ZIP
DESTINATION	REASON
SSN - -	MEDICARE # MEDICAID #
INSURANCE CO	INSURANCE # GROUP #
RESPONSIBLE PARTY	ADDRESS
CITY STATE ZIP	PHONE ( ) -
EMPLOYER	

EN-ROUTE		
ON SCENE		
TO HOSPITAL		
AT HOSPITAL		
IN-SERVICE		

CREW	CERT	STATE #

TIME	ON SCENE (1)	ON SCENE (2)	ON SCENE (3)	EN-ROUTE (1)	EN-ROUTE (2)	AT DESTINATION
BP						
PULSE						
RESP						
SpO$_2$						
ETCO$_2$						
EKG						

IV THERAPY
SUCCESSFUL Y N # OF ATTEMPTS _____
ANGIO SIZE _____ga.
SITE _____
TOTAL FLUID INFUSED _____ cc
BLOOD DRAW Y N INITIALS _____

INTUBATION INFORMATION
SUCCESSFUL Y N # OF ATTEMPTS _____
TUBE SIZE _____ mm
TIME _____ INITIALS _____

MEDICAL HISTORY

CONDITION CODES

⬤ CATIONS

TREATMENTS

TIME	TREATMENT	DOSE	ROUTE	INIT

ALLERGIES

C/C

EVENTS LEADING TO C/C

ASSESSMENT

TREATMENT

GCS	E___ V___ M___	TOTAL =			
GCS	E___ V___ M___	TOTAL =			

HOSPITAL CONTACTED

CPR BEGUN BY   B   P   TIME BEGUN

EMS SIGNATURE

AED USED   Y   N   BY:

RESUSCITATION TERMINATED - TIME

⬤

(   ) OSHA REGULATIONS FOLLOWED

The Combat Veteran

STANDARD

Special Patient Populations

OBJECTIVES

After reading this chapter, you should be able to:

41-1. Define key terms introduced in the chapter.
41-2. Discuss the psychophysiology of stress response.
41-3. Define Post-Traumatic Stress Disorder (PTSD).
41-4. Describe the four essential features of PTSD.
41-5. Recognize signs and symptoms of PTSD.
41-6. Discuss the difference between traumatic brain injury (TBI) and PTSD.
41-7. Discuss the assessment and emergency care for a returning combat veteran exhibiting signs and symptoms of PTSD.

KEY IDEAS

Veterans represent a small number of the potential patients that you will be managing, but they have unique patient care requirements. This chapter reviews the fundamental management techniques for these types of patients.

- Post-traumatic stress disorder (PTSD) occurs when normal people are exposed to abnormal stressors or dangerous conditions. It does not indicate a personality flaw or a "weak mind."

- Clues to help you identify patients of this type include a military haircut, the wearing of military clothing, the presence of tattoos, war memorabilia displayed in the home, use of military vocabulary, and respect for authority.

- Questions posed to the patient must be carefully phrased. "Were you in the military?" or "Where did you see combat?" should be used rather than "Did you ever kill anyone?"

- PTSD has four primary features: response, reliving, avoiding, and anxiety or anger.
- The associated signs and symptoms of PTSD include guilt, shame, depression, avoidance of others, hostility, agitation, and anger. Physical responses include pain of an origin that is difficult to determine.
- About 40 percent of these types of patients engage in pathological alcohol and drug use.
- Several factors can help determine whether patients are a danger to themselves or others. Things to focus on include ensuring your own safety at all times, involving others when possible, determining if there is a history of past violence, finding out if the patient has ever talked about suicide or homicide, removing any weapons, taking action if the patient exhibits excessive behaviors, using care with restraints, paying attention to the "gut test," determining if the patient fits the "suicide formula," paying attention to "anniversary reactions," and taking suicide threats seriously.
- A traumatic brain injury (TBI) is a mild concussion. Its signs and symptoms can overlap with PTSD and may occur in the same person.
- Veterans are used to structure. Provide organization and limits during contact with the patient. Reassure the patient that you are there to help by transporting him or her to a medical facility. Don't say that you understand what the person is going through. Instead, build rapport by focusing on the patient's needs, not assuming PTSD, confirming that any weapons are secure, giving the patient personal space, and recognizing potential triggers.

TERMS AND CONCEPTS

1. Write the number of the correct term next to each definition.
   1. PTSD
   2. TBI

   _____ a. Develops from the extreme stress of combat

   _____ b. A concussion

CONTENT REVIEW

1. What percentage of the total U.S. population do veterans comprise?
   a. 10
   b. 8
   c. 6
   d. 1

2. PTSD has existed for many years. Which term was used to describe it during World War II and in the Korean War?
   a. Combat neurosis
   b. Soldier's heart
   c. Nostalgia
   d. Shell shock

3. PTSD
   a. is recognized by most mental health professionals to be an indicator of a "weak mind."
   b. results from contact with environmental substances that are common in a war zone.
   c. only occurs in combat veterans involved in close-contact battlefield conditions.
   d. occurs when individuals are exposed to an abnormal stressor or a dangerous situation.

4. An era veteran is one who
   a. was trained for combat but never went to war.
   b. went to war and was injured.
   c. served in the military prior to 1980.
   d. served in the military prior to 1945.

5. Which of the following is an inappropriate question to ask the patient?
   a. Were you in the military?
   b. Have you ever killed anyone?
   c. Where did you see combat?
   d. In which branch did you serve in the military?

6. The four essential features of PTSD are
   a. reclusive behavior, response, reliving, and depression.
   b. response, reliving, regression, and excessively social behavior.
   c. response, reliving, avoiding, and anxiety/anger.
   d. depression, reliving, avoiding, and anxiety/anger.

7. What percentage of combat veterans experience flashbacks or sleep disturbances?
   a. 100
   b. 50
   c. 40
   d. 10

8. PTSD
   a. results in a normal aging process.
   b. can present with pain that is difficult to substantiate.
   c. never presents with vague or unfocused pain.
   d. rarely presents with a guilt complex or shame.

9. Drug and alcohol use in veterans
   a. is uncommon and occurs in only a small percentage of patients.
   b. can be determined by asking the patient, "What's the most you can drink and still walk?"
   c. is common among almost 100 percent of the veteran population.
   d. acts as a stimulant, heightening the impact of PTSD.

10. The "gut test"
    a. is used to determine the patient's gastrointestinal stability.
    b. should not be used in the field on patients.
    c. is used only by military personnel when evaluating veterans.
    d. is a reflection of the EMT's survival instinct.

11. Which of the following is an action that the EMT should take when assessing if the patient is a danger to themselves or others?
    a. Avoid involving others in the incident.
    b. Avoid questions about previous violent episodes.
    c. Always use physical restraints on the patient.
    d. Take threats of suicide seriously.

12. The "signature wound" of the Vietnam conflict was
    a. traumatic brain injuries.
    b. gunshot wounds to the chest.
    c. amputations.
    d. concussions.

13. TBI
    a. is caused by an external force such as a concussion.
    b. occurs in only a very few combat veterans.
    c. and its signs and symptoms are distinct from PTSD.
    d. should be described as being caused by PSTD.

14. Which statement is most correct regarding TBIs in the combat veteran patient?
    a. It is appropriate for the patient to "tough the injury out" or to ignore the disorder.
    b. Repeated TBIs have little to no long-term impact on the patient.
    c. Any patient presenting with signs and symptoms of TBI should be transported.
    d. If a TBI is missed as a diagnosis and further brain injury occurs, permanent brain damage may result.

15. Which of the following is an appropriate action to take when managing a combat veteran patient?
    a. Use a statement like "I understand what you are going through" to help calm the patient.
    b. Always assume that the patient has PTSD.
    c. Avoid giving reassurance and providing the patient with structure and limits.
    d. Ask the patient, "How many weapons do you own, and are they secure?"

CASE STUDY

You and your partner, Nancy Heltman, are enjoying a break in your busy day when the station alerting system sounds, "Unit One respond to a distraught man at 10450 Moulin Ave." You both make your way to the ambulance and mark en route. As you approach the scene, you see many police cars in front of the home. Dispatch advises that the scene is secured and your patient has sustained lacerations to both forearms.

A police officer meets you at the door and directs you to the patient. As you approach the patient, you notice several empty beer cans strewn about the unkempt room. You find a well-groomed young man with a military-style haircut sitting in a chair with superficial weeping lacerations to both forearms. The patient appears to be staring off into space and states, "I just want the pain to stop." Nancy approaches the patient and introduces you both. The patient replies "Yes, ma'am. Good to meet you." She notices a Killed In Action (KIA) black bracelet, with date, on his left wrist.

1. What clues could help you and Nancy determine that the patient has a history in the armed services?

2. When speaking with the patient, which of the following practices is appropriate?
    a. Ask the patient if he has ever killed the enemy.
    b. Reassure the patient in a calm, firm voice. Be soothing, but be in charge.
    c. Reassure the patient by saying that you know how he feels.
    d. Discourage casual talk meant to build rapport, such as talking about news, sports, and weather.

3. After bandaging the wounds on the patient's forearms, you place him in a position of comfort on the stretcher. While gathering your assessment, he states he has a history of PSTD. You know that which of the following is true regarding PSTD?

   a. It is an indication that the patient is mentally weak or disturbed.

   b. It develops from abnormal stressors or dangerous conditions.

   c. It is a short-term phenomenon easily treated with suppression therapy.

   d. It cannot cause any "real" pain or associated medical problems.

4. While gathering an ongoing assessment en route to the hospital, the patient states that he recently experienced blurred vision, numbness, and headaches, and has had trouble swallowing. You know these symptoms may be related to

   a. psychosomatic dysfunction.

   b. PTSD.

   c. a false or phantom psychological disorder.

   d. a concussion or TBI.

Upon arrival at the hospital's emergency room, you give your report to the receiving nurse. You wish your patient well and thank him for his service to the country. He smiles and thanks you for your help.

Ambulance Operations and Air Medical Response

▌ STANDARD

EMS Operations (Content Areas: Principles of Safely Operating a Ground Ambulance; Air Medical)

▌ COMPETENCY

Applies knowledge of operations roles and responsibilities to ensure patient, public, and personnel safety.

▌ OBJECTIVES

After reading this chapter, you should be able to:

42-1. Describe the privileges afforded to EMTs operating emergency vehicles and the precautions that must be observed while using these privileges.

42-2. Give examples of habits and behaviors that improve driving safety.

42-3. Discuss factors that can affect your ability to maintain control while driving an ambulance.

42-4. Explain precautions that should be taken when driving an ambulance in inclement weather.

42-5. Explain precautions that should be taken when driving an ambulance at night.

42-6. Describe the appropriate use of emergency warning devices, such as lights and sirens.

42-7. Describe the safety precautions to be taken when working at scenes on and near roadways.

42-8. Give examples of the EMT's responsibilities during each of the major phases of an ambulance call.

42-9. Describe post-run actions that should be taken to reduce the spread of infection to you, your coworkers, and patients.

42-10. Discuss situations in which air medical transport should be considered, potential disadvantages of air medical transport, and guidelines for setting up a landing zone.

42-11. Describe the recommendations of the National Association of Emergency Medical Technicians with respect to EMT security and safety.

42-12. Explain precautions to avoid exposing yourself or others to increased levels of carbon monoxide associated with ambulance operations.

KEY IDEAS

As an EMT, you have the responsibility of getting safely to the scene of an emergency and transporting your patients safely to medical care. This chapter focuses on the safe and effective operation of an ambulance and describes important aspects of air medical response. It also provides information on how to prepare yourself, your equipment, your medical supplies, and your vehicle for the emergency call.

- Operation of an emergency vehicle gives you certain privileges; however, at no time is it justified to operate an ambulance in a manner that endangers or jeopardizes anyone else. The EMT that fails to exercise due regard for the safety of others incurs personal liability for any consequences that may result from that disregard.

- Operation of an ambulance requires familiarity and compliance with agency guidelines or procedures, state and local laws, and regulations governing all aspects of emergency vehicle operation.

- Practice roadway safety procedures by not trusting oncoming traffic, not turning your back to approaching traffic, positioning the first arriving vehicle to create a barrier, wearing highly visible vests, turning off headlights at night that may blind oncoming traffic, using other emergency vehicles to slow and redirect traffic, using other warning signs and measures to slow traffic (including traffic cones), parking uphill or upwind of potential hazardous materials incidents, and assigning a person to monitor oncoming traffic.

- The major phases of an ambulance call include daily prerun vehicle and equipment preparation, dispatch, en route to the scene, at the scene, en route to the receiving facility, at the receiving facility, en route to the station or response area, and post run.

- Infection control procedures play a crucial role in preparing your unit and yourself to return to service.

- If your EMS agency interacts with or provides aeromedical emergency service, you must be familiar with local protocols, the information that is required for requesting air medical support, and landing zone safety considerations. You must always comply with these protocols when performing your job.

CONTENT REVIEW

1. A "privilege" associated with the operation of an emergency vehicle is
   a. driving the posted speed limit.
   b. stopping at red lights.
   c. parking properly.
   d. passing in a no-passing zone.

2. Which of the following demonstrates a failure to exercise "due regard for the safety of others"?
   a. You are en route to the scene of an emergency and cautiously move through a red light, slowing down as you enter the intersection.
   b. En route to an emergency scene, you drive the wrong way down a one-way street without using any warning devices.
   c. You park your vehicle over the crest of a hill on a busy highway, post flares, and direct traffic around your location.
   d. You exceed the speed limit in accordance with state and local regulations while responding to the scene of an emergency.

3. To be a good emergency vehicle operator, the EMT should
   a. always travel as fast as possible.
   b. hold the steering wheel at the 9 o'clock and 12 o'clock positions.
   c. always travel the shortest route to the emergency scene.
   d. brake into a curve and gradually accelerate when going out.

4. Which of the following *best* describes the appropriate use of escorts?
   a. Since the use of escorts will decrease your response time to the scene of an emergency, they should be used when feasible.
   b. The use of escorts significantly minimizes the dangers associated with emergency driving; the use of escorts is encouraged.
   c. The use of escorts doubles the hazards associated with emergency driving and should only be used as a last resort.
   d. The use of escorts doubles the hazards associated with emergency driving and should never be used.

5. When using a siren,
   a. pull directly behind a car and then initiate use of the siren.
   b. it is safe to assume that drivers are aware of you.
   c. emergency vehicle operators tend to increase their speed by 30 mph.
   d. it creates emotional stress for you and the patient.

6. During your daily inspection of the ambulance, you note that the brakes appear to be unsafe. You discuss this with your supervisor, who tells you to drive the vehicle anyway. You should
   a. document the incident and drive the vehicle.
   b. document the incident and drive the vehicle with extra care.
   c. document the incident and respectfully refuse to operate the vehicle.
   d. drive the vehicle as requested; documentation is not required.

7. Mark an X or check mark to indicate which of the following is information that should be provided by dispatch.

   _____ a. Location of the call

   _____ b. Name of patient's physician

   _____ c. Nature of the call

   _____ d. Name, location, and callback number of the caller

   _____ e. Patient's insurance provider

   _____ f. Location of the patient at the scene

   _____ g. Number of patients and severity of the problem

   _____ h. Patient's height and weight

8. En route to the scene, it is a good practice to do which of the following?
   a. Determine and clarify the responsibilities of each team member.
   b. Prealert medical direction of the nature of the call.
   c. Drive above the posted speed limit to reduce response time.
   d. Check on fuel levels to ensure that you have enough gas for the return trip.

9. The following is an incomplete list of the major phases of an ambulance call. Fill in the blanks with the omitted phases.
   1. Daily pre-run vehicle and equipment preparation
   2. Dispatch
   3. En route to the scene
   4. _____
   5. En route to the receiving facility
   6. _____
   7. _____
   8. _____

10. At the scene of a collision, if no other vehicles are on scene, the EMT should park the ambulance
    a. in such a way as to provide a safety zone.
    b. as close to the patient as possible.
    c. on the opposite side of the roadway.
    d. only where directed by law enforcement.

11. Stay a minimum of _____ feet from wreckage or a burning vehicle and _____ feet from hazardous material spills.
    a. 2,000/100
    b. 100/2,000
    c. 200/1,000
    d. 1,000/200

12. Upon arrival at the emergency scene,
    a. determine the responsibilities of team members.
    b. rapidly move all patients to the ambulance.
    c. carefully observe the complete incident as you approach.
    d. always leave your headlights on to alert oncoming traffic.

13. En route to the receiving facility, conduct an assessment at least every _____ minutes for a stable patient and every _____ minute(s) for an unstable patient.
    a. 5/15
    b. 10/10
    c. 15/5
    d. 20/1

14. Allowing family or friends in the patient compartment during transport to the hospital
    a. may be helpful if the patient is a child.
    b. is prohibited by most states' EMS statutes.
    c. is helpful if the family or friend is emotionally distressed.
    d. is prohibited by federal EMS statutes.

15. A complete oral report should be given to emergency department personnel at the patient's bedside in order to
    a. ensure proper continuity of care.
    b. expedite the patient's admission into the hospital.
    c. reassess the patient's condition and interventions.
    d. reassure the patient.

16. The prehospital care report
    a. is never given to the patient.
    b. may substitute for all other hospital reports.
    c. is not necessary if you have given an oral report.
    d. copy should be left at the emergency department.

17. A post-run activity is
    a. changing a soiled uniform.
    b. washing your hands.
    c. providing an oral report to hospital personnel.
    d. leaving a copy of the prehospital care report at the hospital.

18. A substance or process that kills all microorganisms is called
    a. a low-level disinfectant.
    b. an intermediate-level disinfectant.
    c. a high-level disinfectant.
    d. sterilization.

19. An intermediate-level disinfectant solution for surfaces that come into contact with intact skin is made by using a _____ solution of household bleach to water.
    a. 1:10
    b. 1:20
    c. 1:50
    d. 1:100

20. Write the number of the correct level of disinfection or sterilization next to the surface or equipment for which it is appropriate.
    1. Low-level disinfection
    2. Intermediate-level disinfection
    3. High-level disinfection
    4. Sterilization

    _____ a. Reusable instruments that made contact with mucous membranes

    _____ b. Environmental surfaces with no visible contamination and no suspected tuberculosis (TB)

    _____ c. Instruments that are used invasively

    _____ d. Surfaces that come in contact with intact skin

21. Appropriate guidelines for setting up a helicopter landing zone include
    a. putting a fifth warning device on the upwind side.
    b. designating a 75-by-75-foot area for a nighttime landing zone.
    c. keeping spectators at least 100 feet away.
    d. designating a 50-by-50-foot area for a daytime landing zone.

22. National Association of Emergency Medical Technicians (NAEMT) guidelines for ensuring operational safety and security measures require
    a. security briefings at the end of each shift.
    b. decreased involvement of EMS crews in development of security measures.
    c. never leaving EMS vehicles unattended with the keys in the ignition.
    d. reducing the tracking systems of EMS vehicles.

23. Night driving
   a. results in fewer fatal collisions than do daytime driving conditions.
   b. is more difficult for younger people than older drivers.
   c. can be improved by staring directly at the high beams of oncoming cars.
   d. can be improved by using quartz-halogen headlights in EMS vehicles.

24. A technique for safe driving at night is to
   a. use the high beams when entering a curve.
   b. dim your headlights within 50 feet of an approaching driver.
   c. keep your eyes moving; avoid focusing on one object.
   d. flick high beams up and down to remind a driver to dim his bright lights.

25. When driving in bad weather, be aware that
   a. the roads are most slippery at the end of a rainstorm.
   b. if hydroplaning begins, you should hold the wheel steady.
   c. stopping on ice requires three times the stopping distance.
   d. hydroplaning can begin at speeds of 50 mph.

26. Carbon monoxide in ambulances
   a. is easy to detect due to its distinctive odor.
   b. occurs with greater outside air pressure.
   c. can be reduced by opening the rear windows.
   d. may be harmful in amounts over one part per million.

Gaining Access and Patient Extrication

▎ STANDARD

EMS Operations (Content Area: Vehicle Extrication)

▎ COMPETENCY

Applies knowledge of operational roles and responsibilities to ensure patient, public, and personnel safety.

▎ OBJECTIVES

After reading this chapter, you should be able to:

43-1. Define key terms introduced in this chapter.

43-2. Explain elements of dispatch information, including location and whether it is a motor vehicle collision or other type of emergency, that would indicate possible obstacles to patient access, extrication, and care, and discuss how you can plan for such situations.

43-3. Use scene size-up findings to anticipate and prepare for the following:
   a. Potential problems in accessing patients
   b. Need for additional resources
   c. Appropriate personal protective equipment
   d. Appropriate measures to improve scene safety
   e. Location of all patients
   f. Vehicle safety in a collision situation

43-4. Explain actions that may be required to gain residential access.

43-5. Explain actions that may be required to gain motor vehicle access, including the concepts of simple and complex access.

43-6. Describe the role of the EMT and basic considerations for caring for a patient entrapped in a vehicle.

43-7. Describe equipment and methods for stabilizing an upright vehicle, a vehicle on its side, and a vehicle on its roof.

43-8. Describe various methods of accessing, disentangling, and extricating a patient entrapped in a vehicle.

KEY IDEAS

Your primary role in a rescue situation is gaining access to the patient as quickly as can be safely accomplished in order to perform patient assessment and care. Your two major priorities are to keep yourself and your partner safe and to prevent further harm to the patient.

■ Proper protective clothing and equipment must be used at every incident in which hazards (such as shattered glass, sharp metal, flammable liquids, battery acid, and body fluids) are present.

■ If you are first to arrive at the scene, you may be responsible for scene size-up and scene stabilization until police, fire, and other rescue personnel arrive. The most frequent rescue situations are motor vehicle collisions. Related hazards include downed electrical lines and uncontrolled traffic.

■ After all hazards are addressed and the scene is secure, the vehicles involved must be properly stabilized by specially trained rescue personnel. A vehicle is considered stable when it is in a secured position and can no longer move, rock, or bounce.

■ Most emergency calls do not present access problems. However, when they do, it is best to call for rescuers who have had specialized training. Residential access includes locating the patient first and evaluating the need for a forced entry based on dispatch information, what you observe at the scene, and your conversation with the patient. In a motor vehicle collision, the access of choice is a door.

■ The role of the EMT in vehicle stabilization and patient extrication is that of patient care provider. Once specialized rescue personnel assure you that a vehicle is stabilized and the scene is safe, you may approach the patient to initiate care. Patient care always precedes removal from the vehicle unless delay would endanger the life of the patient, EMS personnel, or other rescuers.

■ After gaining access to a patient, provide the same care that you would provide to any trauma patient. In addition, you are responsible for assisting the patient through the extrication process and preparing him mentally and physically for disentanglement from the wreckage. Be sure to stabilize and, if possible, immobilize the spine securely before you remove the patient from the vehicle by normal or rapid extrication procedures.

CONTENT REVIEW

1. When should you first begin to plan for access and extrication problems?
   a. When receiving dispatch information
   b. While en route to the incident
   c. While you are approaching the scene
   d. After effectively evaluating the scene

2. Which of the following will present the most frequent rescue problems for an EMT-Basic?
   a. Water rescue incidents
   b. Motor vehicle collisions
   c. Partial or complete building collapse
   d. Work-site accidents

3. All ambulances should carry which of the following to assess the scene from a safe distance?
   a. An air-particle sniffer
   b. A cell phone
   c. Powerful binoculars
   d. Protective outerwear

4. Which of the following is the most appropriate equipment for personnel involved in the vehicle extrication process?
   a. Full protective turnout gear
   b. Work uniform with helmet
   c. Protective coveralls, helmet, and work gloves
   d. Safety helmet with safety shield

5. When dealing with electrical power lines, which of the following is correct?
   a. Downed lines are electrically alive only when arcing.
   b. Power lines that are not arcing are considered safe.
   c. Always assume that downed lines are electrically alive.
   d. Remove power lines only when wearing rubber gloves.

6. In general, which of the following is the safest method of traffic control at a serious vehicle collision?
   a. Stop all traffic and turn it around.
   b. Stop all traffic and reroute it to different roads.
   c. Slowly guide the vehicles around the scene.
   d. Hold all traffic in place until the scene is cleared.

7. While working a vehicle collision, you notice a small sweater in the rear seat of one of the vehicles. What might this indicate?

   _____

   _____

8. A vehicle is stable when which of the following takes place?
   a. Cribbing has been placed front and rear.
   b. All four tires are on a flat surface.
   c. It can no longer move, rock, or bounce.
   d. The engine is off, and the parking brake is set.

9. The majority of electric current hazards associated with auto collisions can be most simply and quickly eliminated when someone
   a. disconnects the battery.
   b. pulls the main fuse.
   c. disables the coil wire.
   d. turns off the ignition.

10. Briefly explain what steps should be taken to provide patient access in a vehicle collision before turning off or disconnecting the vehicle's power.

    _____

    _____

    _____

11. If it is necessary to disconnect the car battery, first cut or use a wrench to
    a. remove the negative battery cable first.
    b. disconnect the cable on the starter.
    c. disconnect the positive cable first.
    d. lift the battery out of the engine compartment.

12. You are preparing to gain access to your patient trapped in a vehicle. You determine that you will need to use tools and specialized equipment. This type of access is known as
    a. simple access.
    b. complex access.
    c. special access.
    d. pinned access.

13. Police are on the scene, and you are about to make forcible entry into a residence for a medical emergency. Which of the following is the quickest, easiest, and least costly method of forcible entry?
    a. Breaking a window
    b. Forcing a door open
    c. Cutting a door lock
    d. Calling a locksmith

14. The patient is pinned inside a vehicle involved in a collision. He is in the driver's seat, facing front. How should you approach him?
    a. From the left side
    b. From the right side
    c. From the front
    d. From directly behind

15. Your patient is pinned inside a vehicle involved in a collision. What is the best way to tell him to unlock the door?
    a. "Unlock the door, but please turn your body at the shoulders."
    b. "Turn your body at the shoulders, then try to unlock the door."
    c. "Try to unlock the door, but don't move your head or neck."
    d. "Without moving your head or neck, try to unlock the door."

16. When using a sharp tool like a screwdriver to break a vehicle window, the tool should be placed _____ of the window.
    a. against the direct center
    b. against the upper center
    c. against a lower corner
    d. against an upper corner

17. In which of the following situations would removal from the vehicle precede patient care?
    a. The patient is hysterical and tries to extricate himself.
    b. Delaying removal would endanger the patient or rescue personnel.
    c. The vehicle extrication will take over an hour.
    d. There is minor damage, and the patient can be extricated quickly.

18. To protect yourself, the patient, and other EMTs from the glass and flying debris that commonly result from disentanglement operations, you should do which of the following?
    a. Cover the patient with your body.
    b. Direct the patient to move to the back seat.
    c. Share your personal protective equipment with those at the scene.
    d. Use blankets, a tarp, or a spine board.

19. To help reduce your patient's fears while being extricated, you should do which of the following?
    a. Reassure the patient that you are highly skilled.
    b. Explain the activities, noises, and movements.
    c. Try to have the patient think of pleasant thoughts.
    d. Explain that this is an everyday, routine occurrence.

20. The only exception to the rule that the spine must be stabilized and, if possible, immobilized before removing a patient from a vehicle is when
   a. the patient does not complain of pain or discomfort.
   b. the patient appears intoxicated and adamantly refuses treatment.
   c. the patient is in her last trimester of pregnancy.
   d. another patient blocks access to a critically injured patient.

21. Briefly explain how you should perform a 360-degree assessment of a motor vehicle crash site.

_____

_____

_____

22. The most common and effective way to deactivate the undeployed air bags in the motor vehicle is to
   a. place a safety net over the air bag.
   b. disconnect the vehicle's battery cable.
   c. disconnect the air bag wiring from the fuse block.
   d. place the car in park and turn the ignition key to the off position.

23. You are dispatched to an overturned tractor-trailer on the highway. Upon arrival on the scene, you should position your vehicle
   a. uphill and downwind.
   b. downhill and upwind.
   c. downhill and downwind.
   d. uphill and upwind.

SPECIALIZED STABILIZATION, EXTRICATION, AND DISENTANGLEMENT TECHNIQUES

1. You have responded to a motor vehicle crash. What is the first step of stabilizing an upright vehicle?
   a. Remove the door next to the patient.
   b. Immobilize the suspension.
   c. Disconnect the battery cable.
   d. Let the air out of the tires.

2. You are on the scene of a motor vehicle crash where a vehicle has come to rest on its side. The first step in stabilizing this vehicle is to
   a. immobilize the suspension by placing step chocks or blocks beneath the undercarriage.
   b. cut the "A" and "B" posts, then roll the roof downward toward the ground.
   c. place block cribbing or step chocks into the void below both tires near the ground.
   d. attach a pulling device from the undercarriage of the vehicle to an immovable object.

3. You are on the scene of a crash where a four-door, midsize car has come to rest on its roof. Which of the following could lead to collapse of the car's roof?
   a. Using high-pressure air bags
   b. Immobilizing the suspension
   c. Opening a door
   d. Cribbing the voids

4. You are using the hydraulic spreaders to gain access to a patient in the front seat of a vehicle. You know that the front doors are most easily opened by prying at the latch site on the
   a. "A" post.
   b. "B" post.
   c. "C" post.
   d. "D" post.

5. Your patient is trapped inside a vehicle that is on its side. Access to the patient is best gained by
   a. opening the trunk or rear hatch.
   b. lifting the door on top of the car.
   c. cutting the roof off the car.
   d. removing the rear window.

▌ CASE STUDY

You and your partner, Joe Wilson, are working overtime as a standby crew at a local polo match. The last chukker has been completed when you hear a loud screech, followed by a terrible crash. You both look toward the highway and see a large luxury car wrapped around a utility pole. Joe quickly advises dispatch of the situation, that the match has ended, and that you will be responding. As you approach the scene, you notice an electrical line that is broken 80 feet from the pole and is lying across the hood of the car. A crowd of bystanders has begun to surround the scene. Joe radios dispatch, advises them of the utility line, and requests a priority response from the power company. A polo-grounds security guard tells you that his personnel have shut off the power. You can visualize the patient in the car; the middle-aged man is trying to remove his seat belt.

1. Which of the following is the correct way to secure this scene?
   a. Secure an area that is more than 80 feet in all directions. Do not approach the vehicle. Yell instructions to the patient and advise him to stay in the vehicle.
   b. Secure an area up to 75 feet in all directions in case the power is restored. Approach the vehicle, since the guard advised that the power is off, and begin to assess the patient.
   c. There is no reason to secure a perimeter since the power is off; however, you should advise bystanders to keep back so you can work.
   d. Ask bystanders to keep back at least 40 feet (half the distance from the pole). This will keep them clear of danger. Then yell to the patient to stay in the vehicle.

2. Until you are able to gain access, which of the following is the most appropriate way to keep this patient from moving his head and neck?
   a. Instruct the patient to place his hands on either side of his head and apply manual stabilization.
   b. Instruct the patient to close his eyes and try to block out what is happening around him.
   c. Tell the patient to focus and keep his attention on an object directly in front of him.
   d. Have the patient try to lie down across the front seat and remain absolutely still.

3. Briefly explain how you and your partner can decrease the fears that this patient may experience during the noise and confusion that often accompany disentanglement.

   _____

   _____

   _____

Hazardous Materials

STANDARD

EMS Operations (Content Area: Hazardous Materials)

COMPETENCY

Applies knowledge of operational roles and responsibilities to ensure patient, public, and personnel safety.

OBJECTIVES

After reading this chapter, you should be able to:

44-1. Define key terms introduced in this chapter.

44-2. Explain the U.S. Department of Transportation placard system and the National Fire Protection Association symbols for identifying hazardous materials.

44-3. Explain the purpose of shipping papers and material safety data sheets.

44-4. List sensory indications that a hazardous materials situation may exist.

44-5. Identify resources that can be used in the identification and management of hazardous materials incidents.

44-6. Differentiate between the levels of hazardous materials training identified by the Occupational Safety and Health Administration.

44-7. Explain the general rules of hazardous materials rescue.

44-8. Discuss the components of hazardous materials incident management, including:
   a. Preincident planning
   b. Considerations in implementing the plan
   c. Establishing safety zones
   d. Emergency procedures, including decontamination, that should take place in each zone

44-9. Describe special considerations in responding to and managing patients exposed to or contaminated with radiation.

44-10. Differentiate between radiation sickness, radiation injury, and radiation poisoning.

44-11. List factors that determine the amount of risk posed to patients and rescuers by a source of radiation.

44-12. Describe the importance of being knowledgeable about terrorist attacks involving weapons of mass destruction.

KEY IDEAS

Hazardous materials spills and incidents are increasing in frequency. The EMT's role in such emergencies is to recognize that a hazardous material emergency exists, avoid contact with the substance, isolate the area, and notify the appropriate authorities or response agencies (RAIN). This chapter reviews recognition and EMS management of hazardous material emergencies. The personal safety of the EMT is emphasized.

- The principal dangers from hazardous materials are toxicity, flammability, and reactivity.

- The amount of injury caused by a hazardous material depends on the dose, concentration, route of exposure, and amount of time that the patient is exposed.

- The primary concerns in any hazardous material emergency are rescuer safety, public safety, and patient safety.

- The U.S. Department of Transportation's regulations require vehicles containing hazardous materials to be marked with specific hazard labels or placards and accompanied by shipping papers.

- Resources for hazardous material identification and management include state and local agencies, state and local hazardous material teams, the U.S. Department of Transportation's *Emergency Response Guidebook*, CHEMTREC (1-800-424-9300), Chemtel Inc. (1-800-255-3924), and your regional poison control center.

- Avoid contact with any unidentified material, regardless of the level of protection offered by your clothing and equipment.

- The most essential part of hazardous materials rescue is preincident planning. Plan for the worst possible scenario and tailor the plan to the individual community. As part of your plan, predesignate one command officer, establish a clear chain of command and a system of communications, and predesignate receiving facilities.

- An early priority at the scene of any hazardous material emergency is to establish safety zones in which rescue operations may be carried out. These zones are the hot (exclusion) zone, the warm (contamination reduction) zone, and the cold (support) zone.

- Do not enter the hazardous materials area unless you are trained at least to the hazardous materials technician level and are trained in the use of self-contained breathing apparatus (SCBA) and chemical protective clothing.

TERMS AND CONCEPTS

1. Write the number of the correct term next to each definition.

   1. Warm zone
   2. Cold zone
   3. Hazardous material
   4. Hot zone

   _____ a. Includes chemicals, wastes, and other dangerous products

   _____ b. Area adjacent to the warm zone in a hazardous material emergency; normal triage, treatment, and stabilization are performed here; also called *support zone*

   _____ c. Area where contamination is actually present; it generally is the area that is immediately adjacent to the accident site and where contamination can still occur; also called *exclusion zone*

   _____ d. Area that is established surrounding or immediately adjacent to the hot zone, the purpose of which is to prevent the spread of contamination; also called *contamination reduction zone*

CONTENT REVIEW

1. Which of the following is the primary concern in any hazardous material emergency?
   a. Preservation of property and environment
   b. Rescuer, public, and patient safety
   c. Rapid control and removal of the hazard
   d. Locating placards and shipping papers

2. What factors determine a patient's response to a hazardous material exposure?
   a. Material, concentration, and exposure route
   b. Environment, exposure route, preexisting medical conditions, and material
   c. Dose, concentration, route of exposure, and exposure time
   d. Environment, material, preexisting medical condition, and dose

3. A hazardous material warning placard, required by the U.S. Department of Transportation used to designate hazardous materials, is usually
   a. a circle with a triangle in the center.
   b. two concentric circles.
   c. a four-sided diamond.
   d. a triangle with the point facing down.

4. In the internationally recognized NFPA 704 Hazardous Material Identification System, a blue diamond indicates a(n)
   a. health hazard.
   b. acid/alkali hazard.
   c. fire hazard.
   d. reactivity hazard.

5. An important resource available to rescuers 24 hours a day is a public service division of the Chemical Manufacturer's Association. It is referred to as
   a. Chemical Transportation Emergency Center (CHEMTREC).
   b. Chemical Transportation Awareness Program (CHEMA WARE).
   c. Chemical Emergency Response Guide (CHEMERG).
   d. Chemical Manufacturer's Association Center (CHEMMAC).

6. Hazardous materials
   a. should be detected by relying on your senses.
   b. are always easily detectable.
   c. may create colored vapor clouds.
   d. spills need not be treated as dangerous.

7. The principal dangers that hazardous materials present are
   a. toxicity, flammability, and solubility.
   b. toxicity, flammability, and reactivity.
   c. toxicity, flammability, and carcinogenic properties.
   d. solubility, toxicity, and carcinogenic properties.

8. A concise print reference guide that lists more than 1,000 hazardous materials, each with a four-digit UN identification number that is cross-referenced to complete emergency instructions, is called the
   a. *Emergency Response and HAZMAT Directory.*
   b. *Emergency Response Guidebook.*
   c. *American and International Guidebook.*
   d. *HAZMAT Response Guide.*

9. Which of the following is one of the four levels of training that OSHA and the EPA have identified as necessary for dealing with hazardous material emergencies?
   a. Hazardous Materials Generalist
   b. First Responder Awareness
   c. On-Scene Hazardous Materials Advisor
   d. Hazardous Materials Professional

10. Smoke from a hazardous material fire
    a. is transformed into a harmless state because of the intense temperatures of hazardous material fires.
    b. is transformed into a mildly toxic state because of the intense temperatures of hazardous material fires.
    c. threatens the immediate safety of patients and rescuers and threatens their long-term health.
    d. only threatens the immediate safety of patients and rescuers.

11. Before a hazardous material emergency occurs,
    a. two command officers should be appointed for all decision making.
    b. agencies should develop internal, confidential communications plans.
    c. predesignate the hospital receiving facilities that will be used.
    d. train and prepare for the most likely scenario that may occur.

12. Number the following list in the proper order from 1 to 3 to show the three general priorities in a hazardous material emergency.

    _____ Decontaminate clothing, equipment, and the vehicle.

    _____ Protect the safety of all rescuers and patients.

    _____ Provide patient care.

13. Which statement best describes correct activities or actions in the hot zone?
    a. Bystanders are allowed only in the designated area of the hot zone.
    b. Smoking, eating, and drinking are allowed in some areas of the hot zone.
    c. At least three entry points into and out of the hot zone must be established.
    d. Rescue, initial decontamination, and treatment of life threats take place in the hot zone.

14. Prior to air transport of a contaminated patient, be sure to
    a. establish a landing zone within the hot zone.
    b. decontaminate the patient fully.
    c. contact the patient's family.
    d. contact the receiving facility.

15. If you have no training to handle a hazardous material emergency, radio immediately for help and
    a. keep downhill, downwind, downstream, and away from the danger.
    b. keep downhill, upwind, upstream, and away from the danger.
    c. keep uphill, upwind, upstream, and away from the danger.
    d. keep uphill, downwind, downstream, and away from the danger.

16. Failure to decontaminate equipment and the interior of the vehicle properly can result in
    a. mechanical failure.
    b. chronic chemical exposure.
    c. electronic equipment deterioration.
    d. damage to external surface areas.

17. In a radiation accident, the patient may suffer from
    a. contamination by radiation only.
    b. exposure to radiation only.
    c. both exposure to and contamination by radiation.
    d. immediate cardiac failure due to radiation exposure.

18. Which statement is most correct related to radiation accidents?
    a. Every EMT should quickly decontaminate all patients exposed to radiation.
    b. If a Radiation Safety Officer is not available, transport the patient wrapped in a sheet.
    c. The type of radioactive material involved is the most critical factor in how a radiation emergency will be managed.
    d. Alpha rays can be stopped by clothing.

19. _____ is caused by exposure to large amounts of radiation. It starts anywhere from a few hours to days following the exposure and, depending on the dose, can last from a few days to seven or eight weeks.
    a. Radiation sickness
    b. Radiation injury
    c. Radiation syndrome
    d. Radiation poisoning

20. The Federal Nuclear Regulatory Commission recommends that an individual in an emergency situation not be exposed to more than a one-time, whole-body dose of _____ roentgens.
    a. 10
    b. 15
    c. 20
    d. 25

21. _____ occurs when the patient has been exposed to a dangerous amount of internal radiation that results in a host of diseases, including cancer and anemia.
    a. Radiation sickness
    b. Radiation injury
    c. Radiation syndrome
    d. Radiation poisoning

CASE STUDY 1

You have responded to a call for an overturned tractor-trailer on a remote stretch of highway. From a distance, you observe green smoke escaping from the back of the trailer. A man, standing about 100 yards away, waves you down. You pull over and watch him walk up to you. The man is about 45 years old and looks well. He has a normal gait and does not appear to be injured. You ask him, "Why did you call the ambulance?" He says, "I don't know who called you. I called the police. Hey, I was alone, I fell asleep, and I ran off the road. I bounced around inside the truck, and then I crawled out." While talking to the patient, you use your binoculars and spot a diamond-shaped panel on the back of the truck. You take out your *Emergency Response Guidebook* to look up the UN ID number and determine that the number refers to chlorine gas.

1. What is your next *best* action to take?
    a. Enter the truck cab and search for shipping papers.
    b. Approach from downwind to survey the scene.
    c. Enter the truck cab and search for additional patients.
    d. Quickly request additional assistance.

2. After taking the action in question 1, what is your next *best* action?
    a. Call CHEMTREC for hazard control information.
    b. Enter the trailer and begin decontamination procedures.
    c. Keep uphill and upwind, and protect yourself and the patient.
    d. Crack open the trailer doors to vent and prevent buildup of fumes.

CASE STUDY 2

You have responded to a hazardous material accident. The patient is being decontaminated. You arrive on scene and report to the staging area. Shortly after, you are called to the cold zone to transport the patient.

1. You are accidentally splashed with contamination from an anxious and fatigued rescuer. Contamination can occur most easily in which of the following areas of your body?
    a. Lower legs and feet
    b. Lower arms and hands
    c. Under the arms and in the groin
    d. Back

2. How should you decontaminate yourself?
    a. Wash with green soap and plenty of running water, irrigating skin for at least 20 minutes.
    b. Use high-pressure hoses to wash and irrigate skin for at least 20 minutes.
    c. Use baking soda to neutralize the contaminant, then stand under running water for at least 20 minutes.
    d. Blot your skin with towels and dispose of the towels in a sealed biohazard container.

3. What precautions should be undertaken prior to transport of the decontaminated patient?
    a. Treat the patient's major and minor injuries in the hot zone before moving.
    b. Cover exposed areas of the vehicle with plastic sheeting.
    c. Transport the patient's clothing with the patient and leave it at the hospital.
    d. Transport with the patient any contaminated patient care equipment used in the hot zone.

CASE STUDY 3

You have responded to a call for a man down at a local fertilizer distributor. You arrive on scene and observe smoke billowing from the building. A bystander is preparing to enter the building to put the fire out with a garden hose.

1. What should you do?
    a. You should remove the bystander, evacuate the area, and contact dispatch.
    b. You, the bystander, and your partner should enter to put out the fire.
    c. You should contact dispatch while your partner puts out the fire.
    d. You should contact dispatch and remain near the building to direct firefighters.

CHAPTER 44 SCENARIO: DOCUMENTATION EXERCISE

Read the following scenario and think about how you would document this call if you were the EMT who responded to the scene. Then answer the multiple-choice questions and fill in the sample prehospital care report, basing your documentation on information from the scenario.

It is 1:30 P.M. on an overcast Monday. You have just returned to the station after completing a patient transfer from a nursing home to the local hospital when the station alarm sounds: "Rescue 1, respond to 5243 Old Dixie Highway, the Jasper Refrigerated Storage Company, cross street Highway 17 North, for a suspected ammonia exposure. Multiple patients may be involved. Hazmat is responding. Rescue 2, 7, 5, and 10 are also responding. Report to the staging area in front of the Texaco gas station at Old Dixie and Western Avenue. Time out 1330 hours." You and your partner, Colleen, quickly make your way to the vehicle and advise dispatch that you are responding.

You arrive at the staging area in about 10 minutes. You are met by the staging area officer, who advises you that an ammonia leak occurred and that the hazmat crew is entering the building, looking for victims. Another 20 minutes pass, and the staging officer advises you to respond to the storage company to transport a patient removed from the building. You respond to the storage company.

You arrive at an area that the hazmat team has established as a triage area for patients that have been removed from the building. The triage officer tells you that the patient was exposed to ammonia gas and is experiencing mild respiratory distress. The patient is lying on the ground, and oxygen is being administered via a nonrebreather mask at 15 lpm She is alert and looks at you as you approach. She appears to be about 25 years old and seems to be in minor distress. She appears to be breathing adequately, with no abnormal respiratory sounds present. Her skin color looks good. You reach down and feel her pulse while you introduce yourself and your partner. Her pulse is strong and regular, and her skin is warm and dry. You ask her, "What's your name?" She says, "My name is Jill Epson." You ask, "How do you feel, Jill?" Jill says, "It is difficult to breathe at times. However, it's much better now than it was a few minutes ago."

You auscultate the patient's chest and find the breath sounds to be clear and equal bilaterally. The triage officer hands you a patient care record that has Jill's vital signs and physical evaluation recorded. The vitals are that she is alert and oriented to person, place, and time; her respirations are 16 per minute and normal; her pulse is 90 per minute, strong, and regular; her skin is warm, dry, and normal color; her blood pressure is 130/76; and her SpO_2 is 98%. You place Jill on the stretcher, maintaining the oxygen flow, and place her in the ambulance. Colleen obtains a history while on the way to the hospital, takes a second set of vital signs, and completes a physical exam. The vital signs are stable, and no negative physical findings are observed. Jill tells Colleen that she was trapped in a back area of the building and inhaled only a small amount of ammonia gas. She complains of a sore throat and is having some slight difficulty breathing. She takes no medications, has no prior medical history, and last ate at noontime.

1. Command for this hazmat situation should be assumed by
   a. two command officers.
   b. one command officer.
   c. three command officers.
   d. no one; no command is necessary.

2. The receiving facility to which the patient is transported should be
   a. predesignated.
   b. a level I trauma center.
   c. a burn center.
   d. a respiratory care center.

3. You auscultated Jill's chest for the presence of
   a. pulmonary embolism.
   b. a pneumothorax.
   c. pulmonary edema.
   d. cardiac dysrhythmias.

4. For hazmat responses, you and Colleen are most likely trained to the level of
   a. First Responder Awareness.
   b. EMR Operations.
   c. Hazardous Materials Technician.
   d. Hazardous Materials Specialist.

5. The area where the ammonia contamination is present would be designated the
   a. hot zone.
   b. warm zone.
   c. contamination zone.
   d. control zone.

TRIP #		EMERGENCY TRIP SHEET	BILLING USE ONLY				
MEDIC #							
BEGIN MILES			DAY				
END MILES			DATE				
CODE___/___	PAGE___/___		RECEIVED				
UNITS ON SCENE			DISPATCHED				

NAME		SEX M F DOB ___/___/___	EN-ROUTE		
ADDRESS		RACE	ON SCENE		
CITY	STATE	ZIP	TO HOSPITAL		
PHONE ( ) -	PCP DR.		AT HOSPITAL		
RESPONDED FROM		CITY	IN-SERVICE		
TAKEN FROM		ZIP	CREW	CERT	STATE #
DESTINATION		REASON			
SSN - -	MEDICARE #	MEDICAID #			
INSURANCE CO	INSURANCE #	GROUP #			
RESPONSIBLE PARTY	ADDRESS				
CITY	STATE ZIP	PHONE ( ) -	IV THERAPY		
EMPLOYER			SUCCESSFUL Y N # OF ATTEMPTS ___		

TIME	ON SCENE (1)	ON SCENE (2)	ON SCENE (3)	EN-ROUTE (1)	EN-ROUTE (2)	AT DESTINATION
BP						
PULSE						
RESP						
SpO$_2$						
ETCO$_2$						
EKG						

IV THERAPY
SUCCESSFUL Y N # OF ATTEMPTS ___
ANGIO SIZE ___ga.
SITE ___
TOTAL FLUID INFUSED ___ cc
BLOOD DRAW Y N INITIALS ___

INTUBATION INFORMATION
SUCCESSFUL Y N # OF ATTEMPTS ___
TUBE SIZE ___ mm
TIME ___ INITIALS ___

MEDICAL HISTORY	CONDITION CODES				
	TREATMENTS				
MEDICATIONS	TIME	TREATMENT	DOSE	ROUTE	INIT
ALLERGIES					
C/C					
EVENTS LEADING TO C/C					
ASSESSMENT					
TREATMENT					
	GCS E___V___M___TOTAL =				
	GCS E___V___M___TOTAL =				
	HOSPITAL CONTACTED				
	CPR BEGUN BY B P TIME BEGUN				
EMS SIGNATURE	AED USED Y N BY:				
	RESUSCITATION TERMINATED - TIME				
	( ) OSHA REGULATIONS FOLLOWED				

Multiple-Casualty Incidents and Incident Management

▌ STANDARD

EMS Operations (Content Area: Multiple-Casualty Incidents)

▌ COMPETENCY

Applies knowledge of operational roles and responsibilities to ensure patient, public, and personnel safety.

▌ OBJECTIVES

After reading this chapter, you should be able to:

45-1. Define key terms introduced in this chapter.

45-2. List situations that might result in multiple trauma casualties and situations that might result in multiple medical casualties.

45-3. List aspects important to effective management of an MCI.

45-4. Explain the purposes for establishment of the National Incident Management System (NIMS).

45-5. Describe the purposes and desirable features of the incident command system (ICS).

45-6. Identify responsibilities that may be assigned to EMS (units that might be established) at a multiple-casualty incident.

45-7. Describe the principles of a triage system.

45-8. Describe and contrast primary triage with secondary triage.

45-9. Given a scenario with multiple patients, categorize patients according to a color-coded triage system.

45-10. Explain the principles and assessment categories used in START triage.

45-11. Explain why JumpSTART was developed for triage of pediatric patients, contrast JumpSTART with START, and explain how to identify a "child" for triage purposes at the scene of an MCI.

45-12. Explain the important principles of a patient-tagging system to be used during triage.

45-13. Explain the interrelationship of triage and treatment within the treatment unit at an MCI.

45-14. Discuss the logistics of staging and transport at an MCI.

45-15. Discuss common issues with communications in MCI and disaster situations.

45-16. List measures that can be taken to reduce rescuer stress during and after an MCI response.

45-17. Describe requirements of effective disaster assistance.

45-18. Anticipate psychological reactions of disaster victims and describe ways in which EMS providers can assist disaster survivors.

KEY IDEAS

A multiple-casualty incident (MCI) can occur without warning at any time or place. This chapter reviews fundamental management techniques for MCIs, including the National Incident Management System (NIMS). Be sure to review your local community plans for specific MCI procedures and plans.

■ An MCI is an event that places excessive demands on personnel and equipment. The number of patients required to declare an MCI varies with the jurisdiction and the available resources.

■ In any MCI, call for plenty of help as quickly as possible.

■ The NIMS provides for flexibility and standardization in managing any disaster or MCI.

■ The incident command system (ICS) is effective because it consistently uses standardized, common terminology, adopts a manageable span of control, identifies clear objectives to be accomplished (incident action plans), utilizes an integrated communications system, and uses a system of accountability at all levels.

■ There is only one designated incident commander for large-scale disasters and MCI. The incident commander may appoint finance/administration, logistics, operations, and planning sections and chiefs as necessary. The section chiefs then establish units and unit leaders.

■ Large-scale MCIs may require establishing triage, treatment, transport, staging, and morgue units under the direction of an EMS branch director. The EMS branch director reports to the operations chief, who reports to the incident commander.

■ Triage is a system used for sorting patients to determine the order in which they will receive care. Primary triage is performed at the site of the incident immediately upon arrival of the first EMS crew. Secondary triage, or patient reassessment, is performed in the triage unit.

■ Typically, there are four triage priority levels. Priority 1 (P-1/highest priority/red/immediate) patients require immediate care and transport. Priority 2 (P-2/second priority/yellow/delayed) patients receive delayed emergency care and transport. Priority 3 (P-3/lowest priority/green/minor) patients are those who have minor injuries and are ambulatory. Priority 4 (P-4/black/deceased) patients are deceased or have fatal injuries.

■ Typical patient identification systems use colors to signify priorities of care: highest = red, second = yellow, lowest = green, deceased/mortal injuries = black.

■ To reduce stress on yourself and other rescue personnel who are involved in an MCI, rest at regular intervals. Be aware of your exact assignment. Several workers should watch for signs of physical exhaustion and stress in other rescuers. Plenty of food and drinks should be provided, and workers should be encouraged to talk among themselves.

TERMS AND CONCEPTS

1. Write the number of the correct term next to each definition.

    1. Disaster
    2. Incident commander
    3. Incident command system
    4. Mobile command unit
    5. MCI
    6. Primary triage
    7. Secondary triage
    8. Staging unit
    9. Supply unit
    10. Transportation unit
    11. Treatment unit
    12. Triage unit

_____ a. Monitors, inventories, and directs available ambulances to the treatment unit at the request of the transportation unit leader

_____ b. An event that places excessive demands on EMS personnel and equipment

_____ c. The person responsible for coordinating all aspects of the incident

_____ d. Unit responsible for prioritizing patients for emergency medical care and transport

_____ e. The headquarters for the incident manager; the EMS command post

_____ f. A sudden catastrophic event that overwhelms natural order and causes great loss of property and/or life

_____ g. Unit responsible for inventory and distribution of the medical materials and equipment necessary to render care

_____ h. Evaluation of patients that takes place immediately upon arrival of the first EMS crew to quickly categorize the severity of the patients' conditions and priority for treatment and transport

_____ i. The standardized incident management concept that has become the standard for on-scene management of disasters and MCIs.

_____ j. Unit responsible for collecting and treating patients in a centralized treatment area

_____ k. Reevaluation that occurs in the triage unit to categorize the severity of the patient's condition and priority for treatment and transport

_____ l. Unit that coordinates patient transportation with the triage and staging unit leaders and communicates with the hospitals involved

CONTENT REVIEW

1. Which system provides for a consistent approach to managing disasters by federal, state, or local responders to an incident?
   a. Federal Multiple Command System (FMCS)
   b. National Incident Management System (NIMS)
   c. International Single Command System (ISCS)
   d. Regional Disaster Command System (RDCS)

2. The incident commander is stationed in the
   a. mobile command unit.
   b. supply unit.
   c. transport unit.
   d. triage unit.

3. A child that is breathing adequately with a palpable peripheral pulse and is unresponsive to all stimuli or responds to pain with incomprehensible sounds or inappropriate movement (does not localize pain or has no purposeful flexion or extension) is tagged
   a. red.
   b. yellow.
   c. green.
   d. black.

4. Any patient who is able to walk at the scene of an MCI is initially tagged
   a. red.
   b. yellow.
   c. green.
   d. black.

5. You have responded to a bus crash with many patients. The scene is safe, and the bus is stable. Which best describes "primary triage" at this scene?
   a. Primary triage is conducted by the first-arriving EMS crew after removal of the patients from the bus.
   b. Primary triage is conducted by the first-arriving EMS crew inside the bus before moving the patients.
   c. Primary triage is conducted by the first-arriving EMS crew once patients are placed in the triage sector.
   d. Primary triage is conducted by the second-arriving EMS crew once patients are placed in the triage sector.

6. The primary goal of triage is to accomplish which of the following?
   a. Sort patients according to criticality
   b. Provide comprehensive treatment for each patient
   c. Perform a detailed physical exam on each patient
   d. Transport all patients as rapidly as possible

7. Which of the following best describes secondary triage?
   a. Occurs as the patient is extricated from the hot zone and is designed to evaluate the patient's condition initially
   b. Occurs when the patient is within the actual incident site and is designed to evaluate the patient's condition
   c. Occurs during the transporting of the patient to the receiving facility and is designed to reevaluate the primary patient categorization
   d. Occurs as the patient is brought into the triage unit and is designed to reevaluate the initial patient categorization

8. In the START triage system, you should do which of the following?
   a. Check respirations only.
   b. Check respirations and perfusion only.
   c. Check mental status only.
   d. Check respirations, perfusion, and mental status.

9. When assessing the respirations of a patient using the START triage system, you have opened a patient's airway, but the patient is not breathing and has no respiratory effort. Your next immediate action should be to
   a. tag the patient as "red" and immediately move him to the treatment area.
   b. tag the patient as "black" and move on to the next patient.
   c. tag the patient as "yellow" and move on to the next patient.
   d. tag the patient as "red" and reposition the patient's airway.

10. Patients who are transported first in a four-level priority triage system are which of the following?
    a. Priority 1 (red)
    b. Priority 2 (yellow)
    c. Priority 3 (green)
    d. Priority 4 (black)

11. In the START system, a patient with respirations greater than 30 per minute should be assigned to which of the following priorities?
    a. Priority 1 (red)
    b. Priority 2 (yellow)
    c. Priority 3 (green)
    d. Priority 4 (black)

12. A typical patient-tagging system uses colors to triage and identify patients. Red would be used to signify a
    a. high-priority patient.
    b. second-priority patient.
    c. third-priority patient.
    d. fourth-priority patient.

13. Patients should be organized in the treatment unit according to which of the following?
    a. Approximate age
    b. Order in which they were brought to the treatment area
    c. Kind of injury or condition
    d. Triage or priority level

14. Which of the following will help to reduce stress on rescuers during an MCI?
    a. Have rescuers work in 8- to 10-hour shifts and then perform less stressful tasks.
    b. Give a motivating talk to any rescuer who becomes hysterical.
    c. Provide plenty of nourishing food and drinks.
    d. Encourage rescue workers not to talk among themselves.

15. What age group is the JumpSTART pediatric triage system used for?
    a. Newborns to 5 years old
    b. Newborns to 8 years old
    c. 1 year to 18 years old
    d. For any patient that looks like a child

16. Alerts for evacuation must be repeated often and with clarity to convince people that the disaster is really about to occur. Which of the following is likely to be considered part of the minimum information that must be contained in the evacuation alert message?
    a. Location where federal and state assistance will be available following the incident
    b. Safe routes to take out of the area
    c. The name of the local mayor or political official in charge
    d. Estimated time before the evacuated will be able to return to the area

17. During a disaster, the reactions of children depend on their age, individual disposition, family support, and community support. Which of the following groups is more likely to experience extreme aggression and stress that is severe enough to disrupt their lives?
    a. Infants
    b. Preschoolers
    c. Elementary-school-age children
    d. Preadolescents and adolescents

18. Which of the following is considered appropriate when dealing with the psychological impact of disasters?
    a. Giving assurances to your patients that are not true but are intended to help them deal with the problem
    b. Encouraging your patients to talk about the disaster and its long-term effects
    c. Delaying the reuniting of families to lessen the emotional stress
    d. Discouraging patients from doing necessary chores to help them get over their problems

▌ CASE STUDY

You have been dispatched to the scene of a bus-train collision. You are the senior EMT on the vehicle, and you are the closest responding unit to the scene. Your partner quickly pulls out the local "MCI Response Packet" and reviews the MCI plan. You arrive on scene and observe a large commercial bus that has been struck by a train. The bus has been pushed approximately 50 yards from the crossing. There is extensive damage to the bus. There are many bystanders who are next to the bus waving at you to hurry. Several patients have been removed from the bus and are being treated by bystanders. A law enforcement officer grabs you by the arm as you exit the vehicle and tells you, "You had better get some help out here! There are at least 40 people injured. There are victims lying all over the place. Tell them to hurry!"

1. What is your *best* first action to take?
    a. Establish a triage sector
    b. Request additional help and assistance.
    c. Have the walking wounded patients walk to the treatment area.
    d. Triage all patients to determine the total number of injured patients.

2. During your primary triage, a child patient on scene is breathing adequately, has a peripheral pulse and responds to pain by localizing it. The patient should be tagged
    a. red.
    b. yellow.
    c. green.
    d. black.

3. On this scene, the treatment unit
    a. leader radios the hospital that ambulances are en route.
    b. should be located close to the area where ambulances arrive.
    c. must not be marked in order to limit bystander traffic.
    d. is necessarily limited to only one location or area.

4. Utilizing the START triage system, perform the primary triage on the following adult patients from the bus-train collision. Tag each patient using the appropriate universally recognized categorization color: red, yellow, green, or black. (Red = immediate care and transport, priority 1. Yellow = delayed emergency care and transport, priority 2. Green = minor injuries and ambulatory patients, priority 3. Black = deceased or fatal injuries, priority 4.)

_____ a. An ambulatory patient who has a large, bleeding leg wound

_____ b. A patient who is breathing about 12 times each minute and has a peripheral pulse, but does not follow simple commands

_____ c. A patient who is breathing 22 times each minute, has a radial pulse, has capillary refill less than 2 seconds, and squeezes your fingers on command

_____ d. A patient whose respirations are 20 with a palpable radial pulse and is deeply unresponsive and bleeding from the ears

_____ e. A patient who has no obvious injuries and no respirations or respiratory effort after opening the airway

EMS Response to Terrorism Involving Weapons of Mass Destruction

▌ STANDARD

EMS Operations (Content Area: Terrorism and Disaster)

▌ COMPETENCY

Applies knowledge of operational roles and responsibilities to ensure patient, public, and personnel safety.

▌ OBJECTIVES

After reading this chapter, you should be able to:

46-1. Define key terms introduced in this chapter.

46-2. Explain the mnemonics CBRNE and B-NICE and describe the characteristics of the various types of weapons of mass destruction.

46-3. Explain the importance of preplanning a response to terrorism involving weapons of mass destruction.

46-4. Discuss the components that should be included in a plan for responding to terrorism involving weapons of mass destruction.

46-5. Recognize indications that a response may involve terrorism with weapons of mass destruction.

46-6. Describe the EMT's role when responding to terrorism involving weapons of mass destruction.

46-7. Describe types of injuries that may occur from conventional explosives and incendiary devices.

46-8. Discuss the effects of exposure to, and explain the appropriate medical care for, each of the following types of chemical agents:
   a. Nerve agents
   b. Vesicants
   c. Cyanide
   d. Pulmonary agents
   e. Riot-control agents
   f. Toxic industrial chemicals

46-9. Give examples of biological agents in each of the following categories and the appropriate medical care for exposure to biological agents:
   a. Pneumonia-like agents
   b. Encephalitis-like agents
   c. Biological toxins
   d. Other agents

46-10. Differentiate between the characteristics of the following types of radiation:
  - a. X-ray and gamma radiation
  - b. Neutron radiation
  - c. Beta radiation
  - d. Alpha radiation

46-11. Differentiate between primary exposure and fallout associated with a nuclear explosion.

46-12. Explain blast injuries and thermal burns as mechanisms of injury from nuclear explosions.

46-13. Differentiate between a nuclear weapon and a radiological dispersal device (RDD, or "dirty bomb").

46-14. Discuss assessment and care of patients affected by nuclear detonation and radiation injuries.

46-15. Explain issues of personal protection and patient decontamination in connection with chemical, biological, and radiological/nuclear weapons exposure.

KEY IDEAS

This chapter focuses on EMS preparedness for response to terrorism involving weapons of mass destruction (WMDs), including conventional weapons, explosives, and incendiary devices, as well as chemical agents, biological agents, and nuclear weapons and radiation. Signs and symptoms (how to recognize a WMD attack) and appropriate emergency medical care are discussed for each category, as are personal protection and patient decontamination issues.

- The goal of an EMS response to weapons of mass destruction (WMDs) is to manage patients affected by the attack successfully.

- WMDs include biological, nuclear/radiological, incendiary, chemical, and explosive (B-NICE).

- The general prehospital approach to an incident involving WMDs is similar to that for any event involving multiple casualties. Various factors must be considered and planned for prior to the event, including provisions for supplies and equipment, medical direction, training for providers, response protocols, and issues of scene safety.

- Explosives and incendiary devices are, and will most likely remain, the WMDs most commonly used by terrorists. Explosives and incendiary devices cause primary, secondary, and tertiary effects, inflicting damage on the lungs, abdomen, and ears and causing crush and shrapnel injuries.

- Chemical agents include nerve agents, vesicants, cyanide, pulmonary agents, riot-control agents, and toxic industrial chemicals (TICs).

- Biological agents are classified as pneumonia-like agents, encephalitis-like agents, biological toxins, and other biological agents.

- Nuclear detonation results in three mechanisms of death and injury: radiation, blast injuries, and thermal burns.

- Many of the same principles that are applied to dealing with hazardous materials can be applied to a chemical, biological, or nuclear incident.

TERMS AND CONCEPTS

1. Write the number of the correct term next to each definition.
   1. Biological agents
   2. Nerve agents
   3. Persistence
   4. Vesicants
   5. Volatility
   6. WMDs

_____ a. Agents that block the action of acetylcholinesterase in the plasma of the blood, red blood cells, and nervous tissue

_____ b. A characteristic of agents that do not evaporate quickly and tend to remain as a puddle for a long period of time

_____ c. Chemical agents that most commonly result in damage to exposed skin, lungs, and eyes and that cause blisters, tissue burning, and tissue damage on contact

_____ d. Agents that are made up of living organisms, or the toxins produced by the living organisms, used to cause disease in a target population

_____ e. The tendency of a chemical agent to evaporate

_____ f. Weapons intended to cause widespread and indiscriminate death and destruction

CONTENT REVIEW

1. Which of the following is correct regarding the appropriate prehospital response to an incident involving WMDs?
   a. Coordinated community preplanning for a WMD attack is necessary.
   b. A single EMS agency is likely to have enough equipment to handle a WMD attack.
   c. If a statewide disaster plan is in place, it will be both unnecessary and confusing for regional and local agencies to also develop their own disaster plans.
   d. The general approach is significantly different than that for any disaster involving multiple casualties.

2. Which WMDs are those most widely used by terrorists?
   a. Chemical agents
   b. Nuclear agents
   c. Biological agents
   d. Explosive and incendiary agents

3. Incendiary devices
   a. create similar injury patterns to conventional explosives.
   b. are difficult to improvise and manufacture.
   c. include napalm, thermite, and magnesium.
   d. cause burns that are assessed in a vastly different manner from thermal burns.

4. The mnemonic SLUDGE is used to help remember the signs and symptoms associated with
   a. nerve agents.
   b. cyanide.
   c. vesicants.
   d. pulmonary agents.

5. Two drugs that are used to counteract the effects of nerve agents are
   a. epinephrine and calcium chloride.
   b. atropine and pralidoxime.
   c. calcium chloride and magnesium.
   d. epinephrine and magnesium.

6. These agents cause blisters, burning, and tissue damage on contact and were once called "blistering agents." They are called
   a. nerve agents.
   b. cyanide.
   c. vesicants.
   d. pulmonary agents.

7. A substance that disrupts the ability of the cell to use oxygen and leads to cellular hypoxia and eventually death is
   a. phosgene.
   b. cyanide.
   c. tularemia.
   d. ricin.

8. Phosgene, halogen compounds, and nitrogen-oxygen compounds are examples of
   a. nerve agents.
   b. cyanide.
   c. vesicants.
   d. pulmonary agents.

9. The management for exposure to riot-control agents should focus on
   a. administering activated charcoal.
   b. removing the patient from the environment.
   c. administering amyl nitrite or sodium nitrite.
   d. covering the eyes with moist dressings.

10. Biological agents that can be used as WMDs are categorized into what four groups?
   a. Pneumonia-like agents, encephalitis-like agents, biological toxins, and other biological agents
   b. Biological agents, intestinal agents, viral agents, and bacterial agents
   c. Viral agents, bacterial agents, fungal agents, and other agents
   d. Anthrax agents, plague agents, tularemia agents, and other agents

11. Two common encephalitis-like agents are
   a. smallpox and Venezuelan equine encephalitis.
   b. botulinum and ricin.
   c. staphylococcus and botulinum.
   d. epsilon toxin and cholera.

12. The three primary mechanisms of death or injury associated with nuclear detonation are
   a. alpha radiation, beta radiation, and gamma radiation.
   b. radiation, blast, and thermal burns.
   c. neutron radiation, beta radiation, and alpha radiation.
   d. X-ray radiation, gamma radiation, and neutron radiation.

13. This type of radiation is the most penetrating type and can travel long distances. It is called
   a. gamma radiation.
   b. beta radiation.
   c. alpha radiation.
   d. delta radiation.

14. There are two types of radiation exposure associated with a nuclear explosion. After primary exposure, this is the second form of radiation exposure and contains radioactive dust and particles. It is called
   a. a blast injury.
   b. fallout.
   c. a shock wave.
   d. barotrauma.

15. A conventional explosive attached to radioactive materials is referred to as a
   a. radiological dispersal device.
   b. radioactive weapon.
   c. radioactive-conventional weapon.
   d. weapon of destruction.

▌ CASE STUDY

It is 4:00 P.M. on a cold winter day. You are watching TV and relaxing at home when a newsbreak advises you that a nuclear device has just been detonated in a large city located about 60 miles from the town where you live. A mutual-aid call goes to surrounding emergency service personnel to respond to the disaster area. You pack your bags and quickly head to the EMS station for assignment. As you and a crew of 10 of your fellow EMTs are heading to the disaster site, you try to remember the information that you learned in your multiple-casualty and WMD training.

1. The mechanism that causes most deaths and injury associated with nuclear detonation is the
   a. blast and thermal burns.
   b. neutron and alpha radiation.
   c. radiation.
   d. fallout.

2. Which of the following is correct regarding blast injuries associated with nuclear detonation?
   a. The nuclear ignition produces a small contained-gas cloud.
   b. Shock-wave injuries are of a different nature from those caused by conventional weapons.
   c. The intensity of shock-wave injuries is greater the farther the victim is from ground zero.
   d. The windblast is strong enough to cause structural collapse, crush injuries, and entrapment.

3. Your agency's personnel have all received specialized hazardous materials (hazmat) training. Therefore, your crew is prepared to act as an initial-response crew. Is this true or false?
   a. The statement is true because all the principles of a nuclear and a hazmat emergency are identical.
   b. The statement is true because similar principles apply to dealing with a nuclear and a hazmat emergency.
   c. The statement is false because the procedures for dealing with a nuclear emergency are very different from those for a hazmat emergency.
   d. The statement is false because plenty of trained personnel should be available by the time you arrive on scene.

Course Review Self-Test

1. Which department of the U.S. government was charged with developing an Emergency Medical Services (EMS) system and upgrading prehospital emergency care?
   a. Department of Assessment Standards
   b. Department of Technical Assistance
   c. Department of Labor and Employment
   d. Department of Transportation (DOT)

2. The process of ensuring scene safety is *best* described by which of the following?
   a. Ensuring scene safety is accomplished upon arrival on scene.
   b. Ensuring scene safety is dynamic and ongoing.
   c. Ensuring scene safety begins with patient contact.
   d. Ensuring scene safety is continued until patient contact.

3. You are dispatched to a rock climber injured on a very steep hillside. Knowing that you are not trained in this type of rescue, you should
   a. wait for a trained rescue crew.
   b. climb down to the patient.
   c. secure the patient with ropes.
   d. from below, climb up to the patient.

4. You are dispatched to a residence where all of the family members, including the dog, are experiencing similar signs of disorientation. What should you suspect?
   a. The dog has infected the family.
   b. The patients have the flu.
   c. The patients are suffering from the same virus.
   d. The environment is toxic.

5. The chief complaint is the patient's answer to the question
   a. "Where does it hurt?"
   b. "Why did you call EMS?"
   c. "What do you think is wrong with you?"
   d. "Can you point with one finger to where the pain is?"

6. A life-threatening condition that is found during the primary assessment should be treated
   a. once the primary assessment is completed.
   b. once the patient priorities are established.
   c. immediately as it is found.
   d. after assessing the circulation.

7. Which of the following is a criteria for rapid patient transport?
   a. A responsive patient able to obey commands
   b. A patient with minor chest pain and a systolic blood pressure of 110 mmHg
   c. A patient with a body temperature of 100°F
   d. A patient with cool, clammy skin

8. The secondary assessment is performed to do which of the following?
   a. Identify any additional injuries or conditions that may also be life threatening.
   b. Rapidly make the initial identification of life-threatening conditions.
   c. Identify potential hazards that may be present on the scene.
   d. Rapidly identify the total number of patients ill or injured.

9. An unresponsive, adult trauma patient with a midfacial fracture, unequal pupils, and abnormal posturing to painful stimulus requires
   a. rapid transport without spinal immobilization.
   b. that you consider hyperventilation at 20 breaths per minute with supplemental oxygen.
   c. placement of a nasopharyngeal airway and hyperventilation at 20 per minute.
   d. spinal immobilization and rapid transport only.

10. The "S" in the SAMPLE history represents
    a. signs and symptoms.
    b. symptoms and severity.
    c. signs and setting.
    d. setting and scenario.

11. The chest of the adult patient should be auscultated at which of the following anatomical locations?
    a. Third intercostal space at the midclavicular line and fifth intercostal space at the midaxillary line
    b. First intercostal space at the midclavicular line and sixth intercostal space at the midaxillary line
    c. Second intercostal space at the midclavicular line and fourth intercostal space at the midaxillary line
    d. Sixth intercostal space at the midclavicular line and sixth intercostal space at the midaxillary line

12. The three general components of the secondary assessment are the
    a. physical exam, baseline vitals, and history.
    b. focused physical exam, baseline vitals, and history.
    c. detailed physical exam, baseline vitals, and history.
    d. head-to-toe assessment, baseline vitals, and history.

13. A pupil that is large in size and not responding to light should be referred to as
    a. dilated and glazed.
    b. fixed and dilated.
    c. fixed and constricted.
    d. a consensual reflex.

14. The purpose of the reassessment is to do which of the following?
    a. Determine potential scene hazards and obstacles.
    b. Determine patient changes and assess treatments.
    c. Establish priorities of patient management.
    d. Evaluate system effectiveness and benchmarks.

15. Vital signs in the unstable patient should be reassessed every _____ minutes.
    a. 2
    b. 3
    c. 5
    d. 15

16. You are preparing to treat your patient with a particular drug. Which of the following should alert you to stop the therapy?
    a. A side effect
    b. A therapeutic effect
    c. An indication
    d. A contraindication

17. There are many different routes by which medications may be administered. Which of the following describes the correct route for administration of nitroglycerin spray?
    a. Oral
    b. Sublingual
    c. Inhalation
    d. Intramuscular

18. When you must lift a patient, you should do which of the following?
    a. Keep your back in an unlocked position.
    b. Keep your back in a locked-in position.
    c. Lean backward from the waist and bend your knees.
    d. Lean forward from the waist and lock your knees.

19. When pulling an object, you should keep the load
    a. between your shoulders and hips and close to your body.
    b. between your shoulders and waist and away from your body.
    c. above the shoulders and avoid bending at the waist if possible.
    d. below the waist and avoid bending at the waist when possible.

20. In which of the following circumstances should you perform an emergency move?
    a. The patient is unresponsive but is breathing and has a pulse.
    b. It is necessary to gain access to a patient who needs spinal immobilization.
    c. The patient is responsive but has an obvious head injury.
    d. It is necessary to gain access to other patients who display immediate life threats.

21. In which of the following situations when would the use of a stair chair be inappropriate?
    a. The corridors and stairway are narrow.
    b. The patient has an injury to the chest.
    c. The patient weighs more than 200 pounds.
    d. The patient has an altered mental status.

22. To help take the weight of the fetus off the large blood vessels and nerves, a woman in advanced pregnancy should be placed in which position?
    a. On her side
    b. Trendelenburg
    c. Supine
    d. Prone

23. Each three-month period of the approximately nine-month pregnancy is referred to as a
    a. trimester.
    b. trigeminal.
    c. stage.
    d. period.

24. The third stage of labor is the period during which
   a. complete cervical dilation occurs.
   b. the placenta is expelled.
   c. the infant moves through the birth canal.
   d. the amniotic sac ruptures.

25. Which of the following is the organ that contains the developing fetus?
   a. Perineum
   b. Cervix
   c. Placenta
   d. Uterus

26. The first stage of labor ends when contractions are
   a. 6 to 7 minutes apart and last from 15 to 20 seconds.
   b. 4 to 5 minutes apart and last from 15 to 25 seconds.
   c. 3 to 4 minutes apart and last 60 seconds each.
   d. 2 to 3 minutes apart and last from 60 to 90 seconds.

27. When suctioning the newborn's airway during birth, which of the following should you do?
   a. Suction the nose first, then the mouth.
   b. Suction the mouth first, then the nose.
   c. Turn the head to the side to expel the contents.
   d. Suction either the nose or the mouth first.

28. What three criteria are used to rapidly identify intervention beyond normal care?
   a. Term gestation, APGAR score, good muscle tone.
   b. Term gestation, good cry or breathing adequately, good muscle tone.
   c. SpO_2, APGAR, good muscle tone.
   d. Poor peripheral circulation, APGAR, good muscle tone.

29. Which of the following describes a difference found in the infant's or child's airway that is not found in the adult?
   a. The tongue is smaller and takes up less space in the pharynx.
   b. The smallest area of the upper airway is at the level of the vocal cords.
   c. The epiglottis is much lower in the airway.
   d. The trachea is very pliable.

30. A "patent airway" is
   a. partially obstructed by a foreign body.
   b. an airway that is open.
   c. also called an *oropharyngeal airway.*
   d. completely obstructed by the tongue.

31. You are preparing to use an oropharyngeal airway on your patient. You know that
   a. it is available in adult sizes only and contraindicated in the child.
   b. it passes through and extends below the larynx to hold the tongue in position.
   c. it can be used on partially responsive patients.
   d. it is rotated 180 degrees in the adult patient while inserting.

32. Which of the following is true about the nasopharyngeal airway?
    a. It is available in one adjustable size.
    b. It is more likely to stimulate vomiting than an oropharyngeal airway.
    c. It may injure the nasal mucosa.
    d. It must be inserted in the smaller nostril.

33. The depth of a patient's breathing may also be referred to as which of the following?
    a. Chest ventilation
    b. Tidal volume
    c. Total volume
    d. Breathing capacity

34. Excessively rapid breathing is referred to as which of the following?
    a. Tachypnea
    b. Eupnea
    c. Dyspnea
    d. Bradypnea

35. Your patient's minute volume is inadequate. Which of the following should you use to correct this problem?
    a. Nonrebreather mask
    b. Bag-valve mask (BVM)
    c. Nasal cannula
    d. Oxygen by blow-by

36. The preferred method for ventilation of a patient using the bag-valve-mask (BVM) device requires that
    a. one EMT should ventilate the patient.
    b. the EMT who ventilates should be positioned at the patient's side.
    c. the EMT squeezing the bag should also hold the mask.
    d. two EMTs should ventilate the patient.

37. The flow-restricted, oxygen-powered ventilation device provides
    a. a flow rate of more than 50 lpm of 60 percent oxygen.
    b. a reduction in potential gastric distention.
    c. 100 percent oxygen with each ventilation.
    d. positive pressure ventilation for the adult or child patient.

38. A full oxygen cylinder will generally read
    a. 1,000 psi.
    b. 1,500 psi.
    c. 1,750 psi.
    d. 2,000 psi.

39. The safe use of oxygen includes
    a. use of oil-based lubricants on the regulator.
    b. keeping cylinders secured when in transit.
    c. use of a valve that has been modified from another gas cylinder.
    d. storing cylinders below 200°F.

40. The preferred method for the delivery of high-concentration oxygen in the prehospital setting is with which of the following?
   a. Nasal cannula
   b. Simple face mask
   c. Nonrebreather mask
   d. Partial rebreather mask

41. Which statement is most correct with regard to a transient ischemic attack (TIA)?
   a. Patients typically develop only one symptom that is similar to a stroke.
   b. The TIA always resolves within 72 hours.
   c. A TIA that lasts longer than 10–15 minutes is usually a small stroke.
   d. A TIA typically resolves within 3 hours.

42. Before oral glucose may be administered, which of the following criteria must first be met, in addition to an on-line or off-line order from medical direction?
   a. Unresponsiveness; history of diabetes controlled by diet; ability to swallow
   b. Altered mental status; history of diabetes controlled by medication or a blood glucose reading less than 60 mg/dL; ability to swallow
   c. Altered mental status; history of diabetes controlled by medication or a blood glucose reading less than 90 mg/dL; ability to swallow
   d. Open airway; history of diabetes controlled by exercise; present gag reflex

43. When assessing pulse quality, the term *thready* refers to which of the following?
   a. Strong pulse
   b. Regular pulse
   c. Weak pulse
   d. Irregular pulse

44. To determine the chief complaint during the secondary assessment of your alert patient, you should
   a. ask open-ended questions.
   b. ask "yes" or "no" questions.
   c. question a family member.
   d. ask challenging questions.

45. Which of the following sets of vital signs is considered normal for a 42-year-old male?
   a. Pulse 82, blood pressure 154/72, breathing rate 28
   b. Pulse 112, blood pressure 146/92, breathing rate 18
   c. Pulse 78, blood pressure 138/68, breathing rate 12
   d. Pulse 48, blood pressure 122/54, breathing rate 10

46. Which of the following is a meeting that may precede a critical incident stress debriefing (CISD) to allow the rescuers to vent their emotions and get information before the larger group meeting?
   a. Defusing
   b. Critiquing
   c. Teaching
   d. Debriefing

47. Which of the following is the single most important way that you can prevent the spread of infection?
   a. Wearing gloves
   b. Wearing a mask
   c. Hand washing
   d. Cleaning equipment

48. When might it be appropriate to apply a surgical mask to the patient?
    a. When blood may be splashed into the patient's face
    b. When you suspect an airborne infectious disease
    c. When the patient is suspected of having AIDS
    d. When transporting more than one patient at a time

49. Dark red blood that flows steadily from a wound usually indicates a severed or damaged
    a. artery.
    b. vein.
    c. capillary.
    d. arteriole.

50. Your patient has a large laceration to the forearm. After you have applied direct pressure, the wound continues to bleed profusely. You should
    a. apply a tourniquet.
    b. compress the femoral pressure point.
    c. compress the brachial pressure point.
    d. compress the carotid pressure point.

51. Which of the following is a sign of shock?
    a. Constricted pupils
    b. Absent peripheral pulses
    c. Red, warm, dry skin
    d. Slow, deep breathing

52. A child from 1 to 3 years old is referred to as which of the following?
    a. A neonate
    b. An infant
    c. A toddler
    d. A preschooler

53. Which of the following is the primary goal in treating any infant or child patient?
    a. To recognize and treat respiratory problems
    b. To provide rapid transport to the medical facility
    c. To reduce pain and suffering
    d. To determine the cause of the illness or injury

54. Which of the following is an indication of respiratory arrest in the infant or child patient?
    a. Regular respirations
    b. Respiratory rate less than 10 per minute
    c. Hyperactive patient
    d. Strong peripheral pulses and an elevated heart rate

55. Which of the following is the *best* indication of a complete airway obstruction in the infant or child patient?
    a. Crying or talking
    b. Stridor upon inspiration
    c. Pale, cool, clammy skin
    d. Ineffective or absent cough

56. The normal ranges of respirations in the newborn to 1-year-old, and in the 4-year-old to 12-year-old, are, respectively,

    a. 30/minute and 10/minute.

    b. 40/minute and 20/minute.

    c. 50/minute and 30/minute.

    d. 60/minute and 40/minute.

57. Which of the following is a sign of hypoperfusion in the infant or child patient?

    a. Warm, pink, dry skin

    b. Rapid, bounding pulse

    c. Capillary refill under 2 seconds

    d. Absence of tears when crying

58. Sudden infant death syndrome (SIDS) has a peak incidence at around _____ old.

    a. 2 weeks

    b. 1 month

    c. 4 months

    d. 1 year

59. A gastrostomy is performed for patients needing

    a. long-term drainage of cerebrospinal fluid.

    b. long-term nutritional support.

    c. long-term intravenous access.

    d. long-term airway access.

60. You are the primary triage officer at a multiple-casualty incident (MCI). The first patient you triage is not breathing. You take steps to open the airway and speak to the patient, but the patient is still not breathing. You would tag this patient as

    a. red/first priority.

    b. black/no priority.

    c. yellow/second priority.

    d. green/third priority.

61. In triage tagging, which of the following injuries would indicate a yellow or priority 2 patient?

    a. Able to walk; minor injuries

    b. Respirations < 30/minute, follows simple commands

    c. Respirations > 30/minute; unresponsive

    d. Does not obey commands; exhibits signs of shock

62. A patient is found in severe respiratory distress, sitting upright and leaning slightly forward, supporting himself with his arms. This position is called the

    a. Trendelenburg position.

    b. tripod position.

    c. distress position.

    d. trapezoid position.

63. A cough that produces mucus is known as which of the following?

    a. Diminished cough

    b. Productive cough

    c. Paradoxical cough

    d. Wet cough

64. What is cyanosis?
   a. An early sign of hypoperfusion
   b. An early sign of hyperglycemia
   c. A late sign of hypoxia
   d. A late sign of altered mental status

65. An infant with cyanosis, an altered mental status, and bradycardia should be provided
   a. positive pressure ventilation with supplemental oxygen.
   b. oxygen via a simple face mask.
   c. oxygen via a nonrebreather mask.
   d. oxygen via the "blow-by" method.

66. Which of the following is an "S" question in the OPQRST questions used to evaluate a patient with respiratory distress?
   a. "When did the difficulty in breathing start?"
   b. "Does lying flat make the breathing more difficult?"
   c. "How bad is this breathing difficulty on a scale of 1 to 10?"
   d. "What were you doing when the breathing difficulty started?"

67. A patient with difficulty in breathing is considered which of the following?
   a. A high-priority patient
   b. A low-priority patient
   c. A medium-priority patient
   d. A patient not assigned to a priority

68. A loose flap of skin and soft tissue that has been torn loose or pulled completely off is known as an
   a. articulation.
   b. amputation.
   c. avulsion.
   d. abrasion.

69. You are treating a patient who has an abdominal injury with exposed organs. Which treatment is most appropriate?
   a. Apply a sterile dressing moistened with saline, then an occlusive dressing.
   b. Apply an occlusive dressing, then sterile gauze moistened with saline.
   c. Apply a dry, sterile cotton dressing, and then use direct pressure to help control bleeding.
   d. Apply a dry gauze dressing to control bleeding, and then cover with an occlusive dressing.

70. Which of the following is the most appropriate way to transport an amputated body part?
   a. Place the body part in a plastic bag, label the bag, and immediately place the bag on ice.
   b. Immediately immerse the body part in a bag of ice water, label the bag, and transport.
   c. Wrap the body part in a dry sterile dressing, place it in a plastic bag, label the bag, and keep the part cool.
   d. Do not delay to wrap or label the part; transport the part immediately.

71. Which of the following is a common symptom of a hemorrhagic stroke?
   a. Severe headache
   b. Bilateral numbness to hands
   c. Stiff back
   d. Loss of vision in one eye

72. Which of the following is the *most* appropriate means of managing an unresponsive stroke patient with unequal pupils or posturing?
    a. Nasal cannula with a flow of 4–6 lpm
    b. Nonrebreather mask with a flow of 15 lpm
    c. Positive pressure ventilation at 8 per minute
    d. Positive pressure ventilation at 20 per minute (or per protocol)

73. Implied consent applies to which of the following?
    a. The patient adamantly refuses treatment, then becomes unresponsive.
    b. The patient is of legal age and able to make rational decisions.
    c. The parent or legal guardian has consented to treatment and transport.
    d. The patient consents orally or by a nod or an affirming gesture.

74. In a malpractice suit, injuries to the patient are deemed to be the direct result of negligence by the EMT. This is called
    a. battery.
    b. damages.
    c. secondary negligence.
    d. proximate cause.

75. Which chamber of the heart receives oxygen-rich blood from the lungs?
    a. Left ventricle
    b. Right ventricle
    c. Left atrium
    d. Right atrium

76. Which of the following is the most appropriate emergency medical treatment for a responsive patient suffering from a cardiac emergency with an SpO_2 reading of 88?
    a. Administer oxygen at 10 lpm via a nonrebreather mask and consider calling for ALS backup.
    b. Administer oxygen at 15 lpm via a nonrebreather mask and call for ALS backup.
    c. Administer oxygen at 10 lpm via a nasal cannula and consider calling for ALS backup.
    d. Administer oxygen at 6 lpm via a nasal cannula and consider calling for ALS backup.

77. You are preparing to administer nitroglycerin. Which of the following statements is correct regarding nitroglycerin?
    a. It constricts the coronary arteries, increasing the blood flow to the heart.
    b. A second dose can be administered two minutes after the first dose.
    c. The patient's systolic blood pressure must be above 90 mmHg.
    d. Nitroglycerin is indicated in patients suffering from a head injury.

78. When using the automated external defibrillator (AED), the decision to transport the patient to the emergency facility should occur after which of the following conditions is met?
    a. The transport decision is based upon local protocol.
    b. The AED has given a "no shock" message.
    c. The patient regains a pulse and then slips back into cardiac arrest.
    d. The patient has been shocked four times and remains pulseless.

79. Which of the following statements is correct regarding the AED?
    a. After depressing the shock button, you should say, "Clear the patient."
    b. Always minimize the delay to defibrillation and interruptions of chest compression.
    c. The AED cannot be used on a patient who has an implanted pacemaker.
    d. Shocking a patient who has taken nitroglycerin sublingually is contraindicated.

80. You are treating an adult patient who has partial-thickness burns that encircle the right arm and cover the anterior trunk. What is the total body surface area (BSA) burned and the severity?
    a. 36 percent; critical burns
    b. 27 percent; critical burns
    c. 36 percent; moderate burns
    d. 27 percent; moderate burns

81. Electrical current or lightning
    a. damages tissue only in the area immediately surrounding the point of contact.
    b. seldom requires transport to the hospital unless external signs of injury are present.
    c. damages only soft tissue, not organs or other body systems.
    d. can cause irregular heartbeat or cardiac arrest.

82. When dealing with a patient suffering from a behavioral emergency, which of the following statements to the patient would be *most* appropriate?
    a. "You have nothing to worry about; everything will be better before long."
    b. "Trust me; things will be all right after we go to the hospital and see the doctor."
    c. "I'm sensitive to your problems, and I'm sure you can be cured."
    d. "Even with all of your problems, you seem to have people who care about you."

83. Which of the following restraints are considered humane and should be used when restraining a patient who may be a danger to you or himself?
    a. Metal police handcuffs
    b. Soft leather restraints
    c. Disposable flex cuffs
    d. Wide adhesive tape

84. When an error is made on a written prehospital care report, how should you correct the mistake?
    a. Use a commercially available correction fluid.
    b. Erase the mistake, then write over the error.
    c. Draw a single line through the error and initial it.
    d. Blacken out the mistake completely and initial it.

85. Your patient is adamantly refusing treatment and transport to a medical facility. The patient is also refusing to sign a refusal-of-care form. Which of the following should you do?
    a. Have the police respond to the scene, and force the patient to sign the form.
    b. Advise the patient that if the form is not signed, he will have to be transported.
    c. Have someone else sign the form, verifying that the patient refused to sign.
    d. If the patient refuses to sign the form, there is nothing you can do. Clear the scene.

86. According to the National Fire Protection Association (NFPA) 704 system, a diamond-shaped symbol identifies potentially dangerous cargo. Which color and number represent an extreme health hazard?
    a. Red diamond with the number 1 inside the triangle
    b. Red diamond with the number 4 inside the triangle
    c. Blue diamond with the number 1 inside the triangle
    d. Blue diamond with the number 4 inside the triangle

87. At a hazardous materials scene, the zone where contamination is actually present or that is immediately adjacent to the accident site and where contamination can still occur is the
   a. safety zone.
   b. hot zone.
   c. warm zone.
   d. cold zone.

88. While you are waiting for specially trained personnel to arrive to handle a hazardous materials scene, you should protect yourself and bystanders by
   a. keeping downhill and upwind from the scene.
   b. keeping uphill and downwind from the scene.
   c. keeping downhill and downwind from the scene.
   d. keeping uphill and upwind from the scene.

89. Which of the following is a division of the nervous system that influences the activities of skeletal muscles and movements throughout the body?
   a. Automatic nervous system
   b. Voluntary nervous system
   c. Autonomic nervous system
   d. Involuntary nervous system

90. A spinal injury resulting from hanging would be caused by which of the following mechanisms of spine injury?
   a. Flexion
   b. Extension
   c. Lateral bending
   d. Distraction

91. Manual stabilization of the potentially spine-injured patient's neck should
   a. not be released until the cervical spine immobilization collar (CSIC) is applied.
   b. be released if the patient complains of discomfort.
   c. not be released until the patient is completely immobilized to a backboard.
   d. be released if the patient's level of responsiveness deteriorates.

92. A patient who is walking around at a collision scene
   a. does not have a spinal injury.
   b. should not be immobilized.
   c. may have a spinal injury.
   d. should always be immobilized.

93. Paralysis to all four extremities is called which of the following?
   a. Quadriplegia
   b. Paraplegia
   c. Biplegia
   d. Hemiplegia

94. Your patient has ingested a poisonous plant and will respond only to painful stimuli. In which position should you place the patient?
   a. Lateral recumbent
   b. Supine
   c. Fowler's
   d. Trendelenburg

95. Activated charcoal
   a. is commonly used in a wide variety of prehospital toxicologic emergencies.
   b. is rarely used in the emergency medical treatment of ingested poisonings.
   c. is contraindicated in opioids, anticholinergics, or medications with sustained release.
   d. has been demonstrated to provide better patient outcomes from ingested poisons.

96. When treating a patient who has inhaled a poisonous gas, your *first* treatment priority is to
   a. administer high-concentration oxygen.
   b. place the patient on his side.
   c. start positive pressure ventilation.
   d. move the patient out of the toxic environment.

97. The four essential features of post traumatic stress disorder (PTSD) are response, avoiding, anxiety/anger and
   a. rejecting.
   b. escapism.
   c. reliving.
   d. relectance.

98. A full ___ percent of those who successfully commit suicide have told at least one other person of their intention or ideation before they killed themselves.
   a. 40
   b. 50
   c. 60
   d. 70

99. Which of the following terms means "toward the center of the body"?
   a. Superior
   b. Medial
   c. Dorsal
   d. Lateral

100. Which of the following terms refers to the center of each of the collarbones?
   a. Midclavicular
   b. Distal
   c. Midanterior
   d. Midaxillary

101. In this body position, the patient is lying on his back with his head elevated at a 45-degree to 60-degree angle.
   a. Supine position
   b. Lateral recumbent position
   c. Fowler's position
   d. Trendelenburg position

102. Which heart valve is located between the left atrium and the left ventricle?
   a. Mitral valve
   b. Aortic valve
   c. Pulmonary valve
   d. Tricuspid valve

103. Which organ is solid, is located in the left upper quadrant of the abdominal cavity, and aids in the filtration of blood?
    a. Gallbladder
    b. Spleen
    c. Ileum
    d. Duodenum

104. The five vertebrae that form the lower back and are located between the sacral and the thoracic spine form the
    a. iliac spine.
    b. humeral spine.
    c. cervical spine.
    d. lumbar spine.

105. When the amount of heat the body produces or gains exceeds the amount the body loses, the result is which of the following?
    a. Heat stroke
    b. Hyperthermia
    c. Heat cramps
    d. Hypothermia

106. Coma and severely depressed vital signs occur when the body reaches approximately what core temperature?
    a. 70°F
    b. 79°F
    c. 89°F
    d. 90°F

107. A bite from a _____ is often painless at first and then several hours later becomes bluish surrounded by a white periphery, with a red halo or "bull's-eye" pattern.
    a. scorpion
    b. black widow spider
    c. brown recluse spider
    d. fire ant

108. A hyperthermic patient with moist, pale skin that is normal to cool in temperature should be
    a. placed in a bath filled with ice water.
    b. moved to a cool environment.
    c. placed in a supine position with the head elevated.
    d. given fluids if unresponsive.

109. A patient has been stung by a bee. Which of the following methods is the *best* way to remove the stinger?
    a. Use tweezers.
    b. Use your fingers.
    c. Use forceps.
    d. Scrape it gently.

110. You are treating a patient who has been struck in the head with a baseball bat. Clear fluid is draining from the patient's nose. How can you determine if the fluid is cerebrospinal fluid (CSF)?
   a. Taste the fluid. If it has a sour taste, it is CSF.
   b. Dip your finger in the fluid. If it has a low viscosity, it is CSF.
   c. Dip the fluid on paper to see if it has a slight yellow color.
   d. Check the fluid for glucose.

111. Your patient responds to painful stimuli by extending both arms down to his sides and extending his legs, then arching his back. Which of the following describes this response?
   a. Lowest level of purposeful response, known as *flexion* or *decorticate posturing*
   b. Indicates a lower-level brain stem injury, known as *extension* or *decerebrate posturing*
   c. Second-lowest level of nonpurposeful response, known as *flexion* or *decorticate posturing*
   d. Second-lowest level of purposeful response, known as *extension* or *decerebrate posturing*

112. Which of the following signs and symptoms best describes those that may be found in a patient who is suffering from an abdominal aortic aneurysm?
   a. Sudden onset of tearing pain felt in the chest and left arm; pale, cool skin
   b. Abdominal pain with pale skin above the chest and normal color below
   c. Constant, severe abdominal pain and a pulsating abdominal mass
   d. Sudden onset of intermittent abdominal pain that radiates to the neck

113. Which is the correct way of performing the physical assessment of a patient with acute abdominal pain?
   a. Have the patient first point to the area that is most painful; then palpate each quadrant, beginning with the area farthest from the pain.
   b. Palpate the lower two quadrants first; next, palpate the upper two quadrants; then have the patient point to the area that is most painful.
   c. Have the patient first point to the area that is most painful; palpate that area first, moving toward the less painful areas.
   d. Palpate all four quadrants to find the area that is most painful.

114. Which of the following is the main purpose for assessing the elderly patient's mental status?
   a. To determine the degree of senility
   b. To determine if circulation is adequate
   c. To determine if a stroke has occurred
   d. To determine a baseline level of consciousness

115. Which of the following is correct regarding an altered mental status in an elderly patient?
   a. An altered mental status is not caused by a chronic condition such as Alzheimer disease.
   b. An altered mental status never results from the use of drugs and medications.
   c. An altered mental status is normal and to be expected in an elderly patient.
   d. An altered mental status may be the result of the acute onset of an emergency such as a stroke.

116. Nearly one-third of all elderly heart attack patients never experience pain. This is widely known as
   a. an atypical heart attack.
   b. a painless heart attack.
   c. a false heart attack.
   d. a silent heart attack.

117. Which of the following is the route of choice to gain access to the passenger compartment of a car?
    a. Driver's window
    b. Passenger's window
    c. Door
    d. Back window

118. Which of the following is a makeshift tool that can be used in an emergency to gain access through a car's window?
    a. The car's whip antenna
    b. The car's hubcap
    c. The car's seat belt
    d. The car's rear door handle

119. In a vehicle collision, the up-and-over or the down-and-under pathway commonly occurs with which of the following?
    a. Lateral impact
    b. Rear-end impact
    c. Rollover
    d. Frontal impact

120. A "whiplash" injury is commonly caused by which of the following?
    a. Lateral impact
    b. Rear-end impact
    c. Rollover
    d. Frontal impact

121. Which of the following is the most common mechanism of injury?
    a. Motor vehicle collisions
    b. Motorcycle collisions
    c. Gunshot wounds
    d. Falls

122. Penetrating injuries are classified as which of the following?
    a. Hollow, solid, and mixed
    b. Open, closed, and mixed
    c. Low, medium, and high velocity
    d. Partial, complete, and closed

123. Which of the following is called "pathway expansion" and is caused by a pressure wave resulting from the kinetic energy of the bullet?
    a. Cavitation
    b. Profile
    c. Drag
    d. Trajectory

124. Which of the following are the three phases of an explosion that cause specific injury patterns?
    a. First, second, and third phase
    b. Initial, medial, and final phase
    c. Preliminary, general, and specific phase
    d. Primary, secondary, and tertiary phase

125. You are treating a patient with an injured forearm and no other apparent or suspected injuries. There is no distal pulse, and the extremity appears cyanotic. Which of the following is correct?
    a. Complete the initial assessment and transport immediately.
    b. Align the limb with gentle traction; stop only when the pulse returns.
    c. Transport immediately, align the limb, and stop only when the pulse returns.
    d. Align the limb with gentle traction; stop if pain or crepitus occurs.

126. Which of the following describes the correct way to immobilize long-bone injuries?
    a. Immobilize the joint above the injury.
    b. Immobilize the joint below the injury.
    c. Immobilize the joints above and below the injury.
    d. Immobilize the injured long bone only, not the joints.

127. Use of the traction splint is inappropriate in which of the following circumstances?
    a. When the pelvis has also been injured
    b. When the injury is within 3 inches of the hip
    c. When the injury is to the middle of the thigh
    d. When the injury is within 6 inches of the knee

128. After receiving an on-line order from medical direction, you should do which of the following?
    a. Tell medical direction that you have received the order.
    b. Repeat the order back to medical direction, word for word.
    c. Have medical direction repeat the order at least twice.
    d. Write the order on a notepad.

129. In radio terms, which of the following means "message received and understood"?
    a. Copy
    b. Over
    c. Clear
    d. Break

130. When trying to rescue a responsive patient who is struggling in water near the shore of a lake, which order of rescuing the patient is preferred?
    1. Swim to the patient by using a flotation device.
    2. Reach to the patient by holding out an object.
    3. Throw a weighted polypropylene rope to the patient.
    4. Row a boat to the patient if one is immediately available.
    a. 3, 2, 1, 4
    b. 2, 3, 4, 1
    c. 3, 2, 4, 1
    d. 2, 4, 3, 1

131. You are treating a suspected spine-injured patient who is still in the water. Which of the following is correct?
    a. If the patient is found face down, roll the patient over quickly and remove from the water, using any available resources.
    b. To prevent any movement of the head and neck, avoid rescue breathing until the patient is removed from the water.
    c. Slide a long backboard under the patient, secure the torso and legs, then place a cervical spine immobilization collar (CSIC).
    d. Place a CSIC, slide a long backboard under the patient, then secure the torso and legs.

132. When operating an emergency vehicle, you must exercise "due regard for the safety of others." Which statement is true regarding this concept?
    a. You will not be held responsible for your actions if your emergency lights and siren are operating.
    b. Even under the special laws that apply in cases of true emergency, you can be held liable if you do not exercise reasonable care for the safety of others.
    c. You will not be held responsible for your actions if you exceed the speed limit by no more than 10 miles per hour over the posted speed limit.
    d. You must slow down only at red lights, stop signs, or school crossings.

133. Using a police escort is
    a. appropriate in a dangerous neighborhood.
    b. appropriate when high-speed transport is required.
    c. appropriate in a high-traffic area.
    d. a last resort, and usually not a good idea.

134. Which of the following is the first major phase of an ambulance call?
    a. Arrival at scene
    b. Dispatch
    c. Equipment preparation
    d. Post-run

135. A daytime landing zone for a small helicopter requires an area of
    a. 30 × 30 feet.
    b. 40 × 40 feet.
    c. 50 × 50 feet.
    d. 60 × 60 feet.

136. The four corners of a helicopter landing area should be marked. Where should a fifth device be positioned?
    a. On the approach side of the landing area
    b. At the location of the patient
    c. On the upwind side of the landing area
    d. At the location of the ambulance

137. Which of the following, a chronic brain disorder, is the most common cause of seizures?
    a. Diabetes
    b. Stroke
    c. Head injury
    d. Epilepsy

138. Which of the following conditions is a dire medical emergency that requires aggressive airway management?
    a. Postictal state
    b. Status epilepticus
    c. Tonic-clonic seizure
    d. Simple partial seizure

139. Which of the following drugs is considered to be a central nervous system depressant?
    a. Alcohol
    b. Cocaine
    c. LSD
    d. Ephedrine

140. In which of the following overdose cases (in which the drug taken is known) would the talk-down technique *not* be appropriate?
   a. PCP
   b. LSD
   c. Heroin
   d. Cocaine

141. The patient with an eye injury should be asked to follow your finger as you move it left and right, up and down, in order to evaluate
   a. ability to focus on a far object.
   b. ability to focus on a near object.
   c. abnormal gaze.
   d. reactivity to light.

142. Removal of a foreign particle from the eye should not generally be attempted in the field. If required, you should attempt removal of a particle only if
   a. it is lodged on the conjunctiva.
   b. it is lodged on the globe.
   c. it is lodged on the cornea.
   d. it is lodged on the iris.

143. An injury to the globe of the eye should be treated with
   a. patches applied lightly to both eyes.
   b. a firm compress applied to both eyes.
   c. firm hand pressure to the globe of the injured eye.
   d. direct pressure to the globes of both eyes.

144. When a patient has suffered an injury to the face, which of the following *best* states the other areas or structures to which compromise or injury should be suspected?
   a. The airway, spine, and skull
   b. The airway and spine
   c. The spine and skull
   d. The airway and skull

145. Which of the following is the correct way to dress and bandage a bleeding neck wound?
   a. An occlusive dressing covered by a regular dressing and a circumferential bandage
   b. A bulky dressing covered by an occlusive dressing and a circumferential bandage
   c. An occlusive dressing covered by a regular dressing and direct pressure
   d. A regular dressing covered by an occlusive dressing and a self-adhesive bandage

146. When administering an epinephrine auto-injector to a patient who is experiencing a severe allergic reaction, which of the following is the correct injection site?
   a. Any of the large arm veins
   b. Right or left buttocks
   c. Anteriolateral portion of the thigh
   d. Deltoid or shoulder muscle

147. Which of the following key categories of signs and symptoms specifically indicates a severe allergic reaction (anaphylaxis) and indicates immediate intervention and administration of epinephrine?
    a. Itchy, watery eyes with a slow heart rate
    b. Intense itching; increased blood pressure
    c. Respiratory or airway compromise and shock (hypoperfusion)
    d. Hives with a warm, tingling feeling to the hands

148. Your patient has been stabbed in the chest. You quickly expose the chest and find an open wound to the anterior chest. Which of the following is your correct *first* action?
    a. Perform a focused history and physical exam.
    b. Perform a rapid trauma assessment.
    c. Seal the wound with a nonocclusive dressing.
    d. Seal the wound with a gloved hand.

149. Which of the following is an *early* sign or symptom that indicates a complication associated with the sealed chest wound and a developing tension pneumothorax?
    a. Signs and symptoms of respiratory distress
    b. A heart rate that is slower than normal
    c. High blood pressure with a widening pulse pressure
    d. Tracheal deviation away from the injured side

150. You are treating a patient with an abdominal injury but no suspected spinal injury. Which of the following is the *best* position in which to place the patient?
    a. On the left side with the legs straight
    b. Supine with the legs flexed at the knees
    c. Fowler's position with the legs flexed
    d. Trendelenburg position with the legs straight

151. The mnemonic CBRNE is sometimes used to remember types of weapons of mass destruction (WMDs). It stands for
    a. chemical, biological, radiological, nuclear, and explosive.
    b. concussion, biochemical, radiological, nitroglycerin, and environmental.
    c. chemical, bacterial, radioactive, neurological, and extractive.
    d. corrosive, biochemical, radio, nuclear, and environmental.

152. Many of the same principles that apply to hazardous material emergencies also apply to weapons of mass destruction (WMD) emergencies. Which of the following is one of these principles?
    a. All rescuers will be involved in the decontamination of patients.
    b. Zones must be established to limit exposure to rescuers.
    c. Rescuers will not require specialized suits and breathing apparatus.
    d. Preplanning and coordination of agencies is not important or imperative.

Answers to Chapter Exercises

The number(s) following each answer refer to the textbook page(s) where the answer can be found or supported.

Chapter 1: Emergency Medical Care Systems, Research, and Public Health

TERMS AND CONCEPTS

1. a. 4 b. 5 c. 1 d. 6 e. 3 f. 2. *(p. 2)*

CONTENT REVIEW

1. **b.** The other items are AEMT or paramedic skills. *(p. 6)*
2. **a.** *Your* safety first and always; then the safety of other rescuers/bystanders. When the scene is secure, you may then provide care for the patient. *(p. 7)*
3. **c.** It is the EMT's responsibility to maintain certification or licensure to practice. *(p. 10)*
4. **c.** The risk of being struck by traffic at night-time scenes is reduced by wearing reflective clothing and providing adequate scene lighting. Being struck by traffic on nighttime scenes is a key threat to all on-scene personnel. All responders must take precautions to protect and ensure a visible and safe working area. It is never considered "just part of the job," and don't hold a lighted flare in your hand. *(p. 7)*
5. **b.** The best answer, given the situation described, is to move or retreat to an area where you can observe the scene and await the arrival of law enforcement. You should not approach until law enforcement tells you the scene is safe. *(p. 7)*
6. **b.** Quality improvement. *(p. 11)*
7. **b.** Evidence-based medicine (1) formulates a question about emergency care that needs to be answered, (2) uses the medical literature for research data that are related and applicable to the question, (3) appraises the evidence for validity and reliability, and (4) if the evidence supports a change in practice, changes protocols and implements the change in prehospital emergency care. There is currently very little research in prehospital care. It is the responsibility of every EMT to participate in every way possible so that EMS can develop its own evidence to change and support its own profession. *(pp. 12–13)*
8. **c.** The medical director is responsible for clinical and patient care aspects of the EMS system, including both on-line and off-line medical direction and significant involvement in educational programs and refresher courses. The medical director's primary responsibility is to develop and establish guidelines under which emergency service personnel function. *(p. 11)*
9. **b.** The EMT functions as a designated agent of the system medical director. *(p. 11)*
10. Answers will vary. Be honest in your rankings. Ask a friend to rank you on these items; then compare the results. Nobody's perfect, but you must recognize your limitations so you can improve. *(p. 10)*
11. **d.** Patient advocacy includes actions such as collecting patient valuables (if time permits), protecting patients from onlookers, and honoring the patient's requests (if possible). *(p. 14)*
12. All items listed are considered high-risk activities that put the patient at greater risk for injury, medical mistakes, or furthering an existing injury. *(p. 12)*
13. The following are common health prevention and promotion activities EMS has been involved with: (1) primary prevention (vaccinations, education), secondary prevention of complications of disease, and health screening; (2) disease surveillance through identifying and reporting certain diseases or conditions that are identified as a public health issue; and (3) injury prevention through the promotion of the use of safety equipment, education (seat belt use, helmet use, falls, fire prevention), and injury surveillance. *(p. 13)*
14. **c.** The primary responsibilities of the state EMS agency are: Overall planning of the statewide EMS system, coordination of the statewide EMS system, regulation of the statewide EMS system, licensing local EMS agencies and personnel. *(p. 10)*
15. **d.** The FCC currently estimates that wireless (cell) phones are responsible for placing approximately 70 percent of 911 calls. *(p. 4)*

CASE STUDY

1. **d.** Law enforcement has the primary responsibility for traffic control. At this scene, the car was just over the crest of a hill. This could create a potential hazard to rescuers while working this scene. If law enforcement is not on scene when you arrive, you (or others) will need to control traffic until they arrive.
2. **a.** The fire department has the primary responsibility for extrication and hazard control at this scene. The fire/rescue department, if properly trained, may need to secure

downed power lines in emergency situations when the power company is not on scene. Otherwise, the power company would deal with electrical hazards.

3. b. EMS/ambulance service has the primary responsibility for patient care and transport. In many areas, the fire service also provides EMS.

4. d. Do what you can, when you can, for the patient. Patient advocacy requires doing what is in the patient's best interest.

5. a. Prehospital care reports are the most commonly used instruments. Feedback from crews, patients, and family are other instruments that may be used but are not as common as the use of the prehospital care report.

6. c. The correct answer in this case is based on personal judgment. Traffic is certainly a hazard given that the accident occurred on a steep hill at night. The danger of fire is a possibility at any vehicle accident, and the vehicle could have been in an unstable position. Downed power lines in this case are the greatest potential threat because of the nighttime conditions and the frequent difficulty in seeing downed lines.

Chapter 2: Workforce Safety and Wellness of the EMT

TERMS AND CONCEPTS

1. a. 1 **b.** 3 **c.** 2 **d.** 5 **e.** 4. *(p. 18)*

CONTENT REVIEW

1. b. The five emotional stages associated with death and dying are denial, anger, bargaining, depression, and acceptance. *(pp. 18–19)*

2. a. A **b.** I **c.** I **d.** A (Talk to the unresponsive patient as if he is alert because many unresponsive patients are able to hear. Family members, *if cooperative and not preventing appropriate treatment,* should be allowed to remain in the room during resuscitation efforts. Never offer false reassurance. Try saying instead that you are "doing everything possible." Listen to the patient carefully, and deliver any messages to family members.) *(p. 19)*

3. a. Irritability, loss of appetite, and loss of interest in work are signs of stress. The others are signs of normal adaptation responses. *(p. 21)*

4. a. Defusing *(p. 23)*

5. a. "Pathogens" describe microorganisms that spread disease. Viruses, bacteria, and fungi are three specific types of pathogens. *(p. 24)*

6. a. Hand washing *(p. 26)*

7. c. Before attempting any rescue situation involving specialized threats such as hazardous materials, biological agents, high-angle rescue, or white-water rescue, specialized rescue teams should be requested. *(p. 32)*

8. a. 5 **b.** 2 **c.** 3 **d.** 1 **e.** 4. Identify hazards with binoculars and a guidebook, await scene control by hazmat team, put on necessary protective clothing, and then (and only then) provide patient assessment and emergency care. *(p. 31)*

9. a. Call for police assistance before entering a potentially violent scene. *(p. 33)*

10. b. Avoid disturbing a crime scene when possible, but remember that your priority as an EMT is patient care. *(p. 34)*

11. d. Hepatitis B may cause no signs or symptoms at all. (If they do occur, they may include fatigue, nausea, abdominal pain, headache, fever, and/or jaundice.) Hepatitis B is commonly transmitted by contact with a chronic carrier's blood or body fluids. It is a serious disease that may occur over weeks or months. The infection may be prevented by obtaining a vaccination. *(pp. 28–29)*

12. c. The best action to take, given the responses provided, is to contact your supervisor for specific instructions. The supervisor will implement your organization's exposure control policy. *(p. 29)*

13. c. Tuberculosis is a highly communicable disease spread by droplets from coughing and from direct contact with sputum. This disease is making a dramatic comeback. Researchers are concerned because new drug-resistant strains of tuberculosis are developing. Wearing a HEPA or N-95 respirator is recommended (not SCBA). *(p. 29)*

14. c. HEPA or N-95 respirators provide sufficient respiratory protection. Surgical face masks provide limited protection from tuberculosis. An SCBA is not necessary. *(p. 29)*

15. d. AIDS is chiefly spread by sexual contact involving the exchange of semen or blood or through contact with vaginal or cervical secretions, infected needles, infected blood or blood products, or transmission between an infected mother and her child. *(p. 29)*

16. b. AIDS is caused by a virus that destroys an infected individual's immune system. This disease process generally presents without signs and symptoms. AIDS is more difficult than hepatitis B to contract. *(p. 29)*

17. b. Hepatitis C is not prevented by a vaccine, is the most common bloodborne infection in the United States, is not easily transmitted, and causes no symptoms in about 80 percent of all cases. *(p. 29)*

18. c. The actions you can take to prevent exposure are to leave the surgical mask on the patient (if one is not in place, you should place one on the patient) to prevent droplet spread; to look for signs of fever and respiratory symptoms for up to 10 days following contact with the patient; to avoid touching your eyes, nose, or mouth with your gloved hands; and to wash your hands after glove removal. *(p. 30)*

19. a. The severe signs and symptoms of West Nile virus include high fever, headache and stiff neck, confusion and disorientation, seizures, muscle weakness, paralysis, and vision loss. *(p. 30)*

20. d. Multidrug-resistant organisms are commonly encountered during patient transport from hospital intensive care units, in burn units, and in long-term-care facilities. They are considered a significant threat to the EMT and are commonly transmitted by person-to-person contact. The organisms include methicillin/oxacillin-resistant *Staphylococcus aureus* (MRSA), vancomycin-resistant enterococci (VRE), penicillin-resistant *Streptococcus pneumoniae* (PRSP), and drug-resistant *Streptococcus pneumoniae* (DRSP). *(pp. 30–31)*

CASE STUDY

1. d. Acceptance. The patient has obviously accepted his death and is dealing rationally with his very difficult situation.

2. a. The situation is considered a high-stress incident and may require CISM.

3. d. Police, communications, EMS, and emergency department personnel are all involved in defusing. The patient's family should not be involved.

4. a. I **b.** I **c.** I **d.** I. All choices are inappropriate. Don't mask the symptoms and results of stress by using alcohol or drugs. Exercise should be encouraged along with sharing events with coworkers and requesting a slower-duty station rather than a busier station.

Chapter 3: Medical, Legal, and Ethical Issues

TERMS AND CONCEPTS

1. a. 5 **b.** 4 **c.** 3 **d.** 1 **e.** 2 **f.** 6 **g.** 11 **h.** 7 **i.** 8 **j.** 10 **k.** 9 **l.** 12. *(p. 40)*

CONTENT REVIEW

1. c. The EMT's scope of practice is defined by the National EMS Scope of Practice Model, by the *National EMS Education Standards,* and by state laws, regulations, and local policies. A national EMS act does not exist. Just because an EMT has the knowledge to perform certain skills does not permit the EMT to use those skills on a patient. *(p. 41)*

2. d. Battery. *(p. 49)*

3. c. Good Samaritan law. The Good Samaritan law protects a person who is not being paid for his services from liability for acts performed in good faith unless those acts constitute gross negligence. *(p. 42)*

4. a. Standard of care. *(p. 41)*

5. b. The patient's expressed or implied consent. *(p. 43)*

6. a. Implied consent. (It is not minor consent, which must be given by a parent or guardian.) *(p. 42)*

7. a. To refuse care, a patient must be mentally competent and informed. He is not legally required to sign a release, although the EMT should attempt to get a signed and witnessed release for the legal protection of the EMT and the EMS system. *(pp. 44–47)*

8. b. Pushing away or any other indication that care is not welcome—before or after care is begun—constitutes valid refusal if the patient is a competent adult. *(p. 45)*

9. b. Abandonment. *(p. 48)*

10. d. Patient information may not be given to an off-duty EMT, your spouse, or any other person without a legitimate need for the information. A health care provider needs to know this information in order to continue medical care. *(p. 49)*

11. b. The duty to act refers to your obligation to provide care to the patient while you are on duty. Some states require EMTs to stop and render aid even when off duty. *(p. 41)*

12. c. When you are not sure whether the patient can make a rational decision, you should consult medical direction. *(p. 46)*

13. d. A willful threat to a patient that can occur without actual touching is called assault. *(p. 49)*

14. b. The HIPAA, as it relates to the EMT, includes limits on disclosure of patient information, training on specific policies, obtaining patient signatures, and the assignment of an EMS privacy officer. *(p. 50)*

15. c. COBRA and EMTALA are both federal regulations designed to ensure public access to emergency care regardless of ability to pay. *(p. 50)*

16. d. Baby Safe Haven Laws. *(p. 53)*

CASE STUDY 1

1. b. The most important concerns you should have relating to this patient's refusal of treatment is the patient's understanding of the possible consequences of his refusal. He appears to have a hearing problem that may affect his ability to completely understand the ramifications of his actions. The patient seems to be mentally competent. You should also be concerned that the patient quickly signed the release without reading it. Do not let your partner or others influence what you know to be proper patient care decisions.

2. d. The other choices should be pursued only when all efforts to persuade the patient have failed.

CASE STUDY 2

1. a. Y **b.** Y **c.** Y **d.** Y (This situation meets all four criteria for a successful negligence suit.)

Chapter 4: Documentation

TERMS AND CONCEPTS

1. **a.** 4 **b.** 2 **c.** 1 **d.** 3. *(p. 56)*

CONTENT REVIEW

1. **c.** To ensure high-quality patient care. *(p. 57)*
2. **a.** The documentation provided in the PCR typically becomes a part of the patient's permanent medical record, is of great benefit in a lawsuit brought against the EMT, is frequently created in an electronic form, and is commonly used for preparation of bills and for submission to insurance companies. *(p. 58)*
3. **b.** The use of accurate and synchronous clocks is critical for proper EMS documentation of both dispatch needs and medical information needs. *(p. 61)*
4. **b.** Physical assessment findings and pertinent information about the scene should be included in the narrative section (include only objective and pertinent subjective information). *(p. 62)*
5. **c.** The patient denies back and neck pain. (These are symptoms that would be expected in this kind of accident, so the denial is a pertinent negative.) *(p. 62)*
6. **b.** At least two sets of vital signs should be obtained. Be sure to document the time taken and the patient's position when taken. Serial vital signs provide a trend in the patient's condition. *(p. 62)*
7. **b.** State law and the federal HIPAA require that patient information must not be given out to friends, reporters, or others who are merely curious. *(p. 66)*
8. **a.** When dealing with a patient who has refused treatment, document your explanation of possible consequences of failing to accept care, and have the patient sign the form acknowledging refusal of treatment. Discuss the situation with medical direction, complete as much of the assessment as the patient will permit, and ensure that the patient is not under the influence of drugs or alcohol. Documentation of the call is generally more involved and frequently will require more documentation. The issue of patient competency is a primary concern in issues of patient refusal of care. *(p. 66)*
9. **a.** Objective information is measurable or verifiable in some way. A sign is an objective observation. A symptom is a subjective observation based on the individual's perception. A symptom a patient denies having is a pertinent negative. *(p. 62)*
10. **c.** Draw a single line through the incorrect entry and initial it. If the error is discovered after the report is submitted; using different colored ink, draw a single line through the error and initial and date the correction. *(p. 67)*
11. **a.** Triage tags. *(p. 68)*
12. **a.** Additional special documentation by the EMT is required for suspected abuse of a child or an elderly patient, possible exposures to communicable diseases, injury to a member of the EMS crew, and for other situations the EMT believes might require special documentation. *(p. 68)*
13. **c.** Next of kin (usually the immediate family) is not included in the DOT minimum data set and does not usually appear on PCR forms. *(p.60)*
14. **a.** QID (four times a day) **b.** x (times) **c.** $\bar{a}$ (before) **d.** Pt (patient) **e.** Rx (prescription) **f.** q (every) **g.** Tx (treatment) **h.** $\bar{c}$ (with) **i.** Stat (immediately) **j.** $\bar{s}$ (without) **k.** PO (orally, by mouth) **l.** TID (three times a day) *(p. 62)*
15. **d.** The mnemonics SOAP, CHART, and CHEATED all help to organize information on the PCR. Regarding response a., the mnemonic for the level of responsiveness is AVPU. *(p. 68)*
16. **d.** The "A" in the mnemonics SOAP, CHART, and CHEATED stands for "assessment" in each case, representing the assessment portion of patient assessment. *(p. 68)*

CASE STUDY

1. Patient care report narrative section for this call: Fifty-year-old male complains that his right ankle is "a little sore" after slipping on a wet floor approximately a half-hour ago. Patient found to be alert and oriented, having no apparent difficulty breathing, and in no apparent distress. No signs of bleeding. Pulse is strong and regular. Skin is pink, warm, and dry. Focused physical exam reveals that right ankle is markedly swollen, discolored, and very tender to gentle palpation. Pedal pulse is present. Good motion and sensation in injured extremity. Foot is slightly pale but warm to touch. Denies any other injuries. Denies neck and back pain. Vital signs: BP 138/78 mmHg, pulse 68, respirations 18 and adequate, SpO$_2$ on room air is 96 percent. Pupils normal. No allergies or medications. Patient denies any medical problems. Last meal (soup and a sandwich) about a half-hour earlier. States he felt fine all day but slipped on some water on the floor and twisted his ankle. Patient advised that ankle should be splinted for transport to the hospital for evaluation and X-rays. Patient refuses, stating that his wife is already en route to take him to the doctor. Advised against weight bearing on injured ankle until evaluated by doctor. Encouraged to call 911 should any problems arise. B. Jones, EMT
2. **a.** The patient should review the PCR and sign a refusal-of-treatment form. Be prepared to answer any questions that the patient may have.
3. **a.** You must not share any information pertaining to this patient with the safety officer. You should briefly and politely explain that

legally, you cannot discuss this case with him. Even giving what might seem like general information may be a violation of the patient's rights.

Chapter 5: Communication

TERMS AND CONCEPTS
1. **a.** 3 **b.** 1 **c.** 4 **d.** 2 **e.** 5 **f.** 8 **g.** 6
   h. 10 **i.** 9 **j.** 7 **k.** 11. *(p. 73)*

CONTENT REVIEW
1. **d.** The base station generally uses a high output of between 80 and 150 watts of transmission power, should be located in a high area to improve signal transmission, should be located in close proximity to the hospital that serves as the medical command center, and serves as a dispatch and coordination area that is in contact with other system elements. *(p. 74)*
2. **a.** Allow communications over a wide area. *(p. 74)*
3. **d.** Cell phones within an EMS system usually have excellent sound quality, may become overwhelmed during disaster situations, are usually easily maintained, are cost efficient, and often improve communication privacy. *(p. 76)*
4. **b.** License base stations. *(p. 76)*
5. **b.** Radio use must be brief, efficient, and professional, *not* as if talking on the telephone. Always listen for other radio traffic before transmitting, and use the "echo method" by repeating information when receiving orders or information. *(p. 78)*
6. **c.** Provide instructions about what to do until help arrives. *(p. 79)*
7. **1.** Announce arrival on scene. **2.** Announce departure from scene and ETA. **3.** Announce arrival at hospital. **4.** Announce that you are clear and available for another call. **5.** Announce arrival back at base. *(p. 79)*
8. **d.** The patient's mental status and, additionally, baseline vital signs, pertinent physical exam findings, description of care provided, the patient's response to the treatment provided, the patient's current condition, and the estimated time of arrival. *(pp. 79–80)*
9. **b.** Repeat instructions back word for word. *(p. 80)*
10. **a.** Question the order. *(p. 80)*
11. **c.** It is not necessary to obtain permission from police and fire personnel before beginning patient care. Obtain information while going to or at the side of the patient, and always ask for information about what happened and what care has been given. *(p. 81)*
12. **a.** See if a companion or a bystander can interpret or utilize a toll-free interpreter line; talking loudly and slowly does not help if the person doesn't understand English, although talking slowly might help if the person has limited English. *(p. 82)*
13. **a.** Radio codes provide clear, concise information that shortens radio airtime. These codes are not regulated by the FCC and are generally not understood by the patient. *(p. 82)*
14. **d.** Ten-Codes, as well as other codes, have been abandoned by many EMS agencies in favor of the use of standard English. Ten-Codes are published by the APCO, primarily for use by dispatch, although they are also sometimes used by other EMS personnel. *(p. 82)*
15. **c.** 2032 hours represents 8:32 P.M. (Hours from 1:00 A.M. to noon = 0100 to 1200 hours; hours from 1:00 P.M. to midnight = 1300 to 2400 hours. To arrive at the military time representing 8:32 P.M., add 832 to 1200 hours.) *(p. 82)*

CASE STUDY
1. Report on arrival at the scene: "Unit 3 to Dispatch. We are on the scene at the playground at 1031 Bruce Road. Over."
2. Report en route to the hospital: "Washington Memorial, this is Green County BLS Unit 3 en route to you with an ETA of 12 minutes. We have a 3-year-old male with a 1-inch laceration to his chin due to a fall on the playground. He is alert and oriented. Mother reports no allergies. His vital signs are blood pressure 80/68 mmHg, pulse strong at 80, respirations 28 and of good quality with an SpO_2 of 96% on room air. His skin is flushed, warm, and moist. Capillary refill is less than 2 seconds. Pupils are normal. The wound has been dressed and bandaged. The bleeding is controlled. Patient reports injury 'hurts bad.' Over."
3. Report to the hospital personnel when transferring care: "This is Mikey Smith. He has a 1-inch laceration to his chin. Mrs. Smith reports that he has no allergies. We applied a dressing and a bandage. The bleeding is controlled. Current vitals: blood pressure is 80/68 mmHg, pulse 80, respirations 28, skin normal, pupils normal, SpO_2 of 96% on room air."

Chapter 6: Lifting and Moving Patients

TERMS AND CONCEPTS
1. **a.** Lordosis is when the stomach is too anterior and the buttocks are too posterior. *(p. 94)*
   b. A nonurgent move is performed when no immediate threat to life exists. *(p. 97)*
   c. A power grip is when the palm and fingers are in complete contact with the object and the fingers are bent at the same angle. *(p. 96)*
   d. Kyphosis is when the shoulders are rolled forward, which results in fatigue on the lower back. *(p. 94)*
   e. An emergency move is performed when there is an immediate danger to the patient or rescuer. *(p. 97)*

CONTENT REVIEW

1. **a.** Reaching a great distance to lift a light object. *(p. 93)*
2. **a.** Leg, hip, and gluteal muscles (avoid lifting with your back muscles; avoid reaching). *(p. 97)*
3. **b.** Keeping your shoulders, hips, and feet in vertical alignment. *(p. 94)*
4. Flexibility training, cardiovascular conditioning, strength training, and nutrition. *(p. 94)*
5. **c.** Always try to lock the back. Lifting the upper body first reduces movement of the back. *(p. 95)*
6. **b.** Place the weaker leg slightly forward of the good leg. *(p. 96)*
7. **a.** Leaning to the opposite side. *(p. 96)*
8. **d.** Use a spotter to direct and navigate. *(p. 109)*
9. **c.** 20 inches. *(p. 97)*
10. **b.** Push rather than pull; keep the load between hips and shoulder. *(p. 97)*
11. **a.** The patient that presents with neurological deficit should be carefully extricated from the vehicle; there were no other hazards in this case. All of the others should have been rapidly extricated from the vehicle to protect the patient and rescuers. The last patient stopped breathing and needed immediate treatment after rapidly extricating the patient from the vehicle. *(p. 100)*
12. **b.** The EMT at the foot faces the other EMT while walking backward. The stronger of the two EMTs should be placed at the head because there is more weight at this point. The EMT at the foot is required to walk backward, not forward. The EMT at the head walks forward, thus moving the patient feet first. *(p. 109)*
13. **a.** While carrying the patient up stairs, the EMT at the head leads and must walk backward up the steps. Never carry a patient headfirst down steps. This patient was a supine patient and should not be placed in a stair chair. You should restrain the patient's hands and secure them to the stretcher or backboard to prevent the patient from reaching and grabbing. *(p. 104)*
14. **d.** Decrease the spinal loading associated with repetitive movements. They typically weigh more than traditional stretchers and are capable of being outfitted with a power loading system. *(p. 103)*

CASE STUDY

1. **b.** Keep their backs locked and stay as close to the stretcher as possible, avoiding leaning.
2. **c.** Lower the stretcher onto its wheels so the stretcher does part of the work, with the rescuers at the back pushing it along the boardwalk.
3. All of these.
4. **a.** The power lift is recommended for *all* patients, especially heavy patients.

Chapter 7: Anatomy, Physiology, and Medical Terminology

MEDICAL TERMINOLOGY

1. **a.** Nature. *(p. 144)*
2. **c.** Between; *intervertebral* means "between the vertebrae." *(p. 125)*
3. **b.** Over, above. *(p. 122)*
4. **a.** Study of. *(p. 156)*
5. **d.** Skin; *subcutaneous* means "below the (dermis) skin." *(p. 150)*
6. **a.** perfusion **b.** my/o **c.** glottis **d.** vertebra **e.** hypo **f.** card/ium **g.** peri **h.** axil **i.** pleur **j.** inter. *(pp. 158–160)*

TERMS AND CONCEPTS

1. **a.** transverse line **b.** posterior **c.** prone **d.** superior **e.** normal anatomical position **f.** midaxillary **g.** inferior **h.** lateral **i.** anterior **j.** distal **k.** midline **l.** sagittal or lateral plane **m.** midsagittal plane **n.** frontal or coronal plane **o.** transverse or horizontal plane. *(pp. 157–160)*

CONTENT REVIEW

1. **c.** The patient's right. *(p. 122)*
2. **a.** midline **b.** proximal **c.** distal **d.** medial **e.** lateral **f.** palmar **g.** plantar **h.** anterior **i.** posterior **j.** superior **k.** midaxillary **l.** inferior. *(pp. 122–123)*
3. **a.** *Bilateral* refers to right and left; the femur is the thigh bone. *(p. 122)*
4. **a.** Posterior means "toward the back." *(p. 122)*
5. **c.** Lateral means "toward or on the side"; recumbent means "lying down." *(p. 122)*
6. **d.** Thoracic spine. *(p. 125)*
7. **a.** Cervical spine (the neck). *(p. 136)*
8. **d.** Ball-and-socket joints. *(p. 129)*
9. **c.** Skeletal muscles can be consciously controlled; involuntary muscle movements are automatic. *(p. 132)*
10. **b.** The unresponsive patient may not be able to protect his airway, partly because the epiglottis fails to close over the trachea. *(p. 133)*
11. **b.** The thoracic cavity increases, creating lower pressure inside the chest than in the atmosphere, causing air to flow into the lungs. *(p. 136)*
12. **b.** The infant's or child's tongue takes up proportionately *more* space in the smaller mouth. *(p. 136)*
13. **d.** Use of accessory muscles (e.g., muscles of the neck, above the clavicles, below the ribs) to aid in breathing is a sign that normal breathing mechanisms are not functioning adequately. The other choices are signs of adequate breathing. *(pp. 137–138)*
14. **A.** cranium **B.** zygomatic bone **C.** maxilla **D.** cervical vertebra **E.** sternum **F.** xiphoid process **G.** iliac crest **H.** ilium **I.** pelvic girdle **J.** greater trochanter **K.** symphysis pubis **L.** frontal bone **M.** parietal bone **N.** occipital bone **O.** temporal bone **P.** mandible **Q.** clavicle **R.** scapula **S.** ribs

T. humerus   U. elbow   V. ulna
W. radius   X. sacrum   Y. coccyx
Z. carpals   AA. metacarpals   BB. phalanges
CC. femur   DD. patella   EE. tibia
FF. fibula   GG.   tarsals   HH. metatarsals
II. calcaneus. *(pp. 125–127)*

15. a. Gas exchange takes place between capillaries and alveoli and between capillaries and the body's cells. *(p. 132)*

16. d. Atria, ventricles. *(p. 138)*

17. d. The white blood cells. *(p. 142)*

18. c. The carotid (in the neck) is a central pulse. The radial (wrist), brachial (upper arm), and tibial (ankle) are considered peripheral pulses (away from the center). *(p. 141)*

19. d. Perfusion. ("Hypo" in hypoperfusion means "low," so hypoperfusion is low, or inadequate, perfusion.) *(p. 144)*

20. a. Brain and spinal cord. *(p. 146)*

21. b. Pituitary. *(p. 144)*

22. d. Largest organ, protects against bacteria, regulates temperature. *(p. 150)*

23. d. In the semi-Fowler's position, the patient is placed on his back with the torso elevated less than 45 degrees. In the Fowler position, the patient is placed on his back with the torso elevated 45–60 degrees. *(p. 120)*

24. a. Vasoconstriction, decreasing the diameter of the vessel, and vasodilation, increasing the diameter of the vessel, are controlled by smooth muscle within the vessels. Vasoconstriction will increase the resistance inside the vessel, making it harder for the blood to pass through, and will result in an increase in pressure. Whereas vasodilation will result in a decrease in the resistance inside the vessel, making it easier for the blood to flow through, and decreasing the pressure. *(p. 132)*

25. d. *Ventilation* defines the mechanical process of how air is moved in and out of the lungs. Ventilation is primarily based on changes in pressure inside the chest causing air to flow into or out of the lungs. *Respiration* refers to the process of moving oxygen and carbon dioxide across membranes in and out of the cells, capillaries, and alveoli. Thus, respiration deals with the actual gas exchange process. *Oxygenation* is a form of respiration where the oxygen molecule moves across a membrane from an area of high-oxygen concentration to an area of low-oxygen concentration. Cells are oxygenated when the oxygen moves out of the blood in the vessel and into the cell, where it is used in metabolism. *(p. 133)*

26. b. The diaphragm contributes about 60–70 percent of the effort to breathe, whereas the intercostal muscles contribute the remaining 30–40 percent. *(p. 136)*

27. c. An apical pulse is felt on the left side of the chest over the left ventricle. The pulse being felt is from the mechanical contraction of the left ventricle. Because you are only feeling the mechanical contraction of the heart and not the pressure wave of blood, it does not provide an assessment of the effectiveness of the heart or blood volume. *(p. 142)*

28. d. About 97 percent of the oxygen carried in the blood is attached to the hemoglobin molecule, which is on the surface of the red blood cell. The remaining 3 percent (not enough to survive on alone) is dissolved in the blood. *(p. 144)*

29. a. The main source of energy comes from the cell metabolizing glucose (a simple sugar molecule). *(pp. 144–145)*

30. a. *Alpha 1* causes the vessels to constrict (vasoconstriction), thus shunting blood to the core of the body. This causes the skin to become cool, pale, and diaphoretic. *Alpha 2* is thought to regulate the release of alpha 1. *Beta 1* has all of its effects on the heart. It will increase the heart rate, increase the force of contraction, and will speed up the electrical impulse traveling down the heart's conduction system. *Beta 2* will cause smooth muscle to dilate, especially in the bronchioles and in some vessels. *(p. 148)*

31. b. The phrenic nerve exits the spinal column at C3 to C5, the phrenic nerve may be damaged, and the diaphragm will not receive a nervous impulse to contract the diaphragm. *(p. 136)*

32. d. The components of the nervous system that control consciousness are the cerebral hemispheres and the reticular activating system. *(p. 148)*

33. a. The pancreas is a solid organ located behind the stomach. The pancreas contains small areas of specialized tissue called the islets of Langerhans, which produce the hormones somatostatin, glucagon, and insulin. *(p. 152)*

34. c. The spleen is a solid organ located in the upper left quadrant of the abdomen. It helps to filtrate the blood, and because it contains a dense network of blood vessels, it serves as a reservoir of blood the body can use in an emergency such as a hemorrhage. *(p. 152)*

35. a. Ureters carry the waste from the kidneys to the bladder. The urethra carries urine from the bladder out of the body; the duodenum is the first section of the small intestine that receives partly digested food from the stomach; the hepatic ducts receive bile from the right and left lobes of the liver. *(p. 152)*

CASE STUDY

1. *Supine* means on the back (face up).

2. a. Large laceration to right midclavicular line. (center of right clavicle) superior to (above) the right nipple (right = patient's right).

3. a. Deformity to the proximal (nearest the torso) end of the left (patient's left) humerus (upper arm bone).

4. b. Bilateral (to both legs) femoral region (area around and including the thighbone) deformity with puncture wound to the left (patient's left) lateral thigh (toward the outside of the thigh, away from the body's midline, which runs between the legs) proximal to (nearer the torso in relation to) the patella (kneecap).

Chapter 8: Pathophysiology

TERMS AND CONCEPTS

1. a. 1 b. 7 c. 5 d. 11 e. 2 f. 9 g. 3
   h. 6 i. 8 j. 10 k. 4 l. 12 m. 13.
   (p. 164)

CONTENT REVIEW

1. **d.** The process that occurs when glucose crosses the cell membrane and is broken down into pyruvic acid is called *gylcolysis*. *(p. 165)*
2. **a.** A series of reactions that produce energy in the presence of oxygen within the cell is called *aerobic metabolism*. *(p. 165)*
3. **d.** A series of reactions that produce energy without the presence of oxygen in the cell is called *anaerobic metabolism*. *(p. 166)*
4. **c.** Failure of the intracellular sodium/potassium pump causes water to accumulate within the cell. *(p. 166)*
5. **b.** Perfusion is described as the delivery of oxygen, glucose, and other substances to the cells and the elimination of waste products. *(p. 165)*
6. **c.** Ambient air at sea level contains 21 percent oxygen and has a partial pressure of 159 mmHg. The concentration of oxygen in the ambient air directly affects the amount of oxygen that ends up in the blood. The FDO_2 is the fraction of oxygen delivered to a patient via a ventilation device such as a BVM device. *(p. 168)*
7. **d.** The carina is located at the second intercostal space anteriorly and at the fourth thoracic vertebrae posteriorly. *(p. 170)*
8. I Sternocleidomastoid, E Abdominal muscles, I Scalene muscles, I Pectoralis minor muscles, E Internal intercostal muscles. *(p. 171)*
9. **c.** A concept that states the volume of gas is inversely proportionate to the pressure is called *Boyle's law* and helps explain the mechanics of ventilation. *(p. 170)*
10. **b.** During inhalation, the diaphragm provides approximately 60 to 70 percent of the effort of breathing. *(p. 170)*
11. **d.** Two conditions that may require the use of accessory muscles to generate a greater force to fill and empty the lungs are higher airway resistance and poor compliance. Compliance is a measure of the ability of the chest wall and lungs to stretch, distend, and expand. Airway resistance is related to the ease of air flow down the conduit of airway structures leading to the alveoli. *(p. 171)*
12. **d.** Swelling from edema within the airway structures is the most common cause of increased airway resistance. Mucus and bronchial constriction will also decrease the radius of the airway and increase the airway resistance. *(pp. 171–172)*
13. **a.** A patient who has a tidal volume (minute ventilation) of 500 mL and is breathing at 12 times per minute has a minute volume of 6 liters or 6,000 mL. Minute ventilation = tidal volume (VT) × frequency of ventilation (f/minute). *(p. 172)*
14. **b.** The patient's alveolar ventilation is 4.2 liters or 4,200 mL. Alveolar ventilation = (tidal volume – dead air space) × frequency of ventilation/minute. *(p. 172)*
15. **c.** Ventilatory rates of 40 per minute or greater in the adult patient and greater than 60 per minute in the pediatric patient are considered too fast to be sustainable and allow for adequate time for a normal tidal volume. *(p. 174)*
16. **a.** The central chemoreceptors are located near the respiratory center in the medulla, are most sensitive to changes in the pH of the cerebrospinal fluid, and become insensitive to chronically high CO_2 levels. *(p. 174)*
17. **d.** Hypoxia becomes the main stimulus for ventilation rather than hypercarbia in patients with COPD. *(p. 178)*
18. **a.** The relationship between alveolar blood flow and alveolar airflow is called the *ventilation/perfusion ratio*. *(p. 167)*
19. **d.** Oxygen is transported in the blood dissolved in plasma and attached to hemoglobin, a hemoglobin molecule can carry up to four oxygen molecules, a hemoglobin molecule with oxygen attached is called *oxyhemoglobin*, carbon dioxide is chiefly carried in the blood in the form of bicarbonate. *(p. 179)*
20. **b.** The majority of blood is found within the venous system. *(p. 180)*
21. **c.** Plasma oncotic pressure exerts a "pull" effect on intravascular fluids; if low, will promote a loss of vascular volume, and if high, will draw an excessive amount of fluid into the vessel or capillary. *(p. 180)*
22. 1. An <u>increase</u> in stimulation by the sympathetic nervous system will increase the heart rate. 2. A <u>decrease</u> in stimulation by the sympathetic nervous system will decrease the heart rate. 3. An <u>increase</u> in stimulation by the parasympathetic nervous system will <u>decrease</u> the heart rate. 4. A decrease in stimulation by the parasympathetic nervous system will <u>increase</u> the heart rate. *(p. 182)*
23. **b.** The Frank-Starling law of the heart states that the stretch of the muscle fiber at the end of diastole determines the forces necessary to eject the blood contained within it. *(p. 182)*
24. **c.** *Preload* is the pressure in the left ventricle generated at the end of diastole. *(p. 182)*
25. **d.** *Stroke volume* is the amount of blood ejected by the left ventricle with each contraction. *(p. 182)*
26. 1. A decrease in heart rate will <u>decrease</u> cardiac output. 2. An increase in heart rate, if not excessive, will <u>increase</u> cardiac output. 3. A decrease in blood volume will <u>decrease</u> preload, <u>decrease</u> stroke volume, and <u>decrease</u> cardiac output. 4. An increase in blood volume will <u>increase</u> preload, <u>increase</u> stroke volume, and <u>increase</u> cardiac output. 5. A decrease

in myocardial contractility will <u>decrease</u> stroke volume and <u>decrease</u> cardiac output. **6.** An increase in myocardial contractility will <u>increase</u> stroke volume and <u>increase</u> cardiac output. **7.** Neural stimulation from the sympathetic nervous system will <u>increase</u> heart rate, <u>increase</u> myocardial contractility, and <u>increase</u> cardiac output. **8.** Neural stimulation from the parasympathetic nervous system will <u>decrease</u> the heart rate, <u>decrease</u> myocardial contractility, and <u>decrease</u> cardiac output. **9.** Beta$_1$ stimulation from epinephrine will <u>increase</u> heart rate, <u>increase</u> myocardial contractility, and <u>increase</u> cardiac output. **10.** Beta$_1$ blockade (patient on beta blocker) will block beta$_1$ stimulation, <u>decrease</u> heart rate, <u>decrease</u> myocardial contractility, and <u>decrease</u> cardiac output. **11.** An extremely high diastolic blood pressure will <u>increase</u> the pressure in the aorta, requiring a more forceful contraction to overcome the aortic pressure and a higher myocardial workload, and may <u>decrease</u> the cardiac output and weaken the heart over time. **12.** A reduction in the diastolic blood pressure will <u>decrease</u> the pressure in the aorta, require a less forceful contraction to overcome the aortic pressure, and reduce the myocardial workload, and may improve the cardiac output in a weakened heart. *(pp. 182–184)*

27. **b.** A narrow pulse pressure is defined as being less than 25 percent of the systolic pressure. The pulse pressure is determined by subtracting the diastolic pressure from the systolic pressure. *(p. 184)*

28. **1.** An <u>increase</u> in cardiac output will increase the blood pressure. **2.** A <u>decrease</u> in cardiac output will decrease the blood pressure. **3.** An increase in the heart rate will <u>increase</u> the cardiac output, which will <u>increase</u> the blood pressure. **4.** A decrease in the heart rate will <u>decrease</u> the cardiac output, which will <u>decrease</u> the blood pressure. **5.** An increase in the stroke volume will <u>increase</u> the cardiac output, which will <u>increase</u> the blood pressure. **6.** A decrease in the stroke volume will <u>decrease</u> the cardiac output, which will <u>decrease</u> the blood pressure. **7.** An increase in systemic vascular resistance will <u>increase</u> the blood pressure. **8.** A decrease in systemic vascular resistance will <u>decrease</u> the blood pressure. *(p. 184)*

CASE STUDY 1

1. The following are the *most likely* early physiological responses. Others are also likely.
   - <u>X</u> Composition of ambient air
   - _____ Patent airway
   - _____ Mechanics of ventilation
   - <u>X</u> Regulation of ventilation
   - <u>X</u> Ventilation/perfusion ratio
   - <u>X</u> Transport of oxygen and carbon dioxide by the blood
   - _____ Blood volume
   - _____ Pump function of the myocardium
   - _____ Systemic vascular resistance
   - _____ Microcirculation
   - _____ Blood pressure *(pp. 175–176)*

2. Early effects are described. As the incident progresses, the effects of diminished perfusion will compound into a cascade of multiple body system failures. The effects described here do not represent a complete listing of all possible combinations. Discuss this as a group and see how many more effects you can discover. **Composition of ambient air**—as the patient exhales 17 percent carbon dioxide and uses the ambient oxygen, the reduced oxygen content will result in cellular hypoxia. **Regulation of ventilation**—Central chemoreceptors will sense the increasing blood pH resulting from the increasing carbon dioxide levels, while peripheral chemoreceptors sense the decrease of the blood oxygen concentration. Stimulation of these receptors causes an increase in the rate and depth of the patient's ventilations. **Ventilation/perfusion ratio**—Ventilation to the alveoli is intact for some minutes, but as the oxygen in the environment is depleted, oxygen movement across the capillary membrane is diminished. This creates a ventilation-to-perfusion mismatch. **Transport of oxygen and carbon dioxide by the blood**—A disturbance in oxygen availability leads to cellular hypoxia and the inability of the transport system to transport oxygen to body tissues. *(pp. 167–168)*

CASE STUDY 2

1. **c.** The patient's minute ventilation is 7.2 L/min or 7,200 mL/min and the alveolar ventilation is 4.8 L/min or 4,800 mL/min. (450 mL × 16 = 7,200 mL or 7.2 L) ((450 mL − 150 mL) × 16 = 4,800 mL or 4.8 L). *(p. 172)*

2. **c.** The pulse pressure is 24 (110 − 86 = 24). *(p. 184)*

3. **a.** A normal pulse pressure is greater than 25 percent of the systolic blood pressure. *(p. 184)*

4. The following are most likely, early physiological responses.
   - _____ Composition of ambient air
   - _____ Patent airway
   - _____ Mechanics of ventilation
   - <u>X</u> Regulation of ventilation
   - <u>X</u> Ventilation/perfusion ratio
   - <u>X</u> Transport of oxygen and carbon dioxide by the blood
   - <u>X</u> Blood volume
   - <u>X</u> Pump function of the myocardium
   - <u>X</u> Systemic vascular resistance
   - <u>X</u> Microcirculation
   - <u>X</u> Blood pressure *(pp. 167–168)*

   Early effects are described. As the incident progresses, the effects of diminished perfusion will compound into a cascade of multiple body system failures. The effects described here do not represent a complete listing of all possible combinations. Discuss this as a group and see how many more effects you can discover. **Regulation of ventilation**—as the oxygen level in the blood falls, due to a reduction in oxyhemoglobin transport from blood loss, the peripheral chemoreceptors signal the respiratory center in the brain to increase the rate and depth of respirations. **Ventilation/perfusion ratio**—oxygen is available at the alveolar level for exchange, but the falling pulmonary capillary pressure reduces alveolar blood flow and subsequent oxygen transport. **Transport of oxygen and carbon dioxide by the blood**—the loss of hemoglobin via blood loss leads to cellular hypoxia. **Blood volume**—the venous volume is diminished and reduces the preload, which then reduces the cardiac output. **Pump function of the myocardium**—sympathetic nervous system stimulation will increase the heart rate in order to increase the cardiac output. **Systemic vascular resistance**—sympathetic stimulation creates vascular constriction, decreasing the size of the vascular space, increasing the diastolic pressure. **Microcirculation**—blood is shunted from the microcirculation to the central circulation via sympathetic nervous system stimulation. **Blood pressure**—the systolic blood pressure is reduced, the diastolic pressure is increased. Baroreceptors signal the sympathetic nervous system to increase the heart rate, myocardial contractility, and constrict vessels in order to increase the blood pressure.

Chapter 9: Life Span Development

TERMS AND CONCEPTS
1. a. 2 b. 7 c. 5 d. 3 e. 1 f. 10 g. 9
   h. 4 i. 11 j. 6 k. 8. *(p. 191)*

CONTENT REVIEW
1. **c.** An infant's head is equal to 25 percent of its total body weight, an infant will normally weigh 3.0–3.5 kg, its lung tissue is very fragile and is prone to trauma from excessive pressure during positive pressure ventilation, and infants have fewer alveoli with decreased collateral ventilation. *(p. 192)*
2. **d.** By the age of 2 months, an infant should be able to track objects with his eyes, focus on objects 8–12 inches away, recognize familiar faces, display primary emotions and facial expressions, hear and recognize some familiar sounds and voices, and move in response to stimuli. Items a–c are actions that a 12-month-old should be able to perform. *(p. 193)*
3. **b.** A preschooler is 3–6 years of age, a toddler is a child who is 12–36 months in age; a toddler's normal heart rate is 80–130 beats per minute, and the toddler's normal systolic blood pressure will range from 70–100 mmHg. *(p. 191)*
4. **b.** Items a, c, and d are actions that a 5-year-old should be able to perform, but not a 3-year-old. *(p. 191)*
5. **c.** Take additional time to communicate with the child, allow the parent to be present during the assessment, allow the child to touch

the equipment before you use it, demonstrate its use on the parent, and always tell the truth. *(p. 195)*
6. **b.** Is the stage of development from 20–40 years of age, is a stage with a high childbirth rate, and is a stage associated with fewer psychological problems than the other groups. *(p. 197)*
7. **d.** The characteristics described are related to late adulthood. *(pp. 196–198)*
8. **a.** Depression and suicide are more common for adolescents than any other age group. *(p. 197)*
9. 140–160. *(p. 191)*
10. 70–90. *(p. 191)*
11. 98–100. *(p. 191)*
12. 20–30. *(p. 191)*
13. 70–110. *(p. 191)*
14. 12–20. *(p. 191)*
15. 120/80. *(p. 191)*

CASE STUDY
1. **c.** All the vital signs are appropriate for this patient's stage of development.
2. **d.** The patient is likely to have many family conflicts, to prefer his privacy during assessment and evaluation, to believe that he is the "center of attention," and to participate in risky behaviors.
3. **d.** Move the patient to an area of privacy.

CHAPTER 9 SCENARIO: DOCUMENTATION EXERCISE
1. **c.** Patients in this life stage generally feel ashamed to ask for assistance, experience isolation and feel alone, live on fixed incomes and must make difficult financial decisions, and experience significant gastrointestinal and multiple other body system changes.
2. **c.** Appropriate given Mr. Savage's chief complaint. The dizziness could be a symptom of another medical condition, including but not limited to a stroke, infection, or myocardial infarction.
3. **d.** If the protocol allows and the monitoring equipment is available, you should check Mr. Savage's blood glucose level.

Chapter 10: Airway Management, Artificial Ventilation, and Oxygenation

MEDICAL TERMINOLOGY
1. **a.** Two, double. *(p. 225)*
2. **c.** Dark blue. *(p. 209)*
3. **b.** Surgical incision. *(p. 246)*
4. **b.** Trachea. *(p. 205)*
5. **d.** Opening. *(p. 205)*

TERMS AND CONCEPTS
1. a. 3 b. 1 c. 18 d. 2 e. 5 f. 19 g. 22
   h. 21 i. 20 j. 8 k. 16 l. 10 m. 13 n. 7
   o. 6 p. 14 q. 15 r. 9. *(pp. 205–207)*

CONTENT REVIEW

1. **c.** In the infant and child, the tongue takes up more space in the mouth and thus may occlude the airway. The nose and mouth are proportionately smaller in the infant and child. The cricoid cartilage is narrower and less rigid. The diaphragm and external intercostal muscles do not affect the airway. *(p. 250)*

2. **A.** Mandible   **B.** Thyroid cartilage   **C.** Trachea   **D.** Cricoid cartilage   **E.** Nasal cavity   **F.** Nasopharynx   **G.** Soft palate   **H.** Oropharynx   **I.** Tongue   **J.** Epiglottis   **K.** Vocal cords   **L.** Larynx   **M.** Esophagus. *(p. 205)*

3. **a.** The diaphragm also is responsible for approximately 60–70 percent of the effort involved in breathing. *(p. 207)*

4. **b.** The carina is the point at which the trachea splits and becomes the right and left mainstem bronchi. The bronchi continue to branch into the bronchioles and eventually into the alveoli. *(p. 206)*

5. **c.** Sweep the mouth with your *gloved* index finger. *(p. 215)*

6. To perform the head-tilt, chin-lift maneuver, place one hand on the patient's forehead, apply firm backward pressure, tilt the head backward, place the tips of the fingers of the other hand under the bone of the chin, and lift the chin. *(p. 215)*

7. **a.** Jaw-thrust maneuver. *(p. 217)*

8. **d.** Neutral. *(p. 236)*

9. **d.** All of these. *(p. 239)*

10. **c.** Hard catheter. *(p. 219)*

11. **c.** 15, 5. *(p. 220)*

12. **c.** Suction for 15 seconds, provide positive pressure ventilation for 2 minutes, repeat. *(p. 220)*

13. **c.** Measure from the level of the front teeth to the angle of the jaw. *(p. 221)*

14. **c.** The flange rests on the flare of the nostril. *(p. 222)*

15. **a.** *Hypoxia* is the medical term used to describe the insufficient oxygenation of the cells. *Ventilation* is the term used to describe the mechanical process of moving air into and out of the lungs. *(p. 209)*

16. In a patient who is breathing adequately, **a.** The rate will be within normal limits.   **b.** The rhythm will be a regular pattern, with inhalations and exhalations about equal in length.   **c.** The quality will include breath sounds that are equal and full bilaterally, with the chest rising and falling adequately and equally with each breath and no excessive accessory muscle use (children normally use abdominal muscles in breathing more than adults do).   **d.** The depth, or tidal volume, will seem adequate as you feel and hear the breath with your ear next to the patient's mouth and nose and as you see the chest rise and fall adequately. *(p. 209)*

17. **c.** Cyanotic nail beds, skin, or mucous membranes are a late and severe sign of hypoxia. Restlessness, headache, and an altered mental status are all early signs of hypoxia; these are important to recognize so that immediate treatment can be initiated to prevent severe hypoxia from developing. *(p. 209)*

18. Normal ranges are as follows: adult, 10–24; child, 15–30; infant, 25–50 respirations a minute. *(pp. 225–226)*

19. **a.** Bilateral chest rise. *(p. 226)*

20. **b.** The modified lateral (recovery) position should be used in the patient with an altered mental status in whom you do not suspect a spinal injury. A nonrebreather mask or oropharyngeal airway will not prevent aspiration. *(p. 218)*

21. **c.** Provide positive pressure ventilation. *(p. 229)*

22. **c.** Cricoid pressure helps visualize the vocal cords during endotracheal intubation. According to the American Heart Association guidelines of 2010, cricoid pressure is not recommended for routine use but can be used to facilitate insertion of an endotracheal tube in an adult patient. *(p. 231)*

23. **b.** Exhaled oxygen contains about 16 percent oxygen, which is enough to oxygenate a patient with mouth-to-mouth or mouth-to-nose ventilation. *(p. 232)*

24. **a.** The mask eliminates direct contact with the patient. *(p. 234)*

25. **a.** An adult should be ventilated every 5–6 seconds; an infant or child should be ventilated every 3–5 seconds. *(p. 233)*

26. **A.** Face mask   **B.** Nonrebreathing patient valve   **C.** Bag   **D.** Intake valve/oxygen-reservoir valve   **E.** Oxygen reservoir   **F.** Oxygen-supply connecting tube. *(p. 236)*

27. **c.** 21 percent (the same as atmospheric air). *(pp. 207–208)*

28. **b.** It allows delivery of ventilations enriched from an oxygen source. *(p. 255)*

29. **c.** Establish in-line stabilization and perform a jaw-thrust maneuver, then ventilate. *(p. 217)*

30. **d.** The EMT is unable to feel lung compliance during ventilation. *(p. 240)*

31. **a.** As soon as the chest begins to rise. *(p. 241)*

32. **c.** Reevaluate the position of the head, chin, and mask seal. *(p. 238)*

33. **b.** Consult with medical direction. *(pp. 242, 245)*

34. **b.** Approximately 2 pounds per square inch. *(p. 248)*

35. **b.** Petroleum jelly and some adhesive tape. *(p. 249)*

36. **c.** High-pressure regulator. *(p. 249)*

37. **c.** Quickly open and shut the valve on the cylinder. *(p. 252)*

38. **b.** Remove the mask from the patient's face, and then turn off the oxygen. *(p. 253)*

39. **d.** 15 liters per minute. (A lesser flow may not inflate the reservoir bag and may cause hypoxia.) *(p. 253)*

40. **c.** Have someone familiar with the child hold the mask close to the child's face. *(p. 254)*

41. **d.** External respiration is the gas exchange process that occurs between the alveoli and the surrounding pulmonary capillaries. Pulmonary ventilation is the mechanical process of moving air in and out of the lungs, breathing. *(p. 204)*

42. a. 1–6 liters per minute. *(p. 254)*

43. c. Nonrebreather mask. *(p. 254)*

44. d. Leave them in the mouth for a better mask seal. *(p. 248)*

45. d. A patient stricken by carbon monoxide poisoning may have an abnormally elevated SpO_2 reading, even though the patient is severely hypoxic. This inaccurate reading is due to the pulse oximeter's inability to distinguish between hemoglobin saturated with oxygen and hemoglobin saturated with carbon monoxide. The massive amounts of carbon dioxide attached to the hemoglobin will provide an erroneously high reading. This patient still needs high concentrations of oxygen. He is actually severely hypoxic. *(pp. 209, 250)*

46. b. The respiratory system responds primarily to changes in the carbon dioxide levels. Thus, it is said that healthy people breathe on a hypercarbic (high carbon dioxide) drive. When the carbon dioxide level decreases in the blood, the chemoreceptors sense this and send signals to the respiratory muscles to slow down the respiratory rate and depth, and the respirations return to normal. Oxygen is much less of a stimulus for changes in breathing in healthy people. *(p. 208)*

47. b. Oxygen. Because of the constant high carbon dioxide levels, the chemoreceptors are no longer really sensitive to the changes in carbon dioxide. The COPD patient's chemoreceptors must rely on the oxygen levels in the blood to regulate breathing. *(p. 208)*

48. c. You should immediately provide positive pressure ventilations with the BVM that is attached to supplemental oxygen. Signs of inadequate breathing are tachypnea, bradypnea, or poor tidal volume. *(p. 205)*

49. d. *Never* place a patient in a prone position. Placing a patient in this position may reduce the effectiveness of ventilation by pushing the abdominal contents upward against the diaphragm, limiting its movement. This may lead to inadequate ventilation and severe hypoxia. *(p. 218)*

50. a. The vagus nerve may be stimulated, causing the patient to become bradycardic. *(p. 219)*

51. a. Respiratory rate and tidal volume. *(p. 219)*

52. b. To increase the tidal volume (the amount of air breathed in and out), you should assist the patient's breaths by delivering a breath with the BVM each time the patient begins to breathe in. There is no reason to increase the rate because the patient is breathing 12 times a minute. Increasing the tidal volume will help to reduce hypoxia. *(p. 223)*

53. c. This patient should receive ventilations at a rate of 8–10 breaths per minute because this patient is pulseless, and CPR is initiated using the LMA. *(p. 233)*

54. d. You should immediately ventilate the newborn at a rate of 40–60 times each minute. *(p. 231)*

55. b. If the jaw thrust is ineffective in opening or maintaining an airway, use the head-tilt, chin-lift maneuver to ventilate the patient, even if the potential for a spine injury exists. Opening the airway and providing adequate ventilation is a priority in patients in cardiac arrest and takes precedence over other procedures. *(p. 236)*

56. a. The patient has a respiratory rate that is too fast (tachypnea), which leads to an inadequate tidal volume (hypopnea). You should initially assist the ventilation at the patient's rate by delivering the ventilation with each breath. Over the next 5–10 ventilations, slowly adjust the rate so that you are now ventilating every 5–6 seconds with one of the patient's breaths. Remember to reassure your patient. *(p. 243)*

57. c. You should select an infant or child mask for a good fit over the stoma. Suction should be limited to no more than 3–5 inches. Position the head in a neutral, comfortable position for the patient; position will not affect the airway in a stoma patient. Ventilations should be over 2 seconds; watch for chest rise. *(p. 246)*

58. b. Encourage the patient to cough to try to expel the object. Never perform a blind finger sweep. Do not try to reposition the head or administer abdominal thrusts. *(p. 248)*

59. b. Place the patient in a seated or semi-Fowler's position (head and chest at a 45 degree angle). *(p. 244)*

60. d. Immediately remove the CPAP device and provide positive pressure ventilations with a BVM. If the patient's level of consciousness deteriorates to a GCS < 11, the patient is no longer able to obey or understand your commands, or if any of the other contraindications arise, immediately remove the patient from the CPAP device. *(p. 245)*

61. c. Decrease in the respiratory rate, decrease in heart rate, increase in SpO_2 reading, a reduction in cyanosis, and accessory muscle use are all indicators that your patient's condition is improving. *(p. 245)*

62. d. His blood pressure is 102/88 mmHg, The skin is slightly pale, cool, and clammy. Because there are obvious signs of poor perfusion (narrow pulse pressure, and positive skin signs), this patient is suspected of having poor perfusion (shock) and should receive oxygen via a nonrebreather mask with a liter flow of 15 lpm. *(p. 252)*

CASE STUDY 1

1. Answers should include at least three of these indications: her position (upright, tripod position); that she is obviously anxious; her gasping breaths; her statement, "I can't breathe."

2. d. Nonrebreather mask at 15 liters per minute. Be prepared to assist ventilations with the BVM. (The Venturi and simple face masks are not recommended for prehospital use, and the nasal cannula should be used only if the patient will not tolerate the nonre-breather mask.)

3. a. Use a rigid catheter (with large bore), insert without suction, suction for 15 seconds (more time risks hypoxia). However, it is necessary to provide suction until the substance is cleared from the airway to prevent aspiration from spontaneous or artificial ventilation. Repeat this sequence until the airway is cleared.

4. c. Nasopharyngeal airway (responsive patient can't tolerate oral airway), bevel first (the other is upside down)

5. b. Continue to ventilate at a rate of 10–12 breaths each minute and suction as before. (She has a pulse, so CPR is not appropriate. Suctioning must be done so that ventilations are effective. Check pulse often. If pulse becomes absent, begin CPR or defibrillation if available.)

CASE STUDY 2

1. c. In-line stabilization with jaw thrust. (This patient has a suspected spinal injury from the fall.)

2. d. Suction using the rigid or hard catheter. (Turning the head may compromise the spine. Finger sweeps and soft French catheter are inadequate.)

3. d. Any or all of these could be the cause of the chest failing to rise with ventilations (as well as BVM failure or operator error).

Chapter 11: Baseline Vital Signs, Monitoring Devices, and History Taking

MEDICAL TERMINOLOGY

1. a. systol **b.** sphygm/o **c.** diastol **d.** tachy **e.** auscultat **f.** ic **g.** brady **h.** card **i.** cyan **j.** osis. *(p. 267)*

TERMS AND CONCEPTS

1. a. 5 **b.** 1 **c.** 3 **d.** 4 **e.** 7 **f.** 2 **g.** 6 **h.** 10 **i.** 8 **j.** 9. *(p. 267)*

CONTENT REVIEW

1. c. Skin. *(p. 268)*

2. c. Counting the number of respirations in 30 seconds and multiplying by 2. *(p. 269)*

3. a. Normal respirations are described. *(p. 269)*

4. a. In assessing the quality of a patient's respiration, the EMT determines the depth of respirations (how much air the patient is moving in and out, which is known as the *tidal volume*) and how well it is moving (whether there are difficulties moving the air in and out). *(p. 269)*

5. a. carotid **b.** brachial **c.** radial **d.** femoral **e.** posterior tibial **f.** dorsalis pedis. *(p. 270)*

6. c. Count the number of beats in 30 seconds and multiply by 2. *(p. 272)*

7. b. Brachial. *(p. 270)*

8. d. 120–150 beats per minute is the normal range for an infant. *(p. 271)*

9. b. Strong and regular at 70 beats per minute; normal is 60–100. *(p. 272)*

10. a. Pale conjunctiva. *(p. 272)*

11. c. To help assess skin color in dark-skinned people and infants and children, the palms of the hands and the soles of the feet should be checked, in addition to the nail beds, oral mucosa, and conjunctiva. *(p. 272)*

12. c. Relative skin temperature is assessed by using the back of your hand on the patient's skin, in temperature extremes, place your hand on the patient's abdomen. *(p. 273)*

13. d. Dry skin is normal. Wet or moist (clammy) skin may indicate hypoperfusion, heat emergency, or diabetic emergency. *(p. 273)*

14. d. The high limit for capillary refill in infants, children, and adult men is 2 seconds; for females, it is 3 seconds; and for elderly patients, it is 4 seconds. *(p. 274)*

15. d. Pupillary size, equality, and reactivity are initially assessed. *(p. 274)*

16. b. Arteries. *(p. 275)*

17. d. If the pulse pressure (difference between the systolic and diastolic pressures) is less than 25 percent of the systolic pressure, it is considered a narrow pulse pressure. During auscultation of the blood pressure, the systolic pressure is recorded as the first distinct sound of two or more distinct beats. The diastolic pressure is recorded as the last sound heard. When using a sphygmomanometer and stethoscope, the blood pressure is always reported and expressed as an even number. Electronic blood pressure monitors express readings in even and odd increments and should be reported this way. Be sure to document the type of device used to determine the blood pressure. *(p. 276)*

18. a. 124/82 mmHg is considered average for a 34-year-old female. To estimate the systolic pressure in the adult female patient at rest who is less than 40 years of age, add the patient's age to 90. The normal range for the diastolic pressure is 60–85 mmHg. *(p. 276)*

19. c. A sphygmomanometer and a stethoscope *(p. 276)*

20. a. 6 **b.** 5 **c.** 2 **d.** 4 **e.** 3 **f.** 1. The correct sequence is as follows: 1. Position the patient's arm. 2. Palpate the radial pulse, inflate to 70 mmHg, and increase by 10 mmHg until the radial pulse is no longer palpable. Note the number and deflate the cuff. 3. Place the stethoscope in your ears. 4. Inflate the cuff 30 mmHg above the noted number. 5. Deflate the cuff at 2 mmHg per second. 6. Note the systolic and diastolic sounds. *(pp. 277–278)*

21. c. In the stable patient, vital signs should be checked at least every 15 minutes. *(p. 279)*

22. a. A **b.** L **c.** S **d.** M **e.** P **f.** S **g.** A **h.** E **i.** S **j.** L **k.** M **l.** P. *(pp. 285–286)*

23. c. The orthostatic vital signs (tilt test) are tested by taking the patient's pulse and blood pressure in a supine and then in a standing position. An increase in the patient's pulse by 10–20 bpm and a decrease in the patient's blood pressure by 10–20 mmHg is a positive finding and can indicate significant blood or fluid loss. *(p. 278)*

24. **a.** Pulse oximetry is a method of detecting hypoxia in patients and monitoring the effectiveness of airway and ventilation therapy. A reading of 97 percent does not eliminate the potential of hypoxemia in a patient. Other factors may be creating a false reading, such as in patients with hypoperfusion or hypothermia. Readings are commonly affected if the patient is wearing fingernail polish. *(p. 279)*

25. **c.** Carefully assess patient use of accessory muscles to breathe. Patients that use the accessory muscles in the neck and chest are likely having difficulty inhaling, whereas patients that excessively use abdominal muscles are having difficulty exhaling. *(p. 269)*

26. O—Onset, P—Provocation/Palliation, Q—Quality, R—Region/Radiation, S—Severity, T—Time. *(p. 286)*

CASE STUDY

1. **d.** Mr. Baker is in severe respiratory distress. His respiratory rate is faster than normal at a rate of 26 respirations per minute, and his breathing quality is both labored (using accessory muscles) and noisy (audible wheezing and gurgling); in addition, his SpO_2 is 90%.

2. **d.** His skin is slightly cyanotic, cool, and moist. His bluish skin color indicates he has inadequate oxygenation and poor perfusion. Cool, moist skin also indicates hypoperfusion.

3. **a.** His radial pulse is weak (thready) and irregular, which indicates that he is in shock (hypoperfusion). The rate of 50 beats per minute is slower than normal, which may also point to heart problems. An auscultated blood pressure at 80/50 mmHg also indicates hypoperfusion. Your impression is that his heart is not working very efficiently, and as a result, his circulation is inadequate.

4. **Signs and symptoms:** Mr. Baker states that he can't breathe. Rapid, noisy (audible wheezing and gurgling), labored respirations. Skin is slightly cyanotic, cool, and moist. Weak, irregular pulse. **Allergies:** Mrs. Baker says that her husband has no allergies. **Medications:** Digoxin and Lasix taken daily, nitroglycerin as needed for angina. None today, according to wife. **Pertinent past history:** heart attack 5 years ago. **Last oral intake:** Ate a bowl of soup at lunch; did not eat supper. **Events leading to illness:** shoveled snow this morning, and since then has been increasingly short of breath but denied having chest pain.

5. **a.** Mr. Baker should have his vital signs reassessed every 5 minutes because he is an unstable patient, in severe respiratory distress, and showing signs of inadequate oxygenation.

Chapter 12: Scene Size-Up

TERMS AND CONCEPTS

1. **a.** T **b.** T **c.** M **d.** T **e.** M **f.** M. (A medical condition is one brought on by illness or by substances or by environmental factors that affect the function of the body. Trauma is a physical injury or wound caused by external force or violence.) *(p. 304)*

2. **a.** 5 **b.** 1 **c.** 2 **d.** 4 **e.** 3. *(p. 293)*

CONTENT REVIEW

1. **a.** EMTs, patients, and bystanders. *(p. 303)*
2. **d.** While receiving dispatch information. *(p. 296)*
3. **c.** Protective gloves are required at a minimum for every patient contact when you suspect contact with blood, other body fluids, mucous membranes, a break in the continuity of the skin, or other potentially transmissible exposure. *(p. 295)*
4. **a.** Ask some bystanders to hold up a sheet. *(p. 302)*
5. **d.** Call for additional resources. *(p. 307)*
6. **a.** Consider all power lines to be energized until a power company representative advises you they are not. *(p. 297)*
7. **b.** Notify your dispatcher and wait for a rescue crew. *(p. 298)*
8. **d.** Enter the scene only after it has been secured by police. *(p. 299)*
9. **c.** Knock while standing off to the knob side. *(p. 301)*
10. **a.** A large-caliber gunshot is considered a mechanism of injury, or what caused the injury. A laceration and a deformed and swollen wrist are both the result of a specific mechanism of injury. Hot and dry skin is considered a sign. *(p. 304)*

CASE STUDY 1

1. **d.** While still several blocks from the scene, turn off the siren and emergency lights. By arriving discreetly, you will draw less attention to the scene and minimize the chances of drawing a crowd. This will give you better conditions in which to perform the scene size-up.
2. **b.** Immediately call for additional transporting and ALS units.
3. **c.** The patient is unresponsive. Don't touch the gun; notify the police. (The gun is not interfering with treatment, so there is no need to attempt to move it.)
4. **c.** Retreat temporarily until the police can give you support.

CASE STUDY 2

1. Answers may include any three of the following: the address of the call gives a clue about whether this is or is not generally a safe neighborhood; "elderly" helps you to anticipate a geriatric patient; "cough for months" indicates a medical condition and alerts you to take Standard Precautions; a husband calling about his wife may mean a relatively safe domestic environment;

the fact that no one is presently answering the phone may indicate that the emergency is severe or that the caller is also ill.

2. **d.** Before entering the house, both EMTs should put on gloves, eye protection, and an N-95 or a HEPA respirator.

3. **a.** Because the patient presents signs of TB, you continue to wear the N-95 or HEPA respirator and advise the hospital of the precaution. Additionally, a mask should be placed on the patient.

Chapter 13: Patient Assessment

MEDICAL TERMINOLOGY

1. **a.** pnea **b.** dys **c.** a **d.** icter **e.** ic
   f. quadri **g.** para **h.** hemi **i.** plegia. *(p. 312)*

TERMS AND CONCEPTS

1. **a.** 13 **b.** 2 **c.** 7 **d.** 6 **e.** 4 **f.** 11 **g.** 12
   h. 9 **i.** 10 **j.** 8 **k.** 1 **l.** 5 **m.** 3. *(p. 312)*

CONTENT REVIEW

1. **d.** It is very important that you develop a systematic assessment routine. This will ensure that you assess every patient consistently and appropriately, based on the nature of that patient's illness or injury. The steps of the primary assessment allow a systematic but not a required linear approach to assessment for, and control of, life threats. *(p. 314)*

2. **c.** The scene size-up and the primary assessment are the first two stages of the patient assessment. *(p. 314)*

3. **b.** Any of these techniques might be useful, but given the overt physical threats, the best course is to leave until the scene is controlled. *(p. 314)*

4. **b.** The patient has significant mechanisms of injury (hit by a car, laceration on forehead) for spine trauma. Bring the head to a neutral, in-line position while maintaining in-line stabilization of the head and neck. The patient responds to questioning; therefore, his airway is assumed to be patent. *(p. 319)*

5. **c.** Until the patient is fully immobilized to a backboard with backboard straps and a head immobilization device. *(p. 319)*

6. **c.** *Every* patient must receive a primary assessment. If the patient is unresponsive, pulseless, is not breathing or breathing normally, immediately begin CPR with chest compressions. *(p. 314)*

7. **c.** The primary assessment doesn't have to occur in this linear pattern for every patient. The key to performing the primary assessment is to be sure to assess and manage any immediate life-threats to the airway, breathing, oxygenation, and circulation during the first 60 seconds after encountering the patient. The order is less important and is based on managing obvious presenting immediate life-threats. The steps for the primary assessment are as follows: Form a general impression, assess mental status, assess airway, assess breathing, assess oxygenation, assess circulation, and establish patient priorities. If the patient is unresponsive, pulseless, or is not breathing or not breathing normally, immediately begin CPR with chest compressions. *(p. 314)*

8. **a.** General impression. *(p. 316)*

9. **d.** "Why did you call EMS today?" (or "What seems to be the problem today?") elicits the patient's own statement without suggesting an answer. *(p. 317)*

10. **d.** The patient is not alert but does respond to a verbal stimulus, a subtle yet important difference. *(p. 320)*

11. **c.** This patient responds to a verbal stimulus. Patients a and b respond only to a painful stimulus. Patient d is completely unresponsive. *(p. 320)*

12. **b.** Appropriate methods of eliciting a pain response in an unresponsive patient include the use of central (trapezius pinch, supraorbital pressure, sternal rub, armpit pinch) or peripheral (nail bed pressure; pinching the web between the thumb and index finger; pinching the finger, toe, hand, or foot) stimuli. *(p. 320)*

13. **a.** If the patient is talking to you, he is moving air in and out. Observing the speaking pattern also helps in assessing breathing status. *(p. 322)*

14. **b.** Relaxation of upper-airway muscles. The tongue and other soft tissues tend to fall back and cover the opening to the trachea. *(p. 323)*

15. **b.** Snoring respirations—use a head-tilt, chin-lift, or jaw-thrust maneuver. If gurgling respirations are noted, quickly suction the airway. For snoring respirations, use a head-tilt, chin-lift, or jaw-thrust maneuver. For crowing respirations or stridor, avoid inserting anything in the airway, which could result in dangerous spasm of the airway. *(p. 323)*

16. **b.** Indications of inadequate breathing in an adult patient include retractions; use of neck muscles on inhalation; nasal flaring; excessive abdominal muscle use; tracheal tugging; pale, cool, and clammy skin; cyanosis, deteriorating mental status; and an SpO_2 reading of less than 95%. Be aggressive in your treatment when you observe cyanosis; it is a late sign of hypoxia. *(p. 325)*

17. **c.** Positive pressure ventilation can be delivered by BVM device, by mouth-to-mask, or by a flow-restricted, oxygen-powered ventilation device. The other devices listed are used to deliver oxygen passively to patients who are breathing adequately. Be sure to use an airway adjunct during ventilations (such as an oropharyngeal or nasopharyngeal airway). *(p. 326)*

18. **c.** In a cold environment, the vessels in the skin constrict to decrease the blood flow to the skin. In a hot environment, the vessels in the skin dilate, causing the blood to be shunted

to the skin. The alpha properties of circulating epinephrine cause the vessels in the skin to constrict (shunting blood away from the skin) and are responsible for stimulation of the sweat glands. Epinephrine (adrenalin) is released as a protective mechanism by the body during shock or hypoperfusion. Anemic patients take longer to become cyanotic when hypoxic. *(p. 329)*

19. **b.** When assessing the pulse in the primary assessment, determination of the exact pulse rate is not required. It is important to determine if it is present or not, the approximate heart rate (fast, normal, or slow), and the regularity and strength of the pulse. *(p. 327)*

20. **c.** A peripheral (radial, brachial, or femoral) or central (carotid) pulse will likely not be felt if the systolic blood pressure is less than 60 mmHg. *(p. 328)*

21. **b.** The nail beds. Problems associated with environmental temperature, medical illnesses, and smoking can affect the color of the nail beds. *(p. 329)*

22. **a.** Cyanotic skin indicates reduced tissue oxygenation. Red skin may indicate anaphylaxis, vasogenic shock, poisoning, overdose, or some diabetic or other medical conditions. Yellow skin may result from liver failure (jaundice). Pale or mottled skin may result from a decrease in perfusion, such as might occur from blood loss. *(p. 329)*

23. **d.** Cool, clammy skin is one of the major signs of shock (hypoperfusion). *(p. 330)*

24. **b.** Greater than 2 seconds. (2 seconds can be counted by saying "One one-thousand, two one-thousand" or the words "capillary refill.") *(p. 330)*

25. All require rapid assessment and transport except 3 and 5. *(p. 332)*

26. **b.** Properly performed, the rapid secondary assessment takes only moments and should always be completed before moving the patient to the stretcher. *(p. 345)*

27. All are considered significant mechanisms of injury except 2 and 4. *(p. 345)*

28. **c.** Significant mechanisms of injury for an infant or child include a fall from a height greater than 10 feet (2 to 3 times the height of the child), a vehicle collision at a medium speed, a bicycle collision with a motor vehicle, and a vehicle collision where the infant or child was unrestrained. *(p. 346)*

29. **b.** For a trauma patient with a significant mechanism of injury or altered mental status, perform rapid secondary assessment, baseline vital signs, and history. *(p. 345)*

30. **d.** For a trauma patient with no significant mechanism of injury, no multiple injuries, and no altered mental status, perform the modified secondary assessment, baseline vital signs, and history. *(p. 345)*

31. **b.** The patient's GCS score is 5 [eye opening = 1, verbal response = 1, motor response = flexion (decorticate rigidity) 3, total = 5]. *(p. 349)*

32. **a.** A patient with a GCS score of less than 8 has a severe alteration in brain function. It is an important finding if a patient with a potential head injury is unresponsive, then regains responsiveness for a short time, and then begins to exhibit a deteriorating mental status report. Time is the first orientation to be lost in an altered mental status, and self is the last. *(p. 348)*

33. Deformities, contusions, abrasions, punctures/penetrations, burns, tenderness, lacerations, swelling. *(pp. 385–386)*

34. **d.** The use of your sense of smell is missing from this list. *(p. 350)*

35. **c.** In assessing the neck, in addition to the "DCAP-BTLS" criteria, the EMT should inspect for jugular vein distention, tracheal deviation or tracheal tugging, subcutaneous emphysema, and posterior cervical muscle spasms. JVD is a sign of a possible pneumothorax and pericardial tamponade. In the trauma patient, this should be checked with the patient in a supine position rather than positioned at a 45-degree angle. *(p. 353)*

36. **c.** Determine the presence and equality of breath sounds by auscultating the right and left chest at the apex and base of the lungs. *(p. 356)*

37. **a.** When assessing the abdomen during the rapid trauma assessment, the EMT should palpate for tenderness, guarding, and rigidity. *(p. 357)*

38. **a.** The EMT should not palpate the pelvis when the patient complains of pain in the pelvic region or has obvious pelvic deformity. The other choices are not contraindications to palpating the pelvis. *(p. 358)*

39. **a.** "PMS" refers to indicators that circulation and nerve function to the extremities are intact: pulses, motor function, and sensation. *(p. 358)*

40. **a.** Log-roll the patient while maintaining in-line stabilization. *(p. 359)*

41. **c.** Apply the CSIC after the neck has been assessed. (You can't fully assess the neck with a collar on, although most have holes on the anterior surface to allow later inspection.) Remember that the CSIC does not fully immobilize the head and neck; therefore, manual in-line stabilization must continue to be maintained after CSIC is in place until the patient is fully immobilized to the long spine board. *(p. 354)*

42. **d.** Vital signs should be reassessed every 5 minutes in an unstable patient (every 15 minutes in a stable patient). This applies to both trauma and medical patients. *(p. 361)*

43. Signs and symptoms, allergies, medications, pertinent past history, last oral intake, events leading to the incident *(p. 344)*

44. **c.** If there is a suspicion of other injuries, always perform a head-to-toe rapid secondary assessment. *(pp. 343, 345)*

45. d. The secondary exam in the alert and oriented medical patient should be performed in this sequence: History, modified secondary assessment (focused on the area of the patient's complaint), vital signs. *(p. 369)*

46. b. The secondary assessment in the medical patient with an altered mental status should be performed in this sequence: rapid secondary assessment (head to toe), baseline vital signs, history. *(p. 369)*

47. d. In the rapid medical assessment, palpate the abdomen for tenderness, rigidity, distention, and pulsating masses. *(p. 371)*

48. a. When assessing the extremities during the rapid medical assessment, be sure to check around the hands, feet, and ankles for peripheral edema or swelling that could indicate congestive heart failure, fluid overload, or a clot blocking a vein in that extremity. *(p. 372)*

49. a. The vital signs are respiration, pulse, skin, pupils, blood pressure, and pulse oximetery. *(p. 344)*

50. Onset, provocation/palliation, quality, radiation/region, severity, time. *(p. 344)*

51. c. The recovery position (coma position) permits fluids to drain from the mouth of the unresponsive patient and helps prevent airway blockage or aspiration. *(p. 373)*

52. b. Gather both prescription and over-the-counter medications and carefully document the medications taken. Both will be important clues for hospital personnel. *(p. 375)*

53. c. If the patient doesn't have a specific complaint on which you can focus the physical exam, perform a rapid head-to-toe secondary assessment. *(p. 376)*

54. d. The Markle test is performed by striking the bottom of the heel sharply with your clenched fist, to jar the abdomen. It is positive for abdominal irritation if pain results. *(p. 339)*

55. d. It is important to determine the last oral intake when testing a patient's blood glucose level. A fasting blood glucose in the diabetic patient may be 120–140 mg/dL. If an unresponsive medical patient requires ventilation, put him in a supine position. Pain is typically produced by ischemia, inflammation, infection, and obstruction. *(p. 375)*

CASE STUDY 1

1. c. The patient is exhibiting signs of brain herniation. Provide positive pressure ventilation at 10–12 ventilations per minute (follow local protocol); some EMS systems may ventilate at a rate of 20 ventilations per minute while maintaining in-line stabilization.

2. a. Rapid secondary assessment and rapid transport.

3. c. The presence of a pulse indicates that the patient has a blood pressure of *at least* 60 mmHg.

CASE STUDY 2

1. a. Y **b.** Y **c.** Y **d.** Y **e.** Y. (All are clues to an airway problem in this patient.)

2. c. Head-tilt, chin-lift.

3. a. In all patients, the EMT must assess the adequacy of both the respiratory rate and the tidal volume in order to determine if the patient is moving enough air per minute to sustain life. Either an inadequate respiratory rate or an inadequate tidal volume will require administration of positive pressure ventilation.

4. c. Rapid secondary assessment for a medical patient.

5. a. 3 (eye opening = 1, verbal response = 1, motor response = 1, total = 3).

CASE STUDY 3

1. b. Suggest a task for the girlfriend.

2. c. Apply direct pressure, then a pressure dressing.

3. c. Modified secondary assessment (focused on the injury), vitals, history.

CASE STUDY 4

1. b. SAMPLE history, including OPQRST questions to get a full description of the chest pain.

2. d. Ask an open-ended question.

3. a. A rapid secondary assessment.

4. b. The patient is responsive and has adequate breathing, so CPR and positive pressure ventilation are obviously inappropriate. The patient did not refuse treatment; he gave consent by saying, "As long as you're here, you may as well check me out." If he had refused, you would have tried to persuade him to accept treatment and transport. Administer oxygen to maintain an SpO_2 of > 94%.

CASE STUDY 5

1. b. Capillary refill should be checked in a child.

2. d. Complete a rapid secondary assessment.

3. b. The patient displays classic signs of shock (hypoperfusion), including a weak, rapid pulse and pale, cool, and clammy skin. A child with these signs is likely to deteriorate quickly. He is a high priority for rapid transport.

4. b. Oxygen by nasal cannula to maintain an SpO_2 at > 94%.

Chapter 14: Pharmacology and Medication Administration

TERMS AND CONCEPTS

1. a. 2 **b.** 1 **c.** 3 **d.** 9 **e.** 6 **f.** 10 **g.** 8 **h.** 7 **i.** 5 **j.** 4 **k.** 11. *(p. 396)*

CONTENT REVIEW

1. c. Identified in local protocols. *(p. 397)*

2. b. Carried on the unit. *(p. 398)*

3. a. Epinephrine. *(pp. 399–400)*

4. **c.** Ask a family member to retrieve the medication. (Never ask a patient to retrieve his medication. This activity could aggravate his condition.) *(p. 399)*
5. **a.** The brand name is also known as the *trade name*. *(pp. 400–401)*
6. **b.** Isoetharine is also known by the trade name Bronkosol. *(p. 400, Table 14-1)*
7. **b.** The trade name of salmeterol is Serevent. *(p. 400, Table 14-1)*
8. **d.** The sublingual route. *(p. 401)*
9. **a.** Shaken. (The solids in a suspension will settle to the bottom.) *(p. 402)*
10. **b.** Contraindications. *(p. 403)*
11. **a.** The six essential items of information are indications, contraindications, dose, administration, actions, and side effects. *(p. 403)*
12. **b.** Epinephrine is given by injection with a spring-loaded auto-injector. (Be careful to avoid a needlestick.) *(p. 401)*
13. The correct sequence is 8, 1, 2, 4, 6, 3, 5, 7. The correct sequence for administering a medication is: **1.** Obtain an order from medical direction. **2.** Ensure selection of the proper medication. **3.** Verify the patient's prescription. **4.** Check the expiration date. **5.** Check for discoloration or impurities. **6.** Verify the form, route, and dose. **7.** Administer medication. **8.** Document medication administration. *(pp. 404–406)*
14. **a.** Package inserts, *AMA Drug Evaluation*, the *Physician's Desk Reference*, poison control centers, EMS pocket drug reference guide, and ePocrates for the PDA are common sources of medication information. *(p. 406)*
15. No trade name for oxygen *(p. 400, Table 14-1)*
16. Oral glucose. *(p. 400, Table 14-1)*
17. Altered mental status with diabetic history. *(p. 400, Table 14-1)*
18. Poisoning, overdose. *(p. 400, Table 14-1)*
19. Chest pain. *(p. 400, Table 14-1)*
20. Nitroglycerin spray. *(p. 400, Table 14-1)*
21. Chest pain. *(p. 400, Table 14-1)*
22. Adrenalin. *(p. 400, Table 14-1)*
23. Proventil, Ventolin. *(p. 400, Table 14-1)*
24. Alupent, Metaprel. *(p. 400, Table 14-1)*
25. Breathing difficulty associated with respiratory conditions. *(p. 400, Table 14-1)*
26. Isoetharine. *(p. 400, Table 14-1)*
27. Breathing difficulty associated with respiratory conditions. *(p. 400, Table 14-1)*
28. Serevent. *(p. 400, Table 14-1)*
29. Bitolterol. *(p. 400, Table 14-1)*
30. Breathing difficulty associated with respiratory conditions. *(p. 400, Table 14-1)*
31. Xopenex®. *(p. 400, Table 14-1)*
32. Maxair®. *(p. 400, Table 14-1)*
33. Breathing difficulty associated with respiratory conditions. *(p. 400, Table 14-1)*
34. Brethaire®. *(p. 400, Table 14-1)*
35. Bayer®, Ecotrin®, Empirin®, Ascriptin®, Bufferin®, Buffex®. *(p. 400, Table 14-1)*
36. Patient experiencing chest pain or chest discomfort suggestive of an acute coronary syndrome. *(p. 400, Table 14-1)*

CASE STUDY

1. **c.** Never administer medication unless prescribed to the patient and/or you are ordered to do so by medical direction.
2. **b.** False. The medications should not be administered to a patient who has an altered mental status.
3. **c.** Chest pain or chest discomfort suggestive of an acute coronary syndrome.

Chapter 15: Shock and Resuscitation

MEDICAL TERMINOLOGY

1. **d.** Tension.
2. **b.** Contraction.
3. **d.** Vessel.
4. **d.** Without.

TERMS AND CONCEPTS

1. **a.** 4 **b.** 8 **c.** 1 **d.** 10 **e.** 7 **f.** 5 **g.** 2 **h.** 11 **i.** 13 **j.** 9 **k.** 3 **l.** 12 **m.** 6. *(p. 425)*

CONTENT REVIEW

1. **b.** The three base etiologies of shock are inadequate volume, inadequate pump function, and inadequate vessel tone. *(p. 410)*
2. **b.** BP (Blood Pressure) = CO (Cardiac Output) × SVR (Systemic Vascular Resistance). *(p. 413)*
3. **c.** Anaphylactic shock is a type of distributive shock that is caused by the release of chemical mediators that cause massive systemic vasodilation. These chemical mediators also cause the capillaries to become very permeable and to leak. *(p. 413)*
4. **a.** The first stage of shock, in which the body is able to maintain cardiac output, is called compensated shock. *(p. 419)*
5. **a.** The geriatric patient does not compensate well for shock. In addition, some medications that the elderly patient may be taking may prevent some signs or symptoms from appearing, such as an elevated heart rate. An altered mental status and tachypnea may be the most profound signs of shock in the elderly. *(p. 424)*
6. **a.** The compensatory mechanisms of shock are initiated and maintained through two major pathways: direct sympathetic nerve stimulation and the release of hormones. *(p. 442)*
7. **b.** Hyperventilation of the shock patient makes the blood alkalotic and will reduce the offloading of oxygen from the hemoglobin and promote further cellular hypoxia. Also, increasing the pressure inside the chest in a poor volume and perfusion state may decrease preload and cardiac output further. *(p. 424)*
8. **d.** As the systolic blood pressure drops from the decrease in blood volume, the systemic vasoconstriction causes the diastolic blood

pressure to be maintained or to increase, creating a narrow pulse pressure. *(p. 421)*

9. **d.** Certain medications, such as beta blockers or calcium channel blockers, can keep the heart rate from dramatically increasing, making it appear that the patient is not in a compensatory stage of shock. *(p. 422)*

10. **c.** In early distributive shock, the skin is typically flushed and warm. *(p. 423)*

11. **c.** For children less than 10 years of age, a systolic blood pressure of 70 mmHg plus 2 times the age in years is a lower limit of normal. A systolic blood pressure less than the lower limit would be considered hypotensive. Hypotension is a late finding in pediatric patients and often leads to cardiac arrest. *(p. 424)*

12. **a.** The requirements for placement of the AED are patients who are older than 1 year of age (for patients 1–8 years of age, a dose-attenuator system is preferred, but the adult AED may be applied) in cardiac arrest (no breathing, no pulse, and unresponsive to verbal or pain stimuli). The AED is not intended for cardiac arrest resulting from trauma. *(p. 427)*

13. **a.** The components of the chain that are *most critical* to patient survival from cardiac arrest are early high-quality cardiac compressions and early defibrillation. *(p. 442)*

14. **c.** Defibrillation. *(p. 425)*

15. **c.** Ventricular fibrillation is the most common initial rhythm in sudden cardiac arrest. *(p. 427)*

16. **c.** The AED, not the operator, administers the defibrillation. *(p. 428)*

17. **a.** It takes several minutes for a perfusing rhythm to return. Resume CPR with chest compressions and check the pulse in 2 minutes. *(p. 427)*

18. **d.** The AED is not generally indicated for use in the cardiac arrest patient due to trauma. According to 2010 AHA guidelines, the AED may be used in all age groups. However, a dose-attenuating system is preferred for patients less than 8 years of age, and manual defibrillation is preferred in patients less than 1 year of age. *(p. 430)*

19. **d.** Firmly press down on the pad in an attempt to stick it to the chest wall skin. If this does not work, pull the original set of electrodes off. This will remove some of the hair in the area. Apply a second, new set of electrodes with firm pressure applied to the pad. If the AED continues to give you a "check electrode" message, consider shaving the area's chest hair, and then apply a third, new set of electrode pads. *(p. 437)*

20. **a.** Quickly start CPR and proceed with the AED protocol as soon as the AED is ready. *(p. 437)*

21. **d.** Don't place the AED pad directly over the ICD; the AED may be used in the patient with an ICD, and you may touch the ICD patient without fear of harm. Place electrodes

1 inch to the side of the ICD or use an alternative pad placement. *(p. 438)*

22. **d.** Battery failure. *(p. 437)*

23. **b.** Refresher training and practice is recommended every 90 days, or 3 months. *(p. 437)*

24. **d.** Contact with water, ice/snow, metal, and nitroglycerin patches are all safety hazards during AED operation. *(pp. 435–437)*

26. **b.** Prevention of arrest is the first link in the pediatric chain of survival. *(pp. 426, 437)*

CASE STUDY 1

1. **d.** CPR is being performed adequately by the bystander. The next best action is to quickly attach the AED and begin analysis of the patient's rhythm.

2. **c.** Minimize any and all interruptions to CPR.

3. **c.** After any no shock message, immediately begin CPR for 2 minutes (begin with compressions).

CASE STUDY 2

1. **a.** Verify the patient is unresponsive and has no pulse and is not breathing.

2. **a.** If EMS has not been notified, do so now.

3. **c.** Ventilate at 10–12 pm.

CHAPTER 15 SCENARIO 1: DOCUMENTATION EXERCISE

1. **b.** In a severe state of hypoperfusion, the body shunts blood from the extremities to the core by constricting peripheral blood vessels, making it hard or impossible to find a peripheral pulse.

2. **c.** A late sign of decompensated shock is loss of peripheral pulses. Other signs are tachycardia (abnormally fast heart rate), tachypnea (abnormally fast breathing rate), narrowing pulse pressure, unresponsiveness, and a significant drop in blood pressure.

CHAPTER 15 SCENARIO 2: DOCUMENTATION EXERCISE

1. **b.** Ventricular tachycardia (V-Tach) with a rate greater than 180 beats per minute will usually make the AED respond with a shock-advise message. However, some patients in V-Tach remain responsive. Because they are responsive, they are not appropriate candidates for defibrillation

2. **d.** The AED is a very sensitive instrument and can sense spontaneous patient movement and movement of the patient by others. This movement can make the AED report inaccurately. Therefore, you should ensure that no one is touching the patient during this time. Another reason to clear the patient is that anyone in contact during shock delivery may be injured.

3. **a.** According to the American Heart Association, the links in the chain of survival are immediate recognition and activation, early CPR, rapid defibrillation, effective ACLS, and integrated post-cardiac arrest care. All are necessary if rates of patient survival from cardiac arrest are going to improve.

Chapter 16: Respiratory Emergencies

MEDICAL TERMINOLOGY

1. **b.** Breathing. *(p. 448)*
2. **d.** Fast. *(p. 477)*
3. **a.** No, not, without, lack of. *(p. 448)*
4. **d.** Bad, difficult, painful. *(p. 448)*
5. **b.** Absence of breathing; respiratory arrest. *(p. 448)*

TERMS AND CONCEPTS

1. **a.** 2 **b.** 7 **c.** 3 **d.** 6 **e.** 9 **f.** 1 **g.** 5 **h.** 8 **i.** 4 **j.** 10. *(p. 446)*
2. Apnea and respiratory arrest. *(p. 448)*

CONTENT REVIEW

1. **d.** A patient who is having difficulty breathing but has an adequate tidal volume and respiratory rate is in respiratory distress. Because the tidal volume and respiratory rate are still adequate, the patient is compensating and is in need of supplemental oxygen to maintain the SpO_2 at 94% or higher. *(p. 449)*
2. **c.** Hypoxia will cause the patient to become agitated and aggressive. Hypercarbia will cause the patient to become confused. *(p. 458)*
3. **b.** Pale, cool, clammy skin is an early sign of hypoxia in the patient. Cyanosis is a clear but late sign of hypoxia. *(p. 456)*
4. **a.** Severe respiratory distress. *(p. 456)*
5. **a.** Speaking a couple of words between breaths. *(p. 461)*
6. **d.** Patient will be confused and disoriented. *(p. 472)*
7. **a.** Crowing, gurgling, snoring, and stridor all indicate a possible partial obstruction from secretions, blood, vomitus, or a foreign body. Clear the airway with suction, manual maneuvers, and utilize airway adjuncts as needed. *(p. 469)*
8. **b.** May be in an acute state of hypoxia. *(p. 472)*
9. **a.** Immediately begin positive pressure ventilation. (A respiratory rate of 14 is below the normal respiratory range of 15–30 breaths per minute for children.) *(p. 473)*
10. **c.** Apply oxygen and maintain the SpO_2 at 94% or greater. *(p. 473)*
11. **d.** This patient is presenting with obvious signs of imminent respiratory failure and should be treated immediately with positive pressure ventilation. *(p. 472)*
12. **a.** Following the primary assessment. *(p. 468)*
13. **a.** A patient complaining of respiratory difficulty who is breathing 20 times a minute with adequate tidal volume should be administered oxygen to maintain an SpO_2 of greater than 94%. Patients b, c, and d should all receive immediate positive pressure ventilations. Simply put, any patient whose breathing is too fast (tachypnea) or too slow (bradypnea), or who has a poor tidal volume (amount of air moved in and out of the lungs, shallow breathing) in any combination

must receive positive pressure ventilations immediately. *(p. 469)*
14. **c.** The patient is working so hard to breathe that the tissues are being pulled inward. *(p. 469)*
15. **b.** Impending respiratory failure, poor oxygenation, and possible cardiac arrest. Immediate and aggressive treatment is required. *(p. 476)*
16. **c.** Paradoxical motion (can cause ineffective ventilation). *(p. 478)*
17. **c.** When in doubt, provide positive pressure ventilation with supplemental oxygen. Delays can permit rapid deterioration and adversely affect the patient's outcome. *(p. 478)*
18. **b.** A pulse oximeter reading (SpO_2) of less than 90% is a significant indication of severe hypoxia. *(p. 476)*
19. 4, 5, 2, 1, 3. Provide oxygen first. Assess vital signs, which may reveal signs of severe respiratory distress, such as elevated pulse or blood pressure. Pursue administration of a prescribed MDI, if the patient has one, to alleviate symptoms. Complete the secondary assessment and physical exam. Place the patient in a position of comfort (most patients will find breathing is easiest in a sitting position) and transport to the hospital. *(p. 478)*
20. **a.** If your patient presents with a sudden onset of shortness of breath with decreased breath sounds to one side of the chest with no evidence of trauma, you should suspect a possible spontaneous pneumothorax. *(p. 458)*
21. **b.** Don't delay transport. Perform the reassessment of the patient en route. *(p. 459)*
22. **b.** After the medication has been delivered, encourage the patient to try to hold his breath as long as possible and to exhale through pursed lips. The canister should be shaken for 30 seconds prior to administration. The patient must inhale while the canister is depressed. Because the medication will be aimed into the mouth, the patient must breathe through the mouth, not the nose, to take the medication into the lungs. *(p. 464)*
23. **a.** Use of accessory muscles, retractions during inspiration, grunting, tachypnea, tachycardia, nasal flaring, grunting, prolonged exhalation, frequent coughing, cyanosis in the extremities, and anxiety are signs of respiratory difficulty. A sore or hoarse throat is not a sign of respiratory difficulty. *(p. 468)*
24. **a.** Seesaw or rocky breathing is a sign of respiratory failure. Loss of muscle tone or a limp appearance is associated with respiratory failure in infants and children. *(p. 469)*
25. **c.** Immediately initiate positive pressure ventilation and transport. This is a dire emergency. *(p. 469)*
26. **c.** Position of comfort to reduce the work of breathing and maintain an open airway. *(p. 470)*
27. **b.** The child usually sits straight up, juts the jaw forward (late sign), and drools (late sign). Do not perform foreign body airway obstruction

maneuvers if epiglottitis or other disease is suspected. These may seriously aggravate the condition. Foreign body maneuvers should be performed only if there is clear evidence that the child is choking and does not seem to be ill. *(p. 460)*

28. d. Croup. *(p. 460)*

29. a. Active exhalation requires the patient to use energy to exhale and force air from the lungs, leading to faster muscle fatigue and early respiratory failure. *(p. 475)*

30. d. Kussmaul sign describes the distention of the jugular veins during inhalation and their return to normal during exhalation. This is an indication of a severely increased pressure in the chest or around the heart. *(p. 475)*

31. b. An extremely fast respiratory rate (tachypnea) will not allow enough time for the lungs to fill adequately. This will lead to an inadequate tidal volume and inadequate breathing. *(p. 468)*

32. c. Subcutaneous emphysema is an indication of an air leak in the chest or neck. Subcutaneous emphysema can be felt much easier than can be seen on inspection. Due to gravity, the air will travel upward toward the neck and head in the patient who is in a seated position. *(p. 476)*

33. a. You should ventilate at 10–12 times per minute, imposing your ventilation over the patient's spontaneous breathing. *(p. 467)*

34. d. Beta$_2$ metered-dose inhalers also have beta$_1$. The beta$_2$ MDI has some beta$_1$ properties, which is a side effect or a nondesired effect that will increase the heart rate. *(p. 479)*

35. b. Pulmonary embolism is caused by an obstruction of blood flow in the pulmonary arteries caused by an occlusion. The reduction in blood flow leads to hypoxia. *(p. 456)*

36. a. A spontaneous pneumothorax is a sudden rupture of the portion of the visceral lining of the lung, causing a partial collapse. This condition occurs without any type of penetrating or blunt trauma as its cause. *(p. 458)*

37. a. Wheezing is best described as a high-pitched, musical whistling sound primarily heard during exhalation. It is best heard initially on exhalation but may also be heard during inhalation in more severe cases. Wheezing is an indication of narrowing of the lower airways, primarily the bronchioles. With severe obstruction of the lower airways by bronchoconstriction and inflammation, wheezing may be significantly diminished or absent because the velocity of air movement through the bronchioles is no longer sufficient to produce the wheezing sound. *(p. 447)*

38. b. The patient diagnosed with emphysema will often appear to have a barrel chest with an otherwise thin physique. These patients are more often males. The disease is characterized by the destruction of the alveolar walls and distention of the alveolar sacs and a gradual destruction of the pulmonary capillary beds with a severe reduction in the alveolar/capillary area for gas exchange to occur. *(p. 452)*

39. d. The patient in acute pulmonary edema should be kept in an upright sitting position and transported without delay. CPAP may be extremely beneficial in the acute pulmonary edema patient in respiratory distress or very early respiratory failure who is awake, alert, oriented, and able to obey commands (GCS >10); is breathing on his own; is able to maintain his own airway; and has an SpO$_2$ reading of < 94%. Laying the patient flat in a supine position could exacerbate the condition, increasing fluid buildup and difficulty with breathing. *(p. 478)*

40. c. Cystic fibrosis is cited as one of the most common life-shortening genetic diseases and is usually found at an early age. This disease affects the mucus-secreting glands of the lungs, thus producing thick tenacious secretions inhibiting airflow. *(p. 461)*

CASE STUDY

1. b. Breathing is adequate, although the respiration rate is at the high end of the normal range. However, the patient is experiencing respiratory distress and so should receive oxygen and maintain the SpO$_2$ at 94% or higher.

2. a. Provocation (what provokes the illness; what makes it better or worse).

3. b. The body attempts to make up for inadequate oxygenation. (Asthmatic attacks are usually sporadic, with no symptoms between attacks; the range of normal respiration rates is the same for all adults; albuterol should reduce a rapid breathing rate by improving oxygenation.)

4. c. Beta agonist, which relaxes the smooth muscle and dilates the airway.

5. The indications for administration of an MDI are as follows: (1) the patient exhibits signs and symptoms of respiratory distress; (2) the patient has a physician-prescribed metered-dose inhaler; and (3) approval has been given by medical direction to administer the medication.

6. b. Consult medical direction to consider readministering.

7. d. Fowler or semi-Fowler's position (sitting up with back straight or at a slightly reclining angle). This is usually the "position of comfort" for the patient, permitting the greatest ease of breathing.

CHAPTER 16 SCENARIO: DOCUMENTATION EXERCISE

1. b. The patient's age does not play a role in whether a patient must be ventilated with positive pressure ventilation. The decision to ventilate is based strictly on the patient's ability to breathe adequately or not. Mrs. Springer had obvious signs of respiratory failure, such as decreased air movement and increasing respiratory rate. She also displayed several signs of hypoxia, such as decreased mental status, cyanosis, and an abnormally low SpO$_2$ reading.

2. a. The bluish gray color of the skin and mucous membranes is known as *cyanosis*. Cyanosis is a good indication of hypoxia and the need for immediate intervention.

3. d. The bubbly, crackling sound produced with inhalation is associated with the alveoli and terminal bronchioles' popping open with each inhalation. Crackles, also called *rales*, are associated with fluid in the lungs and may indicate pulmonary edema or pneumonia.

4. b. P—provocation, or what makes the symptoms worse. Lying flat made Mrs. Springer's breathing worse. Sitting upright on the edge of the bed improved her breathing.

Chapter 17: Cardiovascular Emergencies

MEDICAL TERMINOLOGY

1. a. per **b.** atri **c.** fus **d.** arter **e.** ion **f.** ary **g.** ven **h.** ventriculus **i.** infarct **j.** myo **k.** card. *(p. 490)*

TERMS AND CONCEPTS

1. a. 2 **b.** 7 **c.** 9 **d.** 6 **e.** 10 **f.** 8 **g.** 4 **h.** 5 **i.** 1. *(p. 490)*

CONTENT REVIEW

1. A. Pulmonary artery **B.** Lung capillaries **C.** Pulmonary vein **D.** Veins **E.** Venules **F.** Bronchi **G.** Alveoli **H.** Arteries **I.** Arterioles **J.** Body capillaries. *(p. 492)*

2. b. The heart (pumps the blood); the blood vessels (carry the blood); the blood (the fluid within the system). *(p. 490)*

3. c. Hypoperfusion resulting from nervous system interference (for example, spinal cord damage) creates a vascular system that is too large for the amount of available blood. *(p. 498)*

4. b. Assess airway, breathing, oxygenation, circulation, skin. *(p. 511)*

5. c. Oxygen only be provided to acute coronary syndrome patients with an $SpO_2 < 94\%$, if an SpO_2 is unknown, or the patient is dyspneic, hypoxemic, or has obvious signs of heart failure. In order to limit the concentration in the blood, oxygen should be administered via a nasal cannula starting at 2 lpm and only enough administered to reverse the hypoxia. It may be necessary to increase the liter flow to reach an SpO_2 of 94%. Once the SpO_2 reaches 94%, the liter flow should be maintained or adjusted to keep the SpO_2 at 94%. Hyperoxygenating the acute coronary syndrome patient could lead to greater cardiac cell damage and death. *(p. 503)*

6. c. Severity. *(p. 512)*

7. d. A silent heart attack. *(p. 513)*

8. a. Sublingual. *(p. 508)*

9. d. The patient has extreme bradycardia (<50 bpm). Other contraindications include the following: the patient's baseline systolic blood pressure is below 90 mmHg systolic or the systolic blood pressure has decreased greater than 30 mmHg from the baseline; the heart rate is greater than 100 bpm (tachycardia); the patient is an infant or a child; three doses have already been taken by the patient; or the patient has recently taken tadalafil (Cialis), vardenafil (Levitra), or sildenafil (Viagra). *(p. 508)*

10. b. The EMT's assessment and care is the same, no matter what the cause of the patient's signs or symptoms. (The EMT should not spend time trying to diagnose the cause of chest discomfort or pain. Titrate oxygen administration to maintain a SpO_2 of 94%; administer aspirin if allowed by local protocol; reassure the patient; consult medical direction regarding administering physician-prescribed nitroglycerin and request ALS backup; initiate early transport. Be alert for the occurrence of cardiac arrest, and should this occur, be prepared to perform defibrillation and CPR as appropriate.) *(p. 506)*

11. a. Because of the potential for serious side effects, you should not administer nitroglycerin to a patient who is taking sildenafil (Viagra), tadalafil (Cialis), or vardenafil (Levitra). You should contact medical direction for specific orders. *(p. 508)*

12. d. The primary contributing factor to the development of coronary disease is the development of atherosclerosis. Atherosclerosis results in a reduction in the coronary arteries' internal diameter, a buildup of fatty plaque, and an inability of the coronary vessels to dilate. *(p. 499)*

13. b. Factors that affect the signs and symptoms and severity of acute coronary syndrome include the site of the occlusion, the artery occluded, how much blood the coronary artery supplies to the heart, the size or portion of the heart muscle not being supplied with oxygenated blood, and the length of time that the artery has been occluded. *(p. 499)*

14. d. A key to effective treatment of the patient is early recognition. Time is a critical element in the survival and outcome. Death of a portion of the heart muscle is permanent and irreversible. It is important to recognize the signs and symptoms of the many possible cardiac conditions, referred to collectively as *cardiac compromise*. Some patients may be eligible for drugs (fibrinolytics and antiplatelet agents) or mechanical therapy (angioplasty) that will destroy the clot and restore the blood flow to the heart. *(p. 498)*

15. d. Angina pectoris is a symptom of inadequate blood supply to the heart muscle. *(p. 499)*

16. c. The typical signs and symptoms of angina pectoris include steady discomfort in the chest, pain that rarely lasts longer than 15 minutes, nausea or vomiting, and a complaint of indigestion. *(p. 500)*

17. a. Appropriate emergency medical care for angina pectoris includes administering a patient's prescribed nitroglycerin, establishing an open airway and providing oxygen at 15 lpm, applying the pulse oximeter upon patient contact, and administering 160–325 mg of aspirin, if local protocol permits. *(p. 500)*

18. b. An acute myocardial infarction is infrequently the result of a coronary spasm, is commonly known as a *heart attack*, and involves heart-muscle death in about 20 minutes following occlusion. Myocardial infarction is defined as the death of heart muscle. *(p. 501)*

19. d. In the patient suffering from acute myocardial infarction, ventricular fibrillation is the most common cause of cardiac arrest and usually occurs within the first hour following the onset of symptoms. Thrombolytic drugs will dissolve the clot and restore blood flow to the heart, preventing further damage, but they will not reverse damage that has already occurred, which is why early administration of these drugs is so important. Ischemic heart tissue can cause dysrhythmias. *(p. 501)*

20. The filled-in chart should appear as shown. *(pp. 499–506)*

Sign/Symptoms	Acute Angina Pectoris	Myocardial Infarction	Heart Failure
Steady discomfort usually located in the center of the chest but may be more diffuse throughout the front of the chest	X	X	
Chest discomfort radiating to the jaw, arms, shoulders, or back	X	X	
Nausea or vomiting	X	X	
Severe dyspnea		X	
Cyanosis		X	X
Anxiety	X	X	X
Dyspnea	X	X	X
Signs and symptoms of pulmonary edema			X
Complaint of indigestion pain	X	X	
Distended neck veins—JVD (late sign)			X
Sense of impending doom		X	
Distended and soft, spongy abdomen			X
Tachypnea			X
Diaphoresis	X	X	X
Discomfort usually described as pressure; tightness; or aching, crushing, or heavy feeling	X	X	
Edema in the ankles, feet, and hands			X
Lightheadedness or dizziness		X	X
Fatigue on any exertion			X
Crackles and possibly wheezes on auscultation of the chest			X
Tachycardia			X
Weakness		X	X
Upright position with legs, feet, arms, and hands dangling			X
Decreased SpO_2 (oxygen saturation) reading			X

21. **d.** Heart failure is categorized as right-sided or left-sided failure and can be caused by a valve disorder, hypertension, pulmonary embolism, and certain drugs. Right-sided heart failure frequently results in peripheral or dependent edema or swelling. Heart failure results when the heart no longer has the ability to eject blood adequately from the ventricle. *(p. 504)*

22. **d.** Management of the heart-failure patient with pulmonary edema is similar to the treatment of the patient with an acute myocardial infarction. Treatment infrequently results in the development of a pneumothorax from positive-pressure ventilation treatment, although this may certainly occur. Treatment is not complicated by a common medication that heart-failure patients take, diuretics or "water pills." Drastic improvement following positive-pressure ventilation or with CPAP is possible. *(p. 505)*

23. **b.** Depolarization is the stage when the heart muscle changes from positive to negative and causes the heart muscle to contract. Repolarization is the second stage, in which the electrical charges return to a positive charge and cause relaxation of the heart muscle. *(p. 497)*

24. **c.** The QRS complex is the second waveform and represents the depolarization or contraction of the ventricles. *(p. 497)*

25. **a.** The T wave is the third waveform in the normal ECG and represents the repolarization or relaxation of the ventricles (b is represented by the P wave, c by the QRS complex). (Repolarization of the atria is overshadowed by the QRS complex and so is not visible on the normal ECG.) *(p. 497)*

26. **b.** The PR interval (PRI) is calculated from the beginning of the P wave to the beginning of the QRS complex. The PRI represents the time that it takes the heart's electrical impulse to travel from the atria to the ventricles. *(p. 497)*

27. **a.** There are three pacemaker sites in the heart. The first and primary pacemaker for the heart is the Sinoatrial (SA) node. The second pacemaker is the atrioventricular (AV) node. *(p. 497)*

28. **a.** Cardiogenic shock is a clinical state (not a diagnosis) in which the left or right ventricle fails to pump out enough blood to meet the demands of the body. The most common cause for this is myocardial damage that occurs after a heart attack. *(p. 504)*

29. **c.** A systolic blood pressure of 90 mmHg or 30 mmHg less than the patient's baseline systolic blood pressure is a contraindication to the administration of any additional nitroglycerin. *(p. 508)*

30. **b.** The absolute contraindications for fribinolytic therapy includes a history of prior intracranial hemorrhage, known diagnosis of a cerebral vascular lesion, diagnosis of a malignant intracranial neoplasm, suspected aortic dissection, active bleeding (excluding menstrual cycles), bleeding disorders, closed head trauma or facial trauma within the past three months and ischemic stroke within the past three months (except acute ischemic stroke within the past three hours). *(pp. 512–513)*

CASE STUDY

1. **c.** Nonrebreather mask at 15 lpm.
2. **b.** Mr. Hansen is experiencing cardiac compromise, thus early transport is necessary.
3. **a.** Reassure him that this is a common side effect of nitroglycerin and the headache pain should pass.
4. **b.** Continue to evaluate him and to update the receiving facility.

CHAPTER 17 SCENARIO: DOCUMENTATION EXERCISE

1. **b.** Mr. Auerbach is most likely suffering from an AMI. He is suffering from severe chest discomfort (9 or 10 in severity), pain in the center of his chest that radiates down the left arm that has been ongoing for at least 1 hour.
2. **c.** The timing (over a half-hour in duration) and location of discomfort (midsternal) suggests an AMI.
3. **c.** Mr. Auerbach's clenched fist positioned over the center of his chest is called the *Levine sign*.
4. **c.** The use of the AED on Mr. Auerbach is inappropriate unless he becomes unresponsive. If no signs of life are present, immediately begin chest compressions and apply the AED as soon as it is available.
5. **c.** OPQRST method: onset, provocative/palliative, quality, radiation, severity, and timing.

Chapter 18: Altered Mental Status, Stroke, and Headache

MEDICAL TERMINOLOGY

1. **d.** To speak. *(p. 524)*
2. **b.** Bad, difficult, painful. *(p. 524)*
3. **d.** Hardening. *(p. 524)*
4. **a.** Half. *(p. 524)*
5. **b.** Paralysis, stroke. *(p. 524)*

TERMS AND CONCEPTS

1. **a.** 4   **b.** 2   **c.** 1   **d.** 3. *(p. 524)*

CONTENT REVIEW

1. **a.** Slurred speech. *(p. 528)*
2. **a.** A stroke (which is a nontraumatic, or medical, brain injury) may result from any disruption of blood flow to the brain—for example, from a rupture to or blockage of a blood vessel in the brain. *(p. 529)*
3. **b.** Chronic hypertension. *(p. 530)*
4. **b.** Brain attack. An ischemic stroke is very similar to a heart attack. It has the same general cause (inadequate delivery of oxygenated blood because of a blood vessel blockage) and the same level of seriousness as a heart attack. *(p. 529)*

5. c. Hypotension is a rare finding in the stroke patient. *(p. 538)*

6. b. An embolic stroke is another type of ischemic stroke that results from a piece of plaque or other material that breaks off from inside a vessel or within the heart and travels into the brain circulation until it becomes lodged in a cerebral vessel, cutting off distal circulation to brain tissue. *(p. 529)*

7. a. Weakness or paralysis affecting one side of the body. *(p. 537)*

8. c. Administer oxygen via nasal cannula at 2 to 4 lpm to maintain an SpO_2 reading of > 94%. *(p. 538)*

9. c. Lateral recumbent position. (This will allow secretions to drain from the patient's mouth and help prevent aspiration when the patient cannot protect his airway. If the patient is responsive, place him in a supine position with head and chest elevated no greater than 30 degrees.) *(pp. 528, 532)*

10. d. One arm drifts downward. *(pp. 535–536)*

11. d. Perform a reassessment every five minutes, paying close attention to airway, breathing, circulation, and mental status. *(p. 539)*

12. a. Elderly patients with a history of heart disease. *(p. 531)*

13. a. Approximately one-third of those who suffer a TIA will go on to have a stroke. *(p. 532)*

14. b. Repeating a phrase with wrong or slurred words strongly suggests a stroke. *(p. 534)*

15. d. The elderly patient who has signs and symptoms of a stroke may, instead, be a diabetic who is suffering hypoglycemia. This patient may be a candidate for administration of oral glucose. The history of diabetes will also be important information for the hospital staff. *(p. 536)*

16. d. Time of onset is crucial information that must be relayed to the receiving hospital because clot-dissolving drugs can only be administered within three hours of the onset of the stroke. *(p. 536)*

17. c. Clot-dissolving drugs may be able to be given by the emergency department. *(p. 536)*

18. b. Ischemic stroke is the type of stroke that occurs when a blood clot or other foreign matter blocks a cerebral artery. *(p. 529)*

19. a. Hemorrhagic stroke is the type of stroke that occurs from bleeding within the brain caused by a ruptured cerebral blood vessel. *(p. 529)*

20. d. Severe headache is a very common symptom of the hemorrhagic stroke. Onset is usually sudden, with a rapid deterioration in mental status. Seizures and stiff neck are also common in this type of stroke. *(p. 530)*

21. b. Thrombotic-type stroke is caused by narrowed arteries through a process called atherosclerosis. This type of stroke is the most common, and signs and symptoms are slower to develop. An embolic stroke occurs when a blood clot lodges in the small arteries of the brain. *(p. 529)*

22. b. Cluster headaches. The pain is usually found only on one side of the head or face in the temporal region or around the eye and is excruciating. The patient may also complain of excessive tear production on the side of the pain, nasal congestion or runny nose (rhinorrhea), and nausea. *(p. 539)*

23. d. Tension headaches are thought to be caused by contraction of the muscles found in the neck and scalp. The pain is usually described as being "tight" or "viselike." This is the most common type of recurring headache found in children, adolescents, and adults. The patient may wake in the morning with a headache that worsens throughout the day. *(p. 540)*

CASE STUDY

1. c. Oxygen should only be provided to stroke patients with an SpO_2 < 94%, or if an SpO_2 is unknown.

2. The patient suspected of having a stroke may be suffering paralysis of the throat muscles, which will cause her to be unable to protect her airway, even if the airway is open. Vomiting is also a frequent consequence of a stroke patient. Suctioning may be required to remove secretions or vomitus that the patient might aspirate.

3. b. Administer positive pressure ventilation at 10–12 ventilations per minute for the adult patient and 12–20 for the infant or child.

CHAPTER 18 SCENARIO: DOCUMENTATION EXERCISE

1. d. This is a significant finding according to the Cincinnati Prehospital Stroke Scale. The patient not only slurred his words but used the wrong words. His apparent frustration can be caused by knowing what he wanted to say but being unable to do so.

2. a. A diabetic emergency can present with symptoms similar to those of a stroke. A normal blood glucose level will help to rule out a diabetic emergency.

3. a. A stroke patient who can protect his airway should be placed with head elevated no more than 30 degrees. If the patient's condition worsens so that he cannot protect his airway, he should be placed in the left lateral recumbent position. Also note that Cory has prepared the suction unit and BVM in anticipation that the patient may deteriorate.

4. b. Severe headache, sudden onset of symptoms, and history of hypertension treated by medication are all common indicators of hemorrhagic stroke. Seizures and stiff neck are also common with this type of stroke.

5. c. Establishing time of onset is crucial in order for hospital personnel to decide if clot-dissolving drugs can be administered. Although this patient has indications of suffering a hemorrhagic stroke, for which clot-dissolving drugs cannot be used, this decision must be made by hospital personnel. The EMT's job is to gather appropriate information that can help hospital personnel with the decision process.

Chapter 19: Seizures and Syncope

TERMS AND CONCEPTS

1. **a.** 1 **b.** 5 **c.** 4 **d.** 2 **e.** 6 **f.** 7 **g.** 3.
   (p. 546)

CONTENT REVIEW

1. **a.** A head injury may cause a seizure in patients. *(p. 547)*
2. **a.** Aura—sensory perception that warns a patient a seizure is about to occur, sometimes described as a sensation that rises from the stomach toward the chest. Tonic phase—the patient's muscles become contracted and tense and the patient exhibits extreme muscular rigidity with arching of the back. Hypertonic phase—extreme muscular rigidity with hyperextension of the back. Clonic phase—convulsions; jerky muscle activity. Postictal phase—recovery phase; confusion or disorientation to complete unresponsiveness, exhaustion, possible headache, and weakness. *(p. 549)*
3. **d.** Postictal. *(p. 547)*
4. **a.** You should suspect a patient's seizure is triggered by a hypoglycemic state if the blood glucose level is below 60 mg/dL. *(p. 553)*
5. **b.** Move objects away; guide the patient's movements. (Never place anything in the patient's mouth; it could break and cause airway obstruction. Do not attempt to restrain the patient, as this could cause injury.) *(p. 554)*
6. **c.** Following a generalized seizure, paralysis to one area or one side of the body may occur that may last up to 24 hours. This is known as Todd paralysis and may indicate a space-occupying problem in the brain that is causing the seizure. *(p. 553)*
7. **b.** Positive pressure ventilation and immediate transport are required for the cyanotic status epilepticus patient that has been seizing for longer than five minutes. *(p. 552)*
8. **c.** High fever. *(p. 550)*
9. **c.** The patient who has regained responsiveness between seizures. (This patient still should be transported for evaluation at a medical facility but is not a high priority for immediate transport.) *(p. 552)*
10. **d.** A febrile seizure is caused by a high fever (*febrile* means "feverish") and is most common in children between the ages of six months and six years. *(p. 550)*
11. **d.** The nasopharyngeal airway is soft and can be inserted when the teeth are clenched. A rigid oropharyngeal airway could break the teeth or be bitten off, risking airway obstruction. *(p. 552)*
12. **b.** Lateral recumbent. The lateral recumbent position permits secretions to drain from the mouth and helps protect the airway and prevent aspiration. *(p. 554)*
13. **c.** A generalized seizure typically involves both cerebral hemispheres (large lobes) of the brain and the reticular activating system, or RAS (the wake/sleep system). This is what produces the unresponsiveness during the seizure. *(p. 558)*
14. **d.** The generalized seizure involves both hemispheres of the brain and usually renders the patient unconscious. *(p. 558)*
15. **a.** The simple partial seizure, also known as a *focal motor seizure* or *motor seizure*, produces jerky muscle activity in one specific area. *(p. 550)*
16. **b.** A typical fainting or syncopal episode is usually preceded by the patient's exhibiting yawning, diaphoresis, or nausea, or complaining of dizziness. *(p. 556)*
17. **b.** The skin of a syncope patient is usually cool, pale, and moist. *(p. 556)*
18. **a.** The parasympathetic nervous system causes the vessels to dilate throughout the body. This causes the blood flow to the brain to drop. The hypoperfused brain no longer functions adequately and the patient has a syncopal episode. *(p. 556)*

CASE STUDY

1. **a.** Guide body movements and move obstacles.
2. **d.** Positive pressure ventilation with a nasopharyngeal airway in place and rapid transport. (If Karl is in status epilepticus, positive pressure ventilation is required. A nasopharyngeal airway cannot be bitten off as an oropharyngeal airway can.)
3. The blood could have come from an injury from a fall or other mechanism; however, it often results when a seizing patient bites the tongue or cheek. Treat by suctioning.
4. **c.** Postictal.
5. **d.** Now that Karl is responsive, and since no head or spinal injury is suspected, place in a lateral recumbent position and maintain his SpO_2 at > 94%.

CHAPTER 19 SCENARIO: DOCUMENTATION EXERCISE

1. **b.** The generalized tonic-clonic or grand mal seizure usually presents with whole-body tonic-clonic movement. It is the most common type of epileptic seizure.
2. **b.** An aura is an odd sensation such as a sound, visual disturbance, smell, or taste that often precedes a generalized tonic-clonic seizure and warns the patient that a seizure is about to occur.
3. **c.** *Status epilepticus* is defined as a seizure that lasts longer than five minutes or seizures that occur consecutively without a period of responsiveness between the seizures. This is a dire emergency and requires immediate airway management and transport.
4. **a.** The postictal state is also known as the *recovery stage*, during which the patient may appear extremely tired, sleepy, weak, and disoriented. This stage may last 5–30 minutes or several hours. Supplemental oxygen should be based upon the patient's SpO_2.
5. **c.** Seizures may be caused by hyperglycemia or hypoglycemia. The glucometer will help to determine if the patient's blood glucose

level is too high, too low, or normal, as in this patient. Hypoxia can trigger seizures; the pulse oximeter is used to determine if the patient is hypoxic. Eclampsia is a complication of pregnancy. While seizures may occur with severe anaphylactic reactions, a glucometer would not determine if there has been an anaphylactic reaction.

Chapter 20: Acute Diabetic Emergencies

MEDICAL TERMINOLOGY
1. **d.** Sugar. *(p. 561)*
2. **a.** Blood condition. *(p. 561)*
3. **a.** Many, much, excessive. *(p. 561)*
4. **b.** Urine. *(p. 561)*
5. **c.** To eat, engulf. *(p. 561)*

TERMS AND CONCEPTS
1. **a.** 4 **b.** 6 **c.** 2 **d.** 1 **e.** 5 **f.** 3. *(p. 561)*

CONTENT REVIEW
1. **d.** When the patient suffers from an altered mental status, this is an indication that the central nervous system has been affected. *(p. 563)*
2. **a.** Carbohydrates are the primary energy source for the cells. *(p. 562)*
3. **d.** Blood glucose meters or glucometers analyze glucose levels in the blood by obtaining a drop of capillary blood. Glucometers, widely used in EMS, are cost-effective, compact, and very portable. They measure blood glucose levels in milligrams per deciliter (mg/dL). Glucometers are widely used by diabetics because they are accurate and simple to use. *(p. 566)*
4. **c.** The blood glucose level in a nondiabetic patient following a meal will typically rise to 120–140 mg/dL. *(p. 566)*
5. **d.** Hyperglycemia can be defined as a blood glucose level greater than 120 mg/dL. Hypoglycemia (low blood glucose level) is typically less than 60 mg/dL with signs and symptoms of hypoglycemia, or less than 50 mg/dL without signs and symptoms of hypoglycemia. A normal blood glucose level range is 80–120 mg/dL. *(p. 566)*
6. **c.** It is important to determine when the patient last had something to eat or drink. The blood glucose level in a nondiabetic patient following a meal will typically rise to 120–140 mg/dL. Thus, this is not considered abnormal. Likewise, after an 8- to 12-hour fast, a nondiabetic patient's glucose level will typically read 80–90 mg/dL. However, in the diabetic patient, the blood glucose level may be as high as 120 mg/dL after an 8- to 12-hour fast. Blood glucose readings as high as 200 mg/dL may be normal in a diabetic patient. *(p. 566)*
7. **a.** Ensure an open airway, administer oxygen to attain a SpO$_2$ of > 94%, place him in a lateral recumbent position, and transport. This is the recommended care for a patient with an altered mental status and no known history of diabetes controlled by medication. (Do not administer oral glucose unless the patient meets all three criteria for this medication: altered mental status, history of diabetes controlled by medication, and ability to swallow.) *(p. 570)*
8. **a.** Type 2 diabetes is usually controlled by diet. Only in severe cases must insulin be administered. *(p. 567)*
9. **a.** When the blood glucose level is decreasing, epinephrine (adrenalin) is released. This will produce the tachycardia, diaphoresis, and pale, cool skin typically seen in the hypoglycemic patient. Any of these may be true of the diabetic patient. *(p. 569)*
10. **d.** Your patient has a history of diabetes; asking whether the patient's family has a history of cancer will not likely help you assess this patient. You should ask: Did the patient take his medication the day of the episode? Did the patient eat (or skip any) regular meals on this day? Did the patient vomit after eating a meal on that day? Did the patient do any unusual exercise or physical activity on that day? *(p. 578)*
11. **c.** A diabetic emergency with signs and symptoms that mimic a stroke is a frequent occurrence in elderly patients. *(p. 578)*
12. **a.** A medical identification device, medical alert tag, or tattoo indicating that the patient has diabetes *(p. 577)*
13. **b.** Determine if the patient can swallow. (Never give anything orally to a patient whose mental status is altered severely enough that he cannot swallow or protect his airway.) *(p. 579)*
14. **b.** Improvement after administration of oral glucose may happen quickly or may take 20 minutes or more. However, also be prepared for further deterioration of the patient's condition, and continually monitor the airway and breathing. Never insert anything in the mouth of a seizing patient. If oral glucose was administered with a tongue depressor and the patient seizes, immediately remove the tongue depressor to help prevent damage to teeth, tongue, and gums. *(p. 579)*
15. **b.** Glucagon is a hormone that stimulates the breakdown of glycogen and allows the release of glucose molecules back into the blood. Glucagon does not contain sugar. *(p. 663)*
16. **d.** If a patient presents with signs of dehydration, check the blood glucose level. Diabetic patients with high blood glucose levels will have a tendency to lose large amounts of body water through excessive urination. *(p. 567)*
17. **a.** An altered mental status in the diabetic ketoacidosis patient is not from a lack of glucose to the brain, but from dehydration and acidosis affecting the brain cells and causing dysfunction. *(p. 573)*

18. a. If insulin is not available, glucose will move into the cell at a rate approximately **10 times** slower. This increase will cause glucose to build up in the bloodstream, causing the blood glucose level to increase as well. *(p. 563)*

19. c. A normal blood glucose range is 80–120 mg/dL. A reading of less than 80 mg/dL may indicate a lower-than-normal level of glucose (sugar) in the blood. A reading of greater than 120 mg/dL may indicate a higher-than-normal amount of glucose in the blood. *(p. 668)*

20. d. Beta blockers may hide the signs of hypoglycemia. *(p. 578)*

UNDERSTANDING DIABETES MELLITUS

1. b. Converting other noncarbohydrate substances into glucose is done by the hormone glucagon, not insulin. The other three choices are the main functions of insulin. *(p. 564)*

2. a. Glucagon's major role in the body is to raise and maintain the blood glucose level. Glucagon converts liver glycogen and other substances into glucose to raise and maintain the blood glucose level until the next meal. *(p. 564)*

3. b. In an elevated hyperglycemic state (above a blood glucose level of 225 mg/dL), there is a large amount of glucose spilled into the urine from the kidneys. Glucose, a large molecule, draws water with it into the urine, resulting in the three Ps. *(p. 567)*

4. a. Type 1 diabetes mellitus patients most often have to administer insulin injections because their pancreas does not produce insulin. Typically, these patients are younger in age when diagnosed, most often under 40. They are usually lean from weight loss and are more likely to suffer from DKA and hypoglycemia. *(p. 567)*

5. d. The cells begin to burn fat for energy because glucose has collected in the blood. The blood glucose levels are typically greater than 350 mg/dL, and signs of DKA usually do not occur for several days. Electrolytes in the body become unbalanced. *(pp. 572–573)*

6. c. Coma is a very late sign of DKA. All of the others are fairly early signs. *(p. 573)*

7. c. The cells of the brain are not able to use proteins or fats for energy. Brain cells can only use glucose as fuel and will quickly suffer, shut down, and eventually die without it. *(p. 575)*

CASE STUDY

1. Probably a rapid onset if it occurred during jogging. Patient is anxious, speaks with inappropriate words, and is wearing a medical identification bracelet (insulin-dependent diabetic). Episode follows a period of physical exercise; tachycardia (heart rate 104); skin is cool and moist.

2. a. Nasal cannula at 2 lpm because her SpO_2 is less than 94%. Maintain her SpO_2 at > 94%.

(Her breathing is adequate, so positive pressure ventilation is not necessary at this time.)

3. a. The blood pressure is not one of the criteria for the administration of oral glucose. The three criteria for administration of oral glucose are as follows: (1) The patient must have an altered mental status. (2) The patient must have a history of diabetes controlled by medication. (3) The patient must be able to swallow.

4. a. In some jurisdictions, off-line medical direction allows the EMT-Basic to administer oral glucose without direct consultation with medical direction, on the basis of standing orders or protocols. Some jurisdictions require on-line medical direction for the administration of oral glucose. Approval given by radio or phone is considered on-line medial direction.

CHAPTER 20 SCENARIO: DOCUMENTATION EXERCISE

1. d. If the patient took his insulin and then forgot to eat, this would lead you to suspect the patient is hypoglycemic (low blood glucose level). If the patient ate but did not take his insulin, you would suspect a hyperglycemic state (high blood glucose level).

2. a. Acetone breath forms when the body has a buildup of ketones, which can be smelled in the patient suffering from DKA. The acetone smell may be mistaken for the smell of alcohol, but this patient is not intoxicated. Syrup of ipecac is not appropriate in this situation. DKA develops slowly, so unresponsiveness is probably not immediately impending.

3. c. Lowering the hand and warming the fingertips encourage better blood flow and produce a better blood sample.

4. d. Because the blood glucose level is below 60 with signs and symptoms of hypoglycemia, this patient is considered to be hypoglycemic. A blood glucose level of less than 50 without signs and symptoms of hypoglycemia is considered to be hypoglycemic. The normal range for a blood glucose level is between 80 mg/dL and 120 mg/dL.

5. b. This patient met all three criteria before receiving the oral glucose treatment (altered mental status, history of diabetes controlled by medication, ability to swallow). If your patient does not meet all of these criteria, oral glucose must not be given.

Chapter 21: Anaphylactic Reactions

TERMS AND CONCEPTS

1. a. 10 **b.** 2 **c.** 7 **d.** 5 **e.** 8 **f.** 4 **g.** 1
h. 9 **i.** 6 **j.** 3. *(pp. 585–593)*

CONTENT REVIEW

1. a. M **b.** S **c.** S **d.** M **e.** S **f.** S. *(p. 589)*
2. c. Medications. *(p. 589)*

3. **c.** Allergens may enter the body by injection, ingestion, inhalation, or contact. *(p. 589)*

4. **d.** The first time an antigen is introduced into the body, chemical mediators are released and cause bronchoconstriction, *increased* capillary membrane permeability, and *vasodilation*. The treatment is the same as for anaphylaxis, and the patient will not have had a previous exposure. *(p. 587)*

5. **a.** Stridor or crowing indicates significant swelling to the upper airway, requiring positive pressure ventilation. *(p. 590)*

6. **a.** Deactivate the pop-off valve or cover it with your thumb in order to achieve adequate pressure to force air past swollen airway structures. *(p. 590)*

7. **c.** Hives and itching are the hallmark signs of an anaphylactic reaction. *(p. 590)*

8. **d.** 20 minutes. *(p. 591)*

9. **b.** Respiratory compromise and/or shock must be present for an anaphylactic reaction to be severe enough to be considered anaphylaxis. Respiratory compromise is characterized by partial or complete airway occlusion, breathing difficulties, and wheezing. Shock (hypoperfusion) may be indicated by absent or weak pulses, rapid heartbeat, decreased blood pressure, and deteriorating mental status. *(p. 594)*

10. **a.** Never underestimate the severity of an anaphylactic reaction. Because death can occur within minutes, immediate intervention is imperative. Do not mistake anaphylaxis for conditions with similar signs and symptoms, such as hyperventilation, anxiety attacks, alcohol intoxication, and hypoglycemia. *(p. 593)*

11. **b.** Common substances that cause anaphylactoid reaction include radiopaque contrast media, NSAIDs, aspirin, opiates, and thiamine. *(p. 587)*

12. **b.** Histamine release results in bronchoconstriction, vasodilation, and increased capillary membrane permeability. *(p. 587)*

13. **d.** Anaphylaxis is a major medical condition with a high mortality rate. It causes blood vessels to dilate, which decreases the blood pressure to dangerously low levels. It affects the entire body from the release of histamine by the immune system. Positive pressure ventilation of the patient may be difficult due to severe bronchoconstriction and swelling of the airway. *(p. 587)*

14. **c.** Signs and symptoms of severe anaphylactic reaction include respiratory distress and/or shock (hypotension). *(pp. 590, 593)*

15. **d.** The upper airway is also likely to be swollen. *(pp. 590, 600)*

16. **b.** The type of antibody produced specific to anaphylaxis is called *immunoglobin E* and is abbreviated as *IgE*. *(p. 586)*

17. **b.** Urticaria (hives) is the most common early physical assessment finding in anaphylaxis. Rhinitis (stuffy, runny, itchy nose) is an early sign indicating respiratory involvement. *(pp. 590, 591)*

CASE STUDY

1. **d.** Although she looks well and is not having difficulty breathing, the patient's skin is flushed, she feels a "lump" in her throat, and her stomach "feels upset"—all early signs of anaphylaxis.

2. **d.** Airway and breathing compromise and poor perfusion.

3. **d.** Excessive mucus in the lower airways.

4. **b.** If the anaphylactic reaction is continuing to develop, coughing and hoarseness may occur, along with other signs and symptoms.

CHAPTER 21 SCENARIO: DOCUMENTATION EXERCISE

1. **a.** Hives and itching are the hallmark signs of an anaphylactic reaction.

2. **a.** Bronchoconstriction and swelling in the lower airway cause breathing difficulty and possible hypoxia.

3. **c.** The auto-injector is administered at the midpoint of the lateral thigh.

4. **b.** Headache and nausea are among the common side effects of epinephrine. Headache may also be a symptom of anaphylactic reaction, but since Kyle Patrick has had an injection of epinephrine, a recurrence of anaphylactic symptoms is not likely.

5. **d.** The epinephrine may be administered directly through the patient's clothing if necessary.

Chapter 22: Toxicologic Emergencies

TERMS AND CONCEPTS

1. **a.** 5 (or 6) **b.** 3 **c.** 1 **d.** 2 **e.** 6 **f.** 4 **g.** 11 **h.** 7 **i.** 9 **j.** 10 **k.** 8. *(p. 607)*

CONTENT REVIEW

1. **d.** More than 1 million poisonings occur each year in the United States. Most poisoning emergencies result from accidental exposure and involve young children. Toxicology is the study of toxins, antidotes, and the effects of toxins on the body. Poisoning is commonly defined as an exposure to a substance other than a drug or medication. *(p. 606)*

2. **c.** Poisoning by inhalation produces a more rapid response than by ingestion; will produce a variety of signs and symptoms, not just respiratory related; may cause lung tissue damage that may lead to pulmonary edema; and primarily affects the pulmonary system. *(p. 607)*

3. **d.** This patient is most likely a "huffer" who inhaled paint or some other substance that left a yellow residue on his nose, nose hairs, and mouth. The presence of singed nasal hairs would indicate inhalation of hot, toxic gases. *(p. 613)*

4. **c.** While all of these things might eventually be done at the scene of a poisoning emergency,

the medical priority is to maintain the patient's airway and breathing and to treat for any potential life threats. *(p. 630)*

5. **c.** Poisons may cause airway and breathing compromise as a result of alteration of mental status, respiratory depression, and direct damage to the airway tissues. *(p. 642)*

6. **d.** The most common inhaled poisons include carbon monoxide and carbon dioxide from industrial sites, sewers, and wells. Inhaled poisons cause thousands of deaths each year, not millions, and occur most often as a result of fires. Long exposure times to inhaled poisons are associated with poor, not good, survival rates. *(p. 606)*

7. ING Abdominal pain tenderness and cramping
INJ Pupillary changes
INH Hoarseness
ING Body or breath odor
INH Difficulty breathing
ABS Liquid or powder on skin
ING Diarrhea
INH Copious secretions
ABS Itching and burning
INJ Pain, redness, and swelling at injection site
INH Singed nasal hairs
INJ Fever and chills
ABS Redness or swelling *(pp. 614–619)*

8. **a.** Y **b.** Y **c.** N **d.** Y **e.** N **f.** N. *(p. 620)*

9. **b.** Prevent further injury by rinsing the substance from his mouth and lips. Be careful when rinsing the mouth that the patient does not swallow the liquid. *(p. 611)*

10. **c.** It is rarely used in the emergency medical care of ingested poisonings. *(p. 611)*

11. **a.** Activated charcoal is indicated for ingested poisons, when rarely ordered by medical direction. *(p. 611)*

12. **d.** In some cases of specific medication ingestion that cause a delayed emptying effect such as opioids, anticholinergic drugs, or medications with a sustained release, medical direction may order the administration of activated charcoal if it is shortly after ingestion. *(p. 608)*

13. **c.** If ordered by medical direction, the usual adult dosage of activated charcoal is 30–100 grams (1g/kg of body weight). *(p. 611)*

14. **c.** Actidose is a brand name for activated charcoal. *(p. 611)*

15. **b.** Activated charcoal is contraindicated in a patient with an altered mental status and who ingested ethanol ammonia or is unable to swallow. Medical control may order activated charcoal for a patient who has recently taken an overdose of an anticholinergic drug. *(p. 611)*

16. **a.** Blackened stool. (Common side effects of activated charcoal include blackened stool, nausea, and vomiting. Other side effects are rare.) *(p. 611)*

17. **c.** Fire-related incidents. *(p. 614)*

18. **b.** Respiratory symptoms. *(p. 614)*

19. **b.** An appropriate action in the management of toxic inhalation is to remove the patient to fresh air as soon as possible. This should be done by properly trained and equipped rescuers. *(p. 613)*

20. **a.** Prevent exposure to yourself from any poisons that may be absorbed through the skin. Wear protective gloves and ensure that the patient is properly decontaminated prior to transport. Chemical burns to the eye should be irrigated. Clothing and jewelry should be removed if contaminated. Dry powder should be brushed away. (Contact medical direction to see if this action should be followed by flushing.) *(p. 617)*

21. **d.** Food poisoning does not commonly result in death, is increasing in incidence from prior years in the United States, is often caused by tainted seafood, and is difficult to detect because the signs and symptoms vary greatly. *(p. 621)*

22. **c.** Carbon monoxide poisoning is caused by an odorless gas that is difficult to detect. It decreases the amount of oxygen carried on the hemoglobin, which inhibits the ability of body cells to utilize oxygen. It causes thousands of deaths each year in the United States. *(pp. 613, 621)*

23. **b.** Carbon monoxide poisoning should be suspected if flulike symptoms are shared by people in the same environment. The other choices are not associated with carbon monoxide poisoning. *(p. 621)*

24. **d.** Cyanide can enter the body through inhalation, absorption, injection, or ingestion. It is found in many household products, including rodent poisons and silver polish, and in cherry and apricot pits. Inhalation can occur in fires where plastics, silk, and synthetic carpets are burning. *(p. 622)*

25. **d.** The smell of bitter almonds is most closely associated with cyanide poisoning. *(p. 622)*

26. **c.** Strong acids have an extremely low pH; if ingested, they will cause the most severe burns in the stomach, producing severe and immediate abdominal pain. They will typically burn for only 1–2 minutes. *(p. 623)*

27. **c.** Alkalis have a high pH, will produce burns that are deeper than acid burns, will typically burn for minutes to hours after contact, and, if ingested, will likely injure the stomach tissue. *(p. 623)*

28. **b.** Hydrocarbon poisoning frequently involves children; toxicity is dependent upon the viscosity of the substance; activated charcoal is ineffective in treatment; and examples of products include kerosene, naphtha, turpentine, and mineral oil. *(p. 623)*

29. **d.** Methanol is also known as wood alcohol. It is commonly found in Sterno, paint removers, and windshield washer fluid. Poisoning can occur by ingestion, inhalation, or absorption. Ingestion will produce large amounts of acid in the body. *(p. 624)*

30. **b.** Isopropanol acts as a respiratory depressant. It is also known as *isopropyl alcohol* or

rubbing alcohol, and poisoning occurs most frequently by ingestion. Isopropanol is found in cosmetics, degreasers, disinfectants, and solvents. *(p. 625)*

31. a. Ethylene glycol is commonly found in detergents, radiator antifreeze, and windshield deicers. Poisoning occurs frequently in children due to its sweet taste. Poisoning occurs in three distinct stages, and ethanol (drinking alcohol) may be recommended for treatment. *(p. 625)*

32. d. About 75 percent of all Americans are allergic to urushiol, the poisonous element in poison ivy. For a reaction to occur, contact with poison ivy need not occur directly. Poison sumac is found mostly in the Southeast and West. Stinging nettle, crown of thorns, and buttercup can cause mild to severe dermatitis. *(p. 626)*

33. c. Poison control centers are staffed and available for service 24 hours a day, 7 days a week; are able to provide information on any poisons; provide follow-up telephone calls to patients to monitor progress; and should routinely be consulted by the EMT when poisoning is suspected. Prior to providing treatment, be sure to contact medical direction for approval of treatment. *(p. 626)*

34. b. The goals are to identify and treat the loss of vital functions caused by the drug—especially impairments to the airway, breathing, oxygenation, and circulation—not the specific effects of the drug itself. Treatment should never be delayed to identify the substance. *(p. 627)*

35. a. Three potential dangers at any drug or alcohol emergency scene are communicable disease, violent behavior, and weapons. *(p. 627)*

36. b. Transport the pill bottles to the emergency department with the patient. *(p. 629)*

37. b. You must first identify and treat the loss of vital functions caused by the drug or alcohol. Drug and alcohol emergencies may mimic many different medical and traumatic disorders, not just a few. These scenes are frequently the site of violent acts and physical abuse. Every scene demands the routine use of Standard Precautions. *(p. 624)*

38. d. Of the choices provided, the best answer is to ask bystanders about any events that may have precipitated the episode. *(p. 624)*

39. a. N **b.** Y **c.** N **d.** Y **e.** Y **f.** Y **g.** N **h.** N. *(p. 630)*

40. c. Scene size-up and patient history. *(p. 632)*

41. 2, 5, 3, 1, 4. The emergency care steps for the disoriented patient who reports an overdose (or, in general, for any drug or alcohol emergency patient) are (1) establish and maintain a patent airway; (2) administer oxygen at 15 lpm by a nonrebreather mask if signs of severe hypoxia are present; (3) maintain body temperature; (4) if protocol permits, assess the blood glucose level; (5) transport. *(p. 632)*

42. a. Hallucinogenic substances (PCP, cocaine, amphetamine, and methamphetamines) often produce a psychological emergency that may present as intense anxiety or paranoia ("bad trip"), depression, disorientation, or an inability to differentiate fantasy from reality. They may also present with tachycardia, dilated pupils, motor disturbances, and flushed face. PCP may cause paralysis, violence, rage, and status epilepticus. *(pp. 628, 634)*

43. b. Touch can be comforting, but invading the drug- or alcohol-abuse patient's "personal space" can trigger a violent response. Always establish rapport, and obtain the patient's permission before touching him. *(p. 636)*

44. a. You should first "talk down" the patient and calm them before transporting. Elements of the talk-down technique for the potentially violent patient who is suffering a "bad trip" include the following: (1) Making the patient feel welcome; remaining relaxed and sympathetic. (2) Identifying yourself clearly and establishing rapport before touching the patient. (3) Reassuring the patient that his condition is caused by the drug and will not last forever. (4) Helping the patient verbalize what is happening to him. (5) Making simple statements to help orient the patient to time and place; encouraging him to feel more secure by helping him identify where he is and what is happening. (6) Forewarning the patient about what he may experience as the drug wears off. (7) Transporting the patient after he has been calmed. *(p. 634)*

45. b. CNS stimulant drugs typically cause dilated pupils, while narcotics cause pinpoint pupils. *(p. 631)*

46. c. Bradycardia, hypotension, inadequate breathing rates and volume, cool and clammy skin, constricted pupils, and nausea are most commonly associated with narcotics. *(p. 631)*

47. b. The physically dependent drug user experiences a strong need to use the drug repeatedly, considers the drug constantly, and will experience severe physiological consequences of drug withdrawal. Tolerance of the drug may develop, in which larger and larger doses are needed. *(p. 627)*

48. d. Common signs and symptoms of drug withdrawal include nausea, abdominal cramping, tremors, anxiety, agitation, confusion, hallucinations, and elevated heart rate and blood pressure. *(p. 627)*

49. b. A chronic brain syndrome resulting from the toxic effects of alcohol on the central nervous system combined with malnutrition is called *Wernicke-Korsakoff syndrome*. *(p. 638)*

50. c. The alcoholic syndrome consists of a combination of problem drinking and true addiction to alcohol. *(p. 637)*

51. d. Withdrawal syndrome occurs when the alcoholic's alcohol level falls below the amount usually ingested. The more the alcoholic was drinking, the more severe the syndrome will be. *(p. 638)*

52. d. Stage 1 of alcohol withdrawal occurs within about 8 hours and is characterized by nausea, insomnia, sweating, and tremors. Stage 2 begins within 8–72 hours and is characterized by worsening of stage 1 symptoms and hallucinations. Stage 3 occurs within 48 hours and is characterized by major seizures. Stage 4 is characterized by delirium tremens. *(p. 638)*

53. **b.** Delirium tremens is the last stage of alcohol withdrawal and is a life-threatening condition with a mortality rate between 5–15 percent. *(p. 638)*

54. **b.** Phencyclidine (PCP) is cheap to make and produces horrible psychological effects that can last for years. It is known by multiple names, such as angel dust, killer weed, supergrass, crystal cyclone, and many others. *(p. 640)*

55. **d.** Cocaine is highly addictive. Cocaine may be inhaled through the nose, injected into the veins and muscles, or smoked (crack or freebased). The treatment is generally the same as for PCP use. *(p. 640)*

56. **c.** The first priority of care for a patient under the influence of PCP is to protect the safety of yourself and your response crew. This is also true of cocaine. *(pp. 640–641)*

57. **d.** Poisons intentionally inhaled commonly contain the chemical agent toluene, decrease the movement of oxygen across the alveolar membrane, have a more rapid onset of symptoms than injected poisons, and accumulate in the regions of the brain responsible for feelings of pleasure. *(pp. 640–641)*

58. **c.** Methamphetamine is a stimulant; it is commonly called crystal meth, crank, or go; and it is used by ingestion, inhalation (snorting or smoking), and injection. *(p. 640)*

59. **c.** Scene safety is paramount in any of these suspected situations. If you enter a scene where this type of suicide bag is suspected or recognized, immediately evacuate the room, contact the fire department, and follow their direction. Any person exposed to the helium or nitrogen, whether it is the patient attempting the suicide or an emergency responder entering the scene, he or she must be treated as a toxic inhalation emergency. *(p. 626)*

60. **a.** You would suspect sympathetic effects, including tachycardia, hypertension, hyperthermia, seizures. The effect of the drug is similar to methamphetamine and cocaine and produces similar signs and symptoms. *(p. 640)*

CASE STUDY 1

1. **a.** If you are not wearing an SCBA or have not been properly trained for a hazardous material rescue, withdraw and request assistance. If you are properly trained and equipped, remove Mr. Johnson from the workshop and into fresh air as quickly as possible.

2. **a.** When Mr. Johnson is removed from the area, spinal immobilization should be maintained; an airway ensured; breathing checked;

positive pressure ventilation provided, if needed; and tight clothing loosened.

3. **a.** Y **b.** Y **c.** Y **d.** Y. All the actions are appropriate. A rapid physical exam should be completed to determine if any traumatic injuries are present.

4. **a.** Mr. Johnson requires an ongoing assessment every five minutes during transport to the hospital.

CASE STUDY 2

1. **b.** The first priority is to make sure the airway is clear while simultaneously assessing the breathing.

2. **c.** Even though the literature has suggested activated charcoal reduces absorption of the ingested poison, there is no evidence that suggests a better patient outcome. Thus, activated charcoal is rarely administered by emergency medical service personnel in ingested poisons. This will also require specific approval from medical direction. The patient additionally has an altered level of consciousness that prevents administration.

3. **b.** The patient is a priority transport and requires careful assessment of the patient's respiratory status, a complete physical exam, vital signs, a reassessment every five minutes, and transport of a sample of the vomitus, pill bottles, and the wine bottle to the hospital.

CHAPTER 22 SCENARIO 1: DOCUMENTATION EXERCISE

1. **c.** The blood pressure is not generally assessed in children less than 3 years of age. Better determinants of adequate perfusion in this age group are mental status, pulse, and skin temperature and color.

2. **a.** Watching closely for life threats and providing information to poison control.

3. **b.** There is no one best answer to this question. Mrs. Wilson was clearly upset. Giving Mrs. Wilson a task relieves her of her anxiety and calms the situation. Children at Jimmy's age most commonly will react to strangers and will not want to have the parent leave the room. In this case, a good rapport was established and the mother could be of assistance in treating Jimmy and gathering information.

CHAPTER 22 SCENARIO 2: DOCUMENTATION EXERCISE

1. **b.** The signs or symptoms of potential LSD use that Ed was exhibiting include motor disturbances (shaking hands), dilated pupils, and hallucinations (hearing voices).

2. **c.** The technique you used is called the *talk-down technique*. It is appropriate for patients who have used hallucinogens or marijuana. This technique can help you reduce the patient's anxiety, panic, depression, or confusion.

3. **a.** The talk-down technique should not be used if the patient has taken PCP. PCP causes paralysis, violence, and rage. The talk-down technique would not be useful for managing

these patients and would likely further agitate them.

4. **a.** Y **b.** Y **c.** Y **d.** Y **e.** Y **f.** Y. You accomplished each step with the patient.

5. **a.** Personal safety is of utmost importance. If one is uncomfortable entering a scene or a scene becomes unsafe, evacuate the area and request law enforcement.

Chapter 23: Abdominal, Hematologic, Gynecologic, Genitourinary, and Renal Emergencies

TERMS AND CONCEPTS

1. **a.** 10 **b.** 4 **c.** 6 **d.** 8 **e.** 2 **f.** 3 **g.** 1 **h.** 12 **i.** 5 **j.** 7 **k.** 9 **l.** 11 **m.** 13 **n.** 14 **o.** 16 **p.** 18 **q.** 17 **r.** 19 **s.** 21 **t.** 22 **u.** 20 **v.** 15 **w.** 23 **x.** 24 **y.** 25. (*pp. 648–653*)
2. **a.** 10 **b.** 2 **c.** 8 **d.** 5 **e.** 6 **f.** 3 **g.** 9 **h.** 7 **i.** 4 **j.** 1. (*pp. 649–651*)

CONTENT REVIEW

1. **A.** Diaphragm **B.** Umbilicus **C.** Right upper quadrant (RUQ) **D.** Right lower quadrant (RLQ) **E.** Left upper quadrant (LUQ) **F.** Left lower quadrant (LLQ). (*p. 649*)

2. **A.** Hypogastric region **B.** Umbilical region **C.** Epigastric region **D.** Right iliac region **E.** Right lumbar region **F.** Right hypochondriac region **G.** Left hypochondriac region **H.** Left lumbar region **I.** Left iliac region. (*p. 649*)

3. **d.** The parietal (somatic) nerve fiber stimulation produces a sharp, intense, constant pain that can be pinpointed. The parietal nerve is associated with inflammation of the peritoneal lining of the abdomen. The visceral nerve produces an intermittent, generalized, dull, aching pain that is caused by ischemia, inflammation, or mechanical obstruction of the affecting organ. The phrenic nerve arises from the cervical roots down to the thorax to control breathing. The optic nerve is located behind the eye. (*p. 650*)

4. **a.** Acute abdominal pain, acute abdomen, or acute abdominal distress. (*p. 652*)

5. **b.** Consider the patient with abdominal pain to have a life-threatening condition until proven otherwise. (*p. 657*)

6. **d.** The position with knees drawn up is called a *guarded position* and is typically assumed by a patient with abdominal pain. (*p. 657*)

7. **a.** A criterion for priority transport of the acute abdomen patient is *any* of the following: (1) poor general appearance, (2) unresponsive, (3) responsive but not following commands, (4) shock (hypoperfusion), and (5) severe pain. (*p. 658*)

8. **d.** Certain types of bleeding do have a distinct smell that can sometimes be identified as you arrive at the patient's side. Patients with abdominal pain are likely to faint, usually in the bathroom. You should look for mechanisms of injury to rule out trauma as the cause of the abdominal pain. Bloody vomitus is not always present in the acute abdomen patient. (*p. 657*)

9. **a.** Have the patient point to the area of the pain and palpate this quadrant last. (*p. 651*)

10. **c.** Bloody vomitus or blood in the stool is the most likely sign associated with the acute abdomen patient. (*p. 658*)

11. **d.** Never give anything by mouth (which can be vomited and aspirated) to an acute abdomen patient. A supine position with legs flat is usually not comfortable for the acute abdomen patient. Reassessment should be performed every five minutes for the unstable patient. You should palpate the painful area last. (*p. 658*)

12. **a.** Cholecystitis, which is inflammation of the gallbladder. The other choices are not associated with acute abdomen. (*p. 653*)

13. **a.** Peritonitis. A modified Markle test that elicits a positive response indicates the patient may be suffering from peritonitis. (*p. 652*)

14. **d.** A narrowing pulse pressure (the difference between the systolic and diastolic blood pressure) with an increased heart rate and pale, cool, and diaphoretic skin is a sign of internal bleeding in the abdomen. (*p. 659*)

15. **b.** Esophageal varices are a bulging, engorgement, or weakening of the blood vessels in the lining of the lower part of the esophagus. These abnormalities are common to heavy alcohol drinkers or patients with liver disease and are caused by increased pressure in the venous blood supply system of the liver, stomach, and esophagus. (*p. 654*)

16. **d.** Gastroenteritis, or inflammation of the stomach and small intestines, is commonly associated with the presence of abdominopelvic pain. This condition can be chronic or acute. Chronic gastroenteritis is most commonly a result of an infection. (*p. 648*)

17. **a.** An abdominal aortic aneurysm is a weakened, ballooned, and enlarged area of the wall of the abdominal aorta. Many times this abdominal pain will be described as a tearing pain. If the aortic aneurysm is starting to rupture, the skin below the waistline will become cyanotic, cold, and mottled. This is from a significant drop in blood flow to the extremities. (*p. 656*)

18. **b.** You should not encourage the patient to shower or bathe; this can wash away vital evidence that can help the investigation of the crime. (*p. 664*)

19. **d.** You should apply a pad externally to absorb the blood flow; do not apply direct pressure or pack the vagina. (*p. 667*)

20. **b.** Blood in the urine, hematuria, is a common sign of the patient suffering from a urinary tract infection. (*p. 669*)

21. **a.** Kidney stones, or renal calculi, are crystals of substances like calcium, uric acid, struvite, and crystine that are formed from metabolic

abnormalities. They most frequently occur in men between the ages of 20 and 50. *(p. 670)*

22. a. Almost all sickle cell patients develop kidney damage. Infections occur at higher rates, especially in the kidney, lung, bone, and central nervous system. *(p. 660)*

23. d. Hemophilia is a blood disorder that affects clotting. When a person with hemophilia is injured, it takes longer for the bleeding to stop because clots are unable to form properly. Bleeding that would be considered minor for a non-hemophiliac, such as a nosebleed, is a major emergency for the hemophiliac. *(p. 663)*

CASE STUDY

1. d. Remember the indicators of a serious medical emergency. This patient is displaying a poor general impression, a diminished mental status (slow to respond to questions, does not look at you when you enter), signs of hypoperfusion (rapid, weak pulse; cool, clammy skin; diminished mental status; nausea), and the patient is in severe pain.

2. c. Ask her to point with one finger to the area that is the most painful. Start with the area that is least painful. Palpate each abdominal quadrant of the abdomen, the most painful quadrant last.

3. a. Emesis (vomitus) should be saved for possible testing at the hospital.

4. c. This patient is an unstable patient who requires careful monitoring. Ongoing assessment should be performed at least every five minutes.

CHAPTER 23 SCENARIO: DOCUMENTATION EXERCISE

1. d. Severe "ripping or tearing" abdominal pain radiating to the back, inequality of femoral pulses, and a pulsating mass are all findings associated with an abdominal aortic aneurysm.

2. d. An aortic aneurysm can result in obstruction of blood flow to the femoral arteries, which can yield complete or partial obstruction of blood flow.

3. d. Careful palpation was important in this case as deep or rough palpation could have ruptured the aneurysm.

4. a. Abdominal aortic aneurysm occurs in 20 percent of men over 50 years of age.

Chapter 24: Environmental Emergencies

TERMS AND CONCEPTS

1. a. 1 **b.** 5 **c.** 2 **d.** 7 **e.** 10 **f.** 4 **g.** 13 **h.** 3 **i.** 11 **j.** 14 **k.** 6 **l.** 8 **m.** 9 **n.** 12. *(p. 677)*

CONTENT REVIEW

1. d. The five basic mechanisms by which the body loses heat are radiation, convection, conduction, evaporation, and respiration. Which mechanism commonly leads to the greatest heat loss? Radiation: It accounts for 55–65 percent of heat loss. *(p. 679)*

2. b. Generalized hypothermia (also called *generalized cold emergency*) and local cold injury. *(p. 680)*

3. a. Factors that may place a patient at the greatest risk for developing generalized hypothermia include a cold environment, age (very old and very young), medical conditions (recent surgery, head injury, burns, generalized infections), drugs and alcohol, duration of exposure, clothing, and level of activity. *(p. 681)*

4. a. 3 **b.** 1 **c.** 2 **d.** 4. The correct sequence is (1) Shivering (Mild), (2) Progressive decline in level of responsiveness (Moderate), (3) Pulse rate decreases by 50 percent (Severe), (4) Pulse rate decreases by 80 percent (Profound). *(p. 688)*

5. a. Emergency care for generalized hypothermia includes quickly but carefully removing the patient from the cold environment, administering warmed and humidified oxygen to maintain the SpO_2 at > 94% (or positive pressure ventilation if required), and rewarming the patient as quickly and safely as possible. Do not allow the patient to exert himself in any way (including walking about). A quick clinical check of the patient's temperature is accomplished by the EMT placing the back of her hand on the patient's abdomen. Follow local protocols for specific guidelines. *(p. 688)*

6. b. Appropriate techniques for active rewarming include adding heat to the patient gradually and gently. The body temperature should not be increased by more than 1°F per hour. Never immerse the patient in a hot tub of water or place in a hot shower. Heat is first applied to the torso rather than the extremities. Active rewarming should be applied to patients with a body core temperature less than 34°C or 93.2°F or those in moderate or severe hypothermia. *(pp. 688–689)*

7. a. 10 minutes. (Make sure you familiarize yourself with normal spring, summer, and fall river, lake, and—if nearby—ocean temperatures in your area. Body temperatures can drop rapidly in what you *think* is relatively warm water.) *(p. 683)*

8. d. Guidelines for the emergency medical care of the patient with immersion hypothermia include lifting the patient from the water in a horizontal position (supine), asking the patient to make as little effort as possible to stay afloat until you reach him, and removing the patient's wet clothing carefully and gently. Treatment is similar to generalized hypothermia management. *(p. 690)*

9. b. The stages of local cold injury are early (superficial) and late (deep). *(p. 684)*

10. d. Appropriate management of local cold injuries includes not rubbing or massaging the affected skin, not removing clothing that is frozen to the skin, avoiding the initiation of thawing if refreezing is possible, and carefully removing clothing and jewelry. *(p. 690)*

11. d. Guidelines for the rapid rewarming of local cold injuries includes maintaining the water temperature 104°F (just above body temperature) and dressing the area with a sterile, dry dressing. Rewarming is reserved for those with a delayed transport time with no chance of refreezing of tissue. The tissue should be kept in warm water until it is soft and skin color and sensation return to the affected part. *(p. 691)*

12. b. Hyperthermia. *(p. 693)*

13. a. Factors that increase an individual's reaction to a heat-related injury include heart disease and various medical disorders such as kidney disease, cardiovascular disease, Parkinson's disease, thyroid disease, skin diseases, and dehydration. Hot temperatures, strenuous activity, extremes of age, lack of acclimation, and certain drugs and medications are additional predisposing factors. *(p. 696)*

14. d. Hot skin—either moist or dry—signals a dire medical emergency in a patient who has been exposed to heat. (In early stages of hyperthermia, the skin will be cool to the touch. If the skin is hot, hyperthermia is in an advanced and life-threatening stage. In about half the cases, the patient with hot skin will still be sweating. In the remainder of cases, sweat mechanisms will have shut down.) *(p. 697)*

15. c. When cooling a heat emergency patient with hot skin (that is moist, or dry), cooling takes priority over all other emergency care procedures *except* management of the patient's airway, breathing, and circulation. One cooling method will generally not be effective to cool the patient; multiple methods are required. Be prepared to manage seizures and to prevent aspiration, and place cold packs in the patient's groin, at each side of the neck, in the armpits, and behind each knee to cool using the large vessels close to the skin surface.. *(p. 698)*

16. b. If the patient is unresponsive (or has an altered mental status) or is vomiting, do not give fluids orally. *(p. 698)*

17. d. Most often, the only time a hyperthermic patient with moist, pale skin that is normal to cool in temperature needs transport is if the patient is unresponsive or has an altered mental status, is vomiting or nauseated and will not drink fluids, has a history of medical problems, has a body core temperature above 101°F, or has a temperature that is continuously rising and does not respond to therapy. *(p. 698)*

18. c. The first step for any heat emergency patient with cool or hot skin is to move the patient to a cool place, such as the back of an air-conditioned ambulance, or at least out of the sun and into the shade. *(p. 698)*

19. c. A rapid increase or decrease in the pulse with a decline in the patient's mental status is a grave finding. *(pp. 699–700)*

20. b. Snakebites are uncommon and result in a small number of fatalities each year. Exercise special caution during the scene size-up to protect yourself from a bite or sting. Complications associated with airway and breathing difficulties occur infrequently but do occur. Most insect bites result in minor reactions, not major anaphylactic reactions. *(p. 700)*

21. d. Urban hypothermia occurs in individuals who live outdoors and are unable to escape the cold environment and in the elderly who attempt to reduce their home heating bills. It is not limited to northern climates during the winter months and can occur in indoor temperatures of between 70°F and 72°F. It occurs in individuals with a predisposition, disability, illness, or medication usage that renders them more susceptible to hypothermia. *(p. 681)*

22. c. Approximately 1,000–5,000 people are struck each year in the United States, with 300–500 deaths occurring as a result of the strikes. Strikes occur most frequently on Sundays, occur mostly in recreation and work-related situations, and typically involve one patient rather than multiple patients. *(p. 706)*

23. a. Lightning strike patients are considered both medical and trauma patients, should be routinely spinal immobilized, are infrequently struck while talking on the telephone (2.4 percent of strikes), and can commonly suffer damage to the body's air-containing cavities. *(p. 707)*

24. b. Dislocations and fractures associated with lightning strikes result from the thunder "blast wave," which results in a propelling or throwing of the patient and strong muscular contractions. *(pp. 707–708)*

25. b. Coral snakes and pit vipers contribute to most snakebites in the United States today. Pit vipers include rattlesnakes, copperheads, and water moccasins. *(p. 701)*

26. b. The signs and symptoms of a pit viper bite are immediate and are gauged by how much poison was injected. The patient's size and weight are also factors. *(p. 701)*

27. a. P **b.** P **c.** N **d.** N **e.** N **f.** P. *(p. 701)*

28. a. The black widow spider has a shiny black body, thin legs, and a crimson red hourglass marking on its abdomen. *(p. 703)*

29. a. General signs and symptoms of a black widow spider bite include severe muscle spasms in the shoulders, back, chest, and abdomen. *(p. 703)*

30. c. The brown recluse spider bite is a serious medical condition and can result in severe tissue damage and necrosis at the site of the bite. *(p. 703)*

31. a. Venom of aquatic organisms is destroyed by the application of heat. *(p. 706)*

32. d. Myxedema coma may make a person more susceptible to becoming hypothermic, occurs late in the progression of hypothyroidism, occurs in only about 0.1 percent of all hypothyroidism patients, and is precipitated by exposure to cold, a recent illness, or infection and trauma. *(p. 683)*

CASE STUDY 1

1. **b.** Remove as much clothing as possible, as quickly as possible.
2. **c.** Begin to cool the patient by one or a combination of the following methods: pour tepid water over the patient's body; place cold packs on the patient's groin, on the side of the neck, in the armpits, and behind each knee; wrap the patient in a wet sheet; fan the patient; keep the skin wet.
3. **d.** The use of cold water should be avoided in this patient because it may produce vasoconstriction and shivering.

CASE STUDY 2

1. **b.** Avoid the application of heat packs or cold packs and prevent the patient from moving about. The area should be washed with a mild agent or strong soap solution.
2. **a.** Lower the injection site slightly below the level of the heart and watch closely for signs of anaphylaxis. Cutting and suctioning of the site is not recommended. Epinephrine would not be administered unless the patient had a current prescription for the epinephrine, the patient was showing signs and symptoms of anaphylaxis, and you had authorization from medical direction to administer the medication.
3. **d.** The patient must be observed closely for signs of developing anaphylaxis. These signs include respiratory distress, hives, and hypotension; all are signs of anaphylaxis.

CASE STUDY 3

1. **c.** Take longer than normal to assess the pulse in a hypothermia patient; the pulse may be present but extremely slow.
2. **a.** Some experts advise active rewarming only if you are more than 15 minutes from the receiving facility. According to the AHA 2010 guidelines, active rewarming should be applied to patients with a body core temperature less than 34°C or 93.2°F or those in moderate or severe hypothermia. Seek medical direction and follow local protocols.
3. **d.** Handle the patient gently. Keep the patient supine to improve blood flow to the brain. Ventilation of the patient is indicated at a normal rate; unnecessary hyperventilation can cause cardiac complications.

CASE STUDY 4

1. **c.** The signs and symptoms of early or superficial local cold injury include blanching of the skin, loss of feeling or sensation, continued softness of the skin in the injured area, and a tingling sensation during any rewarming. Swelling and blisters would indicate later or deep cold injury.
2. **a.** Appropriate treatment for this patient includes removal of wet or restrictive clothing, not massaging the area, administering oxygen to maintain a SpO_2 of > 94%, and splinting the area.

3. **b.** You must prevent refreezing of the tissue. Significant tissue loss can occur if the tissue is subjected to refreezing. Use a dry, sterile dressing.

CHAPTER 24 SCENARIO: DOCUMENTATION EXERCISE

1. **c.** Mrs. Holland is most likely suffering from heat stroke, which has a mortality rate that ranges from 20 to 80 percent.
2. **a.** The cooling of Mrs. Holland was appropriately performed.
3. **d.** A combination of factors allowed you to make the decision that Mrs. Holland was a priority transport. The hot air temperature with high humidity; altered mental status; headache; and flushed, hot, and dry skin all played a factor in the decision. However, the presence of hot, dry skin, when combined with the other factors, is most important.
4. **a.** It was appropriate not to provide any cool water for Mrs. Holland to drink. It was contraindicated due to Mrs. Holland's nausea and altered level of consciousness.
5. **b.** An air temperature of 95°F and a relative humidity of 75 percent represent a severe danger on the heat-and-humidity risk scale.

Chapter 25: Submersion Incidents: Drowning and Diving Emergencies

TERMS AND CONCEPTS

1. **a.** 4 **b.** 3 **c.** 1 **d.** 2 **e.** 5. *(p. 713)*

CONTENT REVIEW

1. **b.** Death from drowning is often associated with the use of alcohol. Drowning does not occur only in deep water, and the incidence would be reduced by use of personal flotation devices and supervision at swimming pools. *(p. 714)*
2. **b.** The two major age groups that are at most risk of death from drowning are children less than 5 years of age and teenagers. The third most common group is the elderly. *(p. 715)*
3. **c.** A drowning in which the victim does not aspirate water into the lungs is referred to as a *dry drowning*. *(p. 716)*
4. **b.** The four categories are asymptomatic, symptomatic, cardiac arrest, and obviously dead. A patient with an altered mental status and a persistent cough would be considered symptomatic. *(p. 720)*
5. **c.** Abdominal thrusts should be used on drowning patients only if a foreign body airway obstruction is suspected. *(p. 716)*
6. **c.** Rescue attempts near shore should be tried in this safest-to-riskiest sequence: Reach (by holding out an object), throw (something that floats), row (get a boat), go (wade or swim). Wade or swim only if you meet *all* of the following criteria: You are a good swimmer, you are specially trained in water rescue, you are wearing a personal flotation device, and you are accompanied by other rescuers. *(p. 717)*

7. **a.** An unresponsive patient found in shallow water should be suspected of having a spinal injury. (The other choices are also possible, but spinal injury should be your primary suspicion.) *(p. 728)*

8. **c.** Attempt resuscitation with full efforts. (Young patients submerged in cold water (68°F) for 30 minutes or longer have been resuscitated.) Some experts advise resuscitation for every drowning patient, regardless of water temperature. Resuscitation efforts should always be performed in an "all-or-none" manner. Resuscitate the patient fully or don't resuscitate the patient. So-called "show codes" or "slow codes" are not appropriate. *(p. 719)*

9. **d.** Differences between salt-water and fresh-water drowning play no role in the goals and techniques of resuscitation. Approximately the same amount of surfactant is washed out in either case, and they result in the same incidence of respiratory distress. *(p. 716)*

10. **c.** Mammalian diving reflex. *(p. 718)*

11. **c.** Scuba diving emergencies are increasing in incidence along with the popularity of the sport. They do not occur only near oceans; a diver can be far from the ocean by airplane before symptoms occur. Scuba divers can drown. Scuba emergencies may be managed by the EMT as well as the paramedic. *(p. 723)*

12. **a.** Boyle's law states that at a constant temperature, the volume of a gas is inversely related to the pressure. *(p. 725)*

13. **a.** Decompression sickness results from bubbles formed by the expansion of nitrogen in the blood. These can act as emboli and block circulation but do not reduce oxyhemoglobin loading. Instead, they compress or stretch the blood vessels or nerves. Decompression sickness is exacerbated by high altitudes and is more likely to occur in cold water than in warm water. *(p. 725)*

14. **c.** The joint where the pain associated with decompression sickness is most commonly experienced is the shoulder, beginning as a mild pain and gradually increasing. *(p. 726)*

15. The chart showing signs and symptoms associated with the three categories of decompression sickness should be filled out as follows. *(pp. 726–727)*

Sign or Symptom	Type 1 DCS	Type 2 DCS	AGE
Pain in joints or tendons	X	X	X
Low back pain		X	
Skin rash, itching	X	X	X
Altered mental status		X	
Substernal burning sensation on inhalation		X	
Dyspnea		X	X
Headache, visual disturbance		X	X
Bloody sputum		X	X
Nausea and vomiting		X	X

16. **b.** Occurs during ascent or descent when air pressure in the body's cavities becomes too great. *(p. 727)*

CASE STUDY 1

1. **d.** Begin resuscitation at once! (Let's hope you didn't have to think much about this one!)

2. **b.** All the clues to possible spinal injury are present. You found the patient at the shallow end of the pool. The patient has a laceration on her forehead. These are signs that she may have dived into the pool and struck her head. Observed bleeding is minor. Checking for gastric distention may be necessary if positive pressure ventilations are noted to be ineffective. This patient is not breathing on her own, so administering oxygen by a non-rebreather mask is not appropriate.

3. **d.** Gastric distention occurs when the stomach fills with water (during submersion) or air (during artificial ventilation). The air or water in the stomach may put enough pressure on the diaphragm and lungs to interfere with the ability to ventilate the patient. If the patient is immobilized by this point in treatment, roll the immobilized patient on her side and, with suction equipment immediately available (because the patient is likely to regurgitate stomach contents), gently press on the epigastric region to relieve the distention. Suction the mouth and nose and then

resume ventilation efforts. If the patient is not yet immobilized, roll her on her left side with manual stabilization of her spine and perform the procedures described earlier.

CASE STUDY 2

1. **d.** Complications from near-drowning can occur up to 72 hours after the incident. Even though this patient looks well now, he must be transported for evaluation by a physician.
2. **b.** Administer oxygen to maintain an SpO_2 of > 94%, monitor carefully, and transport on his left side to allow drainage in case he vomits.
3. **b.** This patient would be placed in the symptomatic category.

CHAPTER 25 SCENARIO: DOCUMENTATION EXERCISE

1. **c.** Scene information and primary assessment indicate that treatment and management of this patient should be focused on drowning, hypothermia, and traumatic injuries.
2. **a.** Stimulation of the mammalian diving reflex initiates a protective mechanism that includes spasms of the larynx to inhibit entry of water, or other substances, into the respiratory tract.
3. **c.** As a result of the very cold water, the body temperature was lowered and body processes slowed. This process helps to decrease the damage normally expected in a normothermic patient.
4. **a.** Removing the patient from the cold environment should be included in the initial management steps.
5. **c.** A drowning patient can develop complications that lead to death as long as 72 hours after the incident. Approximately 15 percent of all drowning-related deaths result from secondary complications.

Chapter 26: Behavioral Emergencies

TERMS AND CONCEPTS

1. **a.** 7 **b.** 1 **c.** 9 **d.** 4 **e.** 2 **f.** 3 **g.** 8 **h.** 6 **i.** 5 **j.** 10. *(p. 730)*

CONTENT REVIEW

1. **a.** N **b.** Y **c.** N **d.** Y **e.** N **f.** Y **g.** Y. *(pp. 732–733)*
2. **a.** A panic attack is a discrete period of intense fear or discomfort. Panic attacks often have a sudden onset that rapidly builds to a peak usually lasting 10 minutes or less. Patients often hyperventilate (breathe too deeply), which causes physical symptoms such as dizziness, tingling around the mouth and fingers, spasms of the hands and feet (carpal-pedal spasms), tremors, irregular heartbeat, palpitations (rapid or intense heartbeat), diarrhea, and sometimes feelings of choking, smothering, or shortness of breath. *(p. 733)*
3. **c.** Deep feelings of sadness and worthlessness accompanied by fatigue, loss of appetite,

and a sense of hopelessness may be due to depression. Depression also often causes severe anhedonia, which is a loss of interest in activities of pleasure that the patient may have previously enjoyed. *(p. 734)*
4. **b.** Schizophrenia is a chronic mental illness in which a patient does not return to his or her premorbid level of functioning. Patients with this illness suffer debilitating distortions of speech and thought, bizarre delusions, hallucinations, social withdrawal, catatonic behavior, and lack of emotional expressiveness. *(p. 735)*
5. **a.** Y **b.** N **c.** Y **d.** Y **e.** Y **f.** N **g.** Y **h.** Y. *(p. 735)*
6. **d.** When dealing with behavioral emergencies, it is important to understand that all individuals are susceptible to emotional injury, but each person has the ability to be resilient. All individuals are affected, in some way, by disaster or injury. An emotional injury is just as real as a physical injury. *(p. 736)*
7. **a.** Careful and complete documentation is your best protection against legal problems. *(p. 746)*
8. **b.** Never attempt restraint until you have sufficient help and an appropriate plan. (Effective teamwork is more important than strength. Use only the minimal amount of force needed. Metal cuffs should not be used. Act quickly; surprise is a key element.) *(pp. 743–744)*
9. **c.** The first priority in dealing with a behavioral emergency is to protect yourself and others from harm. Safety is of the utmost importance. *(p. 738)*
10. Only **d, e, f,** and **h** should be marked. Appropriate treatment for a behavioral emergency includes not making quick movements, not playing along with visual or auditory disturbances, letting the patient decide if he wants to involve family or friends, and not leaving the patient alone. The other choices are not appropriate treatments for a behavioral emergency. *(pp. 737–738)*
11. **c.** Agitated delirium is associated with drug use, especially cocaine, methamphetamine, and other CNS stimulants. The patient presents with unusual strength, high tolerance to pain, agitation, hostility, frenzied and bizarre behavior, hot and diaphoretic skin, and unusual speech patterns. *(p. 736)*
12. **c.** Agoraphobia is anxiety about being in places or situations from which escape would be difficult or help may not be available. Just the thought of leaving the home can cause impending fear and often causes individuals to avoid specific social situations. *(p. 733)*
13. **a.** Dystonia is a movement disorder that causes involuntary contractions of muscles resulting in twisting and repetitive movements that are sometimes painful. *(p. 732)*

1. **d.** Your first action should be to scan the scene for potential hazards.
2. **a.** You should always maintain eye contact and speak calmly. Never play along with visual or auditory disturbances or leave the patient alone. Always be truthful.
3. **c.** Your partner should keep you in his line of sight, be alert that the patient may become violent, try to obtain additional information, and try to disperse bystanders.
4. En route to the hospital, you should explain what you're going to do and seek his permission, then obtain vital signs and complete the secondary assessment. Continue talking quietly with Jim, and answer his questions honestly, but do not create false expectations.

CHAPTER 26 SCENARIO: DOCUMENTATION EXERCISE

1. **c.** When managing a patient who has made a suicide attempt, the EMT's primary concern is to manage any injuries or medical conditions related to the suicide attempt.
2. **a.** Yes, Mrs. Raunecker was at great risk for following through on her suicide threat. She had numerous risk factors, including the recent death of her husband, loss of a job, depression, and previous suicide threats.
3. **a.** In questioning Mrs. Raunecker, you avoided the use of "yes" or "no" questions. Instead, you used open-ended questions, which allowed Mrs. Raunecker to express her feelings freely.
4. **d.** The interview with Mrs. Raunecker should have been conducted in a quiet surrounding with limited people present.
5. **c.** The search of Mrs. Raunecker's home was appropriate, given the circumstances.

Chapter 27: Trauma Overview: The Trauma Patient and the Trauma System

TERMS AND CONCEPTS

1. **a.** 1   **b.** 7   **c.** 4   **d.** 6   **e.** 3   **f.** 8   **g.** 5   **h.** 2   **i.** 9. (*pp. 751–753*)

CONTENT REVIEW

1. **d.** Mass and velocity. (*p. 751*)
2. **c.** Velocity is the most significant factor. (Review the formula for calculating kinetic energy. Notice that if you double the mass, you double the amount of kinetic energy. However, if you double the speed, the kinetic energy produced is four times as great.) (*p. 751*)
3. **d.** Acceleration. (Deceleration is the rate at which a body in motion decreases its speed.) (*p. 752*)
4. **c.** The typical vehicular collision involves three impacts: the vehicle collision (it strikes an object), the body collision (it strikes the inside of the vehicle), and the organ collision (they strike the inside surface of the body). (*p. 752*)
5. **b.** Falls account for over half of all trauma incidents. (*p. 762*)
6. **a.** Vehicular collisions account for over one-third of all deaths due to trauma. (*p. 762*)
7. **c.** The groups that are most likely to suffer injury from air bag deployment are short adults (less than 5'2"), older adults, and infants and children less than 12 years of age. (*p. 753*)
8. **a.** In a motor vehicle collision, the "up and over" and "down and under" pathways are examples of injury patterns associated with a frontal impact. (*p. 754*)
9. **c.** When a passenger's head strikes the car windshield, the glass may crack in a typical "spiderweb" pattern. This is the term frequently used to describe the crack pattern caused by a vehicle occupant's head striking the windshield. (*p. 755*)
10. **b.** A rear-end impact. (*p. 757*)
11. **c.** A lateral impact. (*p. 757*)
12. **a.** Injuries due to rotational or rollover impact can create multiple-system injury and possible ejection if the patient was unrestrained. (*p. 754*)
13. **c.** Children turn toward the vehicle; adults turn away. (*p. 759*)
14. **b.** Femur, chest, abdomen, and head. (Because a child is small and has a low center of gravity, he is likely to be struck high on the body, then thrown in front of the vehicle and run over.) (*p. 759*)
15. **d.** In a collision, a seat belt worn too low can cause hip dislocations or fractures, not lower-leg fractures. Properly applied lap belts and shoulder straps don't prevent lateral head movement, and air bags don't work well in multiple-collision events. A deployed air bag should be lifted from the steering wheel so that the steering wheel can be checked for deformity. (*p. 760*)
16. **d.** Leg burns are the most likely injury from the list provided. "Laying the bike down" is an evasive action meant to prevent ejection or separation of a motorcycle rider from his bike. Abrasions and burns are most likely, although a wide variety of injuries is possible. (*p. 761*)
17. **c.** 20, 10. (*p. 761*)
18. **b.** Three times his height. (*p. 762*)
19. **a.** Between the nipple line and the waist. (*p. 764*)
20. **b.** Blasts and explosions. (*p. 764*)
21. **c.** You should have an increased index of suspicion for serious injury when you find intrusion of greater than 12 inches for the occupant site or greater than 18 inches anywhere to the vehicle. Intrusion of the vehicle is deformity occurring to the interior compartment. The occupant site is anywhere in the vehicle where the patient is riding. (*p. 754*)
22. **a.** "Golden period" better reflects a concept that severely injured trauma patients have the

best chance of survival if surgical intervention takes place as quickly as possible from the time of injury. *(p. 765)*

23. **b.** The patient assessment, emergency care for life threats, and patient preparation for transport should all be accomplished within 10 minutes of arriving on the scene. *(p. 766)*

24. **d.** Sensory or motor deficit is an indication for an on-scene time of 10 minutes or less and rapid transport to the trauma hospital. Other indications are a GCS score of less than 14, a respiratory rate less than 10 or greater than 29/minute, and two or more proximal long-bone fractures. *(p. 764, Table 27-1)*

25. **c.** Level I,   **a.** Level II,   **b.** Level III,   **d.** Level IV. *(p. 766)*

26. **a.** Consider the application of the PASG for decompensated shock (SBP 90 mmHg) associated with suspected pelvic fracture, intra-abdominal bleeding, or retroperitoneal bleeding. *(p. 767)*

27. **d.** To prevent or reverse shock, you must stop the bleeding as quickly as possible. This is done by direct pressure. If this is not effective, a tourniquet is then applied. *(p. 769)*

28. **d.** If you identify a major bleed (arterial or venous) during the general impression, you must first control the bleeding prior to moving on in the assessment. Not deviating from a sequence when presented with obvious life threats may contribute to the deterioration of the patient. *(p. 769)*

29. **a.** Backboards can serve to secure suspected fractures in an unstable patient who requires rapid transport. En route, if time or the patient's condition permits, further stabilization of fractures can be accomplished through splinting. Taking the time at the scene to splint suspected fractures will delay transport and may contribute to the deterioration of the patient. *(p. 769)*

CASE STUDY 1

1. **a.** An occupant of the same car was killed. Significant forces are involved in this accident. Carefully assess and monitor this patient for any injuries.

2. **b.** Along with high speed and death of another vehicle occupant, altered mental status is one of the factors that call for a high suspicion of significant mechanism of injury. You need to assess her mental status and monitor it carefully.

CASE STUDY 2

1. **d.** Knowing how the patient struck the ground will help you determine how the energy dissipated and what potential injuries resulted. The severity of trauma depends on the distance of the fall, the type of surface, and the body part that impacted first.

2. **b.** In a feet-first fall with knees locked, energy will travel all the way up the skeleton. When the patient is thrown forward, it may also cause a Colles fracture, a fracture of the wrist that occurs when the patient tries to break his fall.

CASE STUDY 3

1. **c.** The patient with a penetrating injury between the nipple and waist requires evaluation for both a potential abdominal and chest injury. Lung tissue is relatively tolerant of cavitation caused by projectiles, a pneumothorax is a common result of injury to the chest, and the presence of rib fracture is highly likely in this patient.

2. **a.** It is critical to look for an exit wound and treat it if there is one. Obviously, the wound should not be probed, and an antiseptic solution should not be poured into the wound. Provide oxygen to maintain an SpO_2 of > 95%, inspect for a sucking chest wound, and quickly seal the wound.

Chapter 28: Bleeding and Soft Tissue Trauma

MEDICAL TERMINOLOGY

1. **c.** Away from.
2. **a.** To pull.
3. **a.** Skin.
4. **d.** Blood.
5. **b.** Skin.
6. **b.** Dripping, trickling.
7. **a.** Blood.

TERMS AND CONCEPTS

1. **a.** 8 **b.** 6 **c.** 5 **d.** 1 **e.** 10 **f.** 2 **g.** 4 **h.** 7 **i.** 9 **j.** 3. *(pp. 788–791, 793–795)*

CONTENT REVIEW

1. **a.** 2 **b.** 3 **c.** 1. *(p. 772)*

2. **a.** Severe external bleeding should be controlled only after (or simultaneously with) ensuring an airway and breathing. *(p. 773)*

3. **c.** The first step in controlling severe bleeding is to apply direct pressure, then use a tourniquet. *(p. 776)*

4. **a.** A vessel that is cut across (perpendicular to) itself will have a tendency to retract and clot off. A cut along the length of the vessel will have a tendency to open wider when it contracts. *(p. 773)*

5. **d.** A tourniquet is used to control bleeding when direct pressure fails to control the bleeding. *(p. 776)*

6. **c.** If the breathing is adequate, you should provide oxygen via a nonrebreather mask at 15 lpm. If the breathing is inadequate, you should immediately provide positive pressure ventilation with a BVM and supplemental oxygen. Maintain the SpO_2 at 95% or greater. *(p. 778)*

7. Causes of internal bleeding include blunt trauma, abnormal clotting, rupture of a blood vessel or vascular structure, and certain fractures. *(p. 779)*

8. **c.** Estimate the severity of internal bleeding based on the signs and symptoms. *(p. 779)*

9. **d.** Hemostatic agents to control bleeding are designed as a dressing that promotes clotting and as an agent poured directly onto the wound. They have shown dramatic results when applied to wounds with major arterial and venous bleeding. They are used with a pressure dressing to control arterial or venous bleeding and are usually reserved for prolonged transport times. *(pp. 777–778)*

10. **d.** Epidermis, dermis, subcutaneous layer. *(p. 785)*

11. **b.** 1, 2, 4. Aids in the elimination of water and various salts. Serves as a sensory receptor organ (senses heat, cold, touch, pressure, and pain). Protects the body from the environment. The white blood cells are produced by bone marrow. *(p. 785)*

12. **b.** An amputation is an open injury. Contusions and hematomas are closed injuries. A crush injury may be either open or closed. *(pp. 787–790)*

13. **b.** The hemostatic dressing may have fibrinogen and thrombin, chitosan, and other substances on the surface of the dressing, which promotes clotting and stops bleeding when applied to wounds. *(p. 777)*

14. **c.** Take Standard Precautions before approaching any patient. Assess the airway, breathing, oxygenation, and circulation. Treat for shock, if necessary. Then splint fractures. *(p. 786)*

15. **d.** Occlusive. *(p. 793)*

16. **b.** On three sides only, to allow air to escape as the patient exhales. *(p. 793)*

17. **c.** The statement is true. *(p. 793)*

18. **a.** 2, 4, 3, 1. Secure the object manually. Expose the wound area. Control bleeding. Use a bulky dressing to help stabilize the object. (An impaled object should never be removed in the field, unless it is through the cheek or impaled in the neck and is obstructing airflow through the trachea.) *(p. 794)*

19. **a.** Never place the part directly on ice or on an ice pack since this may cause tissue damage to the amputated part. *(p. 794)*

20. **a.** Occlusive dressings will help prevent air from entering the wound and the bloodstream or tissue. *(p. 793)*

21. To apply a pressure dressing: (a) Cover the wound with several sterile gauze dressings. (b) Apply direct pressure until bleeding is controlled. (c) Bandage firmly to create enough pressure to maintain control of bleeding. Check distal pulses to be sure the bandage is not too tight. (d) If blood soaks through the original dressing and bandages, remove and apply direct fingertip pressure. *(p. 775)*

22. **c.** Distal pulses, motor function, and sensory function. (Bandages should be snug, not tight. To be sure the bandage is not interfering with circulation, always check distal pulses and motor and sensory function before and after bandage application.) *(p. 793)*

23. **a.** Sterile, moist gauze and then an occlusive dressing. (Avoid absorbent materials that could adhere to organs.) *(p. 793)*

24. **c.** It reduces the tension on the abdominal muscles and will make the patient more comfortable. *(p. 794)*

25. **c.** The most dangerous bites are those that occur over a vascular area, which can cause major bleeding and serious infections. *(p. 791)*

26. **d.** Breaking the jar may cause a severe laceration and bleeding. All the other answers are appropriate treatments. *(p. 775)*

CASE STUDY 1

1. **c.** Venous bleeding. (The bleeding from the patient's neck is dark red and flows steadily.)

2. **a.** For a large open neck wound, place your gloved hand over the wound, then apply an occlusive dressing, and finally apply a pressure dressing.

CASE STUDY 2

1. **b.** With any penetrating chest injury, also suspect a spinal injury.

2. **d.** Given the number of shots fired, and in any case of a shooting, you need to look for additional entry and exit wounds.

CHAPTER 28 SCENARIO: DOCUMENTATION EXERCISE

1. **c.** The laceration occurred on the right side of the neck and produced dark red blood that flowed steadily. This would likely be from an affected jugular vein in the carotid area. If an artery had been affected, it would likely produce bright red blood that would spurt with each contraction of the heart.

2. **a.** The gloved hand will help prevent air from being sucked into the vein and carried to the heart, which can be lethal. Bleeding control and prevention of an air embolism are major goals when treating this type of injury.

3. **d.** After applying your gloved hand over the wound to control the bleeding, you should apply an occlusive dressing. This dressing should extend beyond all the wound edges and be taped on all four sides. After you have applied the occlusive dressing, you should next apply a regular dressing. Apply only enough pressure to control the bleeding. A circumferential pressure dressing may compress the major blood vessels in the neck.

4. **b.** If blood has soaked through the original pressure dressing, indicating that the severe bleeding has continued, you should remove all of the original bandages and then apply direct fingertip pressure. After the bleeding is controlled, apply a dressing and bandage the wound.

5. **c.** You should immediately wrap the amputated part in sterile gauze. Keep the part dry by placing the part in a plastic bag and keep cool.

Chapter 29: Burns

TERMS AND CONCEPTS

1. **a.** 5 **b.** 3 **c.** 2 **d.** 1 **e.** 6 **f.** 4. *(pp. 811–815)*

CONTENT REVIEW

1. Functions of the skin include (1) providing a barrier against infection, (2) providing protection from harmful agents in the environment and injury, (3) aiding in the regulation of body temperature, (4) sensation transmission (hot, cold, pain, touch), (5) aiding in elimination of some body wastes, and (6) containing fluids necessary to the functioning of other organs and systems. *(p. 812)*
2. **a.** Body surface area. *(p. 813)*
3. **a.** Superficial (first-degree) burn. *(p. 814)*
4. **b.** The patient who has sustained a deep partial-thickness burn will present with red and blanched white skin. Other signs and symptoms may include thick-walled blisters that often rupture. The patient can still feel pressure at the site. There is poor capillary refill to the burn site. All of the other answers in this question are signs and symptoms of superficial partial-thickness burn. *(p. 815)*
5. **b.** Partial-thickness (second-degree) burn. *(p. 815)*
6. **c.** Burns to the face are considered critical because of the potential for respiratory compromise or injury to the eyes. *(p. 815)*
7. **d.** A fourth-degree burn is often caused by electrical injuries and extends completely through the epidermis and dermis and deep into the muscles, blood vessels, and nerves. *(p. 815)*
8. **b.** In a child, partial-thickness burns of 10–20 percent BSA are considered moderate. *(p. 816)*
9. **c.** Children under age 5 and adults over age 55 have less tolerance for burn injuries. Because of relatively larger skin surfaces (in relation to body mass), children have the potential for greater fluid loss. Older adults have prolonged and possibly impaired healing processes. *(p. 816)*
10. Emergency care for burn injuries includes: (a) Remove the patient from the source of the burn, and stop the burning process. (b) Assess airway, breathing, and mental status. (c) Classify the severity of the burn, and transport immediately if critical. (d) Cover the burned area with a dry, sterile dressing (if greater than 10 percent BSA). (e) Keep the patient warm and treat other injuries as needed. (f) Transport to the appropriate facility. *(p. 821)*
11. **a.** The rule of nines is not applied to superficial burns. The rule of nines is applied to superficial partial-thickness burns, deep partial-thickness burns, and full-thickness burns. *(p. 817)*
12. **b.** Separate burned fingers or toes with dry, sterile dressings to prevent adherence of burned areas. *(p. 822)*
13. **c.** Always apply a dry, sterile dressing to *both* eyes because the eyes move simultaneously, and if the patient moves the unburned eye, the burned eye will move, too. (Reassure the patient and keep him informed about what is going on.) *(p. 822)*
14. **b.** Dry chemicals should be brushed off before flushing with water. *(p. 823)*
15. **d.** A contact burn occurs from contact with a hot object like the exhaust pipe of a vehicle. A flame burn occurs when there is contact with an open flame. A flash burn is a type of flame burn that usually results from a flammable gas or liquid that quickly ignites. Hot gases may also cause upper-airway burns when inhaled. *(p. 818)*
16. **c.** In electrical burns, all tissue between entry and exit wounds is suspect for injury. *(p. 829)*
17. **a.** Direct blood loss from an associated external hemorrhage or internal hemorrhage. Fluid losses are usually not critical in the early hours of a burn; this patient was burned minutes prior to your arrival on scene. *(p. 813)*
18. **b.** Burns increase the capillary permeability, which leads to fluid leaking from the cells into the area between the cells, causing an extreme loss in fluid. This loss of fluid can lead to a decreased blood flow to the kidneys, which can cause a buildup of wastes in the blood. *(p. 813)*
19. **d.** Gastrointestinal dysfunction may be caused by decreased, not increased, blood flow to that system. Leakage of fluid from body cells will cause severe edema. Circumferential burns to the chest can prevent the chest from expanding fully. Scarring from burns can cause long-term muscle wasting and joint dysfunction. *(p. 813)*

CASE STUDY

1. **b.** Cut around the area. Do not attempt to remove the adhered portion, since this may cause further damage to the soft tissues.
2. **c.** Singed nasal hair may be an indication of a compromised airway. Provide oxygen via a nonrebreather mask at 15 lpm with an SpO_2 reading of less than 94% if inhalation of toxic gases is suspected. If breathing becomes inadequate, use positive pressure ventilations with supplemental oxygen. (The child's loud crying indicates that breathing is still adequate.)
3. **c.** Using the rule of nines, approximately 14 percent of the child's body surface area is affected by the burn. Any partial-thickness burn affecting from 10 to 20 percent of the body surface area should be considered moderate in a child. It is considered critical because the foot is involved.
4. **b.** Use sterile, dry dressings on the burn, and keep the patient warm. (Remember that the heat regulation function of burned skin is impaired.)

1. **d.** A scald occurs when the patient comes in contact with a hot liquid. The more viscous the liquid, the more severe the burn because of increased contact time. Smothering the flames while the pan was on the stove with a lid or fire extinguisher could have prevented this burn.

2. **b.** The deep partial-thickness burn (second degree) is characterized by thick-walled blisters, of which some may have ruptured. The burned area is red with blanched white patches, and there is poor capillary refill to the burn site. The patient can still feel pressure at the site.

3. **c.** This patient's burns included the anterior trunk, 18 percent; bilateral anterior legs, 18 percent (9 percent for the anterior portion of each leg); and genitalia area, 1 percent, for a total of 37 percent BSA.

4. **a.** This patient's burns are considered critical because they comprise over 20 percent deep partial-thickness burns. This patient's burns are 37 percent deep partial-thickness burns; she should be treated rapidly and transported without delay to an appropriate facility.

5. **b.** A dry, sterile, particle-free dressing should be used on this burn. A wet or moist dressing may cause the patient to become hypothermic. You must not apply creams. Do not apply dressings that are not particle free. Cotton or paper-type dressings may contaminate the burned area with particles and complicate the treatment and healing process.

Chapter 30: Musculoskeletal Trauma and Nontraumatic Fractures

TERMS AND CONCEPTS

1. **a.** 6 **b.** 1 **c.** 3 **d.** 2 **e.** 5 **f.** 4 **g.** 7. (*p. 833*)

CONTENT REVIEW

1. **b.** Produces platelets. (This is a function of the circulatory system.) (*p. 834*)
2. The six basic components of the skeletal system are (1) skull, (2) spinal column, (3) thorax, (4) pelvis, (5) lower extremities, and (6) upper extremities. (*p. 834*)
3. **c.** Direct, indirect, and twisting. (*p. 837*)
4. **d.** Pulselessness and cyanosis. (*p. 840*)
5. **d.** A fracture to the femur or pelvis is considered a critical injury and must be managed to both immobilize the bones and reduce the associated bleeding. (*p. 839*)
6. 4, 3, 1, 2. The additional steps should be performed in the following order of priority: (1) Immobilize the patient to a spine board. (2) Initiate transport. (3) Perform further management of the life-threatening injuries and ongoing assessments every five minutes. (4) Splint the injured extremity. (*p. 842*)

7. **b.** An open injury. (*p. 841*)
8. Signs and symptoms of bone and joint injury include deformity or angulation, pain and tenderness, grating or crepitus, swelling, disfigurement, severe weakness and loss of function, bruising, exposed bone ends, and joint locked into position. (*p. 840*)
9. **c.** A fracture to the femur bleeds heavily. Application of a traction splint will help to pull the bone in line and reduce the diameter of the thigh. This allows less blood to collect, thereby indirectly putting pressure on the bleeding bones. (*p. 839*)
10. **c.** When in doubt, splint. Pain, swelling, and deformity are signs and symptoms of a possible fracture. (*p. 846*)
11. **c.** Check distal pulses, motor function, and sensation before and after splinting and during the ongoing assessment. (*p. 849*)
12. **a.** The joints above and below the injury site. (*p. 840*)
13. **a.** The PASG performs two functions: It stabilizes the fracture, and it decreases the compartment in which the pelvis can bleed. (*p. 848*)
14. **b.** Make one attempt at aligning the extremity. (Follow local protocol.) If pain, resistance, or crepitus increase, stop. (*p. 844*)
15. **b.** Never intentionally replace protruding bones or push them back below the skin. (*p. 844*)
16. **d.** The improvised splint should be padded so that the inner surfaces are not in contact with the skin. It should also be light in weight, firm, and rigid; long enough to extend past the joints above and below the site; and as wide as the thickest part of the injured limb. (*p. 847*)
17. **b.** Shoulder injury. (The sling supports the arm, and the swathe holds it against the side of the chest.) (*p. 856*)
18. **d.** The position of function for a hand is fingers curled as if holding a ball. A roll of bandage in the hand can support this position. (*p. 848*)
19. **c.** Use a traction splint if the thigh is painful, swollen, or deformed. You do not have to be certain that the femur has actually been fractured. However, do not apply a traction splint if there is injury to the hip, pelvis, or knee or within 1–2 inches of the knee because the traction could aggravate these injuries. (*p. 848*)
20. **c.** It pulls on the thigh and realigns the broken femur. This helps relieve pain and reduces movement of the broken bone ends. (*p. 848*)
21. **b.** If the foot or ankle is injured, having the patient push down and pull back with the great (big) toe will give you the same results as if the entire foot was tested. (*p. 848*)
22. **d.** The PASG is an effective device that can be used to splint the pelvis and decrease the compartment size to reduce bleeding. Another splint used for the suspected pelvic fracture is a folded-sheet improvised pelvic wrap. There are also

commercially produced devices used to splint the pelvis in the same manner as the pelvic wrap. *(p. 839)*

23. **a.** If the pressure in the space around the capillaries exceeds the pressure needed to perfuse the tissues, the blood flow is cut off, and the cells become hypoxic, leading to compartment syndrome. *(p. 849)*

24. **d.** A pathologic fracture results from a disease that causes degeneration and weakens the bone and makes it prone to fracture. *(p. 849)*

25. **c.** Osteoporosis is a condition that dramatically weakens the bones and makes them susceptible to fracture. Osteoporosis typically affects women more than men and occurs most often after menopause. *(p. 837)*

26. **a.** A strain usually occurs with overstretching or tearing of muscle fibers and causes pain that typically increases with the muscle use. A sprain is an injury to a joint capsule, with damage to or tearing of the connective tissue and usually involves ligaments. A dislocation is the displacement of a bone from its normal position in a joint. A fracture involves the breaking of a bone. *(p. 837)*

27. Pain—Pain may be on palpation (tenderness), with movement, or without movement.
Pallor—The skin distal to the injury site may be pale and capillary refill delayed if an artery is compressed or torn. If a vein is blocked by the fracture, the distal extremity may appear warm, red (flushed), and swollen.
Paralysis—The patient is unable to move the extremity. This may be from nerve, muscle, tendon, or ligament damage.
Paresthesia—The patient may complain of numbness or a tingling sensation. This may indicate nerve damage.
Pressure—The patient may complain of a pressure sensation within the extremity. This may be associated with swelling from damaged tissue or blood loss within the muscle and surrounding structures.
Pulses—The pulse distal to the injury may be absent or have a decrease in amplitude. This may indicate damage to an arterial vessel. *(p. 841)*

28. **d.** Nontraumatic fractures will not present with obvious evidence of trauma to the area of fracture, such as contusions, abrasions, lacerations, and hematomas. These patients usually have a history of cancer or osteoporosis. *(p. 849)*

CASE STUDY 1

1. **b.** Remember to check pulses, motor function, and sensation before and after splinting. (Apply a sling and swathe after checking PMS.)

2. **c.** Sensation is intact if the patient can tell you, without looking, which finger or toe you are touching.

3. **b.** The energy from the impact of this patient's hand with the ground travels up the arm and causes an injury to the collarbone (clavicle). This is a classic example of an injury caused by indirect force.

CASE STUDY 2

1. **c.** Do not release traction until after the splint has been applied.

2. **a.** Assess the pedal or posterior tibial pulse for a lower extremity, and assess the radial pulse for an upper extremity.

CASE STUDY 3

1. **a.** Paresthesia, or tingling, may indicate some loss of sensation.

2. **b.** The position of function is with the foot bent at the normal angle to the leg, not pushed downward or upward toward the shin or otherwise manipulated into an unnatural position.

3. **c.** If the injury involves a lower extremity, motor function is intact if the patient can tighten the kneecap and move the foot up and down as if pumping a gas pedal.

CHAPTER 30 SCENARIO: DOCUMENTATION EXERCISE

1. **d.** Crepitus is the sound or feeling of broken fragments of bone grinding against each other. Atelectasis is the condition in which the lungs are collapsed or airless. Eupnea describes good or normal breathing. Kyphosis is the exaggerated curvature or "humpback" appearance of the thoracic spine.

2. **a.** Reducing the diameter of the thigh will allow less blood to accumulate, thereby indirectly putting pressure on the bleeding bone ends.

3. **b.** If your patient is unresponsive or becomes unresponsive, you should apply traction until the injured leg length is the same as the uninjured leg.

4. **d.** You should never elevate the extremity if you suspect a spinal injury. Because of the significant mechanism of injury, you should suspect a possible spinal injury. Applying ice packs will help reduce swelling. Although this was an open fracture, the bone ends have slipped back under the skin before you applied traction. Pulling manual traction while your partner readies the splint is appropriate.

5. **d.** You should evaluate the PMS distal to the injury every 15 minutes to ensure that the splint is not impairing circulation to the extremity.

Chapter 31: Head Trauma

TERMS AND CONCEPTS

1. **a.** 8 **b.** 1 **c.** 10 **d.** 2 **e.** 11 **f.** 3 **g.** 4 **h.** 7 **i.** 9 **j.** 6 **k.** 5 **l.** 12. *(p. 862)*

CONTENT REVIEW

1. **a.** Injury to the brain that results from shearing, tearing, and stretching of nerve fibers is called *diffuse axonal injury*. *(p. 866)*

2. **c.** The single most important sign in cases of suspected head injury is a decreasing mental status. *(p. 871)*

3. **c.** A tool that uses numerical values to carefully monitor a patient's level of consciousness is the Glasgow Coma Scale (GCS). *(p. 871)*

4. **b.** Jaw-thrust maneuver. (This maneuver is performed without tilting the patient's head, which might aggravate a potential spine injury.) *(p. 871)*

5. **d.** The lowest level on the AVPU scale is unresponsiveness; that is, the patient does not respond to any stimulus, indicating the most serious injury. *(p. 871)*

6. **c.** Immediate transport and monitoring. *(p. 872)*

7. **d.** A flexion response or decorticate posturing indicates an upper-level brain stem injury, is considered a nonpurposeful response, and results in the flexing of arms across the chest and extension of the legs, and sometimes the arching of the back. *(p. 871)*

8. **c.** When managing a patient with a suspected head injury, oxygenation and ventilation are of critical importance because any alteration in oxygenation or ventilation can make a head injury worse. It is critical to determine a baseline mental status so that subsequent comparisons can be made accurately. Any patient who lost consciousness, even if only for a brief period of time, requires evaluation at a hospital. A lowered SpO$_2$ can be a sign of a variety of disorders that interfere with oxygenation, not typically a head injury. *(p. 871)*

9. a, c, and e. Cushing reflex is a triad of three signs that may signal increasing intracranial pressure. The systolic BP may increase significantly, the pulse rate may slow (bradycardia), and the respiratory pattern may be altered (normal, irregular, decreased, or absent). *(p. 874)*

10. **d.** Emergency care of a patient with a serious head injury should include consideration of controlled hyperventilation at 20 ventilations per minute (this is controversial and may not be included in your protocol), avoidance of direct pressure on the skull, critical attention to airway and breathing status, and anticipation of potential seizure activity. *(p. 874)*

11. The chart showing signs and symptoms associated with the four types of brain injury should be filled out as follows. *(pp. 866–868)*

Sign or Symptom	Concussion	Contusion	Subdural Hematoma	Epidural Hematoma
Momentary confusion	X	X		
Abnormal respiratory pattern			X	X
Retrograde and anterograde amnesia	X	X		
Loss of responsiveness followed by a return of responsiveness and then rapid deterioration				X
Weakness or paralysis on one side of the body			X	
Dilation of one pupil			X	
Fixed and dilated pupil				X
Posturing (withdrawal or flexion)				X
Repeated questioning about what happened	X	X		
Increasing systolic blood pressure			X	X
Decreasing pulse rate			X	X
Seizures			X	X
Cushing reflex			X	X
Vomiting	X	X	X	X
Headache	X	X	X	X

12. **a.** A mild form of diffuse axonal injury that presents with an altered mental status and progressively improves is called a *concussion*. *(p. 866)*

13. **b.** A contusion of the brain is usually caused by one of two types of injuries: coup/contrecoup and acceleration/deceleration. *(p. 867)*

14. **d.** This brain injury is typically the result of low-pressure venous bleeding above the tissue of the brain between the dura mater and the arachnoid layer. It is called a *subdural hematoma*. *(p. 867)*

15. **d.** Subdural hematoma is the most common type of head injury. It occurs in 33 percent of

all severe head injuries, is more common in patients older than 60, and is more likely in patients with abnormally long blood-clotting times. *(p. 867)*

16. **b.** The two types of subdural hematomas are acute (rapid onset) and occult (delayed onset). *(p. 867)*

CASE STUDY 1

1. **c.** This patient is exhibiting Cushing reflex, a sign of severe head injury.
2. **b.** The reflex described in question 1, Cushing reflex, consists of a "triad" of signs. These three signs are an increasing systolic blood pressure, slowing pulse, and alteration in respirations.
3. **c.** Or answer b. This patient may be managed by controlled hyperventilation at a rate of 20 per minute. Hyperventilation is controversial and may not be included in your protocol.

CASE STUDY 2

1. **b.** The bruising around Mrs. McDonald's eyes is a late sign of skull fracture called *raccoon sign*.
2. **a.** The bruising over the mastoid area is also a late sign of skull fracture. It is called *Battle sign*.
3. Only **a, b, d, e, f, g,** and **i** should be marked. Treatments that should be provided for Mrs. McDonald include manual in-line stabilization, a cervical spine immobilization device, an oropharyngeal airway, oxygen at 15 lpm, consideration of controlled hyperventilation at 20 per minute (some protocols will not include controlled hyperventilation), immobilization to a spine board, and ongoing evaluation of mental status. The head-tilt/chin-lift maneuver is not appropriate for a potential head injury (use a jaw thrust). Do not pack anything into the ear or nose to stop fluid flow (place a loose dressing over the area), and do not place pressure on a skull deformity.

CHAPTER 31 SCENARIO: DOCUMENTATION EXERCISE

1. **c.** Rolling the patient quickly on his side to suction his airway was an important and critical action to take. Whenever potential obstructions to the airway are noted, they must be removed rapidly.
2. **a.** This patient is most likely suffering from a high-level brainstem injury, as characterized by the flexion (decorticate) posturing that occurred following the application of pain.
3. **d.** Or answer a. This patient may require controlled hyperventilation at a rate of 20 ventilations per minute (controlled hyperventilation is controversial, so check your protocol).
4. **a.** This patient is likely suffering from hypoperfusion from bleeding in a body cavity, as indicated by the abrasion and distention to the patient's abdomen, skin temperature, rapid pulse rate, and weak radial pulse.
5. **c.** The patient's fractured ankle did not require immediate immobilization. Straps and

padding could have been used to stabilize the ankle, so long as the action would not delay transport to a hospital.

Chapter 32: Spinal Column and Spinal Cord Trauma

TERMS AND CONCEPTS

1. **a.** 4   **b.** 3   **c.** 1   **d.** 2. *(p. 881)*
2. **a.** Cervical spine (first seven vertebrae, which form the neck); **b.** Thoracic spine (the next 12 vertebrae, which form the upper back); **c.** Lumbar spine (the next 5 vertebrae, which form the lower back); **d.** Sacral spine or sacrum (the next 5 vertebrae, which are fused together to form the rigid part of the back side of the pelvis); **e.** Coccyx (the 4 fused vertebrae that form the lower end of the spine). *(p. 883)*

CONTENT REVIEW

1. All should be marked except for **d** and **g**. Assessment findings, mechanisms of injury or types of emergency scenes that should alert you to the possibility of spinal injury include electrical injuries; blunt trauma; falls; motorcycle crashes; gunshot wounds to the head, neck, chest, abdomen, back, or pelvis; hangings; diving accidents; or any unresponsive trauma patient. Heart attacks and asthmatic attacks are medical emergencies unless they also involve a fall or other mechanism of injury. *(p. 888)*
2. **b.** Maintain a high index of suspicion for spinal injury (regardless of the lack of obvious trauma). *(p. 888)*
3. **d.** Distraction is the mechanism of spinal injury that occurs when the vertebrae and spinal cord are stretched or pulled apart, as in a hanging. *(p. 886)*
4. **c.** Priapism (a persistent erection of the penis), if present (in male patients), is a classic sign of cervical spine injury. Diaphragmatic breathing is associated with a cervical spine injury. Never ask a suspected spinal injury patient to move about for any reason. Obvious deformity of the spine upon palpation is an uncommon finding. *(p. 892)*
5. **d.** When assessing for pulse, motor function, and sensory function in the patient with a spine injury, bilaterally check the radial and pedal pulses for presence, strength, and equality. Motor function is assessed in the upper and lower extremities. Upper: flex arms (C6), extend arms (C7), fingers spread (T1), arm push (C7). Lower: push (S1 and S2), pull (L5). Sensory function is tested in each extremity for both pain and light touch. *(p. 891)*
6. **c.** In manual spinal stabilization, the patient's nose is aligned with the navel, with the head neither flexed nor extended. *(p. 893)*
7. **d.** Two rescuers are needed to apply a CSIC, one to stabilize the neck manually and

the other to apply the device. Never use a soft collar; it permits too much movement. The collar by itself does not immobilize the patient. An improperly sized collar can cause more harm to the patient and further aggravate a potential spine injury. *(p. 897)*

8. The chart showing techniques appropriate to immobilizing particular patients should be filled out as shown below. *(pp. 897–898)*

Patient Type	Standing Immobilization Technique	Rapid Extrication	Apply Vest-Type Immobilization Device	Immobilize to Backboard
Standing patient	X			X
Seated patient with critical injuries		X		X
Seated patient with no critical injuries			X	X
Supine or prone patient				X

9. **b, c, d,** and **f** should be marked. Appropriate management techniques for a patient with a spine injury include always immobilizing if in doubt about a spinal injury, establishing manual in-line stabilization as soon as possible, immobilizing the head in the position found if the patient complains of severe neck or spine pain or the head does not easily move, using the jaw-thrust maneuver to initially open the airway, and recording and documenting the pulses and motor and sensory function in all extremities following immobilization. *(pp. 893–894)*

10. **c.** The log roll technique is ideally performed using four rescuers; however, this is not always possible. Padding of all voids between the patient and the board should be performed to avoid extra movement. The CSIC should be placed before moving the patient onto the board. Immobilize the patient's torso to the board before the head. *(p. 898)*

11. 4, 1, 2, 5, 3, 7, 6. (1) Establish and maintain in-line manual stabilization. (2) Apply a cervical spine immobilization collar. (3) Log-roll the patient onto the long spine board. (4) Place pads in the spaces between the patient and the board. (5) Immobilize the patient's torso to the board with straps. (6) Immobilize the patient's head to the board. (7) Secure the patient's legs to the board. *(p. 898)*

12. **b.** Immobilize the patient from a standing position while maintaining alignment. *(p. 898)*

13. **d.** A noncritical seated patient with a possible spine injury should have a CSIC and a short spinal immobilization device applied, and then be transferred to a long spine board. The torso should be secured before the head is secured. *(pp. 898–899)*

14. **c.** Rapid extrication is indicated if the patient's condition is critical, the patient is at a scene that is not safe, or the patient is blocking access to a critical patient. *(p. 899)*

15. **a.** Safe and effective rapid extrication requires constant cervical spine stabilization. *(pp. 899)*

16. **a.** Removal of a helmet should generally not be attempted if the helmet fits well and the patient's condition does not require removal. Removal is obviously necessary if the patient is having breathing difficulties or is in cardiac arrest. Helmet removal can be adequately performed with two rescuers working carefully, and removal is not limited to any specific helmet type. *(p. 900)*

17. **a.** Removing the helmet while leaving the shoulder pads in place may aggravate a cervical spine injury by hyperextending the neck. *(p. 900)*

18. **a.** Spinal shock usually results from injury high in the cervical spine region. *(p. 886)*

19. **b.** Findings associated with neurogenic shock include flushed, dry skin and a pulse rate of 60–80 per minute. *(p. 887)*

20. **a.** Neurogenic shock results in a relative hypovolemia; the same amount of blood is present within a dilated vascular space. The vascular dilation results from the loss of nervous system control. *(p. 887)*

21. **b.** An anterior cord syndrome results in a loss of the ability to feel pain and crude touch and will likely cause the loss of motor function; however, the patient will retain the ability to feel light touch below the site of injury. Central cord syndrome results in a loss of motor function or weakness and loss of pain sensation to the upper extremities while the motor and sensory function may remain normal in the lower extremities. In a case of Brown-Sequard syndrome, the patient will have a loss of motor function and light touch sensation but retain sensation to pain on one side of the body while experiencing a loss of pain on the opposite side but retaining motor function and light touch sensation. *(p. 887)*

22. See the following chart. *(pp. 887–888)*

Findings	Complete Spinal Cord Injury	Anterior Cord Syndrome	Central Cord Syndrome	Brown-Sequard Syndrome
Upper extremity loss of motor and sensory function	X			
Lower extremity loss of motor and sensory function	X			
Loss of bowel and bladder control	X			
Upper extremity weakness or paralysis and loss of pain sensation with motor and sensory functions normal in the lower extremities			X	
Loss of ability to feel pain and crude touch/loss of motor function; retain ability to feel light touch below injury site		X		
Loss of motor function and light touch sensation but retain sensation to pain on one side of the body while experiencing a loss of pain on the opposite side but retaining motor function and light touch sensation				X

CASE STUDY

1. **b.** When immobilizing this patient, prevention of both lateral movement and movement up and down on the board is required. Pad the voids under the head and torso of this patient. A vest-type device is not required, and the EMT should not pad behind the CSIC.
2. **d.** Manual in-line stabilization can be released only after the head has been immobilized properly to the long spine board.
3. **b.** A minimum of three straps should be used to ensure proper immobilization.

CHAPTER 32 SCENARIO: DOCUMENTATION EXERCISE

1. **d.** The injury sustained by Wardell is most likely the result of lateral bending from the car being struck in the passenger side door.
2. **c.** Improper management and stabilization of Wardell's injury could produce three major complications of spinal injury: inadequate breathing effort, paralysis, and inadequate circulation.
3. **b.** The presence of weakness in Wardell's arms when coupled with normal neurological findings in the lower extremities suggests an

incomplete spinal cord injury (central cord syndrome).

4. **c.** Following immobilization with the short spinal immobilization device, Wardell should be placed on the long spine board. You and Carly should reevaluate—for pulse, motor function, and sensory function—following immobilization to the long spine board.
5. **d.** When securing Wardell to the long spine board, straps should be positioned, at a minimum, at the chest, at the hips, and above the knees.

Chapter 33: Eye, Face, and Neck Trauma

TERMS AND CONCEPTS

1. **a.** 3 **b.** 1 **c.** 9 **d.** 7 **e.** 8 **f.** 4 **g.** 2
   h. 6 **i.** 5. *(pp. 924–926)*
2. Labels on the left of the drawing, top to bottom: cornea, conjunctiva, pupil, aqueous humor. Labels in the center, top to bottom: iris, lens, vitreous humor. Labels on the right, top to bottom: retina, sclera. *(p. 925)*

CONTENT REVIEW

1. **c.** When conducting the secondary assessment and physical exam on a patient with an eye injury, check the lids for bruising, swelling, and laceration; the pupils for equality and reactivity to light; and eye movement in all planes of motion (up, down, right, and left). *(p. 928)*

2. **b.** Stabilize the head and neck of the patient with facial trauma before doing anything else. *(p. 934)*

3. **d.** Suspect significant damage to the eye if there is unusual sensitivity to light. Also suspect significant damage if the patient has loss of vision that does not improve with blinking, loses part of the field of vision, has severe pain in the eye, or has double vision. *(p. 928)*

4. **d.** Every patient with an eye injury must be transported (in a supine position) for evaluation by a physician. *(p. 929)*

5. **a.** Attempt to remove foreign objects from the conjunctiva only. All the rest should be removed by a physician. *(p. 929)*

6. **d.** Appropriate management of a lacerated eyelid includes preserving any avulsed skin and transporting with the patient. Cover the eye with a moist, sterile dressing, avoid the application of direct pressure, and cover the uninjured eye as well as the injured eye. *(p. 930)*

7. **b.** A patient with double vision, a marked decrease in vision, and loss of sensation above the eyebrow, over the cheek, or in the upper lip is most likely suffering from an orbital fracture. *(pp. 928, 930)*

8. **a.** Begin treatment of a chemical burn to the eye immediately during the initial assessment. Further delay will increase the injury. *(p. 930)*

9. **d.** Flush for at least 20 minutes. Remember to remove contact lenses, which can trap chemicals. *(p. 929)*

10. **c.** Place the patient with an impaled or extruded eye injury in a supine position with the head immobilized. *(p. 931)*

11. **c.** They can be clearly seen by using a penlight. Contact lenses are worn frequently by people who also wear glasses. They may be worn in one eye only. Contact lenses should be removed in chemical burns of the eyes. *(p. 931)*

12. **a.** Pinch the soft lens between your thumb and index finger, allowing air to get underneath it. (If the lens has dehydrated, run sterile saline across the eye surface, slide the lens off the cornea, and pinch it up.) A suction cup device can be used for hard contacts. *(p. 933)*

13. **a.** When a patient with a painful, deformed, and swollen jaw has dentures that are still intact and in place, the dentures should be left in place. This provides proper alignment of the jaw when treating the injury. *(p. 934)*

14. **a.** Cover the exposed nerves and tendons with a moist, sterile dressing. Any other type of dressing may dry out the nerves and tissues. *(p. 936)*

15. **b.** Rinse an avulsed tooth with saline to remove debris. Never scrub. Transport the tooth in a cup of saline or wrapped in gauze soaked in sterile saline. *(p. 935)*

16. **c.** Push or pull it out in the same direction in which it entered. (If not removed, it could fall into the mouth and obstruct the airway.) *(p. 935)*

17. **c.** Tape it to the outside of the mouth and monitor closely. (Don't insert your fingers; the patient may bite you, and you need your hands for other procedures. Don't have the patient hold the dressing; he may forget or lose responsiveness and let the dressing fall into the airway.) *(p. 935)*

18. **b.** Apply cold compresses to reduce the swelling, and then transport. *(p. 935)*

19. **d.** Clear or bloody fluid draining from the ear may indicate a skull fracture. Place a loose, clean dressing across the opening to absorb the fluids. Do not exert any pressure. *(p. 936)*

20. **c.** To manage a severed blood vessel of the neck, *never* apply pressure to both sides of the neck at the same time; use an occlusive dressing secured with a figure-eight wrap, and position the patient on his left side, head down, for transport. *(p. 942)*

21. **b.** Hyphema is a condition where blood collects in the anterior portion of the eye. *(p. 930)*

22. **c.** Your initial management priorities for injuries to the midface or jaw are to establish manual spinal stabilization, ensure a patent airway, support breathing as necessary, and control life-threatening bleeding. *(p. 935)*

CASE STUDY

1. Yes, paramedic backup should be considered; the patient may need advanced airway procedures.
2. **d.** This is a high-priority patient. Transport immediately and provide emergency care. Meet the paramedics en route.
3. **a.** Immediately begin flushing the eyes with saline. At the same time, place a gloved hand over the neck wound to control bleeding and administer high-concentration oxygen.

CHAPTER 33 SCENARIO: DOCUMENTATION EXERCISE

1. **d.** When assessing Richard's pupils, Prudence should carefully check the pupil in the right eye and then cover both eyes.
2. **b.** The figure-eight bandage, used to hold the occlusive dressing in place, is secured by placing the bandage over the dressing, across one shoulder, across the back, under the opposite armpit, and anchoring it at the shoulder.
3. **b.** Richard's complaints about numbness over his left eye and double vision just after the injury are most likely the result of an injury to the orbit.
4. **d.** Ali should have applied an occlusive dressing to the neck injury to prevent air from being sucked into the wound.
5. **d.** Richard's neck injury is a serious injury and must be carefully observed for swelling and airway compromise.

Chapter 34: Chest Trauma

MEDICAL TERMINOLOGY
1. b. Spitting.
2. d. Good, normal.
3. a. Chest.
4. d. Straight, breathing.
5. b. New opening.

TERMS AND CONCEPTS
1. a. 2 **b.** 4 **c.** 1 **d.** 3 **e.** 5 **f.** 6. *(p. 945)*

CONTENT REVIEW
1. c. The central portion of the chest cavity is called the *mediastinum.* *(p. 946)*
2. a. The parietal pleura is the outermost layer of the pleura and lines the chest cavity. *(p. 946)*
3. b. Jugular vein distention that occurs during inhalation may be a sign of a tension pneumothorax or pericardial tamponade. The increased intrapulmonary pressure created during an inhalation prevents the emptying of the inferior and superior vena cava and results in jugular vein distention during inhalation. *(p. 948)*
4. c. As the pleural space expands, the lung collapses. *(p. 947)*
5. d. A flail segment results from two or more consecutive ribs being fractured in two or more places, creating a freely moving section of the chest wall. *(p. 948)*
6. a. Primary assessment. (Chest injury is potentially life threatening.) *(p. 955)*
7. b. It is an attempt to reduce pain. (Shallow, rapid breathing can be inadequate and can easily lead to hypoxia.) *(p. 955)*
8. d. Subcutaneous emphysema. Gravity pulls fluids and other heavier matter downward, forcing air to flow upward. *(p. 956)*
9. b. When assessing for tracheal deviation, palpate the position of the trachea immediately above the suprasternal notch. Palpation will reveal tracheal deviation before you will be able to notice deviation visually. *(p. 956)*
10. c. By providing positive pressure ventilation, air is forced into the lungs, overriding the need for the patient's chest to create negative pressure to draw the air into the lungs. *(p. 949)*
11. c. In tension pneumothorax, breath sounds will be absent on the injured side and decreased on the uninjured side. (The air on the injured side forces the mediastinum to shift, compressing the cavity on the uninjured side, interfering with inflation of the lung on the uninjured side). *(p. 949)*
12. b. An increasing heart rate, decreasing blood pressure, and increasing respiratory distress *(p. 957)*
13. a. Pulmonary contusion, or bruised lung, is a serious condition usually caused by blunt trauma to the chest, often as a consequence of a flail segment. Bleeding occurs in and around the alveoli and interstitial

space, greatly decreasing the exchange of oxygen and carbon dioxide, leading to hypoxia. *(p. 950)*
14. d. Pericardial tamponade may result from blood filling the sac that surrounds the heart. Since the sac cannot expand, the result is compression of the heart muscle, resulting in the narrowing pulse pressure (the difference between the systolic and diastolic pressures, less than 30 mmHg). *(p. 953)*
15. c. Never completely wrap the chest or apply a swathe snugly. This may hamper normal respiration. Apply a sling and swathe and position the arm over the injured site, have the patient hold a pillow firmly over the injured site, or allow the patient to guard the injury by placing his arm tightly over the injury site. *(p. 954)*
16. b. This condition is referred to as *commotio cordis.* Sudden cardiac arrest from blunt force applied to the precordial area of the anterior chest (center of sternum) is a rare event. It is often seen in young males (mean age is 13 years) with no underlying cardiac disease during sporting events where a projectile such as a baseball strikes the patient in the center of the chest, causing ventricular fibrillation and cardiac arrest (sudden death). *(p. 953)*

CASE STUDY
1. c. Immediately seal the open chest wound with a gloved hand. Any delay will worsen the patient's condition.
2. d. Lift the corner of the occlusive dressing on the chest wound to release air that is potentially trapped and building up in the chest cavity, and transport immediately.

CHAPTER 34 SCENARIO: DOCUMENTATION EXERCISE
1. b. A flail segment is indicated by paradoxical movement.
2. c. Positive pressure ventilations will continue to splint the chest segment by providing internal positive pressure. This patient has a suspected spinal injury and has been placed on a backboard. You should not position the patient on the injured side. Placing a circumferential splint made from a tightly applied swath to the chest may cause more damage and harm the patient by not allowing adequate respirations.
3. c. You should suspect a pneumothorax if resistance develops to positive pressure ventilations. You should ensure that the airway is open by positioning the patient. Other signs that this patient may have developed a tension pneumothorax are that the breathing becomes more labored with severe tachypnea, there is slight cyanosis around his lips, and he has an SpO_2 of 84%.
4. a. A flail segment occurs when two or more consecutive ribs have been fractured in two or more places.

Chapter 35: Abdominal and Genitourinary Trauma

MEDICAL TERMINOLOGY

1. **b.** behind the peritoneum (retro-backward or behind).
2. **a.** body organs.

TERMS AND CONCEPTS

1. **a.** 4, **b.** 1, **c.** 2, **d.** 3 **e.** 5. (*p. 965*)

CONTENT REVIEW

1. H, S, H, S, H, S, H, S. The stomach, gallbladder, Fallopian tubes, and ureters are hollow organs. The others are all solid organs. (*p. 966*)
2. **c.** The duodenum, pancreas, inferior vena cava, aorta, kidneys, and ureters are located in the retroperitoneal space. (*p. 966*)
3. **a.** The major complication associated with the laceration, or tearing, of a solid organ is major bleeding. Remember that a solid organ may bleed into the capsule that surrounds it for some time before the capsule ruptures and allows the blood to spill into the abdominal cavity. (*pp. 967–968*)
4. **c.** The Kehr sign is pain at the tip of the shoulder and occurs in the presence of blood in the peritoneal cavity. (*p. 967*)
5. **c.** Mechanism of injury. (Because signs and symptoms may be subtle, the other choices are less reliable indicators.) (*p. 968*)
6. **d.** Start palpating farthest from the pain. (*p. 969*)
7. **c.** Supine, legs flexed at knees. (*p. 970*)
8. **c.** An appropriate dressing for an abdominal evisceration is a sterile dressing soaked in saline or sterile water, then covered with an occlusive dressing. (*p. 970*)
9. **a.** Apply direct pressure with a moistened sterile compress such as a sanitary pad. (*p. 972*)
10. **a.** Hollow organs contain substances that can be spewed out and cause severe damage or infection. (*p. 966*)
11. **b.** Parietal peritoneum is the outermost layer of the abdominal cavity. (*p. 966*)
12. **c.** The diaphragm separates the abdominal cavity from the thoracic or chest cavity. (*p. 967*)
13. **d.** During exhalation, the diaphragm is located at the nipple line (fourth or fifth intercostal space). Injuries below the nipple line are likely abdominal and not thoracic. (*p. 967*)

CASE STUDY

1. **d.** The best care for the amputated part is to wrap it in a saline-moistened, sterile dressing; put it in a plastic bag; and place the bag on a cold pack or ice that has been wrapped in a towel. (Placing directly on ice may cause tissues to freeze.) Label the bag and transport the part with the patient.
2. **b.** Direct pressure.

CHAPTER 35 SCENARIO: DOCUMENTATION EXERCISE

1. **a.** Treat an abdominal evisceration by applying a saline-soaked sterile dressing first, then covering the dressing with an occlusive dressing or plastic wrap. Aluminum foil should not be used because it may lacerate the protruding organs. Never use absorbent cotton or other material that may cling to the organs.
2. **d.** This patient has a suspected spinal injury and has been placed on a backboard. You should not flex the legs if you suspect a spinal injury.
3. **b.** Bill's shoulder pain may be the result of blood irritating the diaphragm and causing referred pain to the shoulder. This is called the Kehr sign.

Chapter 36: Multisystem Trauma and Trauma in Special Patient Populations

CONTENT REVIEW

1. **c.** Your understanding of the kinematics or the mechanism of injury will help you locate and treat your trauma patient appropriately. (*p. 977*)
2. **a.** Identify and manage life threats. You should control arterial bleeding as soon as you find it, even if it precedes airway and ventilation assessment. (*p. 977*)
3. **d.** You must manage the airway while maintaining cervical spine stabilization. (*p. 984*)
4. **c.** Your immediate action should be to ventilate with the BVM and airway adjunct because this patient is breathing too slow with inadequate tidal volume. (*p. 981*)
5. **a.** Hemoglobin located in the blood carries oxygen to the cells and carbon dioxide from the cell. Loss of blood, and thus hemoglobin, can result in inadequate tissue perfusion and lead to hypoxia and anaerobic metabolism. (*p. 978*)
6. **d.** Any musculoskeletal injuries should be splinted en route if the patient is unstable. Splinting fractures at the scene for a multisystem trauma patient will delay transport to the hospital, which can lead to increased mortality. (*p. 978*)
7. **a.** The pregnant woman's diaphragm elevates, making her susceptible to developing a tension pneumothorax. (*p. 979*)
8. **b.** Supine hypotension can seriously affect the pregnant patient's venous return in the third trimester. This occurs when the fetus presses on the inferior vena cava when the patient is lying supine and flat. To alleviate this from occurring, tilt the backboard to the left. (*p. 979*)
9. **d.** You should immediately assess the pregnant trauma patient for bleeding or crowning. (*p. 979*)

10. **a.** You should transport the mother to the hospital with full resuscitative efforts. Even though the outcome may be poor for the patient in cardiac arrest, it still may be possible to save the fetus. *(p. 979)*

11. **b.** Multiple injuries in different stages of healing may indicate abuse. An isolated fracture, continuous crying, or abrasions to both knees are not indicative of abuse. *(p. 980)*

12. **d.** The pediatric patient's chest wall is more flexible and can mask underlying traumatic injuries. The child's body surface area is greater than the adult's and can lose more heat. The pediatric head is heavy and the neck muscles are less developed. The location of the pediatric patient's internal organs makes them more susceptible to injury. *(p. 978)*

13. **c.** The appearance or consciousness component refers to the child's overall mental status (unresponsive, irritable, alert), body position, and muscle tone. *(p. 981)*

14. **a.** The brachial pulse should be assessed in the pediatric patient less than 1 year of age. *(p. 984)*

15. **c.** Blood pressures are unreliable in pediatric patients if the child is age 3 or less. *(p. 981)*

16. **a.** You should pad the patient who is less than 8 years old. The pad should extend from the shoulders to the hips. This helps prevent flexion of the neck. *(p. 981)*

17. **c.** Stridor or gurgling may indicate an upper airway obstruction. *(p. 981)*

18. **d.** Add padding to fill in the space; this will help support the patient with these special conditions. Never try to force the patient into a neutral position; this can injure the patient further. *(p. 982)*

19. **a.** Including a trusted caregiver may help to gain trust with the patient. Remember that the patient does not know you, but he does have a relationship with his caregiver. *(p. 983)*

CASE STUDY

1. **b.** You must manage the airway while maintaining cervical spinal stabilization. This is most important, and failing to do so may cause further injury and even death.

2. **d.** Your next and best action is to control the profuse bleeding. Quick action is necessary to help prevent further deterioration of the patient's condition.

3. **b.** You must tilt the backboard to the left to help take pressure off the blood vessels that return blood to the heart.

4. **a.** You should immediately start CPR and ventilate the patient. Even though the prognosis is grim, there is a slight chance that the baby can be saved if transported immediately with resuscitative efforts to the hospital. Although it is never wrong to call the hospital or your supervisor for direction, this should be done at the same time that you provide resuscitative treatment for the patient.

Chapter 37: Obstetrics and Care of the Newborn

TERMS AND CONCEPTS

1. **a.** 3 **b.** 8 **c.** 5 **d.** 7 **e.** 1 **f.** 4 **g.** 6 **h.** 2. *(p. 989)*

CONTENT REVIEW

1. **c.** Vagina. *(p. 991)*

2. **a.** Uterine contractions that expel the fetus and placenta are generally referred to as labor. *(p. 1000)*

3. **c.** The placental stage is the last stage. The three stages of labor are dilation, expulsion, and placental. Dilation occurs as the contractions begin and ends when the cervix becomes fully dilated. Expulsion ends with the delivery of the infant. The placental stage ends with the passage of the placenta (afterbirth). *(p. 1003)*

4. **c.** *Gravida* refers to the number of pregnancies, while *para* refers to the number of births. The Roman numeral that follows each reports the numbers of events. *Primigravida* refers to a woman who is pregnant for the first time. *Primipara* refers to a woman who has given birth for the first time. *(p. 997)*

5. **d.** Postmaturity syndrome occurs when the gestation of the fetus extends beyond 42 weeks. At 42 weeks, the placenta begins to decline, leading to a decrease in oxygenation and nutrient delivery to the fetus from decreased placental blood flow. The postmature baby is more prone to insufficient oxygen and nutrient delivery, hypoxia, a hardened skull leading to a more difficult delivery, and the presence of meconium from increased bowel maturity. *(p. 1010)*

6. **a.** Supine hypotensive syndrome is caused by the pressure of the combined weight of the enlarged uterus and fetus pressing on the inferior vena cava. The pressure may cause inadequate venous blood return to the heart and a drop in cardiac output, which may result in hypotension. *(p. 996)*

7. **c.** Transporting the patient in a sitting position, if appropriate, or on her side or with the right hip elevated. This will minimize compression of the vena cava and improve her cardiac output. *(p. 996)*

8. **d.** Avoid packing the vagina, and administer oxygen at 15 lpm. Provide general management for shock. *(p. 998)*

9. **d.** Care of this patient should include minimizing noise, light, and movement to prevent seizures. Administer oxygen at 15 lpm by a nonrebreather mask. If necessary, provide positive pressure ventilation and transport her on her side (to prevent supine hypotensive syndrome). *(p. 995)*

10. **a.** Contractions that occur every two minutes or closer and last 60–90 seconds are a sign of imminent delivery. Other signs include crowning, the patient feeling the infant's

head in the birth canal (sensation of the urge to defecate), strong urge to push down, and the patient's abdomen being very hard. *(p. 1004)*

11. **2, 4, 1, 3, 5.** (1) Support the bony part of the infant's skull and exert gentle pressure against the perineum as the head delivers. Determine the position of the umbilical cord. (2) In the airway, if obvious obstruction to breathing exists, suction the infant's mouth and nose. Support the body as it delivers, then again suction the mouth and nose (if obvious airway obstruction exists). Dry and wrap the infant. (3) Keep the infant level with the vagina. Have your partner assume care of the infant. When the pulsations cease, clamp or tie and then cut the umbilical cord. (4) Observe for the delivery of the placenta. As it delivers, grasp it gently and rotate. Place in a plastic bag for transport to the hospital. (5) Place a sanitary pad at the vaginal opening. Record the time of delivery and transport. Keep mother and infant warm en route. *(p. 1005)*

12. **b.** Emergency care for the patient with excessive postdelivery bleeding should include the administration of oxygen and firm massage of the uterus. If the mother appears to be in shock (hypoperfusion), transport immediately and initiate uterine massage. *(p. 1006)*

13. **d.** Signs of abnormal delivery include any fetal presentation other than the normal crowning of the head, abnormal color or smell of the amniotic fluid, labor before 38 weeks of pregnancy, and recurrence of contractions after the first infant is born (indicates multiple births). *(p. 1007)*

14. **a.** Management of a breech delivery includes positioning the mother in a supine, head-down, pelvis-elevated position to delay movement of the fetus into the birth canal, administering oxygen at 15 lpm, and transporting rapidly to the hospital. *(p. 1008)*

15. **d.** Prolapsed cord. This is a true emergency. *(p. 1007)*

16. **b.** Insert a gloved hand into the vagina to relieve pressure on the cord. The mother should be transported immediately in a knee–chest position with the stretcher in the Trendelenburg position. *(p. 1008)*

17. **c.** Meconium staining of the amniotic fluid in a newborn that is depressed or nonvigorous should be managed by suctioning first the mouth and then the nose before the infant takes a first breath. It is critical to clear the airway before the newborn is stimulated to prevent aspiration of the meconium into the lungs. *(p. 1009)*

18. **d.** In addition to the usual care for a newborn, care of the premature infant requires vigilant attention to prevent heat loss or contamination. Suctioning should be done very gently, and oxygen should be administered using a "blow-by" technique. *(p. 1009)*

19. **a.** The Apgar score ranges from 0 to 10 and is a method to assess the newborn's overall condition at 1 minute and 5 minutes after delivery. Components of the Apgar assessment include appearance, pulse, grimace, activity, and respirations. *(p. 1015)*

20. **c.** The signs of a severely depressed newborn include a respiratory rate of over 60 per minute, an Apgar score of less than 4, a cyanotic body, and a heart rate over 180 per minute or under 100 per minute. *(p. 1016)*

21. **b.** Newborn bradycardia (HR <100 bpm), labored breathing, apnea, or persistent cyanosis will typically respond to BVM ventilations with supplemental oxygen or blow-by oxygen. A small number may require chest compressions, and an even smaller number may require the medications or intubation that an advanced life support team can provide. *(p. 1016)*

22. **a.** Meconium staining that is thick and dark in color is associated with increased fetal risk. *(p. 1009)*

23. **b.** The Apgar score is initially performed at 60 seconds after birth and five minutes following birth. *(p. 1015)*

24. **a.** Braxton Hicks contractions are false labor contractions and are irregular. Interval times vary and the duration and intensity vary. *(p. 1000)*

25. **c.** A placenta previa is associated with an abnormal implantation of the placenta over or near the cervical opening (os). The three types of placenta previa are total, partial, and marginal. *(p. 993)*

26. **d.** Multiparity (more than two deliveries), rapid succession of pregnancies, greater than 35 years of age, previous placenta previa, history of early vaginal bleeding, and bleeding immediately following intercourse are all predisposing factors for placenta previa. *(p. 993)*

27. **c.** The hallmark sign is third-trimester painless vaginal bleeding of any color. *(p. 993)*

28. **b.** Abruptio placentae results from the rupture of blood vessels under the placenta and the subsequent separation from the uterine wall. It may be either a complete or a partial separation. *(pp. 994–995)*

29. **d.** Predisposing factors for an abruptio placentae include hypertension, use of cocaine and other drugs, preeclampsia, multiparity, previous abruption, smoking, a short umbilical cord, premature rupture of the amniotic sac, and diabetes mellitus. *(p. 994)*

30. **a.** Constant abdominal pain associated with vaginal bleeding is the hallmark sign of abruptio placentae. *(p. 994)*

31. **d.** Preeclampsia chiefly affects women who have a history of diabetes, heart disease, kidney problems, or hypertension. It affects about 1 in 20 women and occurs most frequently in women in their 20s in the last trimester of pregnancy. *(p. 996)*

32. **b.** Preeclampsia is chiefly characterized by hypertension and swelling of the extremities. Blood pressure is usually greater than 140/90. *(p. 996)*

33. d. Ectopic pregnancy is the third leading cause of maternal death in women 25–34 years of age. *(p. 995)*

34. c. Predisposing factors for development of an ectopic pregnancy include previous ectopic pregnancies, pelvic inflammatory disease, adhesions from surgery, and tubal surgery. *(p. 995)*

35. b. Signs and symptoms of ectopic pregnancy include a dull, ache-type pain that is poorly localized and then becomes a sudden, sharp, or "knifelike" abdominal pain. Other signs and symptoms include vaginal bleeding; lower abdominal pain that radiates to one or both shoulders; tender, bloated abdomen; decreased blood pressure; a bluish discoloration around the umbilicus (if the rupture occurred hours earlier); and an urge to defecate. *(p. 995)*

CASE STUDY

1. a. Initial management of this patient should first include immediately assisting respirations with a BVM with oxygen attached at 15 lpm.

2. b. This patient is critically injured and requires aggressive resuscitation. The management of supine hypotensive syndrome is of a secondary nature. However, in this patient, it would be managed by placing a blanket or pillow under one side of the spine board. This relieves pressure on the inferior vena cava during transport.

3. a. CPR should be started immediately and continued throughout transport and until the fetus is surgically delivered at the hospital. Vigorous resuscitation of the mother to save the fetus is acceptable and appropriate.

CHAPTER 37 SCENARIO: DOCUMENTATION EXERCISE

1. d. Make sure that no bleeding is taking place. A small amount of bleeding may be life threatening to a newborn. Ensure that the clamps are preventing any bleeding from taking place.

2. b. Crowning and Mary's need to bear down and push are classic indicators that birth is imminent.

3. d. The one-minute Apgar score is 9. *(To check the score, see page 1201.)*

4. d. The five-minute Apgar score is 10. *(To check the score, see page 1201.)*

5. d. 500 mL of bleeding is considered within normal limits. (The measurements mL and cc are approximately synonymous.)

Chapter 38: Pediatrics

TERMS AND CONCEPTS

1. a. Neonate, period of time from birth to 1 month of age: has total dependence on others; birth defects and unintentional injuries are common emergencies. **b.** Infant, 1 month to 1 year: recognizes the caregiver's face and voice; older infants (over 6 months) are stressed by separation; start assessment from a distance and allow caregiver to hold infant for exam; frightened by initial stimulation around face, so begin exam with feet or trunk and end with the head. **c.** Toddler, 1–3 years: "do not like . . ." stage, so limit touch, avoid separation, limit clothing removal or involve caregiver; fear of pain/needles but comforted by security objects; try toe-to-head exam. **d.** Preschooler, 3–6 years: concrete thinkers and literal interpreters, so explain simply and slowly before any action is taken; modest and resistant to attempts to unclothe, so involve caregiver; fear of pain, blood, and permanent injury but comforted by security objects; believe illness or injury is their fault and view it as punishment; allow them to see and "check out" equipment first; be sensitive. **e.** School-age child, 6–12 years: cooperative and curious; usually have understanding of EMS; maturity levels are highly individualized; honesty very important, so seek their cooperation; modesty and body image issues are common, so explanations are critical; fear of blood, pain, death, and permanent injury. **f.** Adolescent, 12–18 years: have concrete and are developing abstract thinking skills, but believe nothing bad can happen to them; respect their privacy; obtain history when alone; peer influence strong; body conscious; may overreact. *(pp. 1026–1028)*

CONTENT REVIEW

1. b. Involve the caregivers if you can; it helps to calm them and acknowledges them as "experts" of what is normal for this child. *(p. 1026)*

2. d. Newborns and infants are obligate nose breathers; infants have proportionally larger tongues than adults as compared to the size of the mouth, which leaves little room for airway swelling; the smallest level of the airway in the child is at the level of the cricoid cartilage. The epiglottis is much higher in the airway than in the adult. *(p. 1029)*

3. c. Hypothermia. *(p. 1032)*

4. b. Metabolic rates. (Infants and children use oxygen and glucose from the bloodstream three times faster, making respiratory difficulties (apnea or hypoventilation) more dangerous.) *(p. 1034)*

5. c. Respiratory system problems. *(p. 1042)*

6. b. The signs of early (compensated) respiratory distress include an increase in the respiratory rate above normal for that child's age; nasal flaring; intercostal, subclavicular, and subcostal retractions on inspiration; neck muscle use; audible breathing noises (stridor, wheezing, or grunting); and "seesaw" respirations. *(p. 1042)*

7. c. Decompensated respiratory failure. (Provide positive pressure ventilation with supplemental oxygen and prompt transport.) *(pp. 1042–1043)*

8. **c.** Respiratory arrest. (Treat the patient aggressively with positive pressure ventilation with a high concentration of oxygen and transport immediately.) *(p. 1044)*

9. **b.** Normal respiration ranges from 25–30/ min in an infant, and 15–30/min in a child. Measure the respiratory rate by counting the respirations for a full minute. Children generally breathe faster than adults. *(p. 1036)*

10. **c.** When assessing breath sounds in an infant or child, auscultate in the midaxillary lines on both sides of the lateral chest. This is necessary since breath sounds are typically transmitted easily from one side of the child's chest wall to the other. *(p. 1036)*

11. **b.** Urinary output. *(p. 1037)*

12. 1, 4, 2, 3. (1) Support in prone, head-down position. (2) Deliver five sharp backslaps. (3) Transfer to supine position and deliver five chest thrusts using two fingertips. (4) Repeat back slaps and chest thrusts until obstruction is dislodged. *(p. 1049)*

13. **d.** Seizures in infants and children are caused by any condition that would produce seizures in adults. The risk of seizures is high among children up to age 2. Seizures are caused by fever in about 3–5 percent of cases, and they can result in loss of bladder and bowel control. *(p. 1062)*

14. **b.** Status epilepticus occurs when a seizure lasts for longer than five minutes without a recovery period. This is a true emergency. Provide positive pressure ventilation with supplemental oxygen. *(p. 1062)*

15. **a.** Management of the infant or child with a fever includes being concerned if the fever is over 104°F–105°F; if cooling is required, use tepid water; the EMT is not authorized to administer an antipyretic medication; all high temperatures do not result in seizures. *(p. 1065)*

16. **d.** Shock or hypoperfusion in children is uncommon because their blood vessels are able to constrict efficiently, but only up to a point; it can occur in newborns due to loss of body heat and an immature thermoregulatory system. Cardiac arrest in infants and children, when it does occur, is generally due to respiratory compromise. The pediatric patient deteriorates faster and more severely than an adult. *(p. 1056)*

17. **a.** Management of an infant or child in shock includes keeping the patient warm and calm, performing an ongoing assessment every 5 minutes, administering oxygen to maintain an SpO_2 of at least 94%, and providing positive pressure ventilation with supplemental oxygen at 12–20/min (if breathing is inadequate). *(p. 1057)*

18. **c.** SIDS is also known as *crib death*, and it is the leading cause of death in infants one month to one year of age. Its occurrence cannot be predicted, and it cannot be diagnosed easily in the field. *(p. 1069)*

19. **b.** Management of SIDS should include immediate resuscitation efforts unless rigor mortis is present. Don't provide false reassurances to the family. Allow the caregivers to talk and tell their stories. Transport immediately. *(p. 1069)*

20. **a.** Assess for capillary refill by compressing the soft tissue of the kneecap or forearm. Do not use distal portions of extremities. It must be used as only one of several indicators when assessing the perfusion status. It alone can't provide a conclusion of poor perfusion. *(p. 1037)*

21. **d.** Trauma in children is most commonly caused by blunt trauma. Trauma in children ages 1–14 is the leading cause of death. It is caused primarily by automobile-related deaths. It results in death within the first hour in 50 percent of all cases. *(p. 1070)*

22. **a.** Mechanisms requiring transport to a Pediatric Trauma Center, if one is available, would include a motor vehicle crash in which the occupant is ejected (partial or complete) from the vehicle or another occupant is killed or a pedestrian/bicyclist is struck at 20 mph or greater or run over by a vehicle, and intrusion of 12 inches on the driver's side or 18 inches on the passenger's side. Other criteria for children include a fall from a height of 10 feet (two to three times the height of the child) or more (not 5 feet). *(p. 1073)*

23. **d.** The National Highway and Traffic Safety Administration (NHTSA) recommendations for the safe transport of children in ground ambulances is divided into five situations, recommends against transporting infants or children on the squad bench, provides ideal and practical recommendations, and does not allow the caregiver to hold the infant/child in his/her arms during transport. *(p. 1074)*

24. **a.** A common cause of hypoxia is the tongue obstructing the airway. Hypoperfusion is typically not a sign of a closed head injury; infants and children have ribs that are more pliable than adults; the capillary refill test is not a reliable assessment of shock in and of itself. *(p. 1071)*

25. **b.** Fluid loss. *(p. 1071)*

26. **d.** In many cases, the child will be the victim of both abuse and neglect. Physical abuse is an improper action that causes an injury or harm. Neglect is the provision of inadequate attention. The abused child will frequently exhibit fear when questioned about the injury. *(p. 1076)*

27. **c.** Record your observations objectively, follow local reporting protocols, and maintain total confidentiality. *(p. 1077)*

28. **a.** The PAT can be performed from across the room before you actually make physical contact. This tool is especially useful because the necessary assessment information is gathered during the general impression. The triangle is composed of three sides: appearance, work of breathing, and circulation to skin. *(p. 1033)*

29. c. The pediatric patient compensates for decreased cardiac output by increasing the heart rate. *(p. 1031)*

30. b. The use of pulse oximetry in children should be cautiously used for anything other than establishing trends in the patient's condition (just as with vital signs) and is highly recommended and is very reliable. *(p. 1038)*

31. c. If your pediatric patient is still maintaining an adequate respiratory depth and rate, the patient is said to be in early respiratory distress, otherwise known as *compensated respiratory distress.* *(p. 1042)*

32. d. If at any time the respiratory rate or tidal volume becomes inadequate, this is an indication that the patient has progressed from compensated respiratory distress to decompensated respiratory failure. This patient requires immediate ventilation with a BVM device or other acceptable ventilation device and supplemental oxygen. *(p. 1042)*

33. a. When treating a patient who has wheezes and then the wheezing resolves without the use of medication, you should suspect the patient has become worse. If the wheezes are no longer heard, this may indicate the lack of adequate air movement. *(p. 1036)*

34. a. You should first open the airway and inspect it for the hot dog. *(p. 1050)*

35. c. Croup produces stridor on inhalation, with a harsh "seal bark." It typically results from a viral infection and has a slow onset of symptoms. Administer humidified oxygen. *(p. 1051)*

36. c. Epiglottitis is a bacterial infection that causes swelling of the epiglottis and most commonly affects adults. It causes drooling, and the patient sits up and leans forward. If left untreated, it has a 50 percent mortality rate. *(p. 1052)*

37. c. Asthma occurs when the bronchioles constrict causing an increase in airway resistance. Patients with acute symptoms may assume a "tripod" position. Asthma generally results in generalized, not localized, wheezes. *(p. 1052)*

38. d. A severe attack of asthma that cannot be managed with medication is known as *status asthmaticus.* *(p. 1054)*

39. c. A condition that affects children less than 2 years of age and is caused when the small bronchi in the lungs become inflamed by a viral infection is called *bronchiolitis.* *(p. 1054)*

40. d. Chest compressions in children may be necessary if the heart rate drops below 60/min. *(p. 1057)*

41. a. An infection of the brain and spinal cord by a virus or bacteria is called *meningitis.* *(p. 1066)*

42. d. All of these items must be met to immobilize the child in the car seat in which the child was riding during the crash. *(p. 1072)*

43. b. Consciousness, breathing, and color. *(p. 1033)*

CASE STUDY

1. a. The infant is exhibiting signs of decompensated respiratory failure.

2. d. The most appropriate immediate treatment for the infant is to provide positive pressure ventilation with oxygen at 15 lpm and then rapidly transport to the hospital.

3. a. In addition to the problem identified in the case, the infant is most likely suffering from dehydration. This is exhibited by the history of vomiting, no urinary output for the past few hours, a depressed fontanelle, delayed capillary refill, and other physical findings of hypoperfusion and shock.

CHAPTER 38 SCENARIO: DOCUMENTATION EXERCISE

1. b. Any fall of greater than 10 feet (or two to three times the patient's height) is a mechanism of injury that requires transport of the pediatric patient to a level 1 Pediatric Trauma Center.

2. c. The average pulse in this 18-month-old patient is 120 per minute.

3. b. When providing spinal immobilization for this patient, a spinal immobilization collar should be used. A quick check for pulses, motor function, and sensory response should be performed prior to and after the patient is immobilized. Place padding under the shoulders to account for the large occiput, and secure the torso to the immobilization device before securing the head.

4. c. The patient in this case can be accurately referred to as a toddler. A neonate is the period of time from birth to 1 month of age, an infant from 1 to 12 months, a toddler from 1 to 3 years of age, a preschooler from 3 to 6 years of age.

5. b. The patient has a pediatric GCS score of 4 (Eyes – 1, Verbal – 1, Motor – decerebrate extension 2 = 4).

Chapter 39: Geriatrics

TERMS AND CONCEPTS

1. a. 7   b. 4   c. 3   d. 5   e. 1   f. 6   g. 8   h. 2   i. 10   j. 9. *(p. 1090)*

CONTENT REVIEW

1. c. Changes in body physiology typically begin at age 30, people are living longer with chronic diseases, and illness is not an inevitable part of aging. However, the aging body does have fewer reserves to combat the diseases and traumas that do occur. *(p. 1091)*

2. d. Cardiovascular system changes associated with aging include decreased arterial elasticity, degeneration of the conduction system that causes changes in rate or rhythm, decreased cardiac output due to cardiac hypertrophy, and an increased systolic blood pressure due to increased vascular resistance. *(p. 1093)*

3. b. Blunted sensitivity to hypoxia. *(p. 1093)*

4. d. Osteoporosis. *(p. 1095)*

5. **a.** Degeneration of nerve cells. *(p. 1094)*
6. **c.** Malnutrition. *(p. 1095)*
7. **c.** The kidneys become smaller in size, and there is a corresponding decrease in nephrons. The elderly patient's renal system is less resistant to failure during an acute illness or injury. The elderly more commonly suffer from drug toxicity when they take too much medication. *(p. 1096)*
8. **a.** You should always wear a HEPA mask when you are in contact with a potential tuberculosis patient. Elderly patients are more, not less, commonly the victims of heat- or cold-related emergencies. In a nursing home or other facility with multiple residents, be aware that a number of them may suffer from the same problem as your original patient, such as environmental temperature problems or toxic inhalation. It is not unlikely that an elderly patient will suffer from trauma and a medical problem at the same time—for example, when a fainting spell causes a fall that results in injury. *(p. 1107)*
9. **d.** Signs of dehydration in the elderly include eyes that appear sunken in the orbits, membranes of the eyes and mouth that appear dry, and a tongue that appears furrowed. *(p. 1110)*
10. **d.** As a group, the elderly abuse alcohol more than other age groups. They deteriorate more quickly, are less sensitive to pain, and suffer more depression. *(p. 1103)*
11. **d.** A sudden onset of an altered mental status cannot be attributed to dementia. Dementia is a chronic condition with a slow rather than an acute onset. Reduced reflexes may cause a higher incidence of choking. Cervical arthritis may make the head-tilt, chin-lift maneuver difficult, so a jaw thrust may provide a better airway. A resting respiratory rate of greater than 20 per minute, which is fast in a younger patient, may be normal for the elderly patient. *(p. 1102)*
12. **b.** Lying on her side (the best way to protect the airway in a patient with an altered mental status). *(p. 1100)*
13. **c.** Immobilized with blankets (to accommodate his spinal curvature). *(p. 1113)*
14. **c.** Weakness and fatigue are common presentations of a silent heart attack in an elderly patient, as are trouble breathing, aching shoulders, and indigestion. The other choices are not common heart attack presentations. *(p. 1096)*
15. **b.** Fowler position (sitting up; usually helps support breathing in the CHF patient). *(p. 1099)*
16. **d.** After consultation with medial direction, the EMT may assist with administering a prescribed metered-dose inhaler. *(p. 1099)*
17. **a.** Administer oxygen to maintain an SpO$_2$ reading of 94% or greater in the patient with adequate breathing. The patient's sudden onset of breathing difficulty and pain that does not radiate may indicate a pulmonary embolism, not a heart attack with pain that typically radiates. *(p. 1098)*
18. **c.** An elderly patient can easily become fatigued from labored breathing and lose the ability to sustain it. In this case, provide positive pressure ventilation to sustain respiration and expedite transport. *(p. 1099)*
19. **a.** An altered mental status in a geriatric patient is usually difficult to manage. The other choices are not true. *(p. 1100)*
20. **a.** Y **b.** N **c.** Y **d.** Y **e.** Y **f.** Y. (Other causes of altered mental status include decreased blood volume, effects of medications, dementia, heart rhythm disturbances, and heart attack.) *(p. 1100)*
21. **a.** A stroke patient requires maintaining oxygen saturation at a SpO$_2$ reading of 94% or greater. *(p. 1101)*
22. **c.** Older patients are more at risk for drug toxicity than younger patients, and older patients buy the greatest number of prescriptions. All medications that the patient is taking, including over-the-counter medications, should be taken to the hospital with the patient. Treatment of the drug toxicity patient is based on treating the drug's effects. *(p. 1096)*
23. **a.** Cardiac hypertrophy is a thickening of the cardiac walls without any increase in atrial or ventricular chamber size, which decreases stroke volume. *(p. 1092)*
24. **d.** Orthostatic hypotension is a drop in the systolic blood pressure and an elevation of the heart rate when the elderly patient goes from a lying to a standing position. *(p. 1095)*
25. **d.** Factors that contribute to the development of environmental emergencies among the elderly include situational factors, such as an inability to afford adequate heating or cooling. Aging, limitations on movement, and medications may all decrease the ability to regulate body temperature. *(p. 1105)*
26. 4, 3, 1, 5, 2. (1) Protect the airway. (2) Maintain normal breathing and circulation. (3) Remove the patient from the environment. (4) Remove wet clothing. (5) Wrap the patient in a dry blanket. *(p. 1105)*
27. **b.** Chemoreceptors become less sensitive in detecting hypoxia or carbon dioxide levels in the blood. *(p. 1093)*
28. **d.** Kyphosis is a curvature of the spine that is caused by narrowing of the vertebral disks in the elderly patient. *(p. 1095)*

CASE STUDY

1. **a.** Establish and maintain stabilization of the head and neck. The patient fell down a flight of stairs. A significant mechanism of injury exists for a potential cervical spine injury. She does not have symptoms that indicate a need for positive pressure ventilation. Splinting and a call to adult protective services, if warranted, can take place later.
2. **c.** Mrs. Walter's skin is cool and pale, which may indicate circulatory compromise and possible hypoperfusion. She must be carefully observed and vitals repeated frequently until a trend can be established. Her pulse, respirations, SpO$_2$, and blood pressure are all within normal limits.

Chapter 40: Patients with Special Challenges

MEDICAL TERMINOLOGY

1. **d.** *Intra-* means within and *ventricul* refers to ventricle, or within the ventricle.
2. **b.** Disease. Diabetic retinopathy damages the small blood vessels of the eye and results from the long-term effects of diabetes mellitus.
3. **c.** Stroke or paralysis; quadriplegia is paralysis from the neck down; paraplegia is paralysis from the waist down.

TERMS AND CONCEPTS

1. **a.** 1 **b.** 5 **c.** 6 **d.** 3 **e.** 4 **f.** 7 **g.** 2 **h.** 9 **i.** 8. *(p. 1117)*

CONTENT REVIEW

1. **c.** Compression of morbidity refers to maximizing the number of healthy years in one's life while simultaneously minimizing the number of years of disease or disability at the end. *(p. 1118)*
2. **b.** Dysarthria is the inability to effectively communicate verbally. *(p. 1119)*
3. **a.** Fluency disorders. *(p. 1119)*
4. **d.** Ask questions that the patient can answer with as few words as possible, don't finish words or statements for the patient, don't pretend to understand what the patient is saying even though you do not understand, and always allow the patient adequate time to respond to your questions. *(p. 1120)*
5. **c.** In many patients with special challenges, it may be difficult to determine what is "normal" for the patient. Presenting signs and symptoms may be categorized as chronic or acute. Obtaining a clear history from the family or health care provider is important. *(p. 1122)*
6. **a.** Respiratory infections, urinary tract infections, bedsores, and infection at the insertion site of feeding tubes are common problems encountered by paralyzed patients. *(p. 1122)*
7. **d.** Bariatrics. *(p. 1123)*
8. **d.** Over 70 percent of all adults in the United States are obese or overweight and it is the leading cause of preventable deaths today, second only to smoking. *(p. 1123)*
9. **d.** A morbidly obese patient weighs 50 to 100 percent more than the ideal body weight or more than 100 pounds over the ideal weight. *(p. 1123)*
10. **d.** There were over 700,000 homeless people in the United States; the health of a person is correlated with the income of the person or family; 10 percent of the people below the poverty level are older than 65 years of age; and patients who live at or near the poverty level are more likely to be subject to accidental trauma, physical abuse, or crimes and to develop chronic medical conditions. *(p. 1125)*
11. **a.** Management of the homeless patient requires the EMT to become familiar with local homeless services in your community that may provide medical care, shelter, food, or other services. The EMT should not request payment prior to providing service, not be judgmental by suggesting that he get a job, and the treatment is the same as you would provide to any patient. *(p. 1127)*
12. **c.** Intraventricular shunts are the fifth area of equipment commonly used for patients with special challenges. *(p. 1128)*
13. **1.** Information **2.** Device **3.** Function **4.** Assess **5.** Problem **6.** Remediate **7.** Movement. *(p. 1128)*
14. **c.** The three sources of oxygen for the patient at home are cylinder, concentrator, and liquid. *(p. 1128)*
15. **c.** The most common cause for an EMS response to a patient dependent upon home oxygen is equipment failure. *(pp. 1128–1229)*
16. **d.** An apnea monitor is commonly found in the homes of infants (especially in premature births) and is designed to monitor the patient's breathing and emit a warning if breathing stops. *(p. 1129)*
17. **b.** A pulse oximeter is most likely to be found in the home of a patient with a chronic pulmonary condition, a medical need to keep the oxygen concentration within a specific therapeutic range, and in order to determine oxygen needs in a patient who has a fluctuating oxygen demand. *(p. 1129)*
18. **c.** The most common problems associated with a tracheostomy tube are the tube becoming plugged with mucus or the tube becoming dislodged. *(p. 1130)*
19. **a.** Continuous positive airway pressure (CPAP) or bilevel positive airway pressure (BiPAP). *(p. 1131)*
20. **a.** They typically have two or three controls: ventilator rate, tidal volume, and oxygen concentration. The high-pressure alarm is active when lung compliance decreases, the low-pressure alarm is usually set to activate when the tidal volume falls 50–100 mL below the tidal volume, and the FiO_2 alarm will sound when the oxygen source is disconnected or is depleted. *(p. 1131)*
21. **b.** Implanted ports, also known as Port-A-Cath, Medi-Port, Microport, Bardport, Passport, and Infuse-a-Port, are disk-shaped devices that can be easily palpated beneath the surface of the skin after placement. *Vascular access device* is a general term that refers to each of the devices described. *(p. 1135)*
22. **d.** The two primary types of dialysis are hemodialysis and peritoneal dialysis. *(pp. 1334–1136)*
23. **c.** The EMT should never attempt to obtain a blood pressure in any extremity with an AV shunt, fistula, or graft. *(p. 1137)*
24. **a.** Patients that are receiving their nourishment by a feeding tube are said to be receiving enteral feeding. *(p. 1137)*

25. c. Orogastric tubes are slightly larger than nasogastric tubes and are inserted through the patient's mouth. *(p. 1137)*

CASE STUDY 1

1. c. The patient is most likely suffering from volume overload or volume deficit.

2. b. Do not take the patient's blood pressure in the same arm as the AV shunt, fistula, or graft.

3. a. The patient is undergoing hemodialysis. An AV shunt, AV fistula, and AV graft are used for hemodialysis.

CASE STUDY 2

1. d. Empty the urinary bag before transporting the patient and document the volume drained and any irregularities in urine color or smell.

2. b. The urinary catheter provides a portal for bacteria to enter the body.

3. c. Don't attempt to replace the catheter. Document the incident and be sure to report the incident to the receiving facility staff.

CHAPTER 40 SCENARIO: DOCUMENTATION EXERCISE

1. b. Determine the length of the catheter by comparing it to the tracheostomy obturator.

2. b. Cloudy, blood-tinged, or tea-colored urine is a sign of a urinary tract infection and should be reported to Lynn's mother and nurse.

3. c. The sore on Lynn's heel is a bedsore resulting from continual pressure on the heel and should be reported to Lynn's mother and caregiver.

4. b. The proximal end of the tracheostomy tube fits a BVM via a standard 15/22 mm adapter.

5. c. Limit suctioning to no more than 10–15 seconds.

Chapter 41: The Combat Veteran

TERMS AND CONCEPTS

1. a. 1 **b.** 2. *(pp. 1146–1150)*

CONTENT REVIEW

1. d. 1 percent of the population is made up of veterans. *(p. 1146)*

2. a. PTSD has existed for many years. The term used to describe it during World War II and the Korean War was combat neurosis. *Soldier's heart and nostalgia* was the term used during the American Civil War, and *shell shock* was its name during World War I. *(p. 1146)*

3. d. PTSD occurs when individuals are exposed to an abnormal stressor or dangerous condition. It is not the sign of a weak mind, does not occur from contact with environmental substances, and may occur in both combat and noncombat veterans. *(p. 1146)*

4. a. An era veteran is one who trained for combat but never went to war. *(p. 1146)*

5. b. Never ask a veteran if he killed anyone or ask any variation of this question. *(p. 1148)*

6. c. The four essential features of PTSD are response, reliving, avoiding, and anxiety/anger. *(p. 1148)*

7. a. At some point in time, all combat veterans will experience flashbacks or sleep disturbances. *(p. 1148)*

8. b. PTSD patients may present with pain of an origin that is unsubstantiated, or it may be difficult to determine the origin. PTSD can accelerate the aging process. Common signs include guilt, shame, avoidance of others, depression, paranoia, hostility, feeling that the prson will not live much longer, agitation, and anger. *(p. 1149)*

9. b. Drug and alcohol use occurs in about 40 percent of all veterans. The level of use can be determined by asking "What's the most you can drink and still walk?" Alcohol and drugs commonly taken act as depressants to help the person feel "more normal." *(p. 1149)*

10. d. The "gut test" is a reflection of the body's way of saying "danger is here" and should be recognized and acted upon. Protect yourself and others. *(p. 1150)*

11. d. Always take a patient's threat of suicide seriously, try to get others involved, determine if the patient has previous episodes of violence and use care with physical restraints. *(p. 1149)*

12. b. The "signature wound" of the Vietnam War was gunshot wounds to the chest. In the Iraq and Afghanistan wars, it was traumatic brain injury and amputations. *(p. 1150)*

13. a. TBI is caused by an external force such as a concussion, occurs more than infrequently (about 300,000 soldiers have been diagnosed), the signs and symptoms are very similar to PTSD, and should be described as a concussion on scene. *(p. 1150)*

14. c. It is not appropriate for a veteran to ignore a TBI; repeated TBIs can have a serious impact on brain injury and subsequent debilitating neurological disorders. Any patient with a TBI should be transported, and if a TBI is misdiagnosed and further brain injury occurs, permanent brain damage may occur. *(p. 1151)*

15. d. Never use a statement like "I understand" because you don't understand what the combat veteran has experienced. Never assume the combat veteran has PTSD, but keep it in mind when assessing the veteran. Provide assurance, structure, and limits and ask the patient, "How many weapons do you have and are they secure?" *(p. 1151)*

CASE STUDY

1. The patient was well groomed with a military style haircut and replied to questioning with a respectful "Yes, ma'am" or "Yes, sir." The KIA (Killed In Action) memorial wristband of a fallen brother.

2. **b.** You should reassure the patient in a calm, firm voice, being in charge but soothing. Never ask the veteran if they have killed anyone. Do not state you know how the patient feels because you do not. You should build a rapport by casual talking about the weather, sports, and news topics.

3. **b.** PTSD is the result of an abnormal stressor or dangerous condition often associated with combat.

4. **d.** All are signs of a possible TBI, or concussion injury.

Chapter 42: Ambulance Operations and Air Medical Response

CONTENT REVIEW

1. **d.** A "privilege" associated with the operation of an emergency vehicle is passing in a no-passing zone. Other privileges include exceeding the posted speed limit, driving the wrong way down a one-way street, turning in any direction at an intersection, parking anywhere, leaving the ambulance standing in the middle of a street or intersection, and going through red lights or red flashing signals. You must avoid endangering life and property by driving with a due regard for the safety of others; otherwise, you are individually and personally responsible for any liabilities that result. *(p. 1156)*

2. **b.** Driving the wrong way down a one-way street without using any warning devices is obviously disregarding the safety of others. *(p. 1156)*

3. **d.** To be a good emergency vehicle operator, the EMT should try to travel the posted speed limit when possible, hold the steering wheel at the 9 o'clock and 3 o'clock positions, travel a route that will ensure the quickest and safest response (which may not be the shortest route), brake into a curve, and then gradually accelerate when going out of the curve. *(p. 1156)*

4. **c.** The use of escorts doubles the hazards associated with emergency driving; they should be used only as a last resort. *(p. 1158)*

5. **d.** When using a siren, never pull directly behind a car and blast your siren; always assume that other drivers are unaware of you. Operators tend to increase their speed by about 15 mph when the siren is in operation. The siren creates emotional stress for you, your partner, and the patient. *(p. 1161)*

6. **c.** Legally, you may be within your rights to refuse to use a vehicle that you have reason to believe is unsafe. You may be legally liable for damage caused by a malfunctioning vehicle. Respectfully refuse to operate the vehicle. *(p. 1163)*

7. Only **a, c, d, f,** and **g** should be marked. The dispatcher should provide the following information: location of the call; nature of the call; name, location, and callback number of the caller; location of the patient at the scene; the number of patients; and the severity of the problem. *(p. 1164)*

8. **a.** Determine and clarify the responsibilities of each team member. *(p. 1164)*

9. The missing phases of the ambulance call are as follows: at the scene, at the receiving facility, en route to the station, and post run. *(p. 1163)*

10. **a.** Position the ambulance to provide a safety zone. *(p. 1164)*

11. **b.** Stay a minimum of 100 feet from wreckage or a burning vehicle and 2,000 feet from hazardous materials spills. *(p. 1164)*

12. **c.** Prior to arrival at the emergency scene, determine the responsibilities of team members. Upon arrival at the emergency scene, carefully observe the complete incident as you approach, turn your headlights off (unless used to illuminate the scene) so that they don't blind oncoming drivers' vision, and rapidly move unstable patients to the ambulance. *(p. 1164)*

13. **c.** Every 15 minutes for a stable patient; every 5 minutes for an unstable patient. *(p. 1167)*

14. **a.** Allowing family or friends in the patient compartment during transport to the hospital may be helpful if the patient is a child. It is not prohibited by state EMS statutes; a federal EMS statute does not exist; and it may be helpful if the patient's family or friend is emotionally stable. Ensure that companions use safety restraints while accompanying the patient. *(p. 1167)*

15. **a.** Ensure proper continuity of care. *(p. 1167)*

16. **d.** It should be left at the emergency department. (Some EMS systems also may require you to leave a copy with the patient.) *(p. 1167)*

17. **a.** Appropriate post-run activities include changing a soiled uniform, completing an inventory of equipment and supplies, leaving the run report at the hospital before departing (and giving a copy to the patient if local protocol requires it), filling the fuel tank if necessary, and cleaning and disinfecting the ambulance after each call and at the end of the shift. Washing your hands and providing oral and written reports to hospital staff are performed while at the hospital. *(p. 1168)*

18. **d.** A process that kills all microorganisms is sterilization. *(p. 1168)*

19. **a.** 1:10 solution of household bleach and water. *(p. 1168)*

20. **a.** 3   **b.** 1   **c.** 4   **d.** 2. *(pp. 1168–1169)*

21. **a.** Guidelines for setting up a landing zone include placing a fifth warning device on the upwind side, establishing a 100-by-100-foot area for a nighttime landing zone (small helicopter), keeping spectators at least 200 feet away, and establishing a 60-by-60-foot area (small helicopter) for a daytime landing zone. Be sure to refer to your local

aeromedical landing zone guidelines for proper landing procedures. *(p. 1171)*

22. **c.** NAEMT guidelines for ensuring operational safety and security measures require security briefings at the beginning of each shift (or information sheets, postings, or supervisor briefings), increased involvement of EMS crews in the development of security measures, never leaving EMS vehicles unattended with the keys in the ignition, and increased tracking systems of EMS vehicles. *(p. 1171)*

23. **d.** Night driving is improved by the use of quartz-halogen headlights. Nighttime driving conditions result in two and a half times more fatal collisions than do daytime driving conditions. It is more difficult for older drivers as compared to younger drivers and is improved by not staring directly at the high beams of oncoming cars. *(p. 1159)*

24. **c.** Keeping your eyes moving and avoiding focusing on one object. Techniques for safe driving at night also include not using your high beams when entering a curve, dimming your headlights within 500 feet of an approaching driver, and not flicking high beams up and down to remind a driver to dim his bright lights. *(p. 1160)*

25. **b.** When driving in bad weather, the roads are most slippery at the start of a rainstorm. If hydroplaning begins, hold the wheel steady, release the accelerator, and gently pump the brake. Stopping on ice requires five times the stopping distance. Hydroplaning can begin at speeds of 35 mph. *(p. 1159)*

26. **b.** It occurs with greater outside air pressure and can be reduced by keeping the rear windows closed. Carbon monoxide in ambulances is difficult to detect due to its being odorless, colorless, and tasteless. It may be harmful in amounts over 10 parts per million. *(p. 1173)*

Chapter 43: Gaining Access and Patient Extrication

CONTENT REVIEW

1. **a.** When receiving dispatch information. *(p. 1180)*
2. **b.** Motor vehicle collisions. *(p. 1180)*
3. **c.** Binoculars can help you assess the scene from a safe distance. *(p. 1181)*
4. **a.** Full protective turnout gear. (This includes coat, bunker pants, steel-toed boots, helmet with ear flaps and wide brim and a face shield, eye protection, and heavy leather gloves over disposable gloves.) *(p. 1181)*
5. **c.** *Always* assume that downed power lines are alive. (Call the electric-service company for assistance.) *(p. 1182)*
6. **b.** Stop all traffic and reroute it to different roads. (Remember, however, that special

prior training in traffic direction and control is necessary.) *(p. 1182)*
7. A child may have been involved. (This clue should prompt you to ask questions and complete a thorough search of the area.) *(p. 1184)*
8. **c.** A vehicle is stable when it can no longer move, rock, or bounce. *(p. 1184)*
9. **d.** Simply turn off the ignition. *(p. 1184)*
10. Before disconnecting the power to the vehicle, you should try to move the seat backward, lower power windows, and unlock power door locks. This will give you greatest access to the patient. *(p. 1184)*
11. **a.** Remove the negative battery cable first. *(p. 1184)*
12. **b.** Complex access requires tools and specialized equipment. Simple access does not require tools. *(p. 1185)*
13. **a.** Breaking a window. *(p. 1185)*
14. **c.** From the front. (Approach facing the patient to keep him from moving his head.) *(p. 1185)*
15. **d.** Start your request by saying, "Without moving your head or neck." (If you wait until the end of your sentence to say this, the patient may move before you can finish.) *(p. 1186)*
16. **c.** Against the lower corner of the window. *(p. 1186)*
17. **b.** Patient care always precedes removal from the vehicle *except* when delay would endanger the patient or rescue personnel. *(p. 1186)*
18. **d.** Use blankets, a tarp, or a spine board. *(p. 1187)*
19. **b.** Explain the activities, noises, and movements. *(p. 1187)*
20. **d.** The only exception to the rule that the spine must be stabilized and, if possible, immobilized before removing a patient from a vehicle is when there is an immediate threat to your patient's life or your own or when another patient blocks access to a critically injured patient. *(p. 1187)*
21. Once on the scene. you should perform a 360-degree assessment of potential hazards, preferably prior to exiting the ambulance. However, to effectively perform the 360-degree assessment, you must look in the front of the vehicle, on both sides, and in the rear of the vehicle. Also, inspect above and below the vehicle. Potential hazards include downed electrical wires; leaking fuels or fluids; smoke or fire coming from the vehicle or near or around the vehicle; and broken glass, jagged metal, or other sharp objects. *(p. 1181)*
22. **b.** Deactivation is usually done by simply disconnecting the car's battery cables. *(p. 1182)*
23. **d.** Upon a arrival on the scene, it is usually best to position your vehicle uphill to avoid the gravity flow of spilled material and fuels. Stay upwind to avoid the wind blowing dangerous fumes and vapors toward your vehicle. *(p. 1181)*

SPECIALIZED STABILIZATION, EXTRICATION, AND DISENTANGLEMENT TECHNIQUES

1. **b.** The first step to properly stabilizing an upright vehicle is to immobilize the suspension. This is most often accomplished by positioning step chocks under the vehicle parallel to each wheel. *(p. 1187)*

2. **d.** The first step to securing a vehicle that is positioned on its side is to place a strong pulling device or chain from the undercarriage of the car to another vehicle or strong immovable object. *(p. 1188)*

3. **c.** Opening or removing doors during patient extrication will reduce the strength of the post and may cause the roof to collapse. *(p. 1189)*

4. **b.** Prying the latch site on the "B" posts most easily opens the front doors of a vehicle. The "A" posts are the front posts supporting the car roof (hinge side). The "C" posts are at the rear and the "B" posts are in the middle. *(p. 1190)*

5. **d.** If the vehicle is on its side, access is best gained through the rear window. Opening the trunk or rear hatch may cause the vehicle to become unstable, and the trunk will not allow access. Lifting the door on the top of the car is difficult and dangerous because of its weight. Removing the roof will likely make the vehicle unstable. *(p. 1190)*

CASE STUDY

1. **a.** Secure an area that is more than 80 feet in all directions. Yell instructions to the patient to stay in the vehicle. Do not approach the car because power can be automatically restored. Trust only the power company or specialized teams trained in electrical hazards to tell you when it is safe.

2. **c.** Tell the patient to focus and keep his attention on an object directly in front of him.

3. Make the patient aware of how long the process may take, explain the activities and movements around him, explain the noises that will be present, ask the patient if he is ready to have the door opened, stay with the patient at all times, and reassure him constantly.

Chapter 44: Hazardous Materials

TERMS AND CONCEPTS

1. **a.** 3 **b.** 2 **c.** 4 **d.** 1. *(p. 1196)*

CONTENT REVIEW

1. **b.** Rescuer, public, and patient safety is always the primary concern at any hazardous material emergency. *(p. 1197)*

2. **c.** The four factors that determine a patient's response to hazardous material exposure are the dose, the concentration, route of exposure, and the time exposed to the material. *(p. 1197)*

3. **c.** A four-sided diamond. The placard contains a four-digit UN identification number and a legend that indicates whether the material is flammable, radioactive, explosive, or poisonous. *(p. 1197)*

4. **a.** A health hazard. The NFPA 704 system, for use in marking hazardous materials located at fixed facilities, identifies potential dangers with the use of background colors and numbers ranging from 0 to 4. Blue identifies a health hazard, red a fire hazard, and yellow a reactivity hazard; the higher the number, the greater the hazard. *(p. 1201)*

5. **a.** The Chemical Transportation Emergency Center, or CHEMTREC, may be reached at 1-800-424-9300 around the clock for advice on how to handle any emergency involving hazardous materials. *(p. 1202)*

6. **c.** Hazardous materials should not be detected by relying on your senses, are not always easily detectable, and may create colored vapor clouds. All spills should be treated as dangerous until proven otherwise. *(p. 1202)*

7. **b.** The principal dangers hazardous materials present are toxicity, flammability, and reactivity. *(p. 1197)*

8. **b.** *Emergency Response Guidebook.* *(p. 1202)*

9. **b.** First Responder Awareness, First Responder Operations, Hazardous Materials Technician, and Hazardous Materials Specialist are the four levels of training that OSHA and the EPA have identified. *(p. 1204)*

10. **c.** Threatens the immediate safety of patients and rescuers and threatens their long-term health. By carrying toxins and particles of hazardous materials through the air, smoke from a hazardous materials fire not only threatens the immediate safety of patients and rescuers, it also may threaten long-term health, in some cases increasing the risk of cancer and chronic poisoning affecting the brain, liver, lungs, and kidneys. *(p. 1197)*

11. **c.** Before a hazardous material emergency occurs, one command officer should be appointed who will make all decisions, and a clear chain-of-command system must be developed. An established system of communications used throughout the emergency should be developed. The system should be one that all rescuers are informed about, know how to use, and have access to. Predesignate the hospital receiving facilities that will be utilized, and train and prepare for the worst possible scenario that may occur in a local community. *(p. 1205)*

12. 3, 1, 2. (1) Protect the safety of all rescuers and patients. (2) Provide patient care. (3) Decontaminate clothing, equipment, and the vehicle. *(p. 1205)*

13. **d.** Correct activities or actions in the hot zone include not allowing anyone (other than trained rescuers) in the hot zone; not allowing smoking, eating, and drinking; and establishing one entry point. Only rescue, initial decontamination, and treatment

of life threats are performed in the hot
zone. *(p. 1211)*

14. **b.** Decontaminate the patient fully. (A contaminated patient in a closed, tight space could affect the breathing or vision of the air transport team.) *(p. 1208)*

15. **c.** Keep uphill, upwind, upstream, and away from the danger. *(p. 1205)*

16. **b.** Failure to decontaminate equipment and the interior of the vehicle properly can result in chronic chemical exposure. *(p. 1209)*

17. **c.** In a radiation accident, the patient may suffer from both exposure to and contamination by radiation. Exposure occurs when the patient is in the presence of radioactive material without any of the radioactive material actually touching his clothing or body. The exposure he receives may be harmful to him, but the patient himself does not become radioactive and does not pose any major threat to rescue personnel. Contamination occurs when the patient has come into direct contact with the source of radioactivity or with radioactive gases, liquids, or particles. *(p. 1209)*

18. **d.** Alpha rays can be stopped by clothing. *(p. 1209)*

19. **a.** Radiation sickness is caused by exposure to large amounts of radiation. It starts anywhere from a few hours to days following the exposure and can last from a few days to seven to eight weeks. *(p. 1210)*

20. **d.** The Federal Nuclear Regulatory Commission recommends that an individual in an emergency situation not be exposed to more than a one-time, whole-body dose of 25 roentgens. *(p. 1211)*

21. **d.** Radiation poisoning occurs when the patient has been exposed to a dangerous amount of internal radiation. It results in a host of diseases, including cancer and anemia. *(p. 1210)*

CASE STUDY 1

1. **d.** Call for additional assistance quickly.
2. **c.** Keep uphill and upwind, and protect yourself and the patient. (Prevent others from approaching the accident site until specialized help arrives.)

CASE STUDY 2

1. **c.** Under the arms and in the groin. (Contamination occurs most easily in areas of your body where the skin is thin or moist.)
2. **a.** Wash with mild detergent or green soap and plenty of running water. Irrigate exposed skin for at least 20 minutes.
3. **b.** Take precautions to protect your equipment and vehicle during transport, since there may still be some contamination on the patient. Cover exposed areas of the vehicle with plastic sheeting.

CASE STUDY 3

1. **a.** Remove the bystander, evacuate the area, and contact dispatch. (Do not attempt or allow other untrained persons to attempt to put out the fire. Do not remain near the building. Because toxic fertilizers may be burning at this fire, evacuate to a safe area until specialized help arrives.)

CHAPTER 44 SCENARIO: DOCUMENTATION EXERCISE

1. **b.** Command for this situation should be assumed by one command officer.
2. **a.** The receiving facility to which the patient is being transported should be predesignated during preincident planning.
3. **c.** Jill's chest was auscultated for the development of pulmonary edema that may be associated with inhalation of ammonia.
4. **a.** You and Colleen are most likely trained to the level of First Responder Awareness.
5. **a.** The area where contamination is present is called the *hot zone*.

Chapter 45: Multiple-Casualty Incidents and Incident Management

TERMS AND CONCEPTS

1. **a.** 8 **b.** 5 **c.** 2 **d.** 12 **e.** 4 **f.** 1 **g.** 9
   h. 6 **i.** 3 **j.** 11 **k.** 7 **l.** 10. *(p. 1215)*

CONTENT REVIEW

1. **b.** The NIMS provides a consistent approach to managing disasters by all responders to an incident. *(p. 1216)*
2. **a.** Early in a developing MCI or disaster, the incident commander is located or stationed in the mobile command unit or what is formally known as the *incident command post*. *(p. 1218)*
3. **a.** If the child is breathing adequately with a palpable peripheral pulse and is unresponsive to all stimuli or responds to pain with incomprehensible sounds or inappropriate movement (does not localize pain or has no purposeful flexion or extension), tag the child "red" and move on to the next patient. *(p. 1222)*
4. **c.** Any patient who is able to walk at the scene of a multiple-casualty incident is initially tagged as a "green" or low-priority patient. *(p. 1221)*
5. **b.** Primary triage is conducted at the actual site of the incident if it is safe—for example, inside the bus before the patients are moved. *(p. 1219)*
6. **a.** Triage is a system used to sort patients according to criticality. *(p. 1219)*
7. **d.** Secondary triage is performed when the patient is moved to the triage unit. It is designed to reevaluate the initial patient categorization, during which the patient may be upgraded, downgraded, or kept the same. *(p. 1220)*

8. **d.** Check respirations, perfusion, and mental status. Patients who can walk are tagged "green." *(p. 1221)*

9. **b.** This patient is deceased. Tag the patient as "black" and move on to the next patient. *(p. 1221)*

10. **a.** Priority 1 patients are transported first, followed by Priority 2, then Priority 3 patients. Priority 4 patients are deceased. *(p. 1220)*

11. **a.** A patient with respirations greater than 30 per minute is assigned to Priority 1 (red). *(p. 1221)*

12. **a.** Red indicates high priority. (Tagging helps arriving EMTs quickly and efficiently identify treatment and transport priorities.) *(p. 1220)*

13. **d.** Triage or priority level. (Color flags or ribbons should be erected at the ends of each row to designate the respective treatment areas. Place the patient in the appropriate row according to the color or level triaged.) *(p. 1225)*

14. **c.** Provide plenty of nourishing food and drinks. Rest every one to two hours; rapidly remove any rescue workers who become hysterical and transport them to the hospital; encourage rescuers to talk among themselves. *(p. 1227)*

15. **d.** Dr. Romig now recommends that Jump-START be used on any patient who appears to be a child and START be used on any patient who appears to be a young adult or older. *(p. 1222)*

16. **b.** Safe routes to take out of the area, the nature of the disaster and its estimated time of impact, a description of the expected severity, and appropriate destinations for those who evacuate are all appropriate. *(p. 1228)*

17. **d.** Preadolescents and adolescents are most likely to experience extreme aggression and stress that is severe enough to disrupt their lives. *(p. 1229)*

18. **b.** Always tell the truth. Giving false assurances to patients does not help them deal with the reality of the event. Encourage patients to talk about the disaster and its potential long-term effects. Reuniting of families should occur as soon as possible to lessen the emotional stress. Encouraging patients to do necessary chores will help them return to normal. *(p. 1229)*

CASE STUDY

1. **b.** Request additional help and assistance *early* in the MCI. It's better to call too many rescuers than too few.

2. **b.** If the child is alert, responds to your voice, or responds to pain by localizing it, withdrawing from it, or trying to push it away, the patient is tagged "yellow."

3. **b.** The transport unit leader is responsible for notification of the hospital; the unit should be located close to where the ambulances stage or arrive; it should be clearly marked; and if necessary, more than one treatment unit may be required.

4. **a.** Green   **b.** Red   **c.** Yellow   **d.** Red   **e.** Black.

Chapter 46: EMS Response to Terrorism Involving Weapons of Mass Destruction

TERMS AND CONCEPTS

1. **a.** 2   **b.** 3   **c.** 4   **d.** 1   **e.** 5   **f.** 6.   *(p. 1233)*

CONTENT REVIEW

1. **a.** Coordinated community preplanning for a WMD attack is necessary, and a single EMS agency is unlikely to have enough equipment to handle a WMD attack. Local, regional, and state disaster agencies should develop WMD disaster plans, and the general approach is similar to that for any disaster involving multiple casualties, with some additional considerations. *(p. 1235)*

2. **d.** Explosive and incendiary agents are the weapons of mass destruction most widely used by terrorists. *(p. 1234)*

3. **c.** Incendiary devices produce a different injury pattern from conventional explosives. They are easy to improvise and manufacture and include napalm, thermite, and magnesium. Incendiary device burns are assessed in the same manner as thermal burns. *(p. 1238)*

4. **a.** The mnemonic SLUDGE (for salivation, lacrimation, urination, defecation, gastric distress, and emesis) stands for the signs and symptoms associated with nerve agent exposure. *(p. 1239)*

5. **b.** Two drugs used to counteract the effects of nerve agents are atropine and pralidoxime (Protopam). *(p. 1239)*

6. **c.** Vesicants cause blistering, burning, and tissue damage on contact. *(p. 1238)*

7. **b.** Cyanide disrupts the ability of the cell to use oxygen and leads to cellular hypoxia and eventually death. The pulse oximeter may provide a false sense of reassurance, since the blood is being oxygenated well, yet the cell cannot use the oxygen. *(p. 1240)*

8. **d.** Phosgene, halogen compounds, and nitrogen-oxygen compounds are examples of pulmonary agents. *(p. 1241)*

9. **b.** The management for exposure to riot-control agents should focus first on removing the patient from the environment and then irrigating the eyes with water or saline. Activated charcoal, amyl nitrite, and sodium nitrite are not administered for this purpose. The eyes should be irrigated. *(p. 1241)*

10. **a.** Biological agents are categorized into four groups: pneumonia-like agents, encephalitis-like agents, biological toxins, and other agents. *(p. 1242)*

11. **a.** The two most common encephalitis-like agents are smallpox and Venezuelan equine encephalitis. *(pp. 1242–1243)*

12. **b.** The three primary mechanisms of death or injury associated with nuclear detonation are radiation, blast, and thermal burns. *(p. 1244)*

13. **a.** Gamma radiation is the most penetrating type of radiation and can travel long distances. *(p. 1244)*

14. **b.** There are two types of radiation exposure associated with a nuclear explosion. After primary exposure, fallout is the second form of radiation exposure, containing radioactive dust and particles. *(p. 1244)*

15. **a.** A conventional explosive attached to radioactive materials is referred to as an RDD or a "dirty bomb." *(p. 1234)*

CASE STUDY

1. **a.** The mechanism that causes most deaths and injury associated with nuclear detonation is the blast wave and thermal burns.

2. **d.** The nuclear ignition produces an explosively expanding gas cloud, and the shock wave injuries from nuclear detonation are similar to shock wave injuries produced by conventional weapons. The intensity of shock wave injuries is greater the closer the victim is to ground zero, and the windblast is strong enough to cause structural collapse, crush injuries, and entrapment.

3. **b.** It's true that personnel with hazardous materials (hazmat) training are prepared to act as an initial response crew in a nuclear event because similar principles apply.

Answers to Course Review Self-Test

The numbers following each answer refer to the textbook page(s) where the answer can be found or supported.

CH 1.	1. d.	(p. 14)			CH 15.	78. a.	(p. 434)	79. b.	(p. 432)

CH 1.   1. d.   (p. 14)
CH 12.   2. b.   (p. 295)   3. a.   (p. 298)
           4. d.   (p. 304)
CH 13.   5. b.   (p. 318)   6. c.   (p. 314)
           7. d.   (p. 393)   8. a.   (p. 332)
           9. b.   (p. 351)   10. a.   (p. 344)
          11. c.   (p. 338)   12. a.   (p. 380)
          13. b.   (p. 336)   14. b.   (p. 365)
          15. c.   (p. 361)
CH 14.   16. d.   (p. 403)   17. b.   (p. 401)
CH 6.   18. b.   (p. 95)   19. a.   (p. 97)
          20. d.   (p. 97)   21. d.   (p. 104)
CH 37.   22. a.   (p. 996)   23. a.   (p. 991)
          24. b.   (p. 1003)   25. d.   (p. 990)
          26. c.   (p. 1000)   27. b.   (p. 1005)
          28. b.   (p. 1016)
CH 10.   29. d.   (p. 213)   30. b.   (p. 213)
          31. d.   (p. 221)   32. c.   (p. 222)
          33. b.   (p. 223)   34. a.   (p. 209)
          35. b.   (p. 223)   36. d.   (p. 230)
          37. c.   (p. 239)   38. d.   (p. 248)
          39. b.   (p. 249)   40. c.   (p. 253)
CH 18.   41. c.   (p. 532)
CH 20.   42. b.   (p. 570)
CH 11.   43. c.   (p. 272)   44. a.   (p. 284)
          45. c.   (p. 268)
CH 2.   46. a.   (p. 23)   47. c.   (p. 25)
          48. b.   (p. 27)
CH 28.   49. b.   (p. 775)   50. a.   (p. 776)
          51. b.   (p. 782)
CH 38.   52. c.   (p. 1026)   53. a.   (p. 1042)
          54. b.   (p. 1044)   55. d.   (p. 1045)
          56. b.   (p. 1030)   57. d.   (p. 1057)
          58. c.   (p. 1069)
CH 40.   59. b.   (p. 1137)
CH 45.   60. b.   (p. 1222)   61. b.   (p. 1221)
CH 16.   62. b.   (p. 450)   63. b.   (p. 477)
          64. c.   (p. 456)   65. a.   (p. 468)
          66. c.   (p. 474)   67. a.   (p. 474)
CH 28.   68. c.   (p. 789)   69. a.   (p. 793)
          70. c.   (p. 794)
CH 18.   71. a.   (p. 530)   72. d.   (p. 538)
CH 3.   73. a.   (p. 43)   74. d.   (p. 48)
CH 17.   75. c.   (p. 492)
          76. b.   (pp. 505–506) 77. c.   (p. 500)

CH 15.   78. a.   (p. 434)   79. b.   (p. 432)
CH 29.   80. b.   (pp. 816–817) 81. d.   (p. 823)
CH 26.   82. d.   (p. 737)   83. b.   (p. 743)
CH 4.   84. c.   (p. 67)   85. c.   (p. 66)
CH 44.   86. d.   (p. 1201)   87. b.   (p. 1206)
          88. d.   (p. 1205)
CH 32.   89. b.   (p. 882)   90. d.   (p. 886)
          91. c.   (p. 889)   92. c.   (p. 889)
          93. a.   (p. 891)
CH 22.   94. a.   (p. 609)   95. b.   (p. 611)
          96. d.   (p. 615)
CH 41.   97. c.   (p. 1148)   98. d.   (p. 1150)
CH 7.   99. b.   (p. 122)   100. a.   (p. 122)
         101. c.   (p. 120)   102. a.   (p. 138)
         103. b.   (p. 152)   104. d.   (p. 126)
CH 24.   105. b.   (p. 680)   106. b.   (p. 680)
         107. c.   (p. 703)   108. b.   (p. 698)
         109. c.   (p. 705)
CH 31.   110. d.   (p. 873)   111. b.   (p. 871)
CH 23.   112. c.   (p. 656)   113. a.   (p. 685)
CH 39.   114. d.   (p. 1100)   115. d.   (p. 1100)
         116. d.   (p. 1096)
CH 43.   117. c.   (p. 1185)   118. a.   (p. 1186)
CH 27.   119. d.   (p. 754)   120. b.   (p. 757)
         121. d.   (p. 762)   122. c.   (p. 762)
         123. a.   (p. 763)   124. d.   (p. 764)
CH 30.   125. d.   (p. 844)   126. c.   (p. 844)
         127. a.   (p. 848)
CH 5.   128. b.   (p. 78)   129. a.   (p. 82)
CH 25.   130. b.   (p. 717)
         131. c.   (pp. 721–723)
CH 42.   132. b.   (p. 1156)   133. d.   (p. 1158)
         134. c.   (pp. 1163–1164)
         135. d.   (p. 1170)
         136. c.   (p. 1171)
CH 19.   137. d.   (p. 547)   138. b.   (p. 548)
CH 22.   139. a.   (p. 628)   140. a.   (p. 636)
CH 33.   141. c.   (p. 928)   142. a.   (p. 929)
         143. a.   (p. 930)   144. a.   (p. 934)
         145. c.   (p. 937)
CH 21.   146. c.   (p. 598)   147. c.   (p. 593)
CH 34.   148. d.   (p. 948)   149. a.   (p. 959)
CH 35.   150. b.   (p. 970)
CH 45.   151. a.   (p. 1233)   152. b.   (p. 1247)

Notes

Notes

Notes

Notes

Notes

Notes

Notes

Medication Cards

In addition to oxygen, there are six medications that the EMT can administer or assist the patient in administering, with on-line or off-line approval from medical direction. They are activated charcoal, aspirin, epinephrine by auto-injector, metered-dose inhaler/small-volume nebulizer, nitroglycerin, and oral glucose. Detailed information on each of these medications is provided on the next cards in a format that you may cut from the book and carry with you for reference.

ACTIVATED CHARCOAL

Medication Name: Activated charcoal, SuperChar, InstaChar, Actidose, LiquiChar.

Indications: Rarely used; may be ordered if it can be administered shortly after ingestion of opioids, anticholinergics, or medications with a sustained release.

Contraindications: (1) Altered mental status (not fully conscious). (2) Swallowed acids or alkalis. (3) Unable to swallow. (4) Cyanide overdose.

Medication Form: 12.5 grams premixed in water; powder form should be avoided.

Dosage: 1 gram of activated charcoal per kilogram of body weight; usual adult dose 25–50 grams, infants and children 12.5–25 grams.

(see over)

© 2014 by Pearson Education, Inc.

ASPIRIN

Medication Name: ASA, Bayer, Ecotrin, St. Joseph's, Bufferin.

Indications: Chest discomfort that is suggestive of a heart attack, and approval from medical direction.

Contraindications: Patient with a known allergy to the drug or a patient with suspected aortic dissection.

Medication Form: Tablet.

Dosage: 160–325 mg; recommended 160–325 mg of a nonenteric aspirin to be chewed and swallowed.

(see over)

© 2014 by Pearson Education, Inc.

Activated Charcoal (continued)

Administration: Requires orders from medical direction; shake container; encourage patient to drink through a straw from a covered container; record time and response; if patient vomits, notify medical direction to authorize a repeat dose.

Actions: Binds with poisons in the stomach and prevents their absorption into the body.

Side Effects: Blackening of the stools, possible vomiting.

Reassessment: (1) Check for abdominal pain or distress upon administration. (2) Watch for vomiting; position the patient and be prepared to suction.

Aspirin (continued)

Administration: Determine the patient is suffering from an acute syndrome suggestive of a heart attack; obtain approval to administer the medication; ensure that the patient is alert and oriented; have the patient chew a 160–325-mg nonenteric tablet; reassess the patient and record the vital signs.

Actions: Decreases the ability of platelets to clump together; this reduces the formation of additional clots at the site of the coronary artery blockage.

Side Effects: Generally few side effects; patients may report stomach irritation or heartburn, nausea, or vomiting.

Reassessment: Perform a reassessment after administration. The aspirin is not being used as a pain reliever, but to prevent platelets from continuing to clump together and occlude the coronary artery. Record any changes in the patient's condition.

EPINEPHRINE AUTO-INJECTOR

Medication Name: Epinephrine (Adrenalin). Epinephrine autoinjectors: EpiPen, EpiPen Jr., and Twinject (adult and child).

Indications: (1) Signs and symptoms of a moderate to severe allergic reaction (anaphylaxis) with respiratory distress and shock. (2) Medication is prescribed to the patient. (3) EMT has received an order from medical direction.

Contraindications: None, when used to treat life-threatening allergic reaction.

Medication Form: Liquid drug contained within an auto-injector.

Dosage: Auto-injectors deliver a single dose; adult (greater than 66 lb) dose 0.3 mg, infant and child (less than 66 lb) 0.15 mg; a second dose may be required; Twinject can deliver a second dose.

Administration: Push the uncapped tip of the auto-injector firmly against the lateral aspect of the midthigh until the needle is deployed and the medication delivered.

(see over)

METERED-DOSE INHALER (MDI)/ SMALL-VOLUME NEBULIZER (SVN)

Medication Name: Albuterol (Proventil, Ventolin), metaproterenol (Metaprel, Alupent), isoetharine (Bronkosol), bitolterol mesylate (Tornalate), salmeterol xinafoate (Serevent), ipratropium (Atrovent), levalbuterol (Xopenex), pirbuterol (Maxair).

Indications: (1) Exhibits signs and symptoms of breathing difficulty. (2) Patient has a physician-prescribed MDI or medication for nebulization. (3) EMT has received medical direction approval.

Contraindications: (1) Patient is not responsive enough to use the MDI/ SVN. (2) MDI/SVN is not prescribed for the patient. (3) Maximum dose allowed is reached prior to your arrival. (4) Permission denied by medical direction.

Medication Form: Aerosolized medication in a metered-dose inhaler or liquid medication poured into the nebulizer chamber.

Dosage: Each depression of the MDI delivers a precise dose. The number of times the medication can be delivered is determined by medical direction. The SVN takes 5–10 minutes and should be inhaled until a mist is no longer produced.

(see over)

Epinephrine Auto-Injector (continued)

Actions: Mimics the response of the sympathetic nervous system:
(1) Constricts blood vessels to improve the blood pressure and reduces swelling and hives (alpha). (2) Relaxes smooth muscles in the lungs to improve breathing (beta$_2$). (3) Stimulates the heartbeat (beta$_1$).

Side Effects: Increased heart rate, pale skin (pallor), dizziness, chest pain, headache, nausea and vomiting, excitability, and anxiousness.

Reassessment: (1) Reassess for decreasing mental status, decreasing blood pressure, increased breathing difficulties, stridor, or increased hoarseness. (2) If condition worsens, you may have to call medical direction for a second dose and treat for hypoperfusion. You may need cardiopulmonary resuscitation (CPR) and use of the automated external defibrillator (AED).

Metered-Dose Inhaler/Small-Volume Nebulizer (continued)

Administration: (1) Ensure the right patient, right medication, right dose, right route, and right date. Determine if any doses have already been administered. (2) Determine if the patient is alert enough to use the MDI or SVN. (3) Obtain order from medical direction. See EMT Skills 16-2 and 16-3 (MDI) and 16-4 (SVN) for specific administration guidelines.

Actions: Beta$_2$ agonist, relaxes the bronchiole smooth muscles, dilates the lower airway.

Side Effects: Tachycardia, tremors, shakiness, nervousness, dry mouth, nausea and vomiting.

Reassessment: Perform a reassessment, reassess vital signs, question patient about effect, conduct focused history and physical exam, monitor airway, record and document.

NITROGLYCERIN

Medication Name: Nitroglycerin, Nitrostat, Nitro-Bid, Nitrolingual Pumpspray.

Indications: (1) Patient exhibits signs and symptoms of chest pain. (2) Patient has physician-prescribed nitroglycerin. (3) EMT has approval from medical direction.

Contraindications: (1) Baseline blood pressure below 90 mmHg systolic or the systolic pressure has decreased more than 30 mmHg from the baseline. (2) Suspected head injury. (3) Patient is a child or infant. (4) Three doses have already been taken. (5) The heart rate is less than 50 or greater than 100 bpm. (6) The patient has recently taken tadalafil (Cialis), vardenafil (Levitra), or sildenafil (Viagra).

Medication Form: Tablet or sublingual spray.

Dosage: One tablet or one spray under the tongue; may be repeated in three to five minutes if (1) patient experiences no relief, (2) blood pressure remains above 90 mmHg systolic or does not fall more than 30 mmHg below the systolic baseline blood pressure, (3) heart rate remains above 50 and below 100 bpm, and (4) medical direction gives approval. The total dose is three tablets (including what the patient took prior to your arrival).

(see over)

ORAL GLUCOSE

Medication Name: Oral glucose, Glutose, Insta-Glucose.

Indications: Must meet all of the following: (1) Altered mental status with (2) history of diabetes controlled by medication or a blood glucose level less than 60 mg/dL and (3) ability to swallow the medication.

Contraindications: (1) Unresponsive. (2) Unable to swallow the medication. (3) Has a blood glucose of greater than 60 mg/dL.

Medication Form: Gel, in a toothpaste-type tube.

Dosage: Typical dose is one tube.

Administration: Obtain order from medical direction; obtain glucose reading; ensure patient is responsive and able to swallow; squeeze or place a small portion between the cheek and gum.

Action: Increases blood- and brain-sugar levels.

(see over)

Nitroglycerin (continued)

Administration: (1) Ensure that medication is the patient's, blood pressure greater than 90 mmHg or does not fall more than 30 mmHg systolic below the baseline, and the heart rate is between 50 and 100 bpm. (2) Obtain approval from medical direction. (3) Ensure that patient is alert; check expiration date; ask patient when he took his last dose. (4) Place or spray medication under the tongue; keep mouth closed. (5) Reassess the blood pressure in two minutes; record your actions.

Actions: Dilates blood vessels, decreases the workload of and oxygen demands on the heart.

Side Effects: Vessel dilation may cause headache, drop in blood pressure, pulse rate changes.

Reassessment: (1) Monitor blood pressure frequently. (2) Question patient about effects. (3) Obtain approval from medical direction before readministering. (4) Record and document all findings and reassessment.

Oral Glucose (continued)

Side Effects: May cause an airway obstruction or be aspirated in the patient without a gag reflex.

Reassessment: Reassess the mental status and blood glucose level to determine if the drug has had an effect; may take up to 20 minutes to see any improvement.

Medication Cards

In addition to oxygen, there are six medications that the EMT can administer or assist the patient in administering, with on-line or off-line approval from medical direction. They are activated charcoal, aspirin, epinephrine by auto-injector, metered-dose inhaler/small-volume nebulizer, nitroglycerin, and oral glucose. Detailed information on each of these medications is provided on the next cards in a format that you may cut from the book and carry with you for reference.

ACTIVATED CHARCOAL

Medication Name: Activated charcoal, SuperChar, InstaChar, Actidose, LiquiChar.

Indications: Rarely used; may be ordered if it can be administered shortly after ingestion of opioids, anticholinergics, or medications with a sustained release.

Contraindications: (1) Altered mental status (not fully conscious). (2) Swallowed acids or alkalis. (3) Unable to swallow. (4) Cyanide overdose.

Medication Form: 12.5 grams premixed in water; powder form should be avoided.

Dosage: 1 gram of activated charcoal per kilogram of body weight; usual adult dose 25–50 grams, infants and children 12.5–25 grams.

(see over)

ASPIRIN

Medication Name: ASA, Bayer, Ecotrin, St. Joseph's, Bufferin.

Indications: Chest discomfort that is suggestive of a heart attack, and approval from medical direction.

Contraindications: Patient with a known allergy to the drug or a patient with suspected aortic dissection.

Medication Form: Tablet.

Dosage: 160–325 mg; recommended 160–325 mg of a nonenteric aspirin to be chewed and swallowed.

(see over)

Activated Charcoal (continued)

Administration: Requires orders from medical direction; shake container; encourage patient to drink through a straw from a covered container; record time and response; if patient vomits, notify medical direction to authorize a repeat dose.

Actions: Binds with poisons in the stomach and prevents their absorption into the body.

Side Effects: Blackening of the stools, possible vomiting.

Reassessment: (1) Check for abdominal pain or distress upon administration. (2) Watch for vomiting; position the patient and be prepared to suction.

Aspirin (continued)

Administration: Determine the patient is suffering from an acute syndrome suggestive of a heart attack; obtain approval to administer the medication; ensure that the patient is alert and oriented; have the patient chew a 160–325-mg nonenteric tablet; reassess the patient and record the vital signs.

Actions: Decreases the ability of platelets to clump together; this reduces the formation of additional clots at the site of the coronary artery blockage.

Side Effects: Generally few side effects; patients may report stomach irritation or heartburn, nausea, or vomiting.

Reassessment: Perform a reassessment after administration. The aspirin is not being used as a pain reliever, but to prevent platelets from continuing to clump together and occlude the coronary artery. Record any changes in the patient's condition.

EPINEPHRINE AUTO-INJECTOR

Medication Name: Epinephrine (Adrenalin). Epinephrine autoinjectors: EpiPen, EpiPen Jr., and Twinject (adult and child).

Indications: (1) Signs and symptoms of a moderate to severe allergic reaction (anaphylaxis) with respiratory distress and shock. (2) Medication is prescribed to the patient. (3) EMT has received an order from medical direction.

Contraindications: None, when used to treat life-threatening allergic reaction.

Medication Form: Liquid drug contained within an auto-injector.

Dosage: Auto-injectors deliver a single dose; adult (greater than 66 lb) dose 0.3 mg, infant and child (less than 66 lb) 0.15 mg; a second dose may be required; Twinject can deliver a second dose.

Administration: Push the uncapped tip of the auto-injector firmly against the lateral aspect of the midthigh until the needle is deployed and the medication delivered.

(see over)

METERED-DOSE INHALER (MDI)/ SMALL-VOLUME NEBULIZER (SVN)

Medication Name: Albuterol (Proventil, Ventolin), metaproterenol (Metaprel, Alupent), isoetharine (Bronkosol), bitolterol mesylate (Tornalate), salmeterol xinafoate (Serevent), ipratropium (Atrovent), levalbuterol (Xopenex), pirbuterol (Maxair).

Indications: (1) Exhibits signs and symptoms of breathing difficulty. (2) Patient has a physician-prescribed MDI or medication for nebulization. (3) EMT has received medical direction approval.

Contraindications: (1) Patient is not responsive enough to use the MDI/SVN. (2) MDI/SVN is not prescribed for the patient. (3) Maximum dose allowed is reached prior to your arrival. (4) Permission denied by medical direction.

Medication Form: Aerosolized medication in a metered-dose inhaler or liquid medication poured into the nebulizer chamber.

Dosage: Each depression of the MDI delivers a precise dose. The number of times the medication can be delivered is determined by medical direction. The SVN takes 5–10 minutes and should be inhaled until a mist is no longer produced.

(see over)

Epinephrine Auto-Injector (continued)

Actions: Mimics the response of the sympathetic nervous system:
(1) Constricts blood vessels to improve the blood pressure and reduces swelling and hives (alpha). (2) Relaxes smooth muscles in the lungs to improve breathing ($beta_2$). (3) Stimulates the heartbeat ($beta_1$).

Side Effects: Increased heart rate, pale skin (pallor), dizziness, chest pain, headache, nausea and vomiting, excitability, and anxiousness.

Reassessment: (1) Reassess for decreasing mental status, decreasing blood pressure, increased breathing difficulties, stridor, or increased hoarseness. (2) If condition worsens, you may have to call medical direction for a second dose and treat for hypoperfusion. You may need cardiopulmonary resuscitation (CPR) and use of the automated external defibrillator (AED).

Metered-Dose Inhaler/Small-Volume Nebulizer (continued)

Administration: (1) Ensure the right patient, right medication, right dose, right route, and right date. Determine if any doses have already been administered. (2) Determine if the patient is alert enough to use the MDI or SVN. (3) Obtain order from medical direction. See EMT Skills 16-2 and 16-3 (MDI) and 16-4 (SVN) for specific administration guidelines.

Actions: $Beta_2$ agonist, relaxes the bronchiole smooth muscles, dilates the lower airway.

Side Effects: Tachycardia, tremors, shakiness, nervousness, dry mouth, nausea and vomiting.

Reassessment: Perform a reassessment, reassess vital signs, question patient about effect, conduct focused history and physical exam, monitor airway, record and document.

NITROGLYCERIN

Medication Name: Nitroglycerin, Nitrostat, Nitro-Bid, Nitrolingual Pumpspray.

Indications: (1) Patient exhibits signs and symptoms of chest pain. (2) Patient has physician-prescribed nitroglycerin. (3) EMT has approval from medical direction.

Contraindications: (1) Baseline blood pressure below 90 mmHg systolic or the systolic pressure has decreased more than 30 mmHg from the baseline. (2) Suspected head injury. (3) Patient is a child or infant. (4) Three doses have already been taken. (5) The heart rate is less than 50 or greater than 100 bpm. (6) The patient has recently taken tadalafil (Cialis), vardenafil (Levitra), or sildenafil (Viagra).

Medication Form: Tablet or sublingual spray.

Dosage: One tablet or one spray under the tongue; may be repeated in three to five minutes if (1) patient experiences no relief, (2) blood pressure remains above 90 mmHg systolic or does not fall more than 30 mmHg below the systolic baseline blood pressure, (3) heart rate remains above 50 and below 100 bpm, and (4) medical direction gives approval. The total dose is three tablets (including what the patient took prior to your arrival).

(see over)

ORAL GLUCOSE

Medication Name: Oral glucose, Glutose, Insta-Glucose.

Indications: Must meet all of the following: (1) Altered mental status with (2) history of diabetes controlled by medication or a blood glucose level less than 60 mg/dL and (3) ability to swallow the medication.

Contraindications: (1) Unresponsive. (2) Unable to swallow the medication. (3) Has a blood glucose of greater than 60 mg/dL.

Medication Form: Gel, in a toothpaste-type tube.

Dosage: Typical dose is one tube.

Administration: Obtain order from medical direction; obtain glucose reading; ensure patient is responsive and able to swallow; squeeze or place a small portion between the cheek and gum.

Action: Increases blood- and brain-sugar levels.

(see over)

Nitroglycerin (continued)

Administration: (1) Ensure that medication is the patient's, blood pressure greater than 90 mmHg or does not fall more than 30 mmHg systolic below the baseline, and the heart rate is between 50 and 100 bpm. (2) Obtain approval from medical direction. (3) Ensure that patient is alert; check expiration date; ask patient when he took his last dose. (4) Place or spray medication under the tongue; keep mouth closed. (5) Reassess the blood pressure in two minutes; record your actions.

Actions: Dilates blood vessels, decreases the workload of and oxygen demands on the heart.

Side Effects: Vessel dilation may cause headache, drop in blood pressure, pulse rate changes.

Reassessment: (1) Monitor blood pressure frequently. (2) Question patient about effects. (3) Obtain approval from medical direction before readministering. (4) Record and document all findings and reassessment.

Oral Glucose (continued)

Side Effects: May cause an airway obstruction or be aspirated in the patient without a gag reflex.

Reassessment: Reassess the mental status and blood glucose level to determine if the drug has had an effect; may take up to 20 minutes to see any improvement.